FIFTH EDITION

OBSTETRICS AND GYNECOLOGY

CHARLES R. B. BECKMANN, M.D., M.H.P.E.
Professor and Director, Division of Ambulatory Medicine
and Academic Affairs
Department of Obstetrics and Gynecology
Albert Einstein Medical Center / Thomas Jefferson University
Philadelphia, Pennsylvania

FRANK W. LING, M.D.
Women's Health Specialists PLLC
Memphis, Tennessee
Clinical Professor
Department of Obstetrics and Gynecology
Vanderbilt University School of Medicine
Nashville, Tennessee

ROGER P. SMITH, M.D.
Professor and Vice Chair
Department of Obstetrics and Gynecology
University of Missouri at Kansas City
Kansas City, Missouri

BARBARA M. BARZANSKY, PH.D., M.H.P.E.
Secretary, Council on Medical Education
The American Medical Association
Chicago, Illinois

WILLIAM N. P. HERBERT, M.D.
Professor and Chairman
Department of Obstetrics and Gynecology
University of Virginia
Charlottesville, Virginia

DOUGLAS W. LAUBE, M.D., M.ED.
Professor and Chairman
Department of Obstetrics and Gynecology
University of Wisconsin Medical School
Madison, Wisconsin

FIFTH EDITION

OBSTETRICS AND GYNECOLOGY

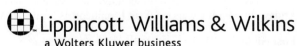
. Lippincott Williams & Wilkins
a Wolters Kluwer business
Philadelphia · Baltimore · New York · London
Buenos Aires · Hong Kong · Sydney · Tokyo

Acquisitions editor: Donna Balado
Developmental editor: Kathleen H. Scogna
Editorial assistant: Tenille Sands
Marketing manager: Emilie Linkins
Production editor: Kevin Johnson
Art Director: Doug Smock

Library of Congress Cataloging-in-Publication Data

Obstetrics and gynecology / Charles R.B. Beckmann ... [et al.].- 5th ed.
    p. ; cm.
    Includes bibliographical references and index.
    ISBN 13: 978-0-7817-5806-2
    ISBN 10: 0-7817-5806-8 (alk. paper)
    1. Gynecology. 2. Obstetrics. I. Beckmann, Charles R. B.
    [DNLM: 1. Genital Diseases, Female. 2. Labor, Obstetric. WP 140 O14 2006]
RG101.O24 2006
618-dc22
                                                        2005029418

First edition, 1992
Second edition, 1995
Third edition, 1998
Fourth edition, 2002

The fourth edition of this excellent text has been the most widely used student text in obstetrics and gynecology. The same educators and authors have prepared this new 5th edition of this popular book with many improvements, including updated information and new features. They have made this valuable text even better than the previous editions.

Each chapter has been reviewed and revised to focus on the "core" material students need to learn in the obstetrics/gynecology clerkship. A larger pool of questions than in previous editions makes it easier for students to perform self-testing and self-evaluation. The questions are now being presented on a CD, which allows students to create custom tests and to track their scoring progress. The educational impact of the book is further enhanced by revised figures and tables that make for better organization of important information. Most important, the superb educational material is based on the latest edition of APGO objectives.

All the authors and editorial advisors are to be congratulated on the production of a medical text based on sound educational principles. This new edition will undoubtedly be the number one text for students on the obstetrics and gynecology clerkship. I strongly recommend it, not only for students, but also for residents, faculty, and other individuals interested in education.

Martin L. Stone, M.D.
Professor and Chairman (Emeritus)
Department of Obstetrics and Gynecology
SUNY at Stony Brook, New York

Obstetrics and Gynecology in this 5th edition is again written specifically for medical students taking their clerkship in obstetrics and gynecology. The goals of the book with respect to medical school education are to provide the basic information about obstetrics and gynecology that medical students need to complete an obstetrics and gynecology clerkship successfully and to pass the national standardized examinations in this content area.

Obstetrics and Gynecology, 5th edition, also provides basic, practical information in obstetrics, gynecology, and women's health needed by physicians and advanced practice nurses in other medical specialties. Family physicians will find this book especially useful in their certification examinations. Nurse midwives will likewise find this book helpful for many practice issues.

Great effort has been made to make each chapter short and concise, written in clear and unambiguous prose, including only the basic information needed. Whenever possible, clear, concise summary tables and figures that teach and illustrate are used. The index has been revised and expanded to facilitate learning.

Obstetrics and Gynecology, 5th edition, is unique in several important ways:

1. This textbook was written to facilitate efficient, focused learning and is based on the "Instructional Objectives for a Clinical Curriculum in Obstetrics and Gynecology, 8th edition" of the Association of Professors of Gynecology and Obstetrics. These national standards are used to organize most Ob–Gyn clerkships in the United States and Canada, and they are used as a guideline in the development of national standardized examinations. An effort has been made to address all the content of these objectives, as the objectives cover basic information that any health-care provider engaged in the primary care of women should know.

2. Each chapter begins with reference to APGO Educational Topics primarily covered in the chapter.

3. Enclosed with this edition of the book is a Brownstone Tutor™ question bank of over 1,400 questions that review the major concepts and facts presented in the chapters. This invaluable study tool allows users to create their own tests by specifying which chapters they are interested in reviewing. The question bank grades each test taken, and users can see their results over time on the "Results" screen. The user can also review the questions in each test by clicking on the "Review Questions" tab.

4. A Contributing Advisory Board of medical educators has been assembled to provide consultation on the updating of the entire book. This has helped to bring a truly national perspective to the content and depth in coverage of various topics.

Obstetrics and Gynecology, 5th edition, was written by leaders in medical education, including obstetrician–gynecologists with additional degrees in education, experience as clerkship and residency program directors, chairs of university departments, national leadership positions in the areas of primary care, and involvement in the preparation of national standardized examinations. The contributing author is a professional educator and anatomist with extensive experience in curriculum development and evaluation.

Other medical school textbooks often contain large amounts of information more useful to advanced practitioners than to medical students and those providing primary women's health care. In contrast, *Obstetrics and Gynecology*, 5th edition, focuses specifically on the basic information medical students need for the primary and obstetric–gynecologic care of women, the same information medical students need during their Ob–Gyn clinical clerkship. The concise and easy-to-read chapters, correlated with national learning objectives, and unique self-evaluation technology for measuring progress, fulfill our intention to provide the fundamental information required for the spectrum of women's health care.

CONTRIBUTING ADVISORY BOARD

ACKNOWLEDGMENTS

We extend our appreciation to Donna Balado, Kathleen H. Scogna, Tenille Sands, Emilie Linkins, and Doug Smock at Lippincott Williams & Wilkins and Anne O'Hearn of the Academic Affairs Division of the Department of OB/GYN, Albert Einstein Medical Center–Philadelphia for their seemingly tireless help and encouragement during the arduous preparation of *Obstetrics and Gynecology*, 5th edition. Likewise, we continue to be grateful for the innovative art provided by Joyce Lavery, which adds so much to the usefulness of the book. We again extend our traditional special thanks to Carol-Lynn Brown, our first editor, for her foresight and support in the early development of this book.

In 2003 and 2004 the Undergraduate Medical Education Committee of the Association of Professors of Gynecology and Obstetrics (UMEC of APGO) revised the objectives listed in the 8th edition to reflect current medical information, and they also substantially updated the document to reflect three priorities of medical student learning: (1) topics all medical student must learn and master; (2) topics medical students should be expected to learn; and (3) topics medical students can be expected to learn. The result was 58 Educational Topic areas containing 267 specific learning objectives (126 considered as Priority 1 and 141 as Priority 2). Finally, best methods of evaluation were reviewed for each.

Each chapter of this 5th edition of *Obstetrics and Gynecology* begins with a listing of the pertinent educational topics. The content is selected to mirror the focus of the 8th edition APGO objectives, as are the questions for each chapter.

CONTENTS

Contents

UNIT III GYNECOLOGY 239

UNIT IV REPRODUCTIVE ENDOCRINOLOGY AND INFERTILITY 339

UNIT I

APPROACH TO THE PATIENT

CHAPTER 1

HEALTH CARE FOR WOMEN: OBSTETRICS AND GYNECOLOGY AS SPECIALTY AND PRIMARY—PREVENTIVE HEALTH CARE

This chapter deals primarily with APGO Educational Topics:

Topic 1: History
Topic 2: Examinations
Topic 3: Pap Smear and Cultures
Topic 4: Diagnosis and Management Plan
Topic 5: Personal Interaction and Communication Skills
Topic 6: Legal and Ethical Issues in Obstetrics and Gynecology
Topic 7: Preventative Care and Health Maintenance

The student should be able to conduct a thorough history, perform an appropriate examination, including obtaining cultures and Pap smear, and generate a problem list leading to a management plan. In addition, the student should be able to explain the importance of health promotion and disease prevention. The student must be able to interact with the patient in a cooperative fashion, recognizing the importance of protecting the patient's interests.

Obstetrician–gynecologists provide obstetric, gynecologic, gynecologic oncology, and reproductive endocrinology and infertility care, as well as a substantial part of the primary care needs for over half of the women in the United States. Thus, the obstetrician–gynecologist must understand the wide range of primary care issues, as well as the specialty of obstetrics and gynecology. He or she must be able to establish a good professional relationship with patients, and must be able to perform an excellent general and woman's health history, review of systems, and physical examination. In addition, the obstetrician–gynecologist must understand the differences between consultation (evaluation and recommendations) and referral (transfer of specific care issues) and when and how to perform and receive each. Finally, as with all physicians, obstetrician–gynecologists must fully understand the concepts of evidence-based medicine and incorporate them into their scholarship and practice.

Part I: Obstetrics and Gynecology Primary and Specialty Care for Women

Obstetrics was originally a separate branch of medicine, and gynecology was a division of surgery. Knowledge of the pathophysiology of the female reproductive tract led to a natural integration of these two areas, and obstetrics and gynecology merged into a single specialty. In the United States, obstetrics is now somewhat indistinctly divided into general obstetrics (dealing with uncomplicated pregnancy) and maternal-fetal medicine (dealing with complicated, or high-risk, pregnancy as well as reproductive genetics). Likewise, gynecology now includes general gynecology (dealing with nonmalignant disorders of the reproductive tract and associated organ systems), gynecologic oncology, reproductive endocrinology–infertility, and the developing area of pelvic reconstructive surgery and urogynecology.

To facilitate the primary–preventive health care responsibility, the Task Force on Primary and Preventive Health Care of the American College of Obstetricians and Gynecologists published *The Obstetrician-Gynecologist and Primary-Preventive Health Care* (1993). This publication contains guidelines for screening, counseling, patient education, behavioral intervention, and consultation related to the major causes of morbidity (Table 1.1) and mortality (Table 1.2; Figure 1.1). Recommendations for screening testing (Table 1.3) and immunizations (Table 1.4) are also included.

Table 1.1. Leading Causes of Morbidity in Women in the United States

Cause of morbidity[a]	Age 12–18	19–39	40–64	>65
HEENT conditions	+	+	+	+
URI	+	+	+	+
Infection (viral, parasites, bacterial)	+	+		
Sexual abuse	+			
Accidental injury	+	+		+
Digestive tract conditions	+			
Acute urinary conditions	+	+		
Osteoporosis/arthritis			+	+
Hypertension			+	+
Orthopaedic conditions		+		
Heart disease			+	+
Hearing and vision impairments			+	+
Urinary incontinence				?

[a]HEENT, head, ears, eyes, nose, and throat; URI, upper respiratory infection.

Table 1.2. Ten Leading Causes of Female Death in the United States

Rank	Age				
	0–14	15–34	35–54	55–74	>75
	Cause[a]				
1	Diseases of infancy	Accidents	Cancer	Cancer	Heart disease
2	Congenital anomalies	Cancer	Heart disease	Heart disease	Cancer
3	Accidents	Homicide	Accidents	COPD	Cerebrovascular disease
4	Cancer	Suicide	Cerebrovascular disease	Cerebrovascular disease	Pneumonia, influenza
5	Heart disease	HIV	Suicide	Diabetes	COPD
6	Homicide	Heart disease	Cirrhosis of liver	Pneumonia, influenza	Diabetes
7	Pneumonia, influenza	Cerebrovascular disease	HIV	Accidents	Accidents
8	Septicemia	Congenital anomalies	Diabetes	Cirrhosis	Arteriosclerosis
9	HIV	Pneumonia, influenza	COPD	Disease of arteries	Alzheimer's disease
10	Cerebral palsy	Diabetes	Homicide	Nephritis	Nephritis

[a]COPD, chronic obstructive pulmonary disease.

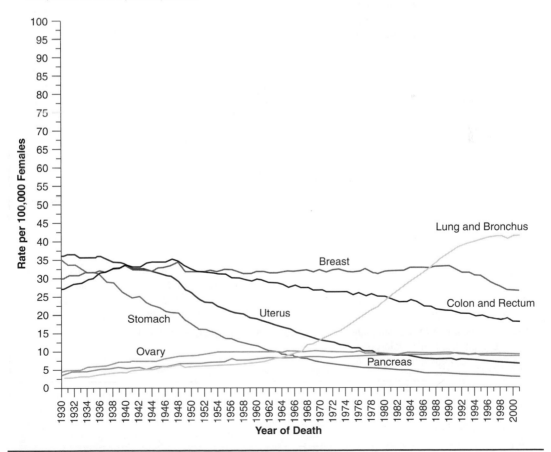

Figure 1.1. Age-adjusted cancer mortality for women in the United States.

Table 1.3. Recommended Screening Testing and Health Care Interventions for Women[a]

Risk Factor/Condition	Screening Test Recommendation or Intervention
Cervical dysplasia/cancer Women with no special risk factors Women considered at high risk (immunosuppression as a result of HIV infection, chronic illness, immunosuppressive therapy for transplant, or chemotherapy; AIDS; multiple STDs; multiple sexual partners or sexual partners in high risk groups such as drug abusers; early sexual activity; smokers)	1. Beginning 3 years after onset of vaginal intercourse, or no later than age 21. Annual screening until age 30, then every 2–3 years if three consecutive tests are negative. Terminate screening at age 70 if uterus intact, three consecutive negative tests, and no positive tests in past 10 years. If using cytology plus HPV DNA testing, screen every 3 years if both tests are negative. 2. Usually yearly, depending on the risk factor and Pap smear history or history of abnormal cervical cytology or histology.
Skin cancer (high risk: extensive sun exposure, family/personal history of skin cancer, suspicious lesions)	Physical examination; counseling about sun exposure; consultation for suspicious lesions
Anemia (high risk: Caribbean, Latin American, Asian, Mediterranean, or African descent or history of menorrhagia)	Hemogram/sickle-cell preparation; quantitative hemoglobin electrophoresis
Hypercholesterolemia, coronary artery disease (high risk: elevated cholesterol; patient or sibling with cholesterol 240 mg/dL or higher; sibling, parent, or grandparent with coronary artery disease, especially at age 55 or under; smoking; diabetes mellitus)	Cholesterol/lipid profile every 5 years from age 19, every 3 to 4 years from age 65
Breast cancer (high risk: first-degree relative with breast cancer, especially if diagnosed premenopausally)	Screening mammography every other year from age 40, every year from age 50; yearly physician breast examination; self-breast examination instruction. Those who fall into high-risk categories may need more frequent studies and from an earlier age. In addition, the role of BRCA evaluation is expanding rapidly and in future years may become a major part of screening for the likelihood of breast (and other) malignancies and the most effective kind and frequency of screening testing for the patient (and for relatives, including specifically children and immediate siblings)
Lung cancer, coronary artery disease	Counseling about smoking; regular blood pressure screening
Colorectal cancer	Colonoscopy every 5–10 years after age 50; fecal occult blood test at physician discretion at the time of annual examinations, or in three sample testings on fecal samples collected by the patient.
Thyroid disease/risk for autoimmune disease (high risk: family history of thyroid disease, autoimmune disease)	TSH every 3 to 5 years after age 65

(continued)

Table 1.3. continued

Risk Factor/Condition	Screening Test Recommendation or Intervention
TB (high risk: patients with AIDS, who are immunosuppressed, or have close contact with those with TB; alcoholics and drug users; inmates of residential care facilities and prisons)	TB skin testing
Sexually transmitted infections	As indicated by history/physical examination: "wet mount" from vaginal fluids, cultures for gonorrhea and chlamydia; RPR/VDRL; hepatitis; HIV; counseling about risk behaviors, safe sex practices
Diabetes mellitus (high risk: family history of diabetes; obesity; personal history of gestational diabetes mellitus)	Fasting blood glucose as indicated
Osteoporosis	Diet and exercise counseling combined with menopausal hormone-replacement therapy and calcium supplementation.
	Bone density studies may play an increasing role in the screening of women, especially those at higher risk for early bone loss, such as women with premature ovarian failure, ovarian removal at surgery, or medical or chemotherapeutic therapy causing oligo-ovulation or anovulation.
Depression (especially women at high risk for depression, including patients who have experienced sexual or domestic abuse, women with chronic emotional illnesses, women in exceptionally stressful psychosocial or economic situations, women who have recently moved from other cultures and/or who are unable to communicate comfortably and effectively in English, or to understand American social systems and to function effectively within them)	Referral to appropriate social help agencies or organizations for women in general, or more specifically focused on an issue or issues faced by a specific patient.
	Referral to religious/pastoral care consistent with the patient's beliefs.
	Referral for psychological or psychiatric evaluation and treatment if the situation requires such action. This is especially true if there is a suggestion or evidence of suicidal ideation or previous or intended action.

[a]BRACA gene, Breast/Ovarian Cancer Susceptibility gene; HPV, Human Papilloma Virus; RPR/VDRL, rapid plasma reagin/Venereal Disease Research Laboratory; STIs, sexually transmitted infections; TB, tuberculosis; TSH, thyroid-stimulating hormone.

By the end of the first half of the 21st century, the number of older women in the United States will double (Figure 1.2) as a result of the increased life span of women. In fact, a female newborn today has a life expectancy of approximately 81 years. With the average age of menopause at 51 to 52 years, most women will spend more than one-third of their lives in menopause. These older women with their special health needs will comprise a significant part of the patients cared for by most general obstetrician–gynecologists. Their age-specific needs will require a still wider range of knowledge and skills than heretofore expected of obstetrician–gynecologists. These women and their families will expect their clinicians to help them maintain an active, healthy, and satisfying lifestyle for most of their lifetime, in addition to the identification and treatment of illness.

Part II: Evaluation and Management

Starting with the first interaction with the patient, the physician strives to establish and

Table 1.4. Immunization Recommendations

Immunization	Recommendations
Tetanus–diphtheria booster	Once between ages 14 and 16
Influenza vaccine	Every 10 years from age 19 to 64 for residents of chronic care facilities; persons with chronic cardiopulmonary disorders; persons with metabolic diseases such as diabetes mellitus, hemoglobinopathies, immunosuppression, or renal dysfunction; annually for women 65 years old
Pneumococcal vaccine	Every 10 years from age 19 to 64 for women with medical conditions that increase the risk of pneumococcal infection (e.g., chronic cardiac or pulmonary disease, sickle-cell disease, nephrotic syndrome, Hodgkin disease, asplenia, diabetes mellitus, alcoholism, cirrhosis, multiple myeloma, renal disease, or other immunosuppression)
Measles, mumps, rubella (MMR)	Rubella titer vaccine for women of childbearing age lacking evidence of immunity; a second measles immunization, preferably as MMR, for all women unable to show proof of immunity
Hepatitis B vaccine	Intravenous drug users; current recipients of blood products; persons in health-related jobs with exposure to blood or blood products; household and sexual contacts of hepatitis B virus carriers; prostitutes; persons with a history of sexual activity with multiple partners in the previous 6 months

develop a professional relationship of mutual trust and respect. At the same time, the patient usually decides if the physician is knowledgeable and trustworthy, and whether she will accept recommendations that are made.

The process begins with an appropriate greeting, which may or may not include a handshake. Surnames should generally be used because the patient–physician relationship, although friendly, is professional. "What brought you to the office today?" or "How may I help you today?" are neutral opening questions

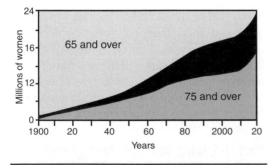

Figure 1.2. Changes of age distributions in American women over time.

that allow the patient to frame a response that includes her problems, concerns, and/or reasons for the visit. If the patient came for a specific issue, e.g., contraception, it is still important to ask about other issues or concerns.

Traditionally, medical education focuses on the "F2 model,"·as described by the Bayer Institute for Healthcare Communication. The F2 model is that of "find it and fix it." However, complete evaluation and management of the patient is best portrayed by the "4 Es" model: engage, empathize, educate, and enlist. This complete model of clinical care actively involves patients as participants and decision makers in their medical treatment.

The first "E," engagement, involves forming and/or strengthening the physician–patient relationship during medical encounters. Successful engagement results in a person-to-person professional partner relationship. Successful engagement is achieved by using a pleasant, consistent tone of voice and by using the first few minutes of the encounter to build a rapport with the patient. Empathy, the second "E," occurs when a patient feels that she is being seen, heard, and accepted for who she is. In short, empathy is being able to view the situation or the encounter truly from the patient's perspective. Empathy differs from sympathy in that empathy involves experiencing the patient's feelings, and sympathy involves your own feelings. Another important component of empathy is the ability to judge the behavior, not the person. Education is the third "E." Educating a patient about her health care and treatment options permits her informed consent as well as your assessment of her understanding of her health status. The final "E" is enlistment, which is an invitation from the clinician to the patient to collaborate in a decision-making process, thereby improving compliance.

In summary, a shift in the paradigm of "find it and fix it" to the model of complete clinical care, which includes find it and fix it, but adds the concepts of engaging the patients, demonstrating empathy, educating patients, and enlisting them as active participants in their health care, will help ensure an accurate evaluation, as well as management and compliance during the medical encounter.

Health Evaluation: History, Physical Examination, and Comprehensive Health Planning

History

Chief Complaint (and Other Problems and Issues)
The chief complaint is the reason for the patient's visit. In sharp contrast to this time-honored concept, it is estimated that the average patient has 3 to 12 complaints that she wishes to have addressed. These complaints may or may not be associated with each other, but adhering strictly to the concept of a single chief complaint may create a frustrating encounter for both the health care provider and the patient. At the end of the encounter, even if a more significant issue is discovered, the patient will expect that her chief complaint, the reason she came in the first place, will be addressed; the clinician will be judged, in part, by whether this happens or not.

Menstrual History
Menstrual history begins with menarche, the age at which menses began. The basic menstrual history should include the duration of bleeding, the interval between the first day of menstrual flow and the first day of the next menstrual flow, the frequency of menses, and the last menstrual period (LMP), dated from the first day of the last normal period. Episodes of bleeding that are "light, but on time" should be noted as such, because they may have diagnostic significance. Estimation of the amount of menstrual flow can be made by asking whether the patient uses pads or tampons, how many are used during the heavy days of her flow, and whether they are soaked or just soiled when they are changed. It is normal for women to pass clots during menstruation, but normally they should not be larger than the size of a dime. Specific inquiry should be made about irregular bleeding, intermenstrual bleeding (bleeding between menses), or contact bleeding (postcoital or postdouching bleeding or spotting). Such abnormal bleeding must be correlated with information about contraceptive method, infections, concurrent gynecologic problems, and sexual practices. Terms describing bleeding abnormalities include:

Amenorrhea–absence of uterine bleeding
Oligomenorrhea–infrequent, often irregular uterine bleeding, intervals more than 34 days
Hypomenorrhea–light, but regular uterine bleeding
Polymenorrhea–frequent, regular uterine bleeding, intervals less than 22 days
Menorrhagia (hypermenorrhea)–heavy, regular uterine bleeding
Menometrorrhagia–heavy, irregular uterine bleeding

The menstrual history may include perimenstrual symptoms (molimina) such as anxiety, fluid retention, nervousness, mood fluctuations, food cravings, variations in sexual feelings, and difficulty sleeping. Crampy pain during the menses is common. It is abnormal when it interferes with daily activities or when it requires more analgesia than provided by nonnarcotic analgesia.

Inquiry about duration, quality, radiation of the pain to areas outside the pelvis, and association with body position or daily activities completes the pain history.

The term menopause refers to the cessation of menses. The climacteric is the time of transition when ovarian function begins to wane. The climacteric history often begins with increasing menstrual irregularity and varying or decreased flow, associated with hot flashes, nervousness, mood changes, and decreased vaginal lubrication. The physician should ask if the patient is taking any menopausal therapy (hormonal or other). A history of medical (radiation or chemotherapy) or surgical oophorectomy should be taken. Any postmenopausal bleeding, defined as bleeding 6 months after cessation of menses, is abnormal because of its association with genital malignancy, especially endometrial carcinoma.

Obstetric History

A basic obstetric history includes the number of pregnancies (gravidity), the number of pregnancies beyond 20 weeks' gestation (parity), and the number of pregnancies that ended prior to 20 weeks' gestation (abortions). The following abbreviations may also be used: gravida (G), para (P), abcde, where

- a = number of pregnancies
- b = number of term pregnancies (beyond 36 weeks)
- c = number of preterm pregnancies (20 through 36 weeks)
- d = number of abortions (spontaneous or induced) and ectopic pregnancies (<20 weeks)
- e = number of living children

For term and preterm deliveries, determine the outcome, any complications, and mode of delivery. For abortions and ectopic pregnancies, determine any known causes, medical therapy and/or surgical procedure(s) done, complications, and feelings about these events. Some key obstetric terms are defined in Table 1.5.

Gynecologic History

The gynecologic history includes information about any gynecologic disease and/or treatment that the patient has had, including the

Table 1.5. Obstetric Definitions

Gravida	A woman who is or has been pregnant
Primigravida	A woman who is in or who has experienced her first pregnancy
Multigravida	A woman who has been pregnant more than once
Nulligravida	A woman who has never been and is not now pregnant
Primipara	A woman who has delivered one pregnancy (regardless of the number of fetuses) that progressed beyond the gestational age of an abortion
Multipara	A woman who has delivered two or more pregnancies that progressed beyond the gestational age of an abortion
Nullipara	A woman who has never had a pregnancy progress beyond the gestational age of an abortion
Parturient	A woman currently in labor
Puerpera	A woman who has just recently given birth

diagnosis, the medical and/or surgical treatment, and the results. Questions about previous gynecologic surgery should include the name of the procedure; indication; when, where, and by whom the surgery was performed; the results; and whether the outcome met her expectations.

The history of a sexually transmitted infection (STI) is particularly germane to women's health. A history of vaginitis or recurrent vaginal discharge may be related to an STI, although not necessarily so. Pelvic inflammatory disease (PID) is a frequently encountered history. Pelvic inflammatory disease is classically characterized by fever, chills, abdominopelvic pain, and an appropriate response to oral or parenteral antibiotic therapy. Pelvic inflammatory disease is often confused with vaginitis, which may be differentiated by the history of vaginal discharge and characterized by local symptoms such as pruritus or irritation. The patient should be asked specifically about a history of sexually transmitted infections such as gonorrhea, herpes, chlamydia, warts (condylomata), hepatitis, acquired immune deficiency syndrome (AIDS), and syphilis. Finally, patients should be asked about behaviors that are high risk for the acquisition of human immunodeficiency virus (HIV) or hepatitis, including parenteral drug use, sexual relationships with drug users or bisexuals, transfusion before approximately 1980, and prostitution or promiscuity.

A history of breast disease and breast cancer should include previous breast biopsy; previous mammography or other imaging study; family history of breast cancer; and appreciation by the patient of a mass, discharge, or painful area. Correlation with the patient's age, menstrual status, and hormonal therapy should be made.

If a patient has a history of infertility (generally defined as failure to conceive for 1 year), questions concerning both partners should cover previous diseases or surgery that may affect fertility, previous fertility (previous children with the same or other partners), duration of time that pregnancy has been attempted, and a history of sexual practices.

Diethylstilbestrol (DES) use by the patient's mother during her pregnancy should be noted because it may be associated with infertility problems and/or vaginal adenosis or clear cell carcinoma in the daughter. A personal hygiene history should address the use of douching and vaginal "feminine sprays," deodorants, or self-medications. A history of gastrointestinal and urinary disorders completes the gynecologic history. If a history of urinary frequency or involuntary urine loss is elicited, consideration should be given to evaluation for urinary tract infection and/or evaluation for urogynecologic issues such as stress urinary incontinence. If a history of chronic constipation or water, blood, or mucus in the stool is elicited, consideration should be given to gastrointestinal evaluation.

Sexual and Contraceptive History

Taking a sexual history is facilitated by behaviors, attitudes, and direct statements by the physician that project a nonjudgmental manner of acceptance and respect for the patient's lifestyle. A good opening question is,

"Please tell me about your sexual partner or partners." This question is gender neutral, leaves the issue of number of partners open, and also gives the patient considerable latitude for response. In the final analysis, however, these questions must be individualized to each patient. Data to be elicited should include age at first intercourse, the patient's present sexual partner(s) (including gender), types of sexual practices, and the patient's level of satisfaction with her sex life. Finally, questions regarding child and/or adult sexual abuse and assault should be asked. The patient may be asked, "Have you ever been touched against your will, either as a child or an adult?"

A patient's contraceptive history should include the method currently used, when it was begun, any problems or complications, and the patient's and her partner's satisfaction with the method. Previous contraceptive methods and the reasons they were discontinued may prove relevant. If no contraceptive actions are being taken, inquiry should be made as to why, which may include the desire for conception or concerns about contraceptive options as understood by the patient. The history concludes with inquiry about the patient's future conceptive or contraceptive plans (Table 1.6).

Physical Examination

Breast Examination

The breast examination by a physician remains the best means of early detection of breast cancer when combined with appropriately scheduled mammography and regular breast self-examination. The results of the breast examination may be expressed by description or diagram, or both, usually with reference to the quadrants and tail region of the breast or by allusion to the breast as a clock face with the nipple at the center (Figure 1.3). Development of the female breast, as described in Tanner's sex maturity ratings, is used in the description of the breast examination (Figure 1.4).

How to Do the Breast Examination The breasts are first examined by inspection, with the patient's

Table 1.6. The Obstetrics–Gynecologic (OB-GYN) History and Physical Examination: Generalized Report Format

I. History
  A. Chief complaint(s)
  B. Menstrual history
    1. Last menstrual period; previous menstrual period
    2. Menarche
    3. Usual menstrual duration; interval between first days of menstrual periods
    4. Menstrual flow
    5. Abnormal menses
    6. Pain
  C. Menopause
    1. Climacteric symptoms, if any
    2. Perimenopausal and postmenopausal history
    3. Postmenopausal bleeding
  D. Obstetric history
    1. Gravidity and parity
    2. Obstetric complications
  E. Gynecologic history
    1. Gynecologic diseases and treatment, including surgery and medical treatment
    2. Sexually transmitted infections
      a. Vaginitis, vulvitis
      b. Local lesions
      c. Pelvic inflammatory disease
    3. Breast disease (history, biopsy information, any family history of breast carcinoma)
    4. Infertility
    5. Urinary tract/bowel complaints
    6. Exposure to diethylstilbestrol (DES)
    7. Personal hygiene
  F. Sexual history (activity, problems, satisfaction)
  G. Sexual assault/abuse, adult and child
  H. Contraceptive history
    1. Present contraception
    2. Past contraception
    3. Conception plans

(continued)

arms at her sides and then with her hands pressed against her hips and/or with her arms raised over her head (Figure 1.5). If the patient's breasts are especially large and pendulous, leaning forward so that the breasts hang free of the chest may facilitate inspection. Tumors often distort the relations of these tissues, causing disruption of the shape, contour, or symmetry of the breast or position of the nipple. Some asymmetry of the breasts is common, but marked differences or recent changes deserve further evaluation.

Table 1.6. continued

II. Physical examination
   A. Height, weight, and blood pressure
   B. Breast examination
   C. Examination of the abdomen, back, and lymphatics
   D. Pelvic examination
      1. Vulva
      2. Clitoris
      3. BUS (Bartholin, urethra, Skene glands)
      4. Vagina
      5. Cervix
      6. Uterus
      7. Adnexa
      8. Rectovaginal examination (guaiac determination, if needed)

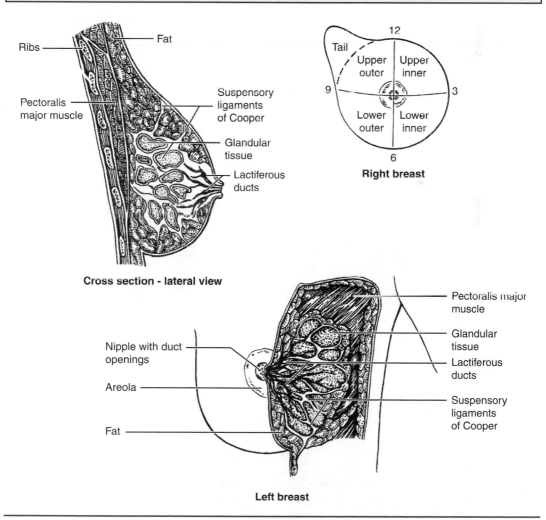

Figure 1.3. Clinical anatomy and associated examination schema of the breast.

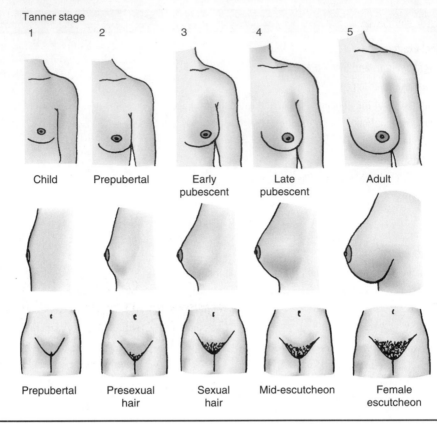

Figure 1.4. Tanner's classification of sexual maturity: breasts and pubic hair.

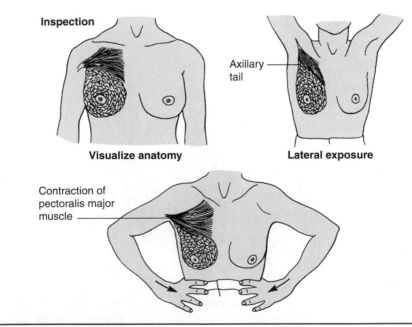

Figure 1.5. Inspection of the breast.

14

Discolorations and/or ulcerations of the skin of the breast or areola/nipple, or edema of the lymphatics, causing a leathery puckered appearance of the skin (like an orange skin, hence called peau d'orange), are abnormal. A clear or milky breast discharge (galactorrhea) requires evaluation. Bloody discharge from the breast is abnormal; it usually does not represent carcinoma, but rather inflammation of a breast structure. Pus usually indicates infection, although an underlying tumor may be encountered.

Palpation follows inspection, first with the patient's arms at her sides and then with the arms raised over her head (Figure 1.6). This is usually done in the supine position, although sometimes use of the sitting position with the patient's arm resting on the examiner's shoulder or over her head for examination of the most lateral aspects of the axilla is helpful. Palpation should be done with slow, careful maneuvers using the flat of the fingers and not the tips. The fingers are moved up and down in a wavelike motion, moving the tissues under them back and forth. By so doing, breast masses are moved so that they may be more easily felt.

A spiral or radial pattern is described over each breast to uniformly cover all of the breast tissue, including that of the axillary tail. If masses are found, their size, shape, consistency (soft, hard, firm, cystic), and mobility, as well as their position, should be determined. Although there are many causes of "lumps," a comparison of three etiologies is presented in Table 1.7. Women with large breasts may demonstrate a firm ridge of tissue found transversely along the lower edge of the breast. This is the inframammary ridge and is a normal finding.

The examination is concluded with gentle pressure inward and then upward at the sides of the areola—a gentle "squeezing" action to express fluid. If fluid is noted on inspection or is expressed, it should be sent for culture and sensitivity and cytopathology (fixed in the same manner as for a slide-technique Pap smear).

How to Teach the Breast Self-Examination Breast self-examination (BSE) is an important part of women's health education. It should be explained that BSE is like the breast examination provided by a clinician as having two

Breast palpation techniques

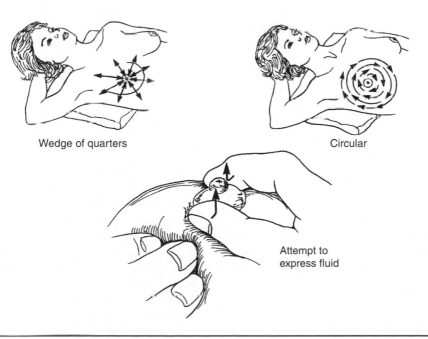

Wedge of quarters

Circular

Attempt to express fluid

Figure 1.6. Palpation of the breast.

Table 1.7. Characteristics of Common Breast Lumps

Characteristic	Fibrocystic disorder	Fibroadenoma	Carcinoma
Incidence with age	25 to menopause, uncommon afterward	Puberty to menopause (peak 20–30)	Increases with age
Number	Usually multiple cysts	Usually one or two	Usually single
Shape and consistency	Well-circumscribed cysts; "sheets" of dense tissue	Smooth, well-circumscribed motile, "rubbery"	Irregular, poorly delineated from other tissue
Mobility	Mobile	Mobile	Mobility limited; often fixed to surrounding skin, tissue
Axillary involvement	No	No	May be present with metastasis
Nipple discharge	No	No	Often

parts–LOOKING and FEELING. The value of performing BSE on a monthly basis and reporting findings to the clinician should be emphasized, specifically including that the treatment of disease detected early in its course is much more likely to be successful compared with treatment started later, after disease had had time to progress. It should be explained that a woman will become expert in knowing her own breast and when something has changed. If something changes, it is then the task of the clinician to determine the significance, if any, of the change.

LOOKING involves observation (inspection) of the breasts in a mirror with arms at the side and then raised over the head (Figure 1.7). Changes in the way the breast or nipples look warrant discussion with the clinician. FEELING involves the systematic examination (palpation) of the entire breast (including up into the area under the armpit) using the flat part of the first three fingers. Lumps, bumps, changes in texture, or unusual discomfort warrant an examination by the clinician. Gentle squeezing of the nipples completes the BSE; if blood, fluid, or pus is expressed, an examination by the clinician is indicated.

Pelvic Examination

How to Do the Pelvic Examination Preparation for the pelvic examination begins with the patient

emptying her bladder and donning an examination gown. An assistant should usually be present, both to prepare specimens and to act as chaperone. Everything that is going to happen should be explained before it occurs. Following the precept "Talk before you touch," avoids anything unexpected.

Abdominal and pelvic examinations require relaxation of the muscles. An abrupt or stern command, such as, "Relax now; I'm not going to hurt you," may raise the patient's fears, whereas a phrase such as, "Try to relax as much as you can, although I know that it's a lot easier for me to say than for you to do" sends two messages: (1) that the patient needs to relax, and (2) that you recognize that it is difficult, both of which demonstrate patience and understanding. A phrase such as, "Let me know if anything is uncomfortable, and I will stop and then we will try to do it differently" tells the patient that there might be discomfort, but that she has control and can stop the examination if discomfort occurs. Likewise, stating, "I am going to touch you now" is helpful in alleviating surprises. Consideration should be given to first touching the inner thigh and not initially touching the genitalia. Few positions leave a woman with such a feeling of helplessness as the lithotomy position; returning a degree of control to her is most helpful.

Using the phrases described here helps demonstrate that the examination is a cooper-

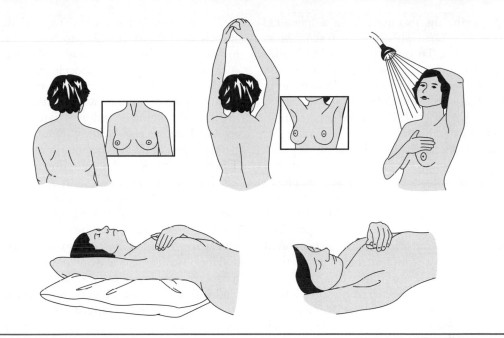

Figure 1.7. Breast self-examination.

ative effort, further empowering the patient in facilitating care. Techniques that help the patient to relax include encouraging the patient to breathe in through her nose and out through her mouth, gently and regularly, rather than holding her breath, and helping the patient to identify specific muscle groups (such as the abdominal wall or the pelvic floor) that need to be made more loose.

The patient is asked to sit at the edge of the examination table and an opened draping sheet is placed over the patient's knees. If a patient requests that a drape not be used, the request should be honored.

Positioning the patient for examination begins with the elevation of the head of the examining table to approximately 30° from horizontal. This serves three purposes: (1) it allows eye contact and facilitates communication between physician and patient; (2) it relaxes the abdominal wall muscle groups, making the examination much easier; and (3) it allows the clinician to observe the patient for responses to the examination, which may provide valuable information (e.g., wincing as evidence of pain on examination). The physician and/or an assistant should help the patient assume the lithotomy position. The patient should be asked to lie back, place her heels in the stirrups, and then slide down to the end of the table until her buttocks are flush with the edge of the table. After the patient is in the lithotomy position, the drape is adjusted so that it does not obscure the clinician's view of the perineum or obscure eye contact between patient and physician.

The physician should sit at the foot of the examining table with the examination lamp adjusted to shine on the perineum. The lamp is optimally positioned in front of the physician's chest a few inches below the level of the chin, at approximately an arm's length distance from the perineum. The physician should glove both hands. This protects the patient's modesty and sense of privacy, and also protects the clinician from any possible sexually transmitted infection. After contact with the patient, there should be minimal contact with equipment such as the lamp.

The pelvic examination begins with the inspection and examination of the external genitalia. The physician may begin by firmly placing the back of his or her hand on the patient's inner thigh, progressing to both hands touching the external genitalia, and thereafter to a sequential inspection and palpation of the external genitalia. Initial touching of the inner thigh begins the examination in a "personal and sensitive" area, although not as sensitive as the perineum. Throughout the pelvic examination, the examiner should make use of the bilateral symmetry of the body. Dissymmetry shows that one side is different from the other, perhaps because of disease, which then requires an explanation.

Inspection should include the mons pubis, labia majora and labia minora, perineum, and perianal area. Inspection continues as palpation is performed in an orderly sequence, starting with the clitoral hood, which may be pulled back to inspect the glans proper. The labia are spread laterally to allow inspection of the introitus and outer vagina. The urethral meatus and the areas of the urethra and Skene glands should be inspected. After forewarning the patient about the possible sensation of having to urinate, the forefinger is placed an inch or so into the vagina to gently milk the urethra. A culture should be taken of any discharge from the urethral opening. The forefinger is then rotated posteriorly to palpate the area of the Bartholin glands between that finger and the thumb (Figure 1.8).

The patient is then asked to bear down slightly as if she were going to have a bowel movement while the vaginal walls are inspected for cystocele or rectocele. Just as with the breast examination, women at different ages demonstrate different stages of development of the genitals and associated hair, as seen in Tanner's classification (Figure 1.4).

The next step is the speculum examination. The parts of the speculum are shown in Figure 1.9. There are two types of specula in common use for the examination of adults. The Pederson speculum has flat and narrow blades that barely curve on the sides. The Pederson speculum works well for most nulliparous women, and for postmenopausal women with atrophic, narrowed vaginas. The Graves speculum has blades that are wider, higher, and curved on the sides; it is more appropriate for most parous women. Its wider, curved blades keep the looser vaginal walls of multiparous women separated for visualization. A Pederson speculum with extra narrow blades may be used for visualizing the cervix in pubertal girls.

Before the examination, the speculum is examined to be sure it is clean and in proper

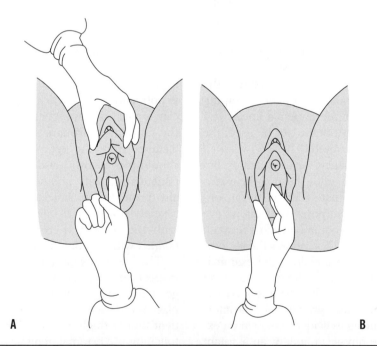

A **B**

Figure 1.8. Palpation of the Bartholin, urethral, and Skene glands. **(A)** Palpation of urethral and Skene glands and "milking" of urethra. **(B)** Palpation of Bartholin glands.

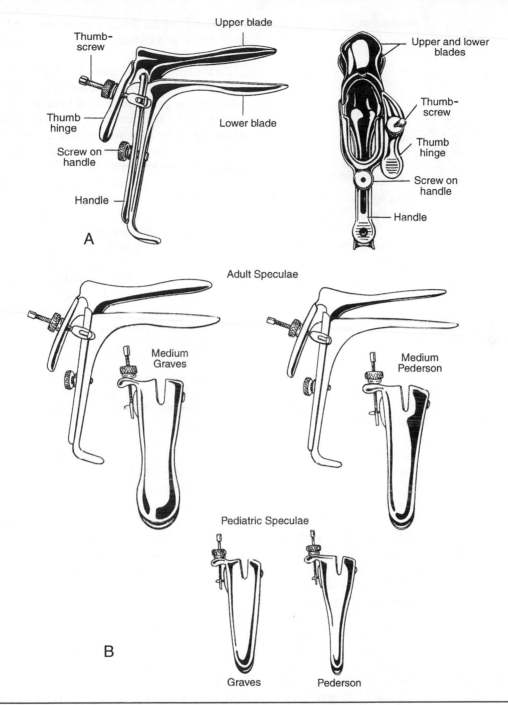

Figure 1.9. The vaginal speculum. **(A)** Parts of the vaginal speculum. **(B)** Types of vaginal specula.

working order. If not already warm, the speculum should be warmed either with warm water or by holding it in the examiner's hand. Warming the speculum is done for the comfort of the patient and to aid with insertion.

Insertion of the speculum should take into account the normal anatomic relations, as illustrated in Figure 1.10. Until recently, use of lubricants was avoided because of interference with cytologic interpretation. With new

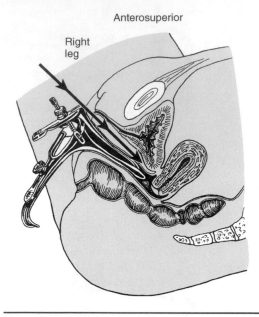

Figure 1.10. Speculum insertion (note the angle of insertion).

liquid-based techniques of obtaining Pap smears, this is now less of a concern. Situations that may require lubricant use are encountered infrequently and include some prepubertal girls, some postmenopausal women, and patients with irritation or lesions of the vagina.

Most physicians find the control of pressure and the movement of the speculum are facilitated by holding the speculum with the dominant hand. The speculum is held by the handle with the blades completely closed. The first two fingers of the opposite hand are placed on the perineum laterally and just below the introitus; pressure is applied downward and slightly inward until the introitus is opened slightly. If the patient is sufficiently relaxed, this downward pressure on the perineum results in an open introitus, into which the speculum may be easily inserted. The speculum is initially inserted in a horizontal plane with the width of the blades oblique to the vertical axis of the introitus. The speculum is then directed posteriorly at an approximately 45° angle from horizontal; the angle is adjusted as the speculum is inserted so that the speculum slides into the vagina with minimal resistance. If the patient is not relaxed,

posterior pressure from a finger inserted in the vagina sometimes relaxes the perineal musculature.

As the speculum is inserted, a slight continuous downward pressure is exerted so that distension of the perineum is used to create space into which the speculum may advance. Taking advantage of the distensibility of the perineum and vagina posterior to the introitus is a crucial concept for the efficient and comfortable manipulation of the speculum examination (and later for the bimanual and rectovaginal examination). Pressure superiorly causes pain in the sensitive area of the urethra and clitoris. The speculum is inserted as far as it will go, which in most women means insertion of the entire speculum length. The speculum is then opened in a smooth and deliberate fashion. With slight tilting of the speculum, the cervix slides into view between the blades of the speculum. The speculum is then locked into the open position using the thumbscrew. Failure to find the cervix most commonly results from not having the speculum inserted far enough. Keeping the speculum fully inserted while opening the speculum does not result in discomfort.

When the speculum is locked into position, it usually stays in place without being held. For most patients, the speculum is opened sufficiently by use of the upper thumbscrew. In some cases, however, more space is required. This may be obtained by gently expanding the vertical distance between the speculum blades by use of the screw on the handle of the speculum.

With the speculum in place, the cervix and the deep lateral vaginal vault may be inspected and specimens obtained.

Before obtaining the Pap smear, the patient should be told that she may feel a slight "scraping" sensation, but no pain. Specimens are collected to fully evaluate the transformation zone, where cervical intraepithelial neoplasia is more likely to be encountered. If a slide is used for the specimen, an endocervical sample and an exocervical sample commonly are obtained, using appropriate sampling devices. The material is thinly smeared on a slide, avoiding large accumulations of mucus and other material. Immediate fixation is important to avoid air drying the artifacts, which compromise cytopathologic evaluation. Slides left in air longer than 10 seconds demonstrate a high incidence of such artifacts. If a liquid-based technique is used, specimens are obtained from the exocervix and endocervix and are placed in a collection medium (Figure 1.11).

Speculum withdrawal also allows for inspection of the vaginal walls. After telling the patient that the speculum is to be removed, the blades of the speculum are opened slightly by putting pressure on the thumb hinge, and the thumbscrew is completely loosened. Opening the speculum blades slightly before starting to withdraw the speculum avoids pinching the cervix between the blades. The speculum is withdrawn approximately 1 inch before pressure on the thumb hinge is slowly released. The speculum is withdrawn slowly enough to allow inspection of the vaginal walls. The blades of the speculum are naturally brought together by vaginal wall pressure. As the end of the speculum blades approaches the introitus, there should be no pressure on the thumb hinge, otherwise the anterior blade can flip up, hitting the sensitive vaginal, urethral, and clitoral tissues.

The bimanual examination uses both a "vaginal" hand and an "abdominal" hand to entrap and palpate the pelvic organs. The bimanual examination begins by exerting gentle pressure on the abdomen approximately halfway between the umbilicus and the pubic hair line with the abdominal hand, while inserting the index finger of the vaginal hand

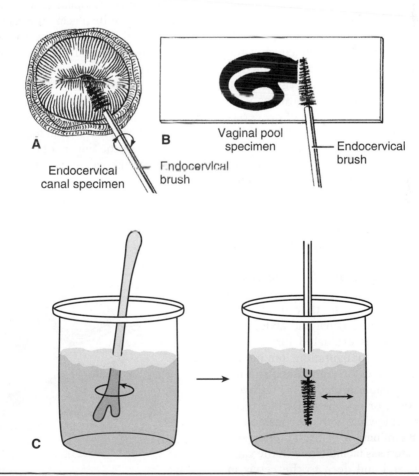

Vaginal pool
specimen

Endocervical
brush

A

Endocervical
canal specimen

B

Endocervical
brush

C

Figure 1.11. Pap smear. **(A)** Obtaining endocervical portion of Pap smear. **(B)** Spread specimen before fixation within 10 seconds. **(C)** Placement of specimens in liquid collection medium.

into the vagina to approximately 2 inches and gently pushing downward, distending the vaginal canal. The patient is asked to feel the muscles being pushed on and to relax them as much as possible. Then both the index and middle fingers are inserted into the vagina until they rest at the limit of the vaginal vault in the posterior fornix behind and below the cervix. A great deal of space may be created by posterior distension of the perineum. Occasionally, only the index finger of the vaginal hand can be comfortably inserted.

During the bimanual examination, the pelvic structures are "caught" and palpated between the abdominal and vaginal hands. Whether to use the dominant hand as the abdominal or vaginal hand is a question of personal preference. The most common error in this part of the pelvic examination is failure to make effective use of the abdominal hand. Pressure should be applied with the flat part of the fingers, not the fingertips, starting midway between the umbilicus and the hairline, moving downward in conjunction with upward movements of the vaginal hand. The bimanual examination continues with the circumferential examination of the cervix for its size, shape, position, mobility, and the presence or absence of tenderness or mass lesions. Cervical position is often related to uterine position. A posterior cervix is often associated with an anteverted or midposition uterus, whereas an anterior cervix is often associated with a retroverted uterus. Sharp flexion of the uterus, however, may alter these relations.

Bimanual examination of the uterus is accomplished by lifting the uterus up toward the abdominal fingers so that it may be palpated between the vaginal and abdominal hands. The uterus is evaluated for its size, shape, consistency, configuration, and mobility, as well as masses or tenderness, and for position (anteversion, midposition, retroversion, anteflexion, or retroflexion). The technique varies somewhat with the position of the uterus. Examination of the anterior and midposition uterus is facilitated with the vaginal fingers lateral and deep to the cervix in the posterior fornix. The uterus is gently lifted upward to the abdominal fingers and a gentle

side-to-side "searching" motion of the vaginal fingers is combined with steady pressure and palpation by the abdominal hand to determine the characteristics of the uterus (Figure 1.12).

Examination of the retroverted uterus is more difficult. In some cases, the vaginal fingers may be slowly pushed below or at the level of the uterine fundus, after which gentle pressure exerted inward and upward causes the uterus to antevert, or at least to move "upward," somewhat facilitating palpation. Then palpation is accomplished as in the normally anteverted uterus. If this cannot be done, a waving motion with the vaginal fingers in the posterior fornix must be combined with an extensive rectovaginal examination to assess the retroverted uterus.

Bimanual examination of the adnexa to assess the ovaries, fallopian tubes, and support structures begins by placing the vaginal fingers to the side of the cervix, deep in the lateral fornix. The abdominal hand is moved to the same side, just inside the flare of the sacral arch and above the pubic hairline. Pressure is then applied downward and toward the symphysis with the abdominal hand, at the same time lifting upward with the vaginal fingers. The same movements of the fingers of both hands used to assess the uterus are used to assess the ad-

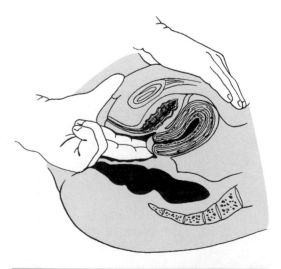

Figure 1.12. Bimanual examination of the uterus and adnexa.

nexal structures, which are brought between the fingers by these maneuvers to evaluate their size, shape, consistency, configuration, mobility, and tenderness, as well as to palpate for masses. Special care must be taken when examining the ovaries, which are sensitive even in the absence of pathology. The ovaries are palpable in normal menstrual women approximately half of the time, whereas palpation of ovaries in postmenopausal women is less common.

The rectovaginal examination is an integral part of the complete pelvic examination on initial and annual examination, as well as at interval examinations whenever clinically indicated. Because patients may have had bad experiences with this part of the pelvic examination, a careful explanation of the value of the examination and reassurance that the examination will be gently done is helpful.

The rectovaginal examination is begun by changing the glove on the vaginal hand and using a liberal supply of lubricant. The examination may be comfortably performed if the natural inclination of the rectal canal is followed: upward at a 45° angle for approximately 1 to 2 cm, then downward (Figure 1.13). This is accomplished by positioning the fingers of the vaginal hand as for the bimanual examination, except that the index finger is also flexed. The middle finger is then gently

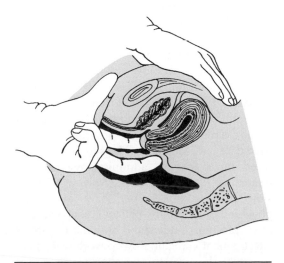

Figure 1.13. Rectovaginal examination.

inserted through the rectal opening and inserted to the "bend" where the angle turns downward. The index (vaginal) finger is inserted into the vagina, and both fingers are inserted until the vaginal finger rests in the posterior fornix below the cervix, and the rectal finger rests as far as it can go into the rectal canal. Asking the patient to bear down as the rectal finger is inserted is not necessary, and may add to the tension of the patient. Palpation of the pelvic structures is then accomplished as in their vaginal palpation. The uterosacral ligaments are also palpated to determine if they are symmetrical, smooth, and nontender (as normally), or if they are nodular, slack, or thickened. The rectal canal is evaluated, as are the integrity and function of the rectal sphincter.

After palpation is complete, the fingers are rapidly but steadily removed in a reversal of the sequence of movements used on insertion. Care should be taken to avoid contamination of the vagina with fecal matter. A guaiac determination is routinely made from fecal material collected on the rectal finger in patients 40 years or older.

At the conclusion of the pelvic examination, the patient is asked to move back up on the table and thereafter to sit up. It is both good manners and helpful to offer a hand to the patient when she sits up. Discussion of the findings and recommendations for further care should be done after the patient has had a chance to clean herself, go to the washroom if needed, and dress.

Comprehensive Health Planning and Patient Management

Obstetrician–gynecologists promote good health, prevent disease, and manage specific disease states or medical conditions. The issues may fall within the scope of the obstetrician–gynecologist's practice, or may require consultation or referral. At times, the obstetrician–gynecologist provides care, and at other times the clinician serves as the coordinator or facilitator of care. When a specific problem is identified, the classic schema of diagnosis and treatment facilitates care. Table 1.8 outlines the five tasks associated with patient management.

> **Table 1.8.** Generalized Patient Management Format
>
> 1. Formulation of differential diagnosis
>   a. Formulate a differential diagnostic list of conditions that reasonably fit history and physical examination findings.
>   b. Use to facilitate consideration of reasonably possible conditions and to provide a list for reconsideration if the presumptive diagnosis proves to be wrong.
> 2. Selection of laboratory testing
>   a. Select tests that are necessary to confirm/rule out elements of the differential diagnosis and to select presumptive diagnosis.
>   b. Tests should be valid and reliable, and present no unreasonable risks or cost relative to the value of the information to be obtained.
> 3. Selection of presumptive diagnosis
>   a. Select a diagnosis that best fits information at hand.
>   b. Remember that a patient may have more than one problem.
> 4. Development of management plan
>   a. Develop a plan that provides proved, effective treatment for presumptive diagnosis.
>   b. Benefits of proposed therapy should outweigh the risk of no treatment.
> 5. Follow-up management
>   a. Follow up on response to therapy to ascertain if the desired outcome is being or has been achieved. If not, the presumptive diagnosis and/or components of the therapy may be in error and reconsideration of both is required.
>   b. This is an iterative process until the desired outcome is achieved.

Part III: The Physician–Patient "Contract"

The relationship between patient and physician should be one founded in mutual trust and respect and with the joint goal of excellent, open, honest communication and decision making free of coercion from the perspective of the patient. The age-old view of the relationship and responsibility of the physician as a sacred trust remains valid and should be a guiding principle in the physician's professional life.

The process of this relationship is often presented in the business/legal language of a "contract." Informed consent, for example, is the specific process used in preparation for some medical and most surgical managements. Special situations such as sexual assault, domestic violence, and child abuse are governed by laws requiring reports to social service or legal authorities, and it is the responsibility of the physician to be aware of these responsibilities and to carry them out as required. As medical technology becomes more powerful, many patients will wish to avail themselves of advance directives so that they are not subject to means of care that go beyond their desires. Using this process to help patients with these decisions is another important responsibility of the physician.

Health care is also an increasingly sophisticated and complicated business. Clinicians practice in different ways (e.g., solo practice, partnerships, as employees of health maintenance organizations or hospitals) and receive patients whose care is paid for by various kinds of health insurance organizations or who will require assistance to enter programs such as Medicare and Medicaid. The systems, in turn, often have special "administrative requirements" for care, sometimes involving "permission" from a "gate-keeper" or primary care physician to whom the patient is assigned. The physician must understand how these systems affect patient care and how to work with them to assure that quality and appropriate care is rendered.

CHAPTER 2

ETHICS IN OBSTETRICS AND GYNECOLOGY

This chapter deals primarily with APGO Educational Topic:

Topic 6: Legal and Ethical Issues in Obstetrics and Gynecology.

Students should be able to recognize and understand the basis of ethical conflicts in women's health care, thereby promoting better patient care and preventing critical errors in treatment planning. Also, legal obligations to protect a patient's interests must be understood to be applied.

Creating an Ethical Framework

Physicians often encounter ethical dilemmas in the context of their dealings with patients. To prepare for these events, it is important to have created a framework within which ethical issues can be addressed. By using the substantial amount of literature that exists on the topic, a health care provider will be able to make choices in a systematic manner rather than those based on emotions, personal bias, or social pressures. A summary of the basic concepts, from the book *Clinical Ethics* (McGraw-Hill, 2002), is included in Table 2.1.

Analysis of Ethical Dilemmas

Consider the hypothetical case of a Jehovah's Witness patient, hemorrhaging from a placenta previa, who needs to have a cesarean section performed. Do we give blood against the patient's expressed wishes (a form of battery), even to save her life? Do we allow her to die while we deliver her child safely but motherless?

How can you use the framework for ethical decision making to identify the basic ethical dilemmas of a complex case? The approach is illustrated by detailed analysis of this case.

The patient's husband, also a Jehovah's Witness, and her mother, who is not a member of that group, accompany her. The patient rapidly loses 1 liter of blood, and evidence of nonreassuring fetal status is found on the electronic fetal monitor. She reaffirms her absolute refusal of blood or blood products, even though an emergency cesarean section is proposed for her own and her fetus's survival. Her blood pressure is dropping, despite rapid hydration. She becomes unconscious. The anesthesiologist says the patient will probably die with the insults of anesthesia and surgery without blood transfusion. The patient's mother demands that you give her daughter blood. The husband refuses. The fetal heart tracing demonstrates increasingly severe nonreassuring fetal status, consistent with impending in utero fetal demise. You begin the cesarean section and deliver a healthy 7-lb girl with Apgar scores of 2 and then 8 with resuscitation. The patient survives the surgery, but in recovery her blood pressure drops to 50/0 postoperatively, and she remains unconscious and on a ventilator with a central venous pressure of 0. The patient's mother screams, "You are killing her! She is my only child!" Her husband firmly reminds you of the religious beliefs he and his wife share, and warns you that his attorney is available if needed. What is the right thing to do?

The first step is to try to separate this complex and emotional case into separate concerns, using the ethical framework. Separating a case into the four areas of concern allows us to fit each particular problem into a group of ethical issues that are associated with particular principles central to medical ethics. This process of systematic analysis and reflection is basic to medical ethics.

Considering this first case, we would ask, "What was the *medical indication* for the cesarean section?" Clearly, both child and

---

Table 2.1. A Functional Scheme for Clinical Ethical Decision Making

Ethical concern: MEDICAL INDICATION	Ethical concern: PATIENT PREFERENCES
What is the best treatment?	What does the patient want?
What are the alternatives?	Ethical principle: AUTONOMY
Ethical principle: BENEFICENCE	Respect for the patient's right to self-determination
The duty to promote the good of the patient	Ethical principle: CONTEXTUAL ISSUES
Ethical concern: QUALITY OF LIFE	What does the patient want? What are the needs of society?
What impact will the proposed treatment or lack of it have on the patient's life	Ethical principle: JUSTICE
Ethical principle: NONMALEFICENCE	The patient should be given what is his or her due.
The duty not to inflict harm or injury	

mother would die without surgery. Continuing acute hemorrhage from placenta previa has no therapy other than surgical delivery and removal of the placenta. Support of the cardiovascular system with blood products is medically indicated. Yet this patient has clearly stated her *preference:* She will, under no circumstances, accept blood products. She believes that receiving blood is directly opposed to God's will and would permanently and negatively affect her spiritual self. She does not believe life under such circumstances, that is, after receiving blood, to be acceptable.

From her physician's viewpoint, blood transfusion is more likely to produce a better quality of life, that is, survival without neurologic or major organ sequelae. Without blood products, her survival is questionable, and even with survival, her risks for prolonged intensive care unit (ICU) stay, cardiac failure, renal failure, and hematologic sequelae are much greater.

Considering *contextual issues,* we wonder how this newborn child will do *without its mother.* In addition, what is the validity of the cost of care in an ICU for the sequelae resulting from the patient's choice when the ICU bed may be needed by other patients? What about the grandmother's concerns? Is the husband coercing the patient not to accept blood? Is he coercing the physician with comments about his attorney, or is that his right to protect his wife? What would the law say if we gave the patient blood without permission?

This case is complex, but it is clear that the patient's choice to refuse blood products is an underlying issue. Does this patient's autonomous refusal constitute a real choice, and, if so, should we accept it? Although the law has much to say about the rights of individuals to choose or refuse care, the choice not to give blood is based on the great respect caregivers must have for the right of patients to determine their care, which medical ethics has supported.

In more general terms, the medical indications for a proposed management always need to be as clear and as "scientific" as possible. Is the benefit of what is proposed clearly greater than the harm that might be caused, or is the benefit at a level that makes the harm acceptable?

Consider a second case: A 33-year-old mother of two, dying of cervical cancer, has been given a high dose of morphine to try to abate her increasing and prolonged pain, but her respirations have dropped to three per minute. Should we give her a narcotic antagonist, or let her die sooner as an effect of the medication for her intractable pain? This patient is at risk from the pain medication needed to alleviate her suffering. Is the relief of pain so great a benefit that the decreased respiratory rate and potential respiratory arrest are acceptable?

Consider a variation on this case. The patient also is unable to eat because of the pain, and the family requests total parenteral nutrition (TPN). It will make them "feel better about things." Many would consider total parenteral nutrition in this case to be medically futile and question the ethics of its continued use. Cases related to *medical indications* involve such concerns as benefit to the patient (or *beneficence*) and the related concept of *futility.*

The cases that can be categorized under *patient preferences* revolve around the principle of *autonomy,* the respect we hold for the patient's right to choose care. It is important to note that the physician–patient relationship emphasizes a relationship between the physician and the patient. Even in obstetrics, in which the consequences of patient choices on another potential life can be significant, the primacy of the physician–patient (versus physician–fetus) relationship is paramount. What the patient wants, and her capacity to make those choices, are in question here.

Consider an additional case: A pregnant woman uses cocaine. Should the mother-to-be who uses cocaine be held accountable for the condition, including death, of her unborn child? Does this drug-using mother have the capacity to make decisions about her unborn child? By reason of the effect of the drugs, has she lost the capacity for acceptable decision making? Is society bound by her choices? What about the rights of the unborn child in this case?

Quality of life issues are always important. The absence of pain in a terminal cancer patient may significantly improve the quality of her living, even if the length of time is shortened. Some patients might consider the diminution of quality of life with potential permanent neurologic damage or loss of time with children arising as a result of blood loss (as in the first case) so significant that they will accept blood despite their religious beliefs. So, the harms of treatment or no treatment viewed in the context of a particular patient's life are what must be considered. In a sense, this deals with *nonmaleficence:* the duty not to harm patients while treating them.

Harm clearly also must be viewed in the patient's framework. In the second case, prolonged life may not be valued if significant pain or a lengthy hospital stay constitutes the quality of life that must be accepted. That becomes unacceptable "harm" to that patient. Yet, in the first case, the quality of life after blood transfusion may be acceptable to the patient because of the added time to be spent with her children and the diminished risk of major organ damage. The benefits of proposed therapy must be framed in the outcome of that therapy for good or ill.

Finally, all the *contextual and socioeconomic issues* that surround a particular case should be considered. It is here that the concerns of the children and mother and father and other relatives, and concerns about legal issues and issues of cost are addressed. Threats to sue, angry families, and "dumping" of patients without health insurance or money to pay for health care, for example, can so overwhelm the health care team that the real ethical issues of a case (e.g., the capacity to choose, or futility) are not considered. Socioeconomic issues, although important in making final choices about care, in general should not override clear medical indications or clear patient preferences.

When socioeconomic considerations are deeply divided from what is medically indicated or what a patient prefers, they cause problems. For example, imagine that the 33-year-old mother cannot die at home near her children because of reimbursement issues. In the first case, the sequelae of refused blood products and prolonged ICU stay deny a bed to a patient with complications of leukemia therapy, so this patient's care must be delivered in another institution away from trusted physicians. These outcomes appear unfair or unjust, and illustrate cases dealing with the ethical principle of justice and how to determine allocation of resources.

What are the unique ethical problems of obstetrics and gynecology? Clearly, maternal and fetal conflicts and how we define procreation and family are uniquely central to obstetrics and gynecology. The primary concern of physicians is the best care of their patients. This has been true since Hippocrates admonished us "to do away with the suffering of the sick." Special-interest groups have variously defined the "rights" of the fetus so that, at times, the primacy of duty to the patient (mother) seems in question. Yet there never has been a time in the development of medical ethics or in the opinions expressed by the American College of Obstetricians and Gynecologists that the fetus has been considered to take precedence over the mother in considerations of medical care or the therapeutic alliance of physician and patient. This is valuable to keep in mind when considering such cases.

Abortion would be a primary example of situations of this type. The controversy can be so emotional and damaging that a discussion based on ethical principles is difficult. Consistent with our primary duty to the patient, circumstances where survival of the mother would be seriously compromised by the maintenance of pregnancy are the least controversial. Clearly, preservation of the patient/mother's life and loss of the fetus would be supported by many viewers. As the "case" gets further away from this relatively clear situation, the discussion becomes more complex. To understand these controversies, it is valuable to explore what elements we use to define life as "human" before we define loss of a fetus as loss of a human life. What are the elements of humanness, and when are they achieved in pregnancy? Is ability to survive independent of the mother significant? Is the potential to achieve those elements defining human pertinent? These are important issues to explore before considering, for example, a case such as elective abortion at 12 weeks, or selective pregnancy reduction in a multifetal gestation.

Defining these issues also helps in consideration of the rights of pregnant women to engage in behavior or activities that put the fetus at some risk, such as use of cocaine, alcohol, smoking, or refusal of cesarean delivery for fetal indications. At what level of human development or potential, if at all, does concern for fetal outcomes override the patient/mother's autonomous choices? In what sort of case might we reasonably override expressed patient wishes to preserve fetal life? For example, how does drug or alcohol use interact with capacity to choose? Consider the case of the cocaine-abusing pregnant woman: Is the drug-using mother's decision to continue to use drugs during pregnancy acceptable? What are the consequences of incarcerating such mothers as a solution? Is an acutely intoxicated mother's decision to refuse cesarean section for fetal indications acceptable?

In looking at the many changes in reproductive endocrinology, the idea of a clearest case, sometimes called a "paradigm" case, may help sort out the ethical discussions. What, for example, is the clearest set of relationships between parents and children? Biologically, the relationship between the mother contributing the egg and the father contributing the sperm *in vivo* without augmentation is the paradigm case. The relationship of this family unit, with the parental responsibilities for financial support, history, culture, and education, has been the traditional paradigm for family in our culture. How these elements change within a group of cases will vary. Adoption by a mother/father pair, adoption by a single parent, adoption by two mothers or two fathers, in vitro combination of egg from mother and father, in vitro combination of unrelated sperm with the maternal egg, and the varieties of gestational patterns with surrogacy and egg and sperm donation are all variations on the original theme.

These questions lead to others. What do we do with the "extra" fertilized or harvested eggs from in vitro fertilization? Is this different or the same as the issue of humanness or potential for humanness in a discussion of abortion? What about the rejuvenation of the menopausal woman so that she can conceive and deliver? She and/or her partner may well not live through the maturation of their child. Who will then assume the parental responsibility, as well as the associated financial and logistic responsibilities? To whom does the child turn to seek redress if these responsibilities are not met, or are met unsatisfactorily?

Professionalism

It is expected that physicians exhibit the highest level of professionalism when dealing with patients and with their colleagues. The Accreditation Council for Graduate Medical Education General Competencies (version 1.3) describes professionalism as commitment to carrying out professional responsibilities, adherence to ethical principles, and a sensitivity to diverse patient populations. The physician must put the interests of the patient above his or her own self-interest (altruism) and demonstrate accountability to patients, to society, and to the profession.

Application of Principles

In obstetrics and gynecology, as in all of medicine, there is potential to use the skills and concepts of medical ethics and of professionalism to help in the management of difficult situations. To do so requires using methods of systematic reflection and analysis to delineate the ethical problems. The analytical framework shown in this chapter helps identify ethical issues, placing them in specific ethical areas, associating them with some principles and families of cases. Further analysis comparing a case to a paradigm case may be helpful. Finally, review of the literature using the National Reference Center for Bioethics Literature ([800]MED-ETHX), the Medline Bioethics search area, or the medical library will bring together various authors' views on the ethical issues surrounding a given clinical situation.

CHAPTER 3

EMBRYOLOGY, ANATOMY, AND REPRODUCTIVE GENETICS

There is no specific educational topic focused exclusively on the understanding of basic embryology, anatomy, and reproductive genetics, which is essential to the study of obstetrics and gynecology and which is the focus of this chapter.

Embryology

A knowledge of the embryology of the female reproductive system is helpful in understanding both normal anatomy and the structural anomalies that can sometimes occur. The genital system develops from embryonic intermediate mesoderm. With the folding of the embryo, the intermediate mesoderm comes to lie as two longitudinal rods on either side of the primitive aorta (the nephrogenic cords [Figure 3.1A]). The *urogenital* ridges are dorsal outgrowths of the nephrogenic cords; they give rise to elements of both the urinary and the reproductive systems (Figure 3.1B).

In general, the elements of the reproductive system pass through an undifferentiated stage in the early embryo; that is, development is identical in the male and female. Later, sex-specific differentiation occurs.

Development of the Ovary

Genetic sex, determined at fertilization, depends on whether the X-bearing oocyte is fer-

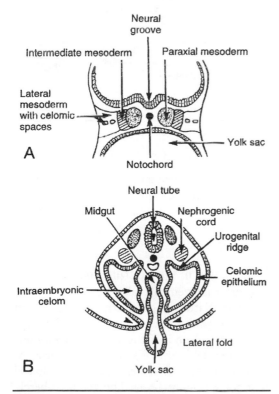

A

B

tilized by an X- or Y-bearing sperm. However, early in development, the gonads are undifferentiated (i.e., the sex of the embryo cannot be determined from the appearance of the gonad).

The gonads begin to develop during the fifth week, when a portion of the urogenital ridge on the medial side of the mesonephric kidney thickens to form the *gonadal ridge*. The celomic epithelium divides to form fingerlike bands of cells (the *primary sex cords*), which project into the underlying mesodermal mesenchyme of the gonadal ridge. This growth results in the creation of a cortex and a medulla in the indifferent (undifferentiated) gonad. In the female, the cortical area predominates in the mature gonad. The follicles are contained in this cortical tissue.

During the fourth week, the *primordial germ cells* (which eventually give rise to the gametes) appear in the yolk sac. As the embryo folds, some of the yolk sac is incorporated into the embryo. During the sixth week, the primordial germ cells migrate into the mesenchyme of the gonadal ridge, where they become associated with the primary sex cords. In the female, the primordial germ cells become oogonia, which divide by mitosis during fetal life. No oogonia form after birth.

In the male, the tunica albuginea of the testis begins to form in the mesenchymal tissue of the medulla during the eighth week. This is the first indication of the sex of the embryo. In the absence of a Y chromosome, the undifferentiated gonad develops into an ovary, which is identifiable by approximately the tenth week of development. In the ovary, the primary sex cords degenerate, and secondary sex cords (cortical cords) appear and extend from the surface epithelium into the underlying mesenchyme. The *oogonia* are incorporated into them, and at approximately 16 weeks of development, the cortical cords organize into *primordial follicles.* Each follicle eventually consists of an oogonium, derived from a primary germ cell, surrounded by a single layer of squamous follicular cells, derived from the cortical cords. *Follicular maturation* begins when the oogonia enter the first stage of meiotic division (at which point they are called oocytes). Oocyte development is then arrested until puberty, when one or more follicles are stimulated to continue development each month (see Chapters 34 and 35).

Figure 3.1. Early development of urogenital system. (**A**) Nephrogenic cords. (**B**) Urogenital ridges.

Development of the Genital Ducts

In both the male and female embryos, two pairs of ducts initially develop, the mesonephric (wolffian) and the paramesonephric (müllerian). As with the gonad, there is an indifferent (undifferentiated) stage in ductal development. During this stage, both sets of ducts are present in both the male and the female embryo.

In the male embryo, the *mesonephric ducts,* which drain the embryonic mesonephric kidneys, eventually form the *epididymis, ductus deferens,* and *ejaculatory ducts.* In the female embryo, the mesonephric ducts almost completely disappear.

In the female embryo, the *paramesonephric ducts* (or müllerian) persist to form major parts of the reproductive tract (the *fallopian tubes, uterus,* and *parts of the vagina*). The paramesonephric ducts start to develop early in the sixth week, beginning as invaginations of the celomic epithelium in the vicinity of the mesonephric kidneys (Figure 3.2A). For each duct, the invagination fuses to form a tube. The cranial end of each duct opens into the celomic (future peritoneal) cavity. The ducts grow caudally, and the caudal segments fuse at approximately the eighth week of development into the Y-shaped *uterovaginal primordium* or *canal* (Figure 3.2B). The cranial (unfused) portion of each duct becomes a fallopian tube, and the fused portions become the uterus and parts of the vagina. This differentiation does not depend on the presence of ovaries.

When the two paramesonephric ducts fuse, two peritoneal folds are brought together. This creates the broad ligaments of the uterus (Figure 3.2C).

Development of the Vagina

Between weeks 5 and 7, the *primitive cloaca,* a pouchlike enlargement of the caudal end of the hindgut, is divided into the *urogenital sinus* (ventral) and the *anorectal canal* (dorsal). The contact of the caudally growing uterovaginal primordium with the urogenital sinus results in the formation of a solid mass of cells called the vaginal plate. The vaginal plate extends from the urogenital sinus into the caudal end of the uterovaginal primordium. The central cells of the vaginal plate disappear, forming the lumen of the vagina. The peripheral cells of the plate

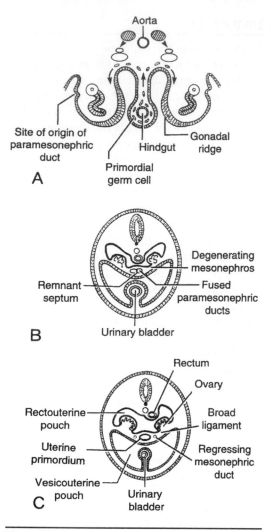

Figure 3.2. Formation of uterus.

persist as the vaginal epithelium. In addition to contributing to the vagina, the urogenital sinus also gives rise to the *epithelium of the urinary bladder,* the *urethra,* the *greater vestibular glands,* and the *hymen.*

Development of the External Genitalia

The external genitalia also pass through an undifferentiated stage. Early in the fourth week, the *genital tubercle,* or phallus, develops at the cranial end of the cloacal membrane. Soon after, labioscrotal swellings and urogenital folds appear at either side of the cloacal membrane (Figure 3.3A). The genital tubercle enlarges in both the male and the female (Figure 3.3B).

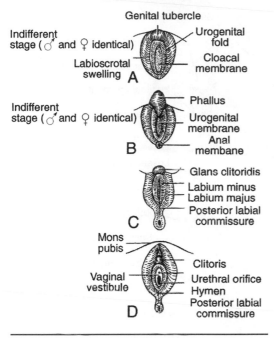

Figure 3.3. Development of the external genitalia.

The division of the cloaca by the urorectal septum divides the cloacal membrane into the dorsal anal membrane and the ventral urogenital membrane. At approximately week 7, these membranes rupture.

At approximately 9 weeks, distinguishing sexual characteristics begin to appear, but the external genital organs are not fully formed until week 12. In the absence of androgens, the external genitalia are feminized (Figure 3.3C). The phallus develops into the relatively small *clitoris*. The unfused urogenital folds form the *labia minora* and the labioscrotal swellings become the *labia majora* (Figure 3.3D).

Anatomy

Bony Pelvis

The bony pelvis is composed of the paired *innominate bones* and the *sacrum*. The innominate bones are joined anteriorly to form the symphysis pubis, and each is articulated posteriorly with the sacrum through the sacroiliac joint (Figure 3.4). The sacrum is composed of five or six sacral vertebrae, which are fused in adulthood. The sacrum articulates with the coccyx inferiorly and with the fifth lumbar vertebra superiorly.

The pelvis is divided into the pelvis major (*false pelvis*) and the pelvis minor (*true pelvis*), which are separated by the linea terminalis. The false pelvis, whose main function is to support the pregnant uterus, is bounded by the lumbar vertebrae posteriorly, an iliac fossa bilaterally, and the abdominal wall anteriorly. The true pelvis is formed by the sacrum and coccyx posteriorly and by the ischium and pubis laterally and anteriorly.

There are *four pelvic planes:* the *pelvic inlet,* the *plane of the greatest diameter,* the *plane of the least diameter* (midplane), and the *pelvic outlet.* The pelvic inlet is bounded posteriorly by the promontory and alae of the sacrum, laterally by the linea terminalis, and anteriorly by the superior surface of the pubic bones. *Thus, the plane of the inlet separates the false pelvis and the true pelvis.* The plane of the greatest diameter is bounded by the junction of the second and third sacral vertebrae posteriorly, the upper part of the obturator foramina laterally, and the midpoint of the pubis anteriorly. The plane of least diameter (the plane of the midplane) extends from the lower border of the pubis anteriorly to the lower sacrum at the level of the ischial spines. This plane is most important clinically because arrest of fetal descent occurs most frequently at this point (midplane arrest). The plane of the outlet consists of two intersecting triangles bounded posteriorly by the tip of the sacrum, laterally by the ischial tuberosities and the sacrotuberous ligaments, and anteriorly by the lower border of the symphysis. There are certain key diameters of the pelvis that are important in assessing the space available during fetal descent (Figure 3.5; Table 3.1).

The female pelvis may be classified into four basic types, according to the scheme of Caldwell and Moloy (Figure 3.6). The most common type of pelvis is the *gynecoid,* occurring in approximately 40 to 50% of women. In general, this pelvic shape is cylindrical and has adequate space along its length and breadth. The *platypelloid* pelvis occurs in only 2 to 5% of women; the *android* pelvis occurs in approximately 30% of all women, but in only 10 to 15% of Black women; and the *anthropoid* type occurs in approximately 20% of all women and in approximately 40% of Black

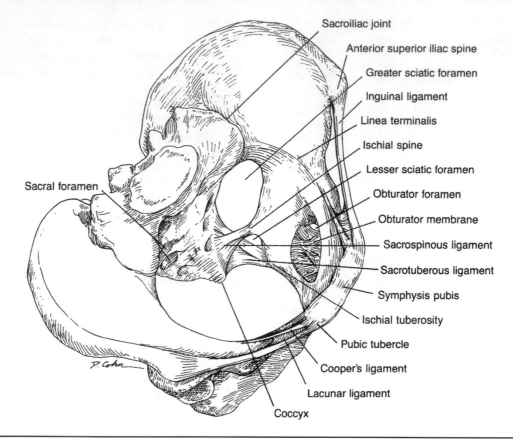

Figure 3.4. View of the pelvis from above, showing bones, joints, ligaments, and foramina.

women. Any female may be of a pure or mixed pelvic type.

Vulva and Perineum

The vulva contains the labia majora, labia minora, mons pubis, clitoris, vestibule, and ducts of glands that open into the vestibule (Figure 3.7). The labia majora are folds of skin with underlying adipose tissue, fused anteriorly with the mons pubis and posteriorly with the perineum. The skin of the labia majora contains hair follicles and sebaceous and sweat glands.

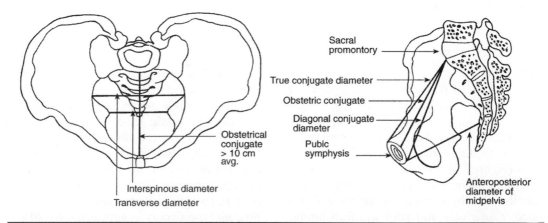

Figure 3.5. Pelvic diameters.

Pelvic Plane	Diameter	Average Length (cm)
Inlet	True conjugate	10.5–11.5
	Obstetric conjugate	10.0–11.0
	Diagonal conjugate	12.5
	Transverse diameter	13.5
	Oblique diameter	12.5
Greatest diameter	Anterior–posterior	12.75
	Transverse	12.5
Midplane	Anterior–posterior	11.5–12.0
	Bispinous (interspinous)	10.0
Outlet	Anterior–posterior	11.5
	Bituberous	8.0–11.0

Table 3.1. Length of Pelvic Plane Diameters

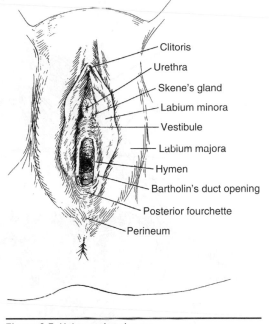

Figure 3.7. Vulva and perineum.

The labia minora are narrow skin folds lying inside the labia majora. The labia minora merge anteriorly with the prepuce and frenulum of the clitoris, and posteriorly with the labia majora and the perineum. The labia minora contain sebaceous and sweat glands but no hair follicles, and there is no underlying adipose tissue. The clitoris, which is located anterior to the labia minora, is the embryologic homolog of the penis. It consists of two crura (corresponding to the corpora cavernosa in the male) and the glans, which is found superior to the point of fusion of the crura. On the ventral surface of the glans is the *frenulum,* the fused junction of the labia minora. The *vestibule* lies between the labia minora and is bounded anteriorly by the clitoris and posteriorly by the perineum. The urethra and the vagina open into the vestibule in the midline. The ducts of *Skene (paraurethral) glands* and *Bartholin glands* also empty into the vestibule.

The *muscles of the vulva* (superior transverse perineal, bulbocavernosus, and ischiocavernosus) lie superficial to the fascia of the urogenital diaphragm (Figure 3.8). The vulva rests on the triangular-shaped *urogenital diaphragm,* which lies in the anterior part of the pelvis between the ischiopubic rami. The urogenital diaphragm surrounds the lower portion of the sacrum. The uterine cervix projects into the upper portion of the vagina. Therefore, the anterior vaginal wall is approximately 2 cm shorter than the posterior wall. The area around the cervix, the fornix, is divided into four regions: the *anterior fornix,* two *lateral fornices,* and the *posterior fornix.* The posterior

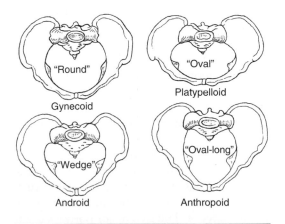

Figure 3.6. Caldwell-Moloy pelvic types.

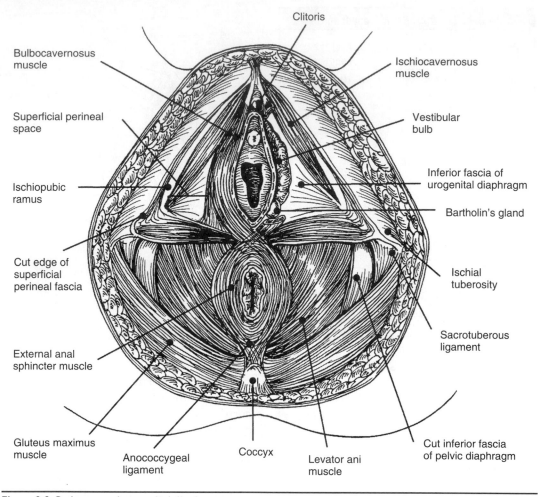

Figure 3.8. Perineum and urogenital diaphragm.

fornix is in close proximity to the peritoneum that forms the floor of the posterior pelvic cul-de-sac (pouch of Douglas).

At its lower end, the vagina traverses the urogenital diaphragm and is then surrounded by the two bulbocavernosus muscles. These act as a sphincter. The *hymen,* a fold of mucosal-covered connective tissue, somewhat obscures the external vaginal orifice in the child. The hymen is fragmented into irregular remnants with sexual activity and childbearing.

The major *blood supply* to the vagina is from the vaginal artery, a branch of the hypogastric artery, and parallel veins.

The *vaginal wall* consists of a mucous membrane and an external muscular layer. The lumen is lined by a stratified squamous epithelium. Beneath this is a submucosal layer of connective tissue, which contains a rich supply of veins and lymphatics. Submucosal rugae throw the lumen of the vagina into the characteristic "H" shape in the young; these folds become less prominent with age. The muscular wall has three layers of smooth muscle. The vaginal wall is extremely distensible, especially under hormonal influences during childbirth.

Uterus

The uterus is covered on each side by the two layers of the broad ligament and lies between the rectum and the bladder (Figure 3.9). The close relation with structures in the broad ligament, especially the uterine arteries and veins and the ureters, has important implications during surgery. The two major portions of the uterus are the *cervix* and the body (*corpus*),

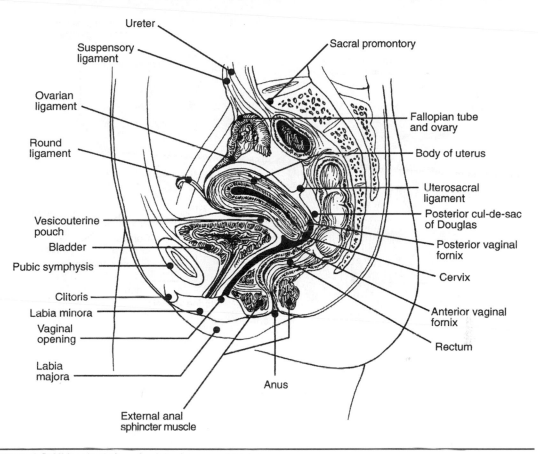

Figure 3.9. Midsagittal view of pelvic viscera and perineum.

which are separated by a narrower isthmus. Before puberty, the length of the cervix and the body are approximately equal; after puberty, the ratio of the body to the cervix is between 2:1 and 3:1. The part of the body where the two uterine (fallopian) tubes enter is called the *cornu*. The part of the corpus above the cornu is called the *fundus*. In the nonparous adult, the uterus is approximately 7 to 8 cm long and 4 to 5 cm wide at the widest part. The cervix is relatively cylindrical in shape and is 2 to 3 cm long. The corpus is generally pear shaped, with the anterior surface flat and the posterior surface convex. In cross section, the lumen of the corpus is triangular.

The position of the uterus is variable. The angle between the long axis of the corpus and the cervix varies from *anteflexion* to *retroflexion*, and the angle between the cervix and the vagina varies from *anteversion* to *retroversion*. The uterus is supported by the following liga-

ments: *uterosacral, cardinal, round,* and *broad.* The *blood supply* to the uterus comes primarily from the uterine arteries, with a contribution from the ovarian arteries, whereas the venous plexus drains through the uterine vein.

The cervix joins the vagina at an angle between 45° and 90°. The opening to the vagina, the external os, is round to oval in nonparous women, but is often a transverse slit after childbirth. The portion of the cervix that projects into the vagina is covered with stratified squamous epithelium, which resembles the vaginal epithelium. The squamous epithelium changes to a simple columnar epithelium in the *transition* (transformation) *zone.* This zone is found at about the level of the external cervical os, although it is found higher in the endocervical canal in postmenopausal women.

There are *three basic layers in the wall of the uterine body* (Figure 3.10). The inner mucosa (the endometrium) consists of the simple

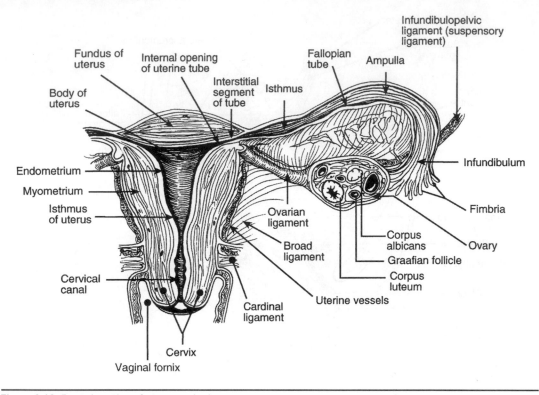

Figure 3.10. Frontal section of uterus and adnexa.

columnar epithelium with underlying connective tissue, changing in structure during the menstrual cycle.

Fallopian Tubes

The fallopian tubes (the oviducts) average approximately 7 to 14 cm in length and are divided into three portions: a narrow and straight isthmus, which adjoins the opening into the uterus; the ampulla, or central portion; and the infundibulum, which is fringed by the finger-shaped fimbriae. The fallopian tubes surround the ovary and help to collect the oocyte at the time of ovulation. The fallopian tubes are supplied by the ovarian and uterine arteries. The epithelial lining of the fallopian tube is ciliated columnar; the cilia beat toward the uterus, assisting in oocyte transport.

Ovaries

Each ovary is approximately 3 to 5 cm long, 2 to 3 cm wide, and 1 to 3 cm thick in the menstrual years. The size decreases by approximately two-thirds after menopause, when follicular development ceases. The ovary is attached to the broad ligament by the mesovarium, to the uterus by the ovarian ligament, and to the side of the pelvis by the suspensory ligament of the ovary (infundibulopelvic ligament), which is the lateral margin of the broad ligament (Figure 3.10). The outer ovarian cortex consists of follicles embedded in a connective tissue stroma. The connective tissue medulla contains smooth muscle fibers, blood vessels, nerves, and lymphatics.

The ovaries are mainly supplied by the ovarian arteries, which are direct branches of the abdominal aorta, but there also is a blood supply from the uterine artery, a branch of the hypogastric artery (or internal iliac artery; Figure 3.11). Venous return via the right ovarian vein is directly into the inferior vena cava, and from the left ovary into the left renal vein.

Anomalies of the Female Reproductive System

Anatomic anomalies, all infrequent, arise from defects during embryologic development.

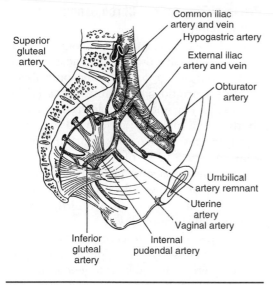

Figure 3.11. Arterial system of the female pelvis.

Absence of the ovary is rare and usually associated with other genital tract anomalies. *Ectopic ovarian tissue* may occur, as supernumerary ovaries or as accessory ovarian tissue. In general, various kinds of uterine and vaginal malformations can arise from incomplete fusion of the paramesonephric ducts, incomplete development of one or both paramesonephric ducts, or incomplete canalization of the vaginal plate.

Absence of the uterus occurs when the paramesonephric ducts degenerate. This condition is associated with vaginal anomalies (such as absence of the vagina) because vaginal development is stimulated by the developing uterovaginal primordium. A double uterus (uterus didelphys) occurs when the inferior parts of the paramesonephric ducts do not fuse; this condition may be associated with a double or a single vagina. A bicornuate uterus results when lack of fusion is limited to the superior portion of the uterine body. If one of the paramesonephric ducts is poorly developed and fusion with the other duct does not occur, the result is a bicornuate uterus with a rudimentary horn. This horn may or may not communicate with the uterine cavity.

Absence of the vagina occurs when the vaginal plate does not develop. It is usually coupled with the absence of the uterus. If the vaginal plate does not canalize, the result is vaginal atresia. Imperforate hymen is a minor example of this.

Reproductive Genetics

Genetics is an integral part of obstetric and gynecologic care. Physicians must be able to identify women at increased risk for fetal abnormalities and to offer appropriate genetic screening and testing to patients based on their personal, family, and medical histories. In addition, physicians are responsible for assessing risk for their patients developing gynecologic or systemic disease.

Genetic Counseling

Genetic counseling serves: (1) to obtain information from the patient to properly assess her risk for developing disease and for conceiving an infant with congenital abnormalities; (2) to provide information to the patient regarding appropriate screening or diagnostic tests. Counseling should be in language understandable to the patient. Genetic counseling is a sensitive area and may evoke anxiety, fear, or denial, even in optimal situations. Counselors should be prepared to repeat all or part of the communicated information, and should check to ensure that patients understand what they have been told.

Information gathering can be accomplished by several methods. Data forms, questionnaires, pedigree construction, and patient interviews are all effective methods for obtaining information concerning personal and family medical history, parental exposure to potentially harmful substances, or other issues that may have an impact on risk assessment. No single method or combination of methods is universally effective in obtaining all appropriate patient information. The specific approaches used to gather information depend on the type of information required and the physician–patient relationship.

Genetic counseling should never be used to coerce a patient to undergo or forgo certain tests or pregnancy-management decisions; information should be obtained and provided in a "nondirective" fashion. *Nondirective counseling* implies that the counselor act in a completely objective manner, never interjecting personal opinions into the counseling session, yet at the same time providing emotional, emphatic support in what are often difficult decision times. It is essential to provide information in this manner so that patients arrive at reproductive decisions based on their own values, ethics, and desires. In addition to decisions concerning genetic screening or testing, such counseling may also involve alternative reproductive options (e.g., pregnancy termination, permanent sterilization, selective pregnancy reduction, donor insemination).

Obstetricians and gynecologists are responsible for determining which women are at increased risk for fetal abnormalities and for describing and offering appropriate prenatal screening or diagnostic tests. Gynecologists and other primary care physicians are responsible for not only providing screening and testing for gynecologic disorders, but also nongynecologic conditions and systemic diseases.

Prenatal Diagnosis—Chromosome Abnormalities

In the United States, the most common indication for invasive prenatal diagnostic testing is increased risk for fetal chromosome abnormalities. Chromosome abnormalities (Table 3.2) also play an important role in spontaneous abortion and infertility; at least 50 to 60% of first-trimester spontaneous abortions, 5% of stillbirths, and 2 to 3% of couples experiencing multiple miscarriage or infertility will have a structural or numerical chromosome alteration. Overall, 0.6% of all live births have a chromosome abnormality.

Couples who desire chromosome analysis because of a history of multiple miscarriage or infertility are evaluated by cytogenetic analysis of cultured lymphocytes obtained from their

Table 3.2. Common Cytogenetic Abnormalities

Chromosome Abnormality	Live Birth Incidence	Characteristics
Trisomy 21 (Down syndrome)	1:800	Moderate to severe mental retardation; characteristic facies; cardiac abnormalities; increased incidence of respiratory infections and leukemia; only 2% live beyond 50 years
Trisomy 18 (Edwards syndrome)	1:8000	Severe mental retardation; multiple organic abnormalities; less than 10% survive 1 year
Trisomy 13 (Patau syndrome)	1:20,000	Severe mental retardation; neurologic, ophthalmologic, and organic abnormalities; <5% survive 3 years
Trisomy 16	0	Lethal anomaly occurs frequently in first-trimester spontaneous abortions; no infants are known to have trisomy 16
45,X	1:10,000	Occurs frequently in first-trimester (Turner syndrome) spontaneous abortions; associated primarily with unique somatic features; patients are not mentally retarded, although IQ of affected individuals is lower than siblings
47,XXX; 47,XYY; 47,XXY (Klinefelter syndrome)	Each approximately 1:900	Minimal somatic abnormalities; individuals with Klinefelter syndrome are characterized by a tall, eunuchoid habitus and small testes; 47,XXX and 47,XYY individuals do not usually exhibit somatic abnormalities, but 47,XYY individuals may be tall
del(5p)	1:20,000	Severe mental retardation, microcephaly, distinctive facial features, characteristic "cat's cry" sound (cri du chat syndrome)

peripheral blood. However, determination of fetal chromosome complement is not simple or safe; obtaining fetal cells involves invasive procedures that increase fetal morbidity and mortality. Fetal chromosome analysis, either of continuing pregnancies or of spontaneous or induced abortions, is currently performed on cells obtained from amniotic fluid, placenta (chorionic villi), or fetal tissue. The procedures used to obtain these specimens are described later in this section.

Indications for Prenatal Cytogenetic Analysis

Advanced Maternal Age

The most common indication for invasive prenatal diagnosis is advanced maternal age. The incidence of *Down syndrome* among newborns is approximately 1:800; however, the incidence of Down syndrome among newborns delivered to 35-year-old women is 1:385, and the incidence among 45-year-old women is 1:33. Down syndrome is not the only chromosome abnormality that increases in frequency with advanced maternal age; other autosomal trisomies and some sex chromosome polysomies (Table 3.2) increase in incidence as women get older. In the United States, it is now standard obstetric practice to offer all women who are 35 years old or older at their estimated day of delivery invasive prenatal diagnostic testing to detect fetal chromosome abnormalities.

Many chromosomally abnormal fetuses are aborted spontaneously after the sixteenth gestational week, resulting in a lower incidence of chromosome abnormalities in newborns than in fetuses evaluated at midtrimester. It is, therefore, important to use consistently either midtrimester or data on live-born infants when counseling patients concerning risks for fetal chromosome abnormalities.

Previous Child With Chromosome Abnormality

Women who have given birth to a child with a numerical chromosome abnormality may be at increased risk for subsequent trisomy. If a woman is younger than 30 years old at the time of delivery, the recurrence risk for a subsequent trisomic newborn is estimated to be 1

to 2%. However, if a woman is 30 years old or older and is delivered of a trisomic infant, the risk for subsequent trisomy is maintained at the estimated maternal age risk. The delivery of a trisomic abortus or stillbirth also confers a similar increased risk of chromosome abnormality; consideration of invasive prenatal testing in future pregnancies is warranted.

Parental Chromosome Abnormality

Although an unbalanced parental chromosome complement is a rare occurrence, a balanced parental chromosome rearrangement is not uncommon. Approximately 4% of Down syndrome children are the result of an unbalanced robertsonian translocation between chromosome 21 and either chromosome 13, 14, 15, 21, or 22. Although 60% of these unbalanced translocations are the result of a *de novo* (i.e., new) rearrangement, the other 40% are the result of an *unbalanced* gamete inherited from a parent with a *balanced* chromosome rearrangement (Figure 3.12).

Three types of *parental chromosome rearrangements* that can result in chromosomally abnormal offspring are robertsonian translocations, reciprocal translocations, and inversions. *Robertsonian translocations* involve the two groups of acrocentric chromosomes, namely the D group (chromosomes 13, 14, and 15) and the G group (chromosomes 21 and 22); it is this type of balanced parental translocation that most frequently results in Down syndrome in offspring. The theoretical risk for a parent who has a balanced robertsonian translocation involving chromosome 21 to have a child with Down syndrome is 33% (Figure 3.13). However, the actual risk for Down syndrome in offspring is dependent on which parent has the translocation, the chromosomes involved, and the fact that many chromosomally abnormal pregnancies spontaneously abort. However, if the balanced translocation involves two number 21 chromosomes, the risk for Down syndrome in live-borns is 100%, irrespective of which parent carries the translocation.

Balanced reciprocal translocations may involve any chromosome, and are the result of a reciprocal "trade" of chromosome material between two or more chromosomes. This results in a re-

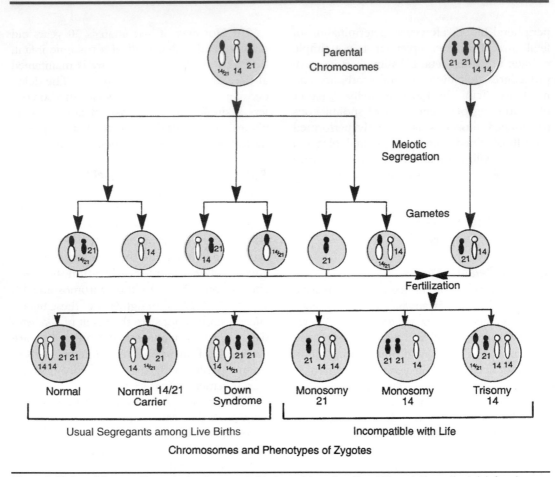

Figure 3.12. Possible gametic products of a parental balanced translocation. Although theoretical risk for abnormal liveborn infants is 33%, the empiric risk is frequently lower.

arranged complement characterized by the same amount of genetic material found in a "normal" complement. Similar to robertsonian translocations, empiric risk for newborn chromosome abnormality is less than the theoretical risk (33%). However, unlike robertsonian translocations, empiric risk of newborn chromosome abnormalities is approximately 11%, irrespective of which parent carries the translocation or the chromosomes involved.

Detection of a *parental inversion* resulting in fetal or newborn chromosome abnormalities is rare, despite the relatively common occurrence of certain specific inversions [e.g., inv9(p13;q21)] in the population. Such commonly occurring inversions do not apparently place couples at increased risk for chromosome abnormalities in offspring. Empiric data

for unique inversions that result in chromosomally unbalanced progeny are unavailable; theoretical risks are dependent on whether the centromere is involved and the size of the inverted portion.

Screening Tests

Screening Genetic Testing

Screening genetic testing is employed on apparently normal individuals to determine the presence or absence, or likelihood, of a given condition. It is routinely offered to all women to detect neural tube defects, to women over 35 years of age to detect Down syndrome, and to certain ethnic groups to identify individuals who are heterogynous for a given autosomal recessive disorder (Table 3.3).

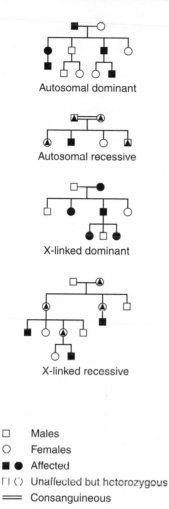

Autosomal dominant

Autosomal recessive

X-linked dominant

X-linked recessive

□	Males
○	Females
■ ●	Affected
⬚ ◯	Unaffected but heterozygous
═══	Consanguineous

Figure 3.13. Patterns of familial transmission expected for autosomal dominant, autosomal recessive, X-linked dominant, and X-linked recessive inheritance.

Maternal serum alpha fetoprotein (MSAFP) screening for neural tube defects serves to detect couples at sufficient risk for a neural tube defect to justify the risk of amniocentesis because only about 5% of neural tube defects occur in families who have had a previously affected child. When performed between 15 and 20 weeks' gestational age and with correction for maternal weight, serum values either 2.0 or 2.5 multiples of the median (MOM) are found in 80 to 90% of pregnancies where there is a neural tube defect. Elevations of MSAFP that do not result from neural tube defects include underestimation of gestational age and multiple gestation. Comprehensive ultrasonographic evaluation follows appreciation of an elevated value.

Low MSAFP levels are associated with trisomy 21 so that such a finding in women under 35 years of age may justify amniocentesis because only 25% of Down syndrome infants are born to women age 35 or older. Other maternal serum analytes are associated with Down syndrome, including *an elevated human chorionic gonadotropin (hCG).*

The combination of maternal age, hCG, and MSAFP using appropriate calculations allows the detection of Down syndrome in 60% of cases with an amniocentesis rate of 5%.

Screening for cystic fibrosis is now offered (CFD heterozygote) to non-Jewish White and Ashkenazi Jews, both of which show carrier frequencies of 1 in 25. In other groups, the carrier frequency is lower and the recommendation is to make the screening test available. Screening is not appropriate for a couple with an affected child.

Table 3.3. Genetic Screening in Ethnic Groups

Ethnic Group	Disease	Screening Test
African Americans	Sickle cell anemia	Quantitative hemoglobin electrophoresis
People of Mediterranean descent	β-Thalassemia	Quantitative hemoglobin electrophoresis
People of Chinese or Southeaast Asian descent	α-Thalassemia	Quantitative hemoglobin electrophoresis
Ashkenazi Jewish descent	Tay–Sachs disease	Decreased serum hemosamidase-A
	Canavans disease	DNA analysis for most common alleles

Mendelian Disorders

Mendelian disorders result from mutations of specific genes. Expression of a disease or trait may result from expression of a single gene at a specific genetic locus on an autosomal chromosome (autosomal dominant; Figure 3.13) or may require expression of two genes at a single autosomal locus (autosomal recessive; Figure 3.13). In addition, X-linked disorders or traits are associated with genes located on the X chromosome. X-linked conditions may also be dominant or recessive. Because males have only one X chromosome, those males possessing a single X-linked gene that is associated with a recessive condition express that condition despite having only a single copy of the gene (hemizygosity). Expression of the same condition in females requires two copies of the same gene.

Many mendelian disorders occur more frequently in certain groups (e.g., sickle-cell disease in African Americans; cystic fibrosis in Whites; Tay-Sachs, Gaucher, and Neimann-Pick disease in Ashkenazic Jews; β-thalassemia in southern Europeans; and α-thalassemia in Asians) and usually have frequencies of less than 1:1000 in the at-risk group. Although screening for certain mendelian disorders is now available (e.g., sickle-cell disease, Tay-Sachs disease, thalassemia), couples at risk for having children affected with most mendelian disorders are usually discovered as a result of information about previously affected offspring or relatives. In addition, advanced paternal age (usually 50 years or older) has been demonstrated to increase risk for certain mendelian disorders characterized by single gene mutations ("new mutations") associated with autosomal-dominant conditions such as Marfan syndrome and achondroplasia. This information is obtained as part of counseling, which plays a critical role in determining risk for a couple having a child with a specific mendelian disorder. Information that better defines a couple's risk for affected offspring includes family history, specifically in regard to mendelian disorders or similar conditions, and the race, religion, and national origin of relatives. This information helps reassess risk and permits couples to further delineate their risk or, in appropriate situations, to undergo invasive prenatal testing.

Genes responsible for many diseases have been located, and tests can be performed for specific mutations. Examples include Tay-Sachs disease, hemophilia A, cystic fibrosis, sickle-cell disease, Duchenne muscular dystrophy, and α-thalassemia. Directly testing for the mutation means that prenatal diagnosis is highly accurate, and testing a proband is not always necessary.

Indirect testing refers to the process of determining DNA sequences of specific length that are linked to the gene. These restriction fragment-length polymorphisms can be tested for by the Southern blot technique. The chromosome carrying the genetic mutation is tracked through the generations and can be tested for prenatally. Indirect testing is not as accurate as direct testing. However, for disorders where mutations causing disease have not been delineated, indirect testing is required.

Certain disorders have eluded characterization by classic mendelian paradigms. Several nontraditional modes of inheritance have been recently described and explain why these diseases are not consistent with conventional mendelian inheritance patterns. This group of nontraditional modes of inheritance includes genomic imprinting, mitochondrial inheritance, and molecular expansion. Understanding these modes has helped delineate the genetics of disorders such as Prader-Willi and Angelman syndromes (genomic imprinting), Kearns-Sayre syndrome (mitochondrial inheritance), fragile X syndrome (CGG [cytosine-guanine-guanine] expansion), and Huntington disease (CAG [cytosine-adenine-guanine] expansion). Of interest is that CGG expansion causes *deactivation* of the FMR-1 gene on the X chromosome and results in fragile X syndrome, whereas CAG expansion causes *activation* of the Huntington disease gene on chromosome 4, and expression of the disease.

Fragile X syndrome is an X-linked disorder and the most common genetic cause of mental retardation. For affected boys, the IQ is similar to Down syndrome. For girls, the IQ may be normal or there may be mild developmental delay. All women who give a family history of boys with developmental delay, extreme hyperactivity, and speech and language problems should be offered fragile X carrier testing.

All DNA tests require recovery of DNA from nucleated cells. For DNA analysis of newborns, children, or adults, nucleated cells are easily available from peripheral blood samples. However, prenatal DNA analyses require fetal nucleated cells, currently obtained by chorionic villus sampling (CVS), amniocentesis, or percutaneous umbilical blood sampling (PUBS).

Polygenic/Multifactorial Disorders

Certain relatively common disorders result in a 2 to 5% recurrence risk if first-degree relatives (parents, siblings, children) are affected. Such recurrence risks suggest a polygenic/multifactorial etiology in which undetermined genes and environmental stimuli are involved in disease expression. Many of these disorders are manifest by anatomic abnormalities. Some examples include cardiac anomalies such as ventricular and atrial septal defects and hypoplastic left heart syndrome; gastrointestinal anomalies, including omphalocele, small bowel atresia, and diaphragmatic hernia; and urologic anomalies, including renal agenesis and ureteropelvic junction obstruction.

Neural tube defects are an example of a polygenic/multifactorial disorder. The spectrum of neural tube defects ranges from anencephaly (absence of a portion or all of the forebrain) to spina bifida (spinal column closure defects). Neural tube defects occur in approximately 1 in 1,500 births in the United States; however, in certain regions of the United States, neural tube defects occur more frequently (1 in 750 live births), whereas in some parts of the United Kingdom, the rate is 1 in 200 live births. Fetal neural tube defects are prenatally diagnosed by ultrasonography and AFP and acetylcholinesterase assays of amniotic fluid obtained by amniocentesis. However, approximately 85% of newborns with neural tube defects are born to women who were not offered amniocentesis because they had no family or medication history that would have indicated them to be at increased risk. Folic acid has been shown to prevent recurrence and occurrence of neural tube defects. All women should be advised to take a

vitamin that contains at least 0.4 mg of folic acid prior to conception. For women who have had a previous child with a neural tube defect, the recommended dose is 4 mg daily.

Fortunately, we are now able to offer all low-risk women, between 15 and 20 weeks' gestation, a screening blood test that measures maternal serum levels of α-fetoprotein (MSAFP). This fetal protein is elevated in the amniotic fluid in open fetal neural tube defects, and also has been found to be elevated in the serum of most women carrying fetuses with open neural tube defects. However, like most screening tests, many women found to have elevated MSAFP levels are not carrying an affected fetus. Accordingly, physicians and health care professionals who provide MSAFP screening must inform their patients of possible false-positive and false-negative results, as well as availability of further diagnostic testing if screening results are abnormal.

Invasive Prenatal Diagnostic Procedures

Amniocentesis involves removing, usually under concurrent ultrasound guidance, 20 to 40 mL of amniotic fluid. Traditionally, amniocentesis is performed between 15 and 20 weeks' gestation. Cytogenetic and DNA analyses of amniotic fluid specimens require culture of amniotic fluid cells because most cells obtained from amniocentesis are not in metaphase and the number of viable cells is relatively small. Direct analysis of the amniotic fluid supernatant (amniotic fluid liquor) is possible for AFP and acetylcholinesterase assays; such analyses permit detection of fetal neural tube defects and other fetal structural defects (e.g., omphalocele, gastroschisis). In addition, some centers have begun to perform amniocentesis before 15 weeks' gestation; however, performing the procedure during the first trimester carries an increased risk of pregnancy loss as compared with second trimester amniocentesis.

CVS was developed to provide early prenatal diagnosis. CVS is performed by transcervical or transabdominal aspiration of chorionic villi (immature placenta) under concurrent ultrasound guidance, usually between 10 and 12 weeks' gestation. Recent multicenter trials have demonstrated transabdominal CVS to have similar safety and accuracy to that of "traditional" (i.e., performed at or after 15 weeks' gestation) amniocentesis; transcervical CVS carries a higher risk of pregnancy loss. Another benefit of CVS is direct and, therefore, rapid cytogenetic and DNA analyses; this is possible because cytotrophoblasts obtained from first-trimester placentas are more likely to be viable and in metaphase than amniotic fluid cells. However, disorders that require analysis of amniotic fluid liquor, such as neural tube defects, are not amenable to prenatal diagnosis by CVS.

PUBS is usually performed after 20 weeks' gestation and is used to obtain fetal blood for blood component analyses (e.g., hematocrit, Rh status, platelets), as well as cytogenetic and DNA analyses. One major benefit of PUBS is the ability to obtain rapid (18 to 24 hours) fetal karyotypes. However, the safety of PUBS remains undetermined; accordingly, PUBS should not be used when amniocentesis or CVS can obtain similar diagnostic results in a timely fashion.

Other prenatal diagnostic procedures include *fetal skin sampling*, *fetal tissue (muscle, liver)*

biopsy, and *fetoscopy*. These procedures are used only for the diagnosis of rare disorders not amenable to diagnosis by less invasive methods.

Teratogenesis

Teratogenesis is the development of fetal defects as a result of maternal exposure to specific compounds (agents) in the environment. Potential teratogenetic agents range from viruses and bacteria to heavy metals and organic compounds.

Teratology is the study of abnormal development of embryos and the causes of congenital malformations. The period of organogenesis, when the embryo is most sensitive to teratogens, is from day 18 to day 60 (embryologic age), although some teratogens also may act at later stages Earlier exposure to teratogens may cause the death of the embryo, and therefore end in spontaneous abortion

The organ system's susceptibility depends on the timing of the exposure. The critical period for brain malformations is 3 to 16 weeks; however, the potential for damage extends throughout fetal development into the first 2 years of life. For the neural tube, the critical period is 2 to 4 weeks (the tube is

Table 3.4. Teratogenic Effects of Drugs at Therapeutic Doses

Drug	Teratogenic Effects
ACE[a] inhibitors (e.g., captopril, enalapril)	Intrauterine growth retardation, fetal hypotension, pulmonary hypoplasia, joint contractures, death
Antiepileptic drugs (e.g., phenobarbitol, phenytoin, valproate)	CNS, cardiac, gastrointestinal, and genitourinary defects; digital hypoplasia, growth retardation
Cyclophosphamide	Skeletal defects, cleft palate
Coumarin derivatives (e.g., warfarin)	Nasal hypoplasia, vertebral abnormalities, CNS malformations
Diethylstilbestrol	Vaginal/cervical carcinoma in females and genital tract abnormalities in males and females
Lithium	Ebstein's anomaly of the tricuspid valve (low risk)
Penicillamine	Connecive tissue abnormalities
Retinoids (Acutane)	CNS and ear defects, cleft lip/palate, cardiac and great vessel defects
Tetracycline derivatives	Staining of teeth (primary dentition)
Thalidomide	Limb reduction, phocomelia, ventricular septal defects, gastrointestinal atresias

[a]Adriamycin, cyclophosphamide, etoposide.

closed by day 28). The heart is vulnerable at 3 to 6 weeks. Insults beyond 9 to 10 weeks lead to functional defects and minor morphologic abnormalities.

A number of drugs have been recognized to have teratogenic effects (Table 3.4), although dosage is a critical factor in some cases. Also, long-term exposure can have an effect at doses that do not cause fetal harm in a single exposure (this is true, for example, in cases of typical fetal alcohol syndrome).

Pregnant women should be advised to consult their physician before ingesting any medication during pregnancy. It is best to avoid using all medication during the first 8 weeks after conception, unless there is a strong medical indication. They should also be advised to discontinue all smoking and alcohol use.

UNIT II

OBSTETRICS

II

CHAPTER 4

MATERNAL-FETAL PHYSIOLOGY

This chapter deals primarily with APGO Educational Topic:

Topic 8: Maternal-Fetal Physiology

Pregnancy profoundly influences maternal health and maternal response to disease, both extrinsic and that associated specifically with pregnancy. Students should be able to explain the maternal anatomic and physiologic changes associated with pregnancy and the physiology of the placenta and fetus, as well as their effect of pregnancy on common diagnostic studies.

Maternal Physiology

Dental Changes

The incidence of dental caries does not change with pregnancy, but that of *gingival disease* does. The gums become more edematous and soft during pregnancy, and bleed easily with vigorous brushing. On occasion, violaceous pedunculated lesions, which bleed very easily, appear at the gum line. These are called *epulis gravidarum* during pregnancy (although they are actually just pyogenic granulomas), and they usually regress within 2 months of delivery. If they bleed excessively, they may need to be excised. Dental care is not contraindicated in pregnancy, and indeed may be requisite to good maternal nutrition. Local anesthetics (preferably without epinephrine) and judicious use of x-rays (with pelvic shielding) are likewise acceptable.

Gastrointestinal Changes

There are several gastrointestinal changes to be expected during pregnancy (Table 4.1). One of the earliest symptoms of pregnancy is *nausea* and *vomiting,* or "morning sickness." Morning sickness typically begins between 4 and 8 weeks of gestational age and abates by the middle of the second trimester, usually by 14 to 16 weeks. The cause of this nausea is unknown, although it appears to be related to elevated levels of progesterone, human chorionic gonadotropin (hCG), and relaxation of the smooth muscle of the stomach. There are usually no significant nutritional deficits or weight loss associated with this distressing but transient symptom complex. Treatment consists primarily of reassurance, frequent small meals, and inclusion of bland foods (such as toast or crackers), as well as avoidance of those foods found to exacerbate the nausea and vomiting.

If symptoms persist beyond the middle of the second trimester or if there is an associated weight loss, ketonemia, or electrolyte imbalance at any time, the diagnosis of *hyperemesis gravidarum* should be considered. Patients with this severe variety of nausea and vomiting in pregnancy often need hospitalization to receive parenteral fluid and electrolyte replacement and aggressive antiemetic therapy. Environmental stressors and/or emotional illness is commonly associated and should be evaluated and treaated if needed.

Despite the gastrointestinal upset seen in early pregnancy, many patients report *dietary cravings* during pregnancy. Some may be the result of the patient's perception that a particular food may help with nausea and heartburn. *Pica* is an especially intense craving for such things as ice, laundry starch, or clay. Other patients develop dietary or olfactory aversions during pregnancy. *Ptyalism* is perceived by the patient to be the excessive production of saliva, but probably represents the inability of a nauseated patient to swallow the normal amounts of saliva that are produced.

Most women increase their caloric intake by about 200 kcal/day, although the recommended dietary allowance in pregnancy is an additional 300 kcal/day. Energy requirements vary from person to person so that clinical dietary management should be individualized.

There is decreased *gastrointestinal motility* during pregnancy because of increasing levels of progesterone. Transit time in the stomach and small bowel increases significantly, 15 to 30% in the second and third trimesters, and more during labor. The *heartburn* experienced so commonly in pregnancy is *gastric reflux* associated with the increased emptying time, as well as re-

Table 4.1.	Key Gastrointestinal Changes in Pregnancy
Gastrointestinal Area	**Change**
Appetite	Usually increases, sometimes with unusual cravings (pica)
Gastric reflux	Results from cardiac sphincter relaxation and anatomic displacement
Gastric motility	Decreases
Intestinal transit time	Decreases
Liver	Does not change functionally; alkaline phosphatase increases
Gallbladder	Dilates
Bile composition	Does not change

duced tone of the sphincter muscle at the gastroesophageal junction and increased intra-abdominal pressure as gestational age increases.

Constipation is common in pregnancy and is associated with mechanical obstruction of the colon by the enlarging bowel, reduced motility as elsewhere in the gastrointestinal tract, and increased water absorption during pregnancy. Increased liquid intake, bowel softeners, and bulk expanders may be helpful.

Gallbladder emptying is also delayed in pregnancy, with the subsequent cholestasis resulting in an increased tendency to form gallstones. Liver function also changes in pregnancy, with alkaline phosphatase elevated as much as twofold during pregnancy. Serum cholesterol levels are increased during pregnancy, whereas serum albumin decreases. Liver-produced proteins such as fibrinogen rise as much as 50% compared with the nonpregnant state, as do the levels of ceruloplasmin and the binding proteins for corticosteroids, sex steroids, thyroid hormones, and vitamin D.

Hemorrhoids are common in pregnancy and are caused by both constipation and elevated venous pressures resulting from increased pelvic blood flow and the effects of the enlarging uterus. The treatment of hemorrhoids during pregnancy is generally reassurance and topical medication for symptomatic relief; surgery is reserved for intractable cases.

Pulmonary Changes

Pregnancy-related changes of the respiratory system result from anatomic and functional changes (Table 4.2). Mucosal hyperemia results in marked nasal stuffiness and an increased amount of nasal secretions. Allergy-like symptoms or chronic colds are often associated with these changes. As the uterus increases in size, the subcostal angle as well as chest circumference and diameter increase slightly. There is increased diaphragmatic excursion and the diaphragm is elevated approximately 4 cm by late pregnancy.

Pulmonary functions are altered in pregnancy. There is a 30 to 40% increase in tidal volume. Inspiratory capacity increases approximately 5%, with respiratory rate, vital capacity, and inspiratory reserve remaining the same as in the nonpregnant state. The functional residual capacity, expiratory volume, and residual volume are all decreased by approximately 20%. The total lung capacity is also decreased by 5%, with a resulting increase in minute ventilation of 30 to 40%. Arterial blood gases reflect these changes in the following ways: oxygen (PO_2) is increased, carbon dioxide (PCO_2) is decreased, and serum bicarbonate is reduced. An especially important change is decreased $PaCO_2$. Because of the increased minute ventilation in pregnancy, $PaCO_2$ levels fall to 27 to 32 mm Hg in the second half of pregnancy compared with the nonpregnant level of 40 mm Hg. This in turn causes an increase in the CO_2 gradient between fetus and mother, facilitating transfer of CO_2 from fetus to mother. Maternal arterial pH is maintained at normal levels (7.40 to 7.45) because the decreased PCO_2 is compensated by increased renal excretion of bicarbonate, yielding normal pregnancy bicarbonate levels of 18 to 31 mEq/L, which are significantly below nonpregnant normal values.

Table 4.2. Key Pulmonary Changes in Pregnancy

Increases	Does Not Change	Decreases
Oxygen requirement	Arterial pH	Carbon dioxide pressure
Oxygen pressure		Expiratory reserve volume
Tidal volume		Residual volume
Inspiratory capacity		Total lung capacity
Vital capacity		PCO_2
Minute volume		Serum bicarbonate
PO_2		

In summary, there is a mild maternal respiratory alkalosis, with the patient aware of dyspnea, hyperventilation, and a relative decrease in exercise tolerance. This sensation of dyspnea (*dyspnea of pregnancy*) is experienced by nearly two-thirds of women starting in the late first or early second trimester.

Cardiovascular Changes

The dramatic changes in the maternal cardiovascular system during pregnancy serve to improve oxygenation and flow of nutrition to the fetus (Table 4.3). Cardiac output increases up to 50% in the first half of pregnancy as a result of increased stroke volume, and in the latter half of pregnancy as a result of increased maternal heart rate as stroke volume returns to near-normal prepregnancy levels. Specifically, the diastolic blood pressure and the mean arterial blood pressure reach their nadir at approximately 16 to 20 weeks, returning to prepregnancy levels by term. Late in pregnancy there may be a decrease in cardiac output when venous return to the heart is decreased because of vena caval obstruction by the enlarging gravid uterus. At times, nearly complete occlusion of the inferior vena cava is common in term pregnancy, especially in the supine position, with venous return from the lower extremities shunted primarily through the dilated paravertebral collateral circulation. Although most women do not become overtly hypotensive when lying supine, perhaps one in 10 have symptoms that include dizziness, light-headedness, and syncope. This is often termed the *inferior vena cava syndrome* and may be related to some extent to the inability of these women to shunt via the paravertebral circulation. The distribution of the cardiac output also varies during pregnancy. The uterus receives about 2% of the cardiac output in the first trimester, increasing to up to 20% at term, mainly by means of a relative reduction of the fraction of cardiac output going to the splanchnic bed and skeletal muscle. The absolute blood flow to these areas is not changed, however, because of the increase in cardiac output in late pregnancy.

Because of the smooth muscle-relaxing effect of increased levels of progesterone during pregnancy, *peripheral vascular resistance* is decreased. Arterial blood pressure decreases during the first 24 weeks of pregnancy with a gradual increase returning to nonpregnant levels by term. Blood pressures higher than the nonpregnant values for a particular patient should be presumed abnormal, pending evaluation. Accurate serial blood pressure measurement during pregnancy is important. To do so, it is useful to remember that measured blood pressure is highest when a pregnant woman is seated, somewhat lower when supine, and lowest while lying on the side. In the lateral recumbent position, the measured pressure in the superior arm is about 10 mm Hg lower than that simultaneously measured in the inferior arm.

Because the cardiovascular system is in a hyperdynamic state, normal physical findings on *cardiovascular examination* during pregnancy include an increased second heart sound split with inspiration, distended neck veins, and low-grade systolic ejection murmurs presumably associated with increased blood flow across the aortic and pulmonic valves. Many normal pregnant women have an S_3 gallop, or third heart sound, after midpregnancy. Diastolic murmurs should not be considered normal findings in pregnancy.

Table 4.3. Key Cardiovascular Changes in Pregnancy	
Increases	**Decreases**
Cardiac output	Systemic vascular resistance
Stroke volume	Pulmonary vascular resistance
Heart rate	Colloid osmotic pressure
Left ventricular stroke work index	
Mean arterial pressure (slight)	
Blood flow:	
Uterus	
Kidney	
Breasts	
Skin	
Brain	

Table 4.4. Key Hematologic and Biochemical Changes in Pregnancy

Increases	Does Not Change	Decreases
Plasma volume	Amylase	Hemoglobin concentration
Total erythrocyte volume	Lactic acid dehydrogenase	Hematocrit
Mean cell volume		Serum iron
Total iron-binding capacity	Glutamic oxaloacetic transaminase	Total protein
Erythrocyte sedimentation rate	Glutamic pyruvic transaminase	Albumin
Alkaline phosphatase		Osmolality

Anatomically, the heart is displaced upward and to the left. Because the diaphragm is elevated and because the heart is in a more horizontal position, chest radiographs might appear to demonstrate cardiomegaly when no such abnormality actually exists.

During the course of labor, cardiac output increases approximately 40% above that in late pregnancy, and mean arterial pressure by approximately 10 mm Hg at contraction. That these findings are significantly reduced when a patient has a labor epidural anesthetic suggests that much of these changes are the result of pain and apprehension during labor. Cardiac output increases significantly immediately after delivery because obstruction of venous return to the heart caused by the gravid uterus is released and because extracellular fluid is quickly mobilized.

Hematologic Changes

Maternal *plasma volume* begins to increase as early as the sixth week of pregnancy and reaches a maximum at 30 to 34 weeks, after which it is stable. The mean increase in plasma volume is approximately 50%. Larger babies are associated with a greater increase of maternal plasma volume, as is multiple gestation, whereas a pregnancy complicated by intrauterine growth restriction is often associated with a less-than-normal increase in blood volume.

Red cell mass begins to increase later in pregnancy, but to a lesser degree than does plasma volume. As a result, there is a "physiologic" anemia caused by dilution of approximately 15% compared with nonpregnancy levels. Whereas erythrocyte volume increases by approxi-

mately 18% without iron supplementation, it can increase up to 30% with iron supplementation. After 30 to 34 weeks, the hematocrit may increase somewhat, as erythrocyte volume continues to increase while plasma volume is stable (Table 4.4).

The normal pregnant patient requires a total of 1,000 mg of additional iron: 500 mg are used to increase maternal red cell mass, 300 mg are transported to the fetus, and the additional 200 mg are used to compensate for normal iron loss. Supplemental iron use in pregnancy is intended to prevent iron deficiency in the mother, not to prevent either iron deficiency in the fetus or to maintain maternal hemoglobin concentration. Because iron is actively transported to the fetus, fetal hemoglobin levels are maintained despite maternal anemia. To supply her needs, 60 mg of elemental iron are recommended daily for the nonanemic patient, which is provided in 300 mg of ferrous sulfate. Patients who are anemic should receive twice this dose.

White blood cell counts also increase slightly in pregnancy, returning to nonpregant levels during the puerperium. During labor, the white blood count may further increase to 30,000/mL, primarily from increased granulocytes. Platelet counts during pregnancy may decline slightly but remain within the normal range of those of nonpregnant patients.

Pregnancy is considered a hypercoagulable state with an increased risk of *venous thromboembolism,* both during pregnancy and the puerperium. The risk of thromboembolism is approximately 2 times normal during pregnancy and increases to 5.5 times normal during the puerperium. Fibrinogen (factor I) increases to a level of 400 to 500 mg/dL. There is an increase in fibrin split products and in factors VII, VIII, IX, and X. Prothrombin (factor II) and factors V and XII remain unchanged during pregnancy. *Bleeding time* and *clotting time* do not change during normal pregnancy.

Renal Changes

Kidneys enlarge approximately 1 cm in size during pregnancy as a result of an increase in interstitial volume as well as distended renal vasculature. Both the renal pelves as well as the ureters are dilated during pregnancy because of the relaxing effect of progesterone. Typically, the right ureter is more dilated than the left. Mechanical compression of the ureters by both the ovarian venous plexus and the enlarging uterus contributes to dilation. Because progesterone also decreases *bladder* tone, there is increased residual volume and, with the dilated collecting system, urinary stasis results, predisposing to an increased incidence of pyelonephritis in patients with asymptomatic bacteriuria. Because of the enlarging uterus, bladder capacity decreases, resulting in urinary frequency (Table 4.5).

Renal plasma flow begins to increase early in the first trimester to as much as 75% over nonpregnant levels at term. Similarly, *glomerular filtration rate* (GFR) increases to 50% over the nonpregnant state. Because of these changes, *creatinine clearance* is markedly increased in pregnancy, with 150 to 200 mL/min considered normal. Serum levels of creatinine, uric acid, and blood urea nitrogen decrease in normal pregnancy. Blood urea nitrogen falls about 25% to levels of 8 to 10 mg/dL at the end of the first trimester and is maintained at these

levels for the remainder of the pregnancy. Likewise, serum creatinine values fall from a nonpregnant level of 0.8 mg/dL to pregnancy levels of 0.5 to 0.6 mg/dL by term. *Plasma osmolality* is decreased, primarily because of reduction in the serum *sodium concentration*. The tendency to lose sodium, as a result of the increased GFR, and the elevated levels of progesterone are compensated for by an increase in renal tubule reabsorption of sodium as well as by the increased levels of aldosterone, estrogen, and desoxycorticosterone. The plasma renin activity is up to 10 times that of the nonpregnant state. Similarly, renin substrate (angiotensinogen) and angiotensin are increased approximately fivefold. Normal pregnant patients are relatively resistant to the hypertensive effects of the increased levels of renin-angiotensin-aldosterone, whereas patients with hypertensive disease and hypertensive disease of pregnancy are not.

Because of the increase in GFR, there is a greatly increased load of glucose presented to the renal tubules. As a result, *glucose excretion* increases in virtually all pregnant patients. Therefore, quantitative urine glucose measurements are not clinically useful in managing patients with diabetes because they do not reflect blood glucose levels.

There is no significant increase in *protein loss* in the urine during pregnancy, the nonpregnant range of 100 to 300 mg per 24 hours being equally valid in pregnancy. There are increases in urinary excretion of vitamin B_{12} and folate.

Skin Changes

During pregnancy, *vascular spiders* (spider angiomata) are most common on the upper torso, face, and arms. *Palmar erythema* occurs in more than 50% of patients. Both are associated with increased levels of circulating estrogen and regress after delivery. *Striae gravidarum* occur in over half of pregnant women and can be either purple or pink initially, and appear on the lower abdomen, breasts, and thighs. They are not related to weight gain, but are solely the result of the stretching of normal skin. There is no effective therapy to prevent these "stretch marks," nor can they be eliminated once they appear. They do eventually become white or silvery in color.

Table 4.5. Key Renal Changes in Pregnancy	
Increases	**Does Not Change**
Renal plasma flow	Urinary output
Glomerular filtration rate	24-hour protein excretion
Renin	
Angiotensin I and II	
Renin substrate	

Hyperpigmentation is believed to be the result of elevated levels of estrogen and a melanocyte-stimulating hormone and a cross-reaction with the structurally similar b-hCG. It commonly affects the umbilicus and perineum, although it may affect any skin surface. The lower abdomen linea alba darkens to become the linea nigra. The "mask of pregnancy," or *chloasma* (melasma), is also common, and may never disappear completely. *Skin nevi* can increase in size and pigmentation but resolve after pregnancy, although the removal of rapidly changing nevi is recommended during pregnancy because of the risk of malignancy. *Eccrine sweating* and *sebum production* are increased during normal pregnancy, with many patients complaining of acne.

Hair growth during pregnancy is maintained although there are more follicles in the anagen (growth) phase and fewer in the telogen (resting) phase. Late in pregnancy, the number of hairs in telogen is approximately half of the normal 20%, so that postpartum, the number of hairs entering telogen increases; thus, there is significant hair loss 2 to 4 months after pregnancy. Hair growth typically returns to normal 6 to 12 months after delivery. Patients are often concerned about this "hair loss" until they are reassured that it is transient and that hair growth will renew.

Breast Changes

The breasts increase in size, rapidly in the first 8 weeks of pregnancy and steadily thereafter. A total enlargement of 25 to 50% is common; in addition, the nipples become larger and more mobile and the areola larger and more deeply pigmented with enlargement of the Montgomery glands. Blood flow increases to the breasts as they change, to support lactation. Some patients may complain of breast or nipple tenderness and a tingling sensation. Estrogen stimulation also results in ductal growth, with alveolar hypertrophy being a result of progesterone stimulation. During the latter portion of pregnancy, a thick yellow fluid can be expressed from the nipples. This *colostrum* is more common in parous women. Ultimately, lactation depends on synergistic actions of estrogen, progesterone, prolactin, human placental lactogen, cortisol, and insulin.

Musculoskeletal Changes

As pregnancy progresses, a compensatory lumbar lordosis (anterior convexity of the lumbar spine) is apparent. This change is functionally useful as it helps keep the woman's center of gravity over the legs as the enlarging uterus would otherwise shift it anteriorly. But, as a result of the change, virtually all women complain of low back pain during pregnancy. Beginning early in pregnancy, the effects of relaxin and progesterone result in a relative laxity of the ligaments. The pubic symphysis separates at approximately 28 to 30 weeks. Patients often complain of an unsteady gait and may fall more commonly during pregnancy than during the nonpregnant state, as a result of both these changes and an altered center of gravity.

To provide for adequate calcium supplies to the fetal skeleton, mobilization of calcium stores occurs. Maternal serum ionized calcium is unchanged from the nonpregnant state, but maternal total serum calcium decreases. There is a significant increase in maternal parathyroid hormone, which acts to maintain serum calcium levels by increasing absorption from the intestine and decreasing the loss of calcium through the kidney. The skeleton is well maintained, despite these elevated levels of parathyroid hormones. This may be because of the effect of calcitonin. Although the rate of bone turnover increases, there is no loss of bone density during a normal pregnancy if adequate nutrition is supplied.

Ophthalmic Changes

The most common visual complaint of pregnant women is blurred vision. This is primarily caused by increased thickness of the cornea associated with fluid retention and decreased intraocular pressure. These changes are manifest in the first trimester and regress within the first 6 to 8 weeks postpartum. Therefore, changes in corrective lens prescriptions should not be encouraged during pregnancy.

Reproductive Tract and Abdominal Wall Changes

The effects of pregnancy on the *vulva* are similar to the effects on other skin. Because of an increase in vascularity, *vulvar varicosities* are very common. These usually regress after delivery. An increase in vaginal transudation as well as stimulation of the vaginal epithelium results in a thick profuse *vaginal discharge.* The epithelium of the endocervix everts onto the ectocervix, with an associated mucous plug being produced. The *uterus* undergoes an enormous increase in weight from the 70-g nonpregnant size to approximately 1,100 g at term, primarily through hypertrophy of existing myometrial cells. Thus, the uterus returns to an only slightly increased size after pregnancy as the actual number of cells comprising it are minimally increased. Similarly, the uterine cavity, which in the nongravid state has a volume of less than 10 mL, increases up to as much as 5 liters. There is also increasing pressure caused by intra-abdominal growth of the uterus, resulting in an exacerbation of *hernia defects,* most commonly seen at the umbilicus and in the abdominal wall (*diastasis recti,* a physiologic separation of the rectus abdominus muscles).

Endocrinologic Changes

Carbohydrate Metabolism

Several hormones secreted by the placenta are responsible for the *diabetogenic effect of pregnancy.* Human placental lactogen increases the resistance of peripheral tissues and liver to the effects of insulin. Because human placental lactogen is secreted in proportion to placental mass, resistance to insulin increases as pregnancy progresses. Progesterone and estrogen also contribute to insulin resistance during pregnancy, and insulin is broken down by the placental production of insulinase. *Pregnancy is characterized by hyperglycemia, hyperinsulinemia, hypertriglyceridemia, and reduced tissue response to insulin.* The typical fasting glucose level is lower than that in the nonpregnant state because the fetoplacental unit serves as a constant drain on maternal glucose levels. As a result, in response to maternal starvation, the patient demonstrates exaggerated hypoglycemia

Table 4.6. Key Endocrine Changes in Pregnancy[a]

Gland/Organ	Increases	Does Not Change	Decreases
Thyroid	Total T_4		
	Total T_3	Free T_3	
	TBG	Free T_4	
Adrenal	CBG		
	Cortisol		
	Androstenedione		
	DOC		DHEAS
	Aldosterone		
Pituitary	Prolactin	TSH	FSH
	ACTH	Oxytocin	
Ovaries and placenta	Progesterone		
	17-Hydroxyprogesterone		
	Estradiol		
	Estriol		
	HPL		
	hCG (peak increase at 8–10 weeks' gestation)		

[a]ACTH, adrenocorticotropic hormone; CBG, corticosteroid-binding globulin; DHEAS, dehydroepiandrosterone sulfate; DOC, deoxycorticosterone; FSH, follicle-stimulating hormone; hCG, human chorionic gonadotropin; HPL, human placental lactogen; T_3, 3,5,3′-triiodothyronine; T_4, thyroxine; TBG, thyroxine-binding globulin; TSH, thyroid-stimulating hormone.

and hypoinsulinemia. Delivery of glucose from the mother to the fetus occurs by facilitated diffusion and, as a result, fetal glucose levels depend on maternal levels. The fetus does not, however, depend on the mother for insulin because fetal insulin is apparent at 9 to 11 weeks of gestation (Table 4.6).

The major change in blood glucose levels in the pregnant woman is a lower fasting level with a prolonged elevation of glucose values after a glucose load is administered. The lower fasting levels result from the constant diffusion to the fetus, where glucose is used as the primary energy source. In addition, there is hypertrophy of the cells of the maternal pancreas, which secrete two to three times the nonpregnant level of insulin late in pregnancy.

Thyroid Function

Several changes in the pregnant patient relate to thyroid function, with the net effect being that the normal pregnant woman remains euthyroid. Estrogen induces an increased level of thyroxine-binding globulin, resulting in an increase in total thyroxine (T_4) and total 3,5,3-triiodothyronine (T_3) beginning early in pregnancy. Free T_4 and free T_3, the active hormones, are unchanged from the normal range for nonpregnant patients (Table 4.6).

Adrenal Function

During pregnancy, there is an estrogen-induced increase in the plasma concentration of corticosteroid-binding globulin, resulting in elevated levels of plasma cortisol. As with thyroid hormone, only the portion of cortisol that is unbound is metabolically active. Unlike thyroid hormone, however, the concentration of free plasma cortisol is elevated, progressively increasing from the first trimester until term. There is also increased plasma concentration of deoxycorticosterone, whereas dehydroepiandrosterone sulfate is decreased (Table 4.6).

Fetal Physiology

Circulation

The umbilical vein, which carries oxygenated blood (80% saturated) from the placenta, enters the portal system of the fetus and gives off branches to the left lobe of the liver (Figure 4.1). It then becomes the origin of the ductus venosus. Another branch joins blood flow from the portal vein that is flowing to the right lobe of the liver. Fifty percent of the umbilical blood supply goes through the ductus venosus. The blood flow from the left hepatic vein is mixed with the blood in the inferior vena cava and is directed toward the foramen ovale. Consequently, the well-oxygenated umbilical vein blood enters the left ventricle and supplies the carotid arteries. The relatively less-oxygenated blood in the right hepatic vein, having entered the inferior vena cava, flows through the tricuspid valve into the right ventricle. Blood from the superior vena cava also preferentially flows through the tricuspid valve to the right ventricle. Blood from the pulmonary artery primarily flows through the ductus arteriosus into the aorta. Less than 10% of cardiac output goes to the lung, with blood flow through the foramen ovale accounting for approximately one-third of the cardiac output. Within a fetal heart rate range of 120 to 180 bpm, the fetal cardiac output remains relatively constant.

The proximal aorta supplies highly saturated blood (65% saturated) to the brain and upper body. It is joined in its descending portion by the ductus arteriosus. The descending aorta then supplies blood to the lower portion of the fetal body, with a major portion of this blood being delivered to the umbilical arteries, which carry deoxygenated blood to the placenta.

The umbilical blood flow represents about 40% of the combined output of both fetal ventricles. In the last half of pregnancy, this flow is proportional to fetal growth (approximately 300 mL/mg per minute) so that umbilical blood flow is a relative constant, normalized to fetal weight. This allows measurement of fetal blood flow to be used as an indirect measure of fetal growth and potentially fetal well-being.

Placenta

Glucose is the primary substrate for placental metabolism. It is estimated that as much as 70% of the glucose transferred from the mother is used by the placenta. The glucose that crosses the placenta does so by facilitated diffusion. Other solutes that are transferred from the mother to the fetus depend on the concentration

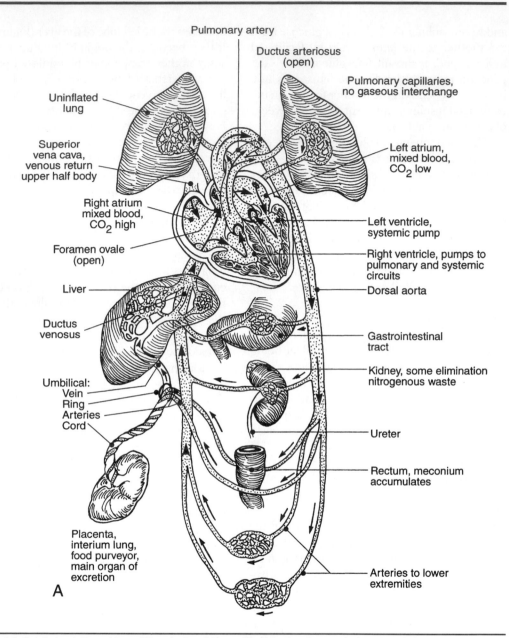

Pulmonary artery

Ductus arteriosus
(open)

Pulmonary capillaries,
no gaseous interchange

Uninflated
lung

Superior
vena cava,
venous return
upper half body

Left atrium,
mixed blood,
CO_2 low

Right atrium
mixed blood,
CO_2 high

Left ventricle,
systemic pump

Foramen ovale
(open)

Right ventricle, pumps to
pulmonary and systemic
circuits

Liver

Dorsal aorta

Ductus
venosus

Gastrointestinal
tract

Umbilical:
Vein
Ring
Arteries
Cord

Kidney, some elimination
nitrogenous waste

Ureter

Rectum, meconium
accumulates

Placenta,
interium lung,
food purveyor,
main organ of
excretion

Arteries to lower
extremities

A

Figure 4.1. Fetal circulation at term (**A**) and after delivery (**B**). Note the changes in function of the ductus venosus, foramen ovale, and ductus arteriosus in the transition from intrauterine to extrauterine existence. Stippling, deoxygenated blood; no stippling, oxygenated blood.

gradient as well as on their degree of ionization, size, and lipid solubility. Fetal uptake of O_2 and excretion of CO_2 depend on the maternal and fetal blood-carrying capacities for these gases and on uterine and umbilical blood flows. There is active transport of amino acids, resulting in levels that are higher in the fetus than in the mother.

Free fatty acids have very limited placental transfer, with resultant fetal levels that are lower than in the mother.

Hemoglobin and Oxygenation

Although the partial pressure of oxygen in fetal arterial blood is only 20 to 25 mm Hg, the

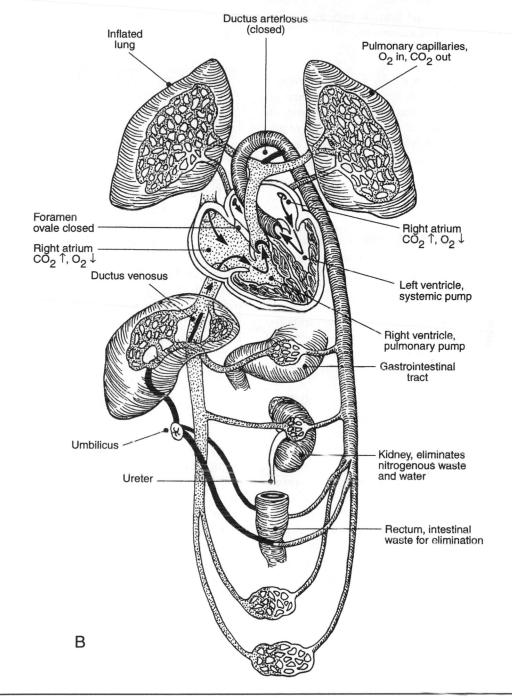

Figure 4.1. *(continued)*

fetus is adequately oxygenated because of its higher cardiac output and organ blood flow. In addition, the higher hemoglobin concentration in the fetus than in the adult and the higher oxygen saturation are responsible for the oxygenation of the fetus. At any given oxy-gen tension, the fetal blood has a higher oxygen saturation than does adult blood.

Kidney
The fetal kidney forms urine at a rate of 400 to 1200 mL/day and is the primary source of the

amniotic fluid. Fetal urine is hypotonic compared with that of a newborn.

Liver

The fetal liver is not fully functional even at term. Bilirubin is primarily eliminated through the placenta. It is this immaturity of function that accounts for the common practice of giving supplemental vitamin K to newborns to prevent bleeding problems.

Thyroid Gland

The fetal thyroid gland develops without direct influence from the mother. The placenta does not transport thyroid-stimulating hormone, and only minimal amounts of T_3 and T_4 cross the placenta.

Gonads

The primordial germ cells migrate during the eighth week of gestation from the endoderm of the yolk sac to the genital ridge. At this point, the gonads are undifferentiated. Differentiation into the testes occurs 6 weeks after conception, if the embryo is 46,XY. This testicular differentiation appears to depend on the presence of the H-Y antigen and the Y chromosome. If the Y chromosome is absent, however, an ovary develops from the undifferentiated gonad. Development of the fetal ovary begins at approximately 7 weeks. The development of other genital organs depends on the presence or absence of specific hormones and is independent of gonadal differentiation. If the fetal testes are present, testosterone and müllerian inhibitory factor inhibit the development of female external genitalia. If these two hormones are not present, the female genitalia develop with regression of the wolffian ducts.

Immunology of Pregnancy

Although the maternal immune system is not altered in pregnancy, the antigenically dissimilar fetus is able to survive in the uterus without being rejected. This fetal allograft appears to be somehow protected in this privileged immunologic site.

The placenta serves as an effective interference between the maternal and fetal vascular compartments by keeping the fetus from direct contact with the maternal immune system. The placenta also produces estrogen, progesterone, hCG, and human placental lactogen, all of which may contribute to suppression of maternal immune responses on a local level. In addition, the placenta is the site of origin for blocking antibodies and masking antibodies, which alter the immune response.

The mother's systemic immune system remains intact as evidenced by leukocyte count, B and T cell count and function, and immunoglobulin (Ig) levels. Because IgG is the only immunoglobulin that can cross the placenta, maternal IgG comprises a major proportion of fetal immunoglobulin, both in utero and in the early neonatal period. It is in this fashion that passive immunity can be transferred to the fetus.

Fetal lymphocyte production begins as early as 6 weeks of gestation. By 12 weeks of gestation, IgG, IgM, IgD, and IgE are present and are produced in progressively increasing amounts throughout pregnancy.

CHAPTER 5

ANTEPARTUM CARE

This chapter deals primarily with APGO Educational Topics:

Topic 9: Preconception Care and Topic 10: Antepartum Care

The student should recognize the relationship between good health prior to and during pregnancy and reduction in maternal and fetal morbidity/mortality.

The purpose of antepartum care is to help achieve as good a maternal and infant outcome as possible. Complete obstetric care includes the correct diagnosis of pregnancy followed by an initial thorough assessment early in pregnancy; periodic examinations and screening tests as appropriate through the course of gestation; patient education addressing pregnancy care, labor and delivery, nutrition, exercise, and early infant care; and management of the patient during labor, delivery, and the postpartum period. Antepartum care ends with a final visit, generally 6 weeks following delivery.

Most pregnant women would deliver healthy infants without any prenatal care. Therefore, *obstetric care is designed to promote good health throughout the course of normal pregnancy, while screening for and managing any complications that may develop.* Specific conditions to which poor maternal and neonatal outcomes are often attributed include:

- Preterm or postterm delivery
- Perinatal infections
- Intrauterine growth restriction
- Hypertension
- Diabetes mellitus
- Birth defects
- Multiple gestation
- Abnormal placentation

Ideally, obstetric care should commence before pregnancy with a *preconception visit,* during which a thorough family and medical history for both parents and a physical examination of the prospective mother is done. Preexisting conditions that may affect conception and/or pregnancy are identified, and appropriate management plans formulated with the goal of a "healthy" subsequent pregnancy. Because neural tube defects are associated with a folic acid deficiency, discussion about folic acid supplementation is an essential component of preconceptual counseling.

Unfortunately, preconceptual counseling is not commonly used; instead, most women seek care only after one or more periods have been missed and pregnancy has already begun. All too many pregnant women have only episodic care, which contributes to increased perinatal and maternal morbidity and mortality. Educating patients on the benefits of regular, early care and motivating them to seek it is one of the most important public health goals of our time. For these reasons, obstetric care should be designed to (1) provide easy access to care, (2) promote patient involvement, (3) provide a team approach to ongoing surveillance and education for the patient and her fetus, and (4) establish protocols for screening for high-risk conditions, along with an organized plan to address any complications that may arise.

Diagnosis of Pregnancy

In a woman with regular menstrual cycles, a history of one or more missed periods (especially if associated with fatigue, nausea/vomiting, and breast tenderness) strongly suggests pregnancy. Urinary frequency caused by the enlarging uterus pressing on the bladder is another common finding.

The *diagnosis of pregnancy* should not be made solely on the basis of nonspecific symptoms and equivocal physical findings that are common in early pregnancy. A pregnancy test is used to make an accurate diagnosis. Once a positive pregnancy test is identified, the physician and patient must be aware of signs and symptoms of *spontaneous abortion, ectopic pregnancy,* and *trophoblastic disease,* which may complicate the early course of what is otherwise expected to be a normal intrauterine pregnancy.

On *physical examination,* softening and enlargement of the pregnant uterus become apparent 6 or more weeks after the last normal menstrual period. A *pelvic examination* in early pregnancy is one of the better ways to establish a due date (estimated date of confinement or estimated date of delivery). Beginning at approximately 12 weeks of gestation (12 weeks from the onset of the last menstrual period), the uterus is enlarged sufficiently to be palpable in the lower abdomen. Other genital tract findings early in pregnancy include congestion and a bluish discoloration of the vagina (Chadwick sign) and softening of the cervix (Hegar sign). Increased pigmentation of the skin and the appearance of striae on the abdominal wall occur later in pregnancy. *Palpation of fetal parts and the appreciation of fetal movement and fetal heart tones* are diagnostic of pregnancy, but at a far more advanced gestational age. The patient's initial perception of fetal movement (called "quickening") is not usually reported before 16 to 18 weeks of gestation, and often as late as 20 weeks in first-time mothers.

Detection of *fetal heart tones* is also evidence of a viable pregnancy. With a traditional, non-electronic fetoscope, auscultation of fetal heart tones is possible at or beyond 18 to 20 weeks of gestational age. The commonly used electronic Doppler devices can detect fetal heart tones at approximately 12 weeks of gestation. With this device, the patient and her family can also hear the fetal heart beat, a strong bonding experience that also can provide reassurance.

Several types of *urine pregnancy tests* are available, all of which measure *human chorionic gonadotropin* (hCG) produced in the syncytiotrophoblast of the growing placenta. Because hCG shares an α-subunit with luteinizing hormone, interpretation of any test that does not differentiate luteinizing hormone from hCG must take into account this overlap in structure. The concentration of hCG necessary to evoke a positive test result must, therefore, be high enough to avoid a false-positive diagnosis of pregnancy, i.e., a positive test result even though the patient is not pregnant. *Standard laboratory urine pregnancy tests become positive approximately 4 weeks following the first day of the last menstrual period* (i.e., around the time of the missed period). Home urine pregnancy tests have a low false–positive rate but a high false–negative rate (the test result is negative even though the patient is pregnant). All urine pregnancy tests are best performed on early-morning urine specimens, which contain the highest concentration of hCG.

Serum pregnancy tests are more specific and sensitive because they test for the unique β-subunit of hCG. This allows detection of pregnancy very early in gestation, even before the patient has missed a period. During the first few weeks, the status of a pregnancy may be evaluated by following serial quantitative hCG levels and comparing them to the expected rise. This can help differentiate normal from abnormal pregnancies. As might be expected,

these more reliable and sensitive serum tests are more expensive to perform.

Progesterone concentrations can also be useful in determining pregnancy viability. Generally, serum progesterone levels <5 ng/mL are not consistent with a viable pregnancy, intrauterine or extrauterine, whereas levels >25 ng/mL are usually consistent with a viable intrauterine pregnancy.

Ultrasound examination can detect pregnancy early in gestation. With abdominal ultrasound, a gestational sac is initially seen 5 to 6 weeks after the beginning of the last normal menstrual period (corresponding to β-hCG concentrations of 5,000 to 6,000 mIU/mL,). Transvaginal ultrasound can detect a pregnancy at 3 to 4 weeks of gestation (corresponding to β-hCG concentrations of 1,000 to 2,000 mIU/mL). If the β-hCG concentration is greater than 4,000 mIU/mL, the embryo should be visualized by all techniques, and cardiac activity is usually detected.

Initial Antenatal Evaluation

At the initial prenatal appointment, a comprehensive history is taken, focusing on past pregnancies, past medical history with specific attention to issues that may affect pregnancy, information pertinent to genetic screening, and information about the course of the current pregnancy. Special attention is also given to diet; the use of tobacco, alcohol, and medications; and substance abuse. Routine laboratory studies are ordered (Table 5.1), and the patient is given instructions concerning routine prenatal care, warning signs of complications, whom to contact with questions or problems, and nutritional and social service information. A complete physical examination is performed, including a Pap test, wet prep for bacterial vaginosis, and a cervical culture for *Neisseria gonorrhoeae* and *Chlamydia trachomatis*.

Risk assessment is an important part of the initial antenatal evaluation. Questions about past medical–surgical and obstetric history are asked, as well as questions designed to learn about the patient's financial status, support mechanism (who will be able to help during and after pregnancy, specifically including the degree of involvement of the father), employ-

Table 5.1. Routine Obstetric Laboratory Tests

Laboratory Tests	Discussion
1. Complete blood count	To determine hematologic status; to rule out anemia
2. Urinalysis and urine culture and sensitivity	To evaluate for UTI and renal function
3. Blood group, Rh	To determine blood type, Rh status, and risk of isoimmunization
4. Antibody screen	To detect maternal antibodies, which may damage fetus or make procurement of compatible blood for transfusion more difficult; the antibody screen is usually negative; anti-I and anti-Lewis are seen in approximately 1% of patients and are of no consequence to the fetus
5. Serologic test for syphilis (RPR, VDRL)	To detect previous or current infection; if positive, specific treponemal test required (e.g., FTA-ABS or MHA-TP)
6. Hepatitis B surface antigen	To detect carrier status or active disease; if positive, further testing indicated
7. Rubella titer	Approximately 85% of mothers have evidence of prior infection; if patient is seronegative, special precautions are needed to avoid infection, which can severely affect the fetus; vaccination is then required postpartum
8. Cervical cytology (Pap smear)	To screen for cervical dysplasia/cancer
9. Cervical culture for *Neisseria gonorrhoeae/Chlamydia trachomatis*	To screen for infection; both cause neonatal and *Chlamydia trachomatis* conjunctivitis; association with premature labor and postpartum endometritis
10. Hemoglobin electrophoresis	To detect sickle-cell trait (HbSA), associated with higher risk for UTI, and sickle-cell disease (HbSS), at risk for multiple fetal and maternal complications
11. HIV titer by ELISA; Western blot if HIV-positive by ELISA	Should be offered to all patients at risk (multiple sexual partners, drug use, or sexual contact with drug users); may be offered to all patients at physician's discretion
12. Glucose screening (usually 1-hour glucola)	To screen for glucose intolerance in high-risk patients; usually at 28 weeks in low-risk patients
13. MSAFP at 15 to 18 weeks (usually with hCG, estriol)	Elevated levels seen with neural tube defects, gastroschisis, and omphalocele; low levels associated with Down syndrome
14. Hematocrit at 25 to 28 weeks	To rule out anemia
15. Glucose screening (usually 1-hour glucola) at 24 to 28 weeks	To screen for glucose intolerance

ELISA, enzyme-linked immunosorbent assay; FTA-ABS, fluorescent treponemal antibody absorption test; hCG, human chorionic gonadotropin; MHA-TP, microhemagglutination assay, *Treponema pallidum;* MSAFP, maternal serum α-fetoprotein; RPR, rapid plasma reagin; UTI, urinary tract infection; VDRL, Venereal Disease Research Laboratory.

ment, transportation for antenatal care, ability to provide for the newborn, and social situation including the use of tobacco, alcohol, and drugs of abuse. Approximately 20% of pregnant women are victims of "battering" and will benefit from counseling and, at times, help in finding shelters and other social supports. Various social service and third-party payers attempt to designate patients "at risk," and inclusion in this category may allow for provision of additional services and support during and after antepartum care. Inclusion in a "WIC" (women, infants, and children) program provides needed support for foodstuffs and other benefits postpartum and for some time into early childhoood. In the United States, suicide, homicide, and trauma associated with vehicular accidents where seat belts were not used account for three-fourths of maternal mortality. Questions about these risks and education about seat belt perinatal/health promotion activities are of great potential value. Finally, an increasing percentage of women seeking antepartum care in the United States speak a language other than English, and provision for accurate translation by qualified professional translators is of great benefit.

Initial Assessment of Gestational Age: The Estimated Date of Confinement

Every effort is made to assess accurately gestational age from which the estimated date of confinement (due date or estimated date of delivery) is calculated. This information is crucial to obstetric management because it is needed to manage possible preterm labor or postdates pregnancy as well as the timing of evaluations (e.g., α-fetoprotein measurement, 1-hour glucose challenge testing). Initial assessment of gestational age is made by obtaining a thorough *menstrual history.* "Normal" pregnancy lasts 40 ± 2 weeks, calculated from the first day of the last normal menses (*menstrual or gestational age*). Calculation of the estimated date of confinement is accomplished by adding 7 days to the first day of the last normal menstrual flow and counting back 3 months. In a patient with an idealized 28-day menstrual cycle, ovulation occurs on day 14, so the *fertilization age* or *conception age* of the normal pregnancy is actually 38 weeks. The use of the first day of the last menses as a starting point for gestational age assignment is standard, and gestational, not conceptional, age is universally used.

To establish an *accurate* gestational age, the date of onset of the last normal menses is crucial. A light bleeding episode should not be mistaken for a normal menstrual period. A history of irregular periods or taking medications that alter cycle length (e.g., oral contraceptives, other hormonal preparations, psychoactive medications) can confuse the menstrual history. If sexual intercourse is infrequent, or timed for conception based on basal body temperature readings, a patient may know when conception is most likely to have occurred, thus facilitating an accurate calculation of gestational age.

Pelvic examination by an experienced examiner is accurate in determining gestational age within 1 to 2 weeks until the second trimester, at which time the lower uterine segment begins to form, thereby making clinical estimation of gestational age less accurate. From 16 to 18 weeks of gestation until 36 weeks of gestation, the fundal height in centimeters (measured from the symphysis to the top of the uterine fundus) is roughly equal to the number of weeks of gestational age in normal singleton pregnancies in the cephalic presentation within an anatomically normal uterus (Figure 5.1). At 20 weeks of gestation, the uterine fundus is at the umbilicus

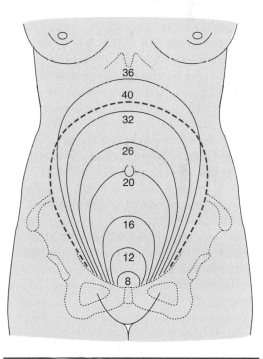

Figure 5.1. Fundal height. In a normal singleton pregnancy in the vertex presentation, fundal height roughly corresponds to gestational age between 16 and 36 weeks of gestation. A convenient "rule of thumb" is 20 weeks equals 20 cm equals fundus at umbilicus in a woman with a normal body habitus. After 36 weeks, the fundal height either grows more slowly, or actually decreases as the uterus changes shape and/or the fetal head engages in the pelvis.

Obstetric ultrasound examination is the most accurate measurement available in the determination of gestational age. In the first trimester, transvaginal and transabdominal techniques allow gestational age determination with ± 1 to 2 weeks' accuracy by using measurements of the gestational sac and embryo/fetus. In the second trimester, accuracy is still high, in the ±2-week range. In the latter portions of the third trimester, however, accuracy decreases to ±2 to 3 weeks.

Subsequent Antenatal Evaluation

For a patient with a normal pregnancy, *periodic antepartum visits* at 4-week intervals are usually scheduled until 32 weeks, at 2-week intervals between 32 and 36 weeks, and weekly thereafter. Patients with high-risk pregnancies or those with ongoing complications are usually seen more frequently, depending on the clinical circumstances. At each visit, patients are asked about how they are feeling and if they are having any problems, such as vaginal bleeding, nausea/vomiting, dysuria, or vaginal discharge. After quickening, patients are asked if they continue to feel fetal movement, and if it is the same or less since the last antepartum visit. Decreased fetal movement is a warning sign requiring further evaluation of fetal well-being.

The only routine laboratory test performed at every prenatal visit is *determination of glucosuria and proteinuria*. A trace of glucosuria is a normal finding in pregnancy and requires no further evaluation. Anything other than the presence of trace proteinuria should be considered abnormal and warrants further evaluation.

Maternal physical findings measured at each prenatal visit include blood pressure, weight, and assessment for edema. *Blood pressure* generally declines at the end of the first trimester, rising again in the third trimester. Compared with baseline levels, however, any increase in the systolic pressure of more than 30 mm Hg or any increase in the diastolic pressure of more than 15 mm Hg suggests pregnancy-associated hypertension. The *maternal weight* is compared with the pregravid weight and to the generally prescribed recommendation of a 25- to 35-pound weight gain through the course of pregnancy. There is usually a 3- to 4-pound increase between monthly visits. Significant deviation from this trend may require nutritional assessment and further evaluation. The presence of significant *edema* in the lower extremities (dependent edema) and/or hands is very common in pregnancy and, by itself, is not abnormal. Fluid retention can be associated with hypertension, however, so that blood pressure as well as weight gain and edema must be evaluated in the clinical context before the findings are presumed to be innocuous.

Obstetric physical findings made at each visit include assessment of the uterine size by pelvic examination or fundal height measurement, documentation of the presence and rate of fetal heart tones, and determination of the presentation of the fetus. Until 18 to 20 weeks, the *uterine size* is generally stated as *weeks* size, such as "12 weeks size," "16 weeks size," and so on. After 20 weeks of gestation (when the fundus is palpable at or near the umbilicus), the uterine size can be assessed with the use of a tape measure, which is the *fundal height measurement*. In this procedure, the top of the uterine fundus is identified and the zero end of the tape measure is placed at this uppermost part of the uterus. The tape is then carried anteriorly across the pregnant uterus to the level of the symphysis pubis.

Until 36 weeks in the normal singleton pregnancy, the number of weeks of gestation approximates the fundal height in centimeters. Thereafter, the fetus moves downward into the pelvis beneath the symphysis pubis ("lightening"), and fundal height measurement is less reliable. If the fundal height measurement is significantly greater than expected, i.e., "large for dates," possible considerations include incorrect assessment of gestational age, multiple pregnancy, macrosomia (large fetus), hydatidiform mole, or excess accumulation of amniotic fluid (hydramnios). A fundal height measurement less than expected, i.e., "small for dates," suggests the possibility of incorrect assessment of gestational age, hydatidiform mole, fetal growth restriction, inadequate amniotic fluid accumulation (oligohydramnios), or even intrauterine fetal demise.

Fetal heart activity should be verified at every visit, by direct auscultation or by the use of a fetal Doppler ultrasound device. The normal fetal heart rate is 120 to 160 bpm, with higher rates found in early pregnancy. The maternal pulse may also be detected with the Doppler device, so simultaneous palpation of maternal pulse and auscultation of fetal pulse may be necessary to differentiate the two. Deviation from the normal rate or occasional arrhythmias must be evaluated carefully.

Several determinations concerning the fetus can be made by *palpation of the pregnant uterus.* The most important of these is identifying the presentation, or "presenting part" of the fetus; i.e., what part of the fetus is entering the pelvis first. This is especially important after 34 weeks. Before that time, breech, oblique, or transverse presentations are not uncommon, nor are they significant because they may vary from day to day. At term, more than 95% of fetuses are in the cephalic presentation (head down), with other presentations rather uncommon: approximately 3.5% are breech (bottom first) and <1% are shoulder first. Unless the fetus is in a transverse lie (the long axis of the fetus is not parallel with the mother's long axis), the presentation will be either the head (vertex, cephalic) or the breech (buttocks).

The head is hard and well defined by ballottement, especially when the head is freely mobile in the fluid-filled uterus; the breech is softer, less round, and, therefore, more difficult to outline. If a breech presentation is noted between 34 and 37 weeks, the option of external cephalic version must be entertained and discussed with the patient. This procedure involves turning the fetus from the breech presentation to a vertex presentation, thereby eliminating the need for a cesarean section resulting from malpresentation, and avoiding the potential adverse consequences of a vaginal breech delivery.

Specific Techniques of Fetal Assessment

Evaluation of the fetus can be conveniently categorized as assessment of fetal (1) growth, (2) well-being, and (3) maturity. The appropriate interpretation of these tests in light of the natural course of any antenatal problem provides a firm basis on which decisions are made.

Assessment of Fetal Growth

Fetal growth can be assessed by fundal height measurement and ultrasonography. The increase in fundal height through pregnancy is predictable. Deviation of more than 2 cm in fundal height measurement from that expected at a particular gestational age between 18 and 36 weeks should prompt repeat measurement and may lead to further evaluation. A deviation of 4 cm or more is of great concern and requires further evaluation, including ultrasound assessment.

Ultrasonography is the most valuable tool in assessing fetal growth. In early pregnancy, determination of the gestational sac diameter and the crown-to-rump length correlates closely with gestational age. Later in pregnancy, measurement of the biparietal diameter of the skull, the abdominal circumference, the femur length, and the cerebellar diameter can be used to assess gestational age and, using various formulas, to estimate fetal weight. The range of normal values for these measurements increases significantly as pregnancy advances so that a specific assessment of gestational age in the third trimester may be ±3 weeks of the actual age. Earlier in pregnancy there is less deviation in normal values and the information derived is of greater accuracy. Measurements in the late first and early second trimesters are most reliable, generally ±1 to 2 weeks. Ultrasound evaluation of the nuchal thickness can be useful in diagnosing Down syndrome between 10 and 13 weeks of gestation. A level II ultrasound examining detailed fetal anatomy and structures (such as cardiac, bowel, cerebellum, cerebral ventricles, and kidneys) can be performed between 18 and 20 weeks, and not only assess fetal growth but assess the presence of anomalies.

Assessment of Fetal Well-being

Assessment of *fetal well-being* includes maternal perception of fetal activity and several tests using electronic fetal monitors and ultrasonography. Tests of fetal well-being have a wide range of uses, including *the assessment of fetal status at a particular time and prediction of fetal status for varying time intervals,* depending on the test and the clinical situation.

An active fetus is generally a healthy fetus, so *quantification of fetal activity* is a common test of fetal well-being. A variety of methods can be used to quantify fetal activity, including the time necessary to achieve a certain number of movements each day, an average of the number of fetal movements in a given period of time repeated several times a day, or counting the number of movements in a given hour. If, for example, the mother detects more than four fetal movements while lying comfortably and focusing on fetal activity for 1 hour, the fetus is considered to be healthy. This type of testing has several advantages: it is reliable, it is inexpensive, and it involves the patient in her own care. For these reasons, fetal movement testing is frequently a part of routine obstetric care late in pregnancy, or earlier if high-risk conditions warrant. A useful qualitative measure is to ask the question, "Is your baby moving more, less, or the same this week compared to last week?" An answer of "more" or "the same" is relatively reassuring, whereas "less" warrants further evaluation.

Techniques using *electronic fetal monitoring* and *ultrasonography* are more costly but also provide more specific information. The most common tests used are the nonstress test, the

contraction stress test (called the oxytocin challenge test if oxytocin is used), and the biophysical profile.

The *nonstress test* (NST) measures the response of the fetal heart rate to fetal movement. With the patient in the left lateral position and the electronic fetal monitor transducer placed on her abdomen to record the fetal heart rate, the patient is asked to note fetal movement, usually accomplished by pressing a button on the fetal monitor, which causes a notation on the monitor strip. Interpretation of the NST depends on whether the fetal heart rate accelerates in response to fetal movement. A *normal, or reactive, NST* occurs when the fetal heart rate increases by at least 15 bpm over a period of 15 seconds following a fetal movement at 32 weeks' gestational age or more; and at least 10 bpm at <32 weeks' gestational age. (Figure 5.2A). Two such accelerations in a 20-minute span are considered reactive, or normal. The absence of these accelerations in response to fetal movement is a *nonreactive NST* (Figure 5.2B). A reactive NST is generally reassuring in the absence of other indicators of fetal stress. Depending on the

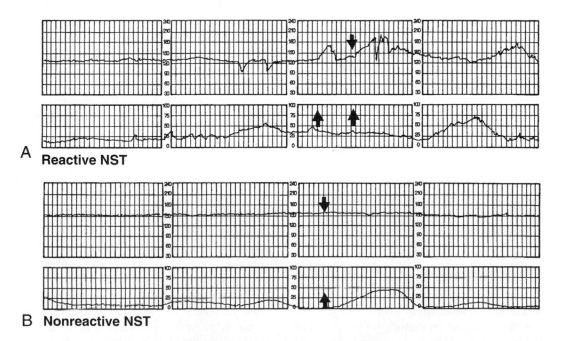

Figure 5.2. Nonstress testing. **(A)** Reactive nonstress test (NST); note fetal heart rate acceleration in response to fetal movement. **(B)** Nonreactive NST; note lack of fetal heart rate acceleration in response to fetal movement.

clinical situation, the test is repeated every 3 to 4 days or weekly. A nonreactive NST is nonreassuring and must be immediately followed with further assessment of fetal well-being.

Whereas the nonstress test evaluates the fetal heart rate response to fetal activity, the contraction stress test (CST) measures the response of the fetal heart rate to the stress of a uterine contraction. With uterine contractions, uteroplacental blood flow is temporarily reduced. *A healthy fetus is able to compensate for this intermittent decreased blood flow, whereas a fetus that is compromised is unable to do so, demonstrating abnormalities such as fetal heart rate decelerations or bradycardia.* To perform a CST, a tocodynamometer is placed on the maternal abdomen along with a fetal heart rate transducer. If contractions are occurring spontaneously, the test is known as a contraction stress test; if oxytocin infusion is required to elicit contractions, the test is called an *oxytocin challenge test* (OCT). The normal fetal heart rate response to contractions is for the baseline fetal heart rate to remain unchanged and for there to be no fetal heart rate decelerations. Decelerations, especially of the late variety (see Chapter 8), are nonreassuring. Repetitive decelerations following each contraction when three contractions occur in a 10-minute window consti-

tute a positive, or abnormal, CST or OCT. This is usually an indication for expedited delivery.

Tests of fetal well-being have a significant incidence of false–positive results, i.e., the test suggests that the fetus is in jeopardy but the fetus is actually healthy. For this reason, these tests must be interpreted together with other assessments and are often repeated within 24 hours to verify the results. In addition, interpretations of the NST and OCT/CST are often combined. Because positive OCTs are common, fetal heart rate reactivity can have a significant impact on the final interpretation of the tests. If an OCT is positive, evidence for "reactivity" is sought (see Chapter 8). If the NST is reactive, the OCT result may be interpreted as a false–positive result. If, however, the positive OCT is accompanied by a nonreactive NST, the combination is considered especially worrisome, and a nonreassuring fetal status is likely to occur when labor begins.

The *biophysical profile* is a series of five assessments of fetal well-being, each of which is given a score of 0 or 2 (Table 5.2). The parameters include a reactive NST, the presence of fetal breathing movements, the presence of fetal movement of the body or limbs, the finding of fetal tone (flexed extremities as opposed to a flaccid posture), and an adequate amount of

Table 5.2. Biophysical Profile

Biophysical Variable	Score	Explanation
Fetal breathing movements (FBM)	Normal = 2	At least 1 FBM of at least 30-sec duration in 30 min
	Abnormal = 0	No FBM of at least 30-sec duration in 30 min
Gross body movement	Normal = 2	At least three discrete body/limb movements in 30 min
	Absent = 0	Two or less discrete body/limb movements in 30 min
Fetal tone	Normal = 2	At least one episode of active extension with return to flexion of fetal limbs/trunk or opening/closing of hand
	Absent = 0	Either slow extension with return to partial flexion or movement of limb in full extension or no fetal movement
Reactive fetal heart rate	Normal = 2	Reactive NST
	Absent = 0	Nonreactive NST
Qualitative amniotic	Normal = 2	At least one pocket of amniotic fluid at fluid volume and at least 1 cm in two perpendicular planes
	Absent = 0	No amniotic fluid or no pockets of fluid greater than 1 cm in two perpendicular planes

NST, nonstress test.

amniotic fluid volume. Perinatal outcome can be correlated with the score derived from these five parameters. A score of 8 to 10 is considered normal, a score of 6 is equivocal and requires further evaluation, and a score of 4 or less is abnormal, usually requiring immediate intervention.

The importance of adequate amniotic fluid volume is well established. Diminished amniotic fluid is thought to represent decreased fetal urinary output caused by chronic stress and shunting of blood flow away from the kidneys. The decreased amniotic fluid provides less support for the umbilical cord, which may be more frequently compressed, reducing blood flow and resulting in chronic fetal stress. Changes in fetal tone, breathing movements, and fetal movements are more likely to be signs of acute stress to the central nervous system.

Assessment of Fetal Maturity

In some high-risk obstetric situations, the maternal or fetal status is so grave that immediate delivery is required, regardless of gestational age; in others, a decision must be made as to whether the mother and fetus are at greater risk by continued antepartum management or whether delivery is best. If the pregnancy is viable but <36 weeks, the questions are, "How premature is the pregnancy?" and, more specifically, "Will the risk of prematurity-associated problems such as respiratory distress syndrome (RDS) be greater than those of continued intrauterine life?"

Because the respiratory system is the last fetal system to mature functionally, many of the *tests available to assess fetal maturity* focus on this organ system. Such tests, termed *direct tests* if they specifically measure substances associated with lung maturity, are routinely used, although not all tests are used in all hospitals. Other tests measure parameters from which the likelihood of maturity can be estimated; these are termed *indirect tests,* the most common being ultrasonography.

Neonatal RDS is the inability of the newborn to ventilate successfully because of the immaturity of the lungs. Respiratory distress syndrome results from lack of a group of phospholipids, collectively known as *surfactant,* which decreases the surface tension within alveolar sacs and thereby promotes easy venti-lation by maintaining patency of these sacs. In utero, production of these phospholipids remains low until 32 to 33 weeks, after which production increases. There is great variation in this process. Gestational age alone does not reliably predict surfactant production or lung maturity. Respiratory distress syndrome is manifest by signs of respiratory failure–grunting, chest retractions, nasal flaring, and hypoxia–possibly leading to acidosis and death. Management consists of skillful support of ventilation and correction of associated metabolic disturbances until the neonate can ventilate successfully without assistance. Recently, administration of synthetic or semisynthetic surfactant to the neonate has been shown to offer additional hope for an improved outcome for these infants.

The fetus breathes in utero, and phospholipids enter the amniotic fluid where they can be obtained by amniocentesis and measured. Direct tests that measure components of surfactant are listed in Table 5.3. Use of fluid obtained vaginally after spontaneous rupture of membranes is not as common, although such fluid can be used for certain tests in some instances.

Ultrasonographic determination of gestational age and estimated fetal weight are common indirect tests performed to help assess maturity. Unfortunately, ultrasonographic assessment of gestational age and fetal size do not sufficiently correlate with maturity to allow for reliable prediction, especially in the marginal maturational period between 28 and 35 weeks of gestation. Performed correctly, any test that indicates fetal maturity is associated with the subsequent development of RDS in 5% or less of cases. The predictive value of these tests is much less helpful. Overall, only 50% of infants who are delivered shortly after test results indicate immaturity develop RDS.

Antepartum Management Plans and Patient Education

Plans for the antepartum, intrapartum, and postpartum periods are iteratively developed during the course of antepartum care and are associated with significant opportunity for patient education. The latter is crucial because it

Table 5.3. Tests of Fetal Lung Maturity

Test	End Point for Maturity	Comment
Lecithin:sphingomyelin (L:S) ratio	≥2.0	Lecithin is the major component of surfactant; this test measures its production compared with sphingomyelin, a substance with constant production throughout pregnancy; the L:S ratio was the first reliable test of fetal lung maturity; the method is methodologically involved and labor-intensive; it has been replaced by less costly tests in many laboratories
Phosphatidylglycerol (PG)	Present	A minor phospholipid that "appears" late in pregnancy; it can be measured by several methods, thus results are reported in different ways
Foam stability index (FSI)	≥47	Measures the ability of amniotic fluid surfactant to maintain foam at the meniscus of a solution of amniotic fluid and alcohol
Fetal lung maturity (FLM)	≥55	Involves fluorescence polarization; measures ratio of surfactant to albumin

may provide new information for the patient or a good review of information already held, in either case necessary to allow informed decision making. Figure 5.3 contains the excellent summary "checklist" portion of the Antepartum Records of the American College of Obstetricians and Gynecologists. It is useful as a reminder of the issues to be discussed during antepartum care and the plans to be made, and as a record of what has been done and what remains to be done. Often, for example as in "labor signs," iterative education is important; in others, such as "newborn car seat," a decision is needed, as many hospitals will not release a newborn unless the parent(s) have a car seat. Many clinicians will write the date tasks are done to help keep track of patient care.

Other Considerations and Common Questions in Pregnancy

Employment
In normal pregnancy there are few restrictions concerning work, although it is beneficial to allow moderate activity and to allow for addi-

---

PLANS/EDUCATION (COUNSELED ☐)

☐ ANESTHESIA PLANS _____
☐ TOXOPLASMOSIS PRECAUTIONS (CATS/RAW MEAT) _____
☐ CHILDBIRTH CLASSES _____
☐ PHYSICAL/SEXUAL ACTIVITY _____
☐ LABOR SIGNS _____
☐ NUTRITION COUNSELING _____
☐ BREAST OR BOTTLE FEEDING _____
☐ NEWBORN CAR SEAT _____
☐ POSTPARTUM BIRTH CONTROL _____
☐ ENVIRONMENTAL/WORK HAZARDS _____

☐ TUBAL STERILIZATION _____
☐ VBAC COUNSELING _____
☐ CIRCUMCISION _____
☐ TRAVEL _____
☐ LIFESTYLE, TOBACCO, ALCOHOL _____
REQUESTS _____
_____
_____

TUBAL STERILIZATION	DATE	INITIALS
CONSENT SIGNED	___/___/___	___ ___

Figure 5.3. Obstetric management plans and patient education. This figure contains the useful management plan and patient education section from the Antepartum Records of the American College of Obstetricians and Gynecologists.

tional periods of rest. Strenuous work is best avoided. A physician's note asking employers to transfer pregnant patients to less physically demanding activities may be needed.

The traditional time designated for maternity leave is approximately 1 month before the expected date of delivery and extending until 6 weeks after birth. This may be modified, depending on complications of pregnancy, the work involved, the employer attitude, the rules of the health care system under which the patient receives care, and the wishes of the patient. Recent trends have shortened this time in many cases.

Exercise

Moderate exercise programs can be continued during pregnancy. During pregnancy regular, nonweight-bearing activity should be maintained on a three-times-a-week schedule, if possible. Overly strenuous exercise, especially for prolonged periods, should be avoided. Patients unaccustomed to regular exercise should not undertake vigorous new programs during pregnancy. Supine exercises should be discontinued after the first trimester to minimize circulatory changes brought on by pressure of the uterus on the vena cava. Any activity should be discontinued if discomfort, significant shortness of breath, or pain in the chest or abdomen appears. Changes in body contour and balance will alter the types of activities practical, and abdominal trauma should be avoided.

Nutrition and Weight Gain

Concerns about adequate nutrition and weight gain during pregnancy are common and appropriate. Poor nutrition, obesity, food faddism, and problems such as *pica* are associated with poor perinatal outcome. Concerns about the retention of weight gained during pregnancy are also common.

A complete nutritional assessment is an important part of the initial antepartum assessment, including history of dietary habits, special dietary issues or concerns, and weight trends. Regular weighing is an important part of antepartum care. Calculation of body mass index is useful because it relates weight to height, allowing a better indirect measurement of body fat distribution than is obtained with weight measurement alone.

Recommendations for total weight gain during pregnancy and the rate of weight gain per month appropriate to achieve it may be made based on a body mass index calculated for the prepregnancy weight (Table 5.4). The "components" of an average weight gain in a normal singleton pregnancy are listed in Table 5.5. The maternal component of this weight gain starts in the first trimester and is most prominent in the first half of pregnancy. Fetal growth is most rapid in the second half of pregnancy, with the normal fetus tripling its weight in the last 12 weeks of pregnancy.

Published recommended daily allowances (RDAs) for protein, minerals, and vitamins are useful approximations. It should be kept in

Table 5.4. Recommended Weight in Pregnancy[a]				
	Weight Gain (kg)		Weight Gain (lb)	
Maternal Classification	**Total**	**Rate (4 weeks)**	**Total**	**Rate (4 weeks)**
Prepregnant BMI[b]				
Underweight (<19.8)	12.7–18.2	2.3	28–40	5.0
Normal weight (19.8–26.9)	11.4–15.9	1.8	25–35	4.0
Overweight (26.1–29.0)	6.8–11.4	1.2	15–25	2.5
Obese (>29.0)	6.8	0.9	15	2.0
Twin gestation	15.9–20.4	2.7	35–40	6.0

[a]Rate has been adjusted to second trimester.
[b]Pregnant weight (kg) Π height (cm) ¥ 100.
BMI, body mass index.
Adapted from *Nutrition during Pregnancy*. Washington, DC: National Academy Press, 1990.

Table 5.5. Components of Average Weight Gain in a Normal Singleton Pregnancy

Organ, Tissue, Fluid	Weight (kg)	Weight (lb)
Maternal		
Uterus	1.0	2.2
Breasts	.4	.9
Blood	1.2	2.6
Water	1.7	3.7
Fat	3.3	7.3
Subtotal	7.6	16.7
Fetal		
Fetus	3.4	7.5
Placenta	.6	1.3
Amniotic fluid	.8	1.8
Subtotal	4.8	10.6
Total	*12.4*	*27.3*

mind, however, that the RDAs are a combination of estimates and clinical research data and are not averages or means; rather, they are values adjusted near the top of the normal ranges to encompass the estimated needs of most women. Thus, many women have an adequate diet for their individual needs, even though it does not supply all the RDAs. Recommended daily allowances are useful guidelines, but they must be considered in the light of individual nutritional assessment.

A balanced, adequate diet usually supplies all the vitamins needed in pregnancy. Vitamin supplementation is appropriate for specific therapeutic indication such as a patient's inability or unwillingness to eat a balanced, adequate diet, or clinical demonstration of specific nutritional risk. Except for iron, mineral supplementation is likewise not required in otherwise healthy women.

Financial problems and the inability to get to a grocery store may prevent some women from obtaining adequate foodstuffs. The WIC federal supplemental food program, food stamp programs, and Aid for Families with Dependent Children are resources that may help in these situations.

Breast-Feeding

Prenatal care is an excellent time to educate the patient about the benefits of breast-feeding, which include, for the newborn, excellent nutrition and provision of immunologic protection, and, for the mother, more rapid uterine involution, economy, maternal–child bonding, and to some extent "natural child spacing." Indeed, these benefits are so great that women should be encouraged to consider breast-feeding, if not for an extended period of time, for at least the first few months of life. However, in balance it should be remembered that breast-feeding is not for everyone, and some women simply cannot breast-feed because of intolerant employment situations and similar constraints. Even in these circumstances, however, the use of breast pumps and milk storage may allow some degree of breast-feeding that is beneficial. In the event that breast-feeding is not possible or chosen, however, care must be taken not to suggest that "bottle-feeding" is somehow equivalent to "inadequate mothering," as adequate nutrition is also attainable by "bottle-feeding."

Tobacco

Smoking should be prohibited during pregnancy because of the established risks to both mother and fetus. In addition to the adverse maternal effects, metabolites from burning tobacco and paper covering are quickly transferred from the patient to her fetus. Infants born to women who smoke weigh less than those born to nonsmokers. Even exposure to passive smoking is associated with high levels of tobacco metabolites. At times, the gastrointestinal discomforts of early pregnancy are associated with a decreased interest in cigarette smoking. The patient should take advantage of this opportunity to cease smoking.

Sexual Intercourse

Sexual activity is not restricted during a normal pregnancy, although advice about more comfortable positions in later pregnancy may be appreciated, i.e., side-to-side, female superior. Sexual activity may be restricted or prohibited under certain "high-risk" circumstances such as known placenta previa, premature rupture of membranes, or actual or history of preterm labor (or delivery). Education of patient (and partner) about safe sex practices is as important in antepartum as in regular gynecologic care.

Travel

Travel is not prohibited during pregnancy, although it is customary and probably advisable for patients to avoid distant travel in the last month of pregnancy. This is not because of substantial risk to either mother or fetus but rather because of the likelihood that labor may ensue away from home and customary health care providers. If a long trip near term is planned, it is useful for the patient to carry a copy of her obstetric record in case she requires obstetric care. When traveling, patients are advised to avoid long periods of immobilization such as sitting. Walking every 1 to 2 hours, even for short periods, promotes circulation, especially in the lower legs, and decreases the risk of venous stasis and possible thromboembolism. Education about the regular use of a seat belt is especially important, with the seat belt worn under the abdomen as pregnancy advances.

Headaches

Headaches are common in early pregnancy and may be severe. The etiology of such headaches is not known. Treatment with acetaminophen in usual doses is recommended and is generally adequate.

Nausea and Vomiting

The majority of pregnant women experience some degree of upper gastrointestinal symptoms in the first trimester of pregnancy. Classically, these symptoms are worse in the morning (the so-called morning sickness). However, patients may experience symptoms at other times or even throughout the day. Treatment consists of frequent small meals, avoidance of an "empty stomach" by ingesting crackers or other bland carbohydrates, and patience. Avoiding spicy or fatty foods may also be beneficial in reducing nausea. Medication specifically for nausea and vomiting during pregnancy (Bendectin) was removed from the market by the manufacturer several years ago because of growing litigation concerning congenital anomalies. This occurred even though the safety of the drug had actually been well established. Components of that drug–pyridoxine (vitamin B_6) and an antihistamine–have subsequently been used successfully to treat nausea and vomiting. A variety of other antinausea agents are sometimes used in patients unresponsive to conservative treatment. Hospitalization with fluid and electrolyte therapy may be required in extreme cases.

Heartburn

Heartburn (gastric reflux) is common, especially postprandially, and is often associated with eating too-large meals or spicy or fatty foods. Patient education about smaller and more frequent meals and blander foods, combined with not eating immediately before retiring, is helpful. Antacids may be helpful and used judiciously in pregnancy.

Constipation

Constipation is physiologic in pregnancy, associated with increased transit time, increased water absorption, and often decreased bulk. Dietary modification including increased fluid intake and increased bulk with such foods as fruits and vegetables is usually helpful. Other useful interventions may include surface-active bowel softeners such as *docusate* (Colace, 100 mg orally, twice daily) and the use of supplemental dietary fibers such as *psyllium hydrophilic mucilloid* (Metamucil).

Fatigue

In early pregnancy, patients often complain of extreme fatigue that is unrelieved by rest. There is no specific treatment, other than adjustment of the patient's schedule to the extent possible to accommodate this temporary lack of energy. Patients can be reassured that the symptoms disappear in the second trimester.

Leg Cramps

Leg cramps, usually affecting the calves, are common during pregnancy. A variety of treatments including oral calcium supplement, potassium supplement, or tonic water have been proposed over the years, none of which are universally successful. Massage and rest are often advised.

Back Pain

Lower back pain is common, especially in late pregnancy. The altered center of gravity caused by the growing fetus places unusual stress on the lower spine and associated muscles and ligaments. Treatment focuses on heat, massage, and limited use of analgesia. A specially fitted maternal girdle may also help, as will avoiding shoes with high heels or platforms in favor of more sensible footwear.

Round Ligament Pain

Sharp groin pain, especially as pregnancy advances, is very common, often quite uncomfortable, and disturbing to patients who fear that it represents preterm labor, labor, or "something is wrong." This pain is often more pronounced on the right side because of the usual dextrorotation of the gravid uterus. Reassurance that this represents stretching and spasm of the round ligaments (with an explanation of what round ligaments are) often suffices. Modification of activity, especially more gradual movement, is often helpful; analgesics are rarely indicated.

Varicose Veins and Hemorrhoids

Varicose veins are *not caused* by pregnancy but often first appear during the course of gestation. Besides the disturbing appearance to many pa-tients, varicose veins can cause an aching sensation, especially when patients stand for long periods of time. Support hose can help diminish the discomfort, although they have no effect on the appearance of the varicose veins. Popular brands of support hose do not provide the relief that prescription elastic hose can provide. *Hemorrhoids* are varicosities of the hemorrhoidal veins. Treatment consists of sitz baths and local preparations. Varicose veins and hemorrhoids regress postpartum, although neither condition may abate completely. Surgical correction of varicose veins or hemorrhoids should not be undertaken for approximately the first 6 months postpartum to allow for the natural involution to occur.

Vaginal Discharge

The hormonal milieu of pregnancy often causes an increase in normal vaginal secretions. These normal secretions must be distinguished from vaginitis, which has symptoms of itching and malodor, and spontaneous rupture of membranes, for which thin, clear fluid appears.

Medications in Pregnancy

The number of medications available for a clinician's use increases every day, and with that increase there is an increase in complexity of ac-

Table 5.6.   Medications in Pregnancy and Breast-Feeding: Pregnancy Risk Factors

Risk Factor Category	Description
A	Controlled human studies demonstrate no evidence of risk in pregnancy in any trimester, and the possibility of fetal harm appears remote.
B	Animal-reproduction studies have not demonstrated fetal risk and there are no controlled human studies, or animal-reproduction studies have demonstrated an adverse effect that was not confirmed in controlled human studies in the first trimester and there is no evidence of a risk in later trimesters.
C	Animal-reproduction studies have demonstrated an adverse fetal effect and there are no controlled human studies, or animal-reproduction and human studies are not available, so drugs should be given only if the potential benefits justify the potential risk to the fetus.
D	Positive evidence of human fetal risk exists, but use may be acceptable despite the fetal risk if the drug is needed in a life-threatening situation, or for a serious disease for which safer drugs cannot be used or are ineffective.
X	Animal-reproductive and/or human studies demonstrate fetal abnormalities such that the risk of the use of the drug in pregnant women clearly outweighs any possible benefit. *Use of class X drugs is contraindicated in women who are or may become pregnant.*

curate prescription. Dosages and schedules vary with indication, age, weight, and physiologic parameters such as renal function; drug interactions are common, often with adverse results; drugs may be toxic, have serious or uncomfortable side effects, and may be contraindicated in pregnancy and/or breast-feeding. The Food and Drug Administration assigns medications a pregnancy risk factor based on extant information about the medication and its risk: benefit ratio. These pregnancy risk factors help guide the appropriate use of medications in pregnancy; they are presented in Table 5.6. Pregnancy category X is especially notable because it indicates a teratogenic association and that the drug is contraindicated in pregnancy.

Obstetric Statistics

The rates of maternal and fetal mortality are important in evaluating the natural history of disease and the quality of obstetric care. Four statistics are commonly used for this purpose. *Maternal death* occurs during pregnancy; it is classified as *direct* if the cause of death is an obstetric disease and *indirect* if the cause of death is a disease made worse by pregnancy. If death is caused by accident, it is classified as *nonmaternal.* The *maternal death rate* is the number of deaths of obstetric cause per 100,000 live births. *Fetal death* is synonymous with *stillbirth* and is the number of infants born without any signs of life. It is expressed as the *fetal death rate,* or *stillbirth rate,* which is the number of stillbirths per 1,000 infants born. *Neonatal death* refers to an infant's death within the first 28 days of life and is expressed as the *neonatal mortality rate* (the number of neonatal deaths per 1,000 live births). *Perinatal death* is the number of fetal deaths plus the number of neonatal deaths and is expressed as the *perinatal mortality rate* (deaths per 1,000 total births).

More pleasant statistics are the *birth rate,* which is expressed as the number of births per 1,000 people in the total population, and the *fertility rate,* which is expressed as the number of live births per 1,000 females aged 15 to 45 in the population.

CHAPTER 6

INTRAPARTUM CARE

The primary focus of this chapter is APGO Educational Topic:

Topic 11: Intrapartum Care

> The student should be able to understand the normal events of labor and delivery, thereby facilitating optimal patient care as well prompt recognition of abnormal events.

Labor is the process by which products of conception (fetus, placenta, cord, and membranes) are expelled from the uterus. It is defined as the progressive effacement and dilation of the uterine cervix, resulting from rhythmic contractions of the uterine musculature. Cervical dilation that occurs without uterine contractions is not considered true labor, but may actually represent cervical incompetency. Uterine contractions without effacement and dilation of the cervix occur normally in the third trimester of pregnancy and are termed "Braxton Hicks contractions," or false labor. Approximately 85% of patients undergo spontaneous labor and delivery between 37 and 42 weeks of gestation.

Changes before the Onset of Labor

As the patient approaches term, there is an increasing number of uterine contractions of greater intensity. Spontaneous uterine contractions, which are not felt by the patient, occur throughout pregnancy. Late in pregnancy they become stronger and more frequent, resulting in the patient's perception of discomfort. These Braxton Hicks contractions (false labor) are not associated with dilation of the cervix, however, and therefore do not fit the definition of labor. It is frequently difficult for the patient to distinguish these often uncomfortable contractions from those of true labor. As a result, it is difficult for the physician to determine the true onset of labor by history alone. Braxton Hicks contractions are typically shorter in duration and less intense than true labor contractions, with the discomfort being characterized as over the lower abdomen and groin areas. It is not uncommon for these contractions to resolve with ambulation, hydration, or analgesia.

True labor, on the other hand, is associated with contractions that the patient feels over the uterine fundus, with radiation of discomfort to the low back and low abdomen. These contractions become increasingly intense and frequent. The ultimate test of whether the contractions are those of true labor is if they are associated with progressive cervical effacement and dilation; i.e., the definition of labor.

Another event of late pregnancy is termed *lightening*, in which the patient reports a change in the shape of her abdomen and the sensation that the baby has gotten less heavy, the result of the fetal head descending into the pelvis. The patient may also report that the baby is "dropping." The patient often notices that the lower abdomen is more prominent and the upper abdomen is flatter, and there may be more frequent urination as the bladder is compressed by the fetal head. The patient may also notice that she has an easier time breathing, because there is less pressure on the diaphragm.

Patients often report the passage of blood-tinged mucus late in pregnancy. This *bloody show* results as the cervix begins thinning out (*effacement*) with the concomitant extrusion of mucus from the endocervical glands. Cervical effacement is common before the onset of true labor because the internal os is slowly drawn into the lower uterine segment. The cervix is often significantly effaced before the onset of labor, particularly in the nulliparous patient. The mechanism of effacement and dilation is shown in Figure 6.1.

Evaluation for Labor

Instruction as to when to report to the hospital when labor is suspected is a routine part of antepartum care. *Patients are told to come to the hospital for any of the following reasons:* if their contractions occur approximately every 5 minutes for at least 1 hour, if there is a sudden gush of fluid or a constant leakage of vaginal fluid (suggesting rupture of membranes), if there is any significant vaginal bleeding, or if there is significant decrease in fetal movement. At the time of initial evaluation at the hospital, the *prenatal records* are reviewed to (1) identify complications of pregnancy up to that point, (2) confirm gestational age to differentiate preterm labor from labor in a term pregnancy, and (3) review pertinent laboratory information. A *focused history* helps in determining the nature and frequency of the patient's contractions, the possibility of spontaneous rupture of membranes or significant bleeding, or changes in maternal or fetal status. A *focused review of systems* should look for common complications of pregnancy resulting in altered labor management. A *limited general physical examination* is performed (with

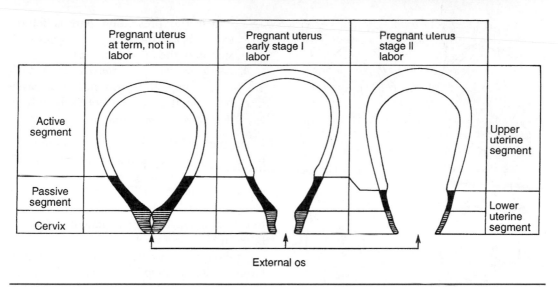

	Pregnant uterus at term, not in labor	Pregnant uterus early stage I labor	Pregnant uterus stage II labor	
Active segment				Upper uterine segment
Passive segment				Lower uterine segment
Cervix				

External os

Figure 6.1. Mechanism of effacement, dilation, and labor. With continuing uterine contractions, the upper uterus (active segment) thickens, the lower uterine segment (passive segment) thins, and the cervix dilates. In this way, the fetus is moved downward, into and through the vaginal canal.

special attention to vital signs) along with the abdominal and pelvic examinations. If contractions occur during this physical examination, they may be palpated for intensity and duration by the examining physician. Auscultation of the fetal heart tones is also of critical importance, particularly immediately following a contraction, to determine the possibility of any fetal heart rate deceleration. A limited transabdominal ultrasound may also be useful, especially if there is a question of fetal lie, placental location, or decreased amniotic fluid volume associated with postdatism or other abnormalities.

The initial examination of the gravid abdomen may be accomplished using *Leopold maneuvers* (Figure 6.2), a series of four palpations of the fetus through the abdominal wall that helps accurately determine fetal lie, presentation, and position. *Lie* is the relation of the long axis of the fetus with the maternal long axis. It is longitudinal in 99% of cases, occasionally transverse, and rarely oblique (when the axes cross at a 45° angle, usually converting to transverse or longitudinal lie during labor). *Presentation* is determined by the "presenting part," i.e., that portion of the fetus lowest in the birth canal, palpated during the examination. For example, in a longitudinal lie, the presenting part is either breech or cephalic.

The most common cephalic presentation is the one in which the head is sharply flexed onto the fetal chest such that the occiput or vertex presents. *Position* is the relation of the fetal presenting part to the right or left side of the maternal pelvis (Figure 6.3). The fetal head may also be turned more or less toward the sacrum or symphysis, termed anterior and posterior *asynclitism,* respectively (Figure 6.4). Persistent asynclitism may affect the ease with which the fetus negotiates the birth canal.

The *four Leopold maneuvers* (see Figure 6.2) include the following:

1. *Determining what occupies the fundus.* In a longitudinal lie, the fetal head is differentiated from the fetal breech, the latter being larger and less clearly defined.
2. *Determining location of small parts.* Using one hand to steady the fetus, the fingers on the other hand are used to palpate either the firm, long fetal spine or the various shapes and movements indicating fetal hands and feet.
3. *Identifying descent of the presenting part.* Suprapubic palpation identifies the presenting part as the fetal head, which is relatively mobile, or a breech, which moves the entire body. The extent to

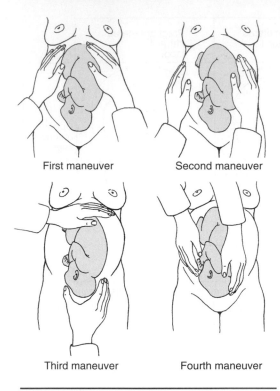

First maneuver   Second maneuver

Third maneuver   Fourth maneuver

Figure 6.2. Leopold maneuvers.

which the presenting part is felt to extend below the symphysis suggests the station of the presenting part.

4. *Identifying the cephalic prominence.* As long as the cephalic prominence is easily palpable, the vertex is not likely to have descended to zero station.

As part of the abdominal examination, palpation of the uterus during a contraction is helpful in determining the intensity of that particular contraction. The uterine wall is not easily indented with firm palpation during a true contraction, but may be indented during a Braxton Hicks contraction.

The *vaginal examination* should be performed using an aseptic technique. If it is unclear whether or not membranes have been ruptured, a sterile speculum examination should be performed before any digital examination of the cervix to ascertain if spontaneous rupture of membranes has occurred (see Chapter 23). If membranes are ruptured and the patient is not in labor, digital cervical examination is often delayed until labor ensues. Visualization of the

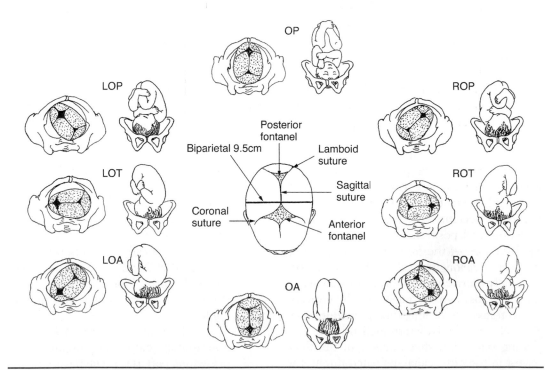

Figure 6.3. Various positions in vertex presentation. LOP, left occiput posterior; LOT, left occiput transverse; LOA, left occiput anterior; ROP, right occiput posterior; ROT, right occiput transverse; ROA, right occiput anterior.

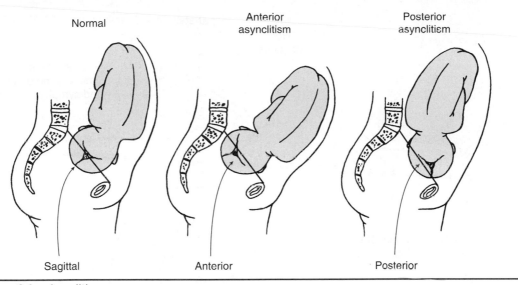

Normal Anterior asynclitism Posterior asynclitism

Sagittal Anterior Posterior

Figure 6.4. Asynclitism.

cervix through the speculum allows for better identification of the source of any bleeding. In the presence of significant bleeding, every effort should be made to identify placental location (previous ultrasound report or concurrent bedside sonogram). The vaginal examination should be done with extreme care, if at all, because of the risk of disrupting a placenta previa (see Chapter 20). These strategies are intended to reduce the risk of uterine infection if membranes are ruptured.

The digital portion of the vaginal examination allows the examiner to determine the consistency and degree of *effacement of the cervix*. *Effacement* is the degree to which the cervix has thinned, and is expressed as a number of centimeters of cervical length in which 4 cm is considered uneffaced, or as a percent of thinning from a perceived uneffaced state (Figure 6.5). A cervix that is not effaced, but is softened, is more likely to change with contractions than one that is firm, as it is earlier in pregnancy. If the cervix is not significantly effaced, it may also be evaluated for its *relative position*, i.e., anterior, midposition, or posterior in the vagina. A cervix that is palpable anterior in the vagina is more likely to undergo change in labor sooner than one found in the posterior portion of the vagina. This suggests that the presenting part has descended into the pelvis, creating more pressure on the cervix, thereby

rotating it anteriorly. With more effective force on the lower uterine segment, contractions would cause a greater change in dilation and effacement of the cervix.

The cervix is also palpated for *cervical dilation*, described as centimeters of dilation. The individual examiner uses one or two fingers to identify the diameter of the internal os of the cervix.

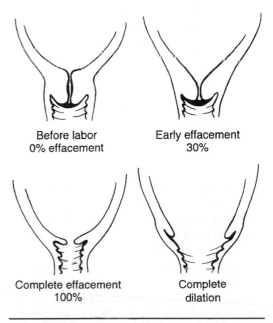

Before labor 0% effacement

Early effacement 30%

Complete effacement 100%

Complete dilation

Figure 6.5. Effacement and dilation.

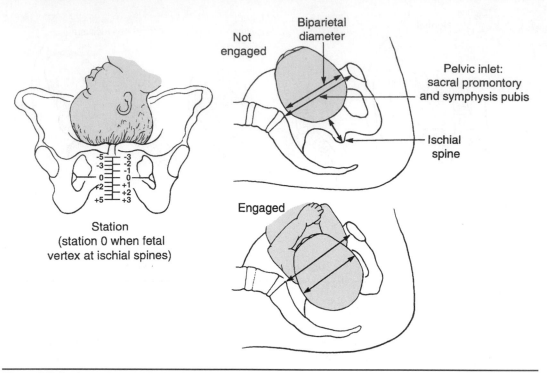

Figure 6.6. Station and engagement of the fetal head.

Fetal *station* is also determined by identifying the relative level of the foremost part of the fetal presenting part relative to the level of the ischial spines (Figure 6.6). If the presenting part has reached the level of the ischial spines, it is termed *zero station*. The distance between the ischial spines to the pelvic inlet above and the distance from the spines to the pelvic outlet below are divided into thirds or fifths (depending on which nomenclature is being used), and these measurements are used to further define station. If the presenting part is palpable at the pelvic inlet, it is called −3 or −5 station; if it has descended one-third of the way to the ischial spines, it is called −2 or −4 station; and so on. Descent of the fetal presenting part below the spines is similarly defined using "+" signs before the number. Zero station is the level of the ischial spines in both nomenclatures. *The clinical significance of the fetal head presenting at zero station is that the biparietal diameter of the fetal head, the greatest transverse diameter of the fetal skull, is assumed to have negotiated the pelvic inlet. The fetal head is said to be engaged at zero station.*

If the patient is found not to be in active labor, i.e., <4 cm dilated, and there are no confounding medical or obstetric problems, she may be sent home to await the onset of true labor. If there is a question as to whether or not true labor has commenced, the patient may be reevaluated after approximately 1 hour. In some cases, patients are encouraged to ambulate to differentiate Braxton Hicks contractions (which may resolve) from true labor (which will continue). If the patient is in labor, she is admitted to the labor area of the hospital and active management of labor is undertaken.

Stages of Labor

Although labor is a continuous process, it is divided into four functional stages. The *first stage* is the interval between the onset of labor and full cervical dilation (10 cm). The first stage is further divided into two phases. The *latent phase* encompasses cervical effacement and early dilation. The second is the *active phase*, during which more rapid cervical dilation

Table 6.1. Mean Duration of the Various Phases and Stages of Labor with Their Distribution Characteristics

Parity	Latent Phase (hr)	Active Phase (hr)	Maximum Dilation (cm/hr)	Second Stage (hr)
Nulliparous				
Mean	6.5	4.5	3.0	1.0
Upper limit[a]	20.0	12.0	1.0	3.0
Multiparous				
Mean	5.0	2.5	6.0	0.5
Upper limit[a]	13.5	5.0	1.5	1.0

[a]Fifth or 95th percentile.

occurs, usually beginning at approximately 4 cm. The *second stage* encompasses complete cervical dilation through the delivery of the infant. The *third stage* begins immediately after delivery of the infant and ends with the delivery of the placenta. The *fourth stage* is defined as the immediate postpartum period of approximately 2 hours after delivery of the placenta, during which time the patient undergoes significant physiologic adjustment. Table 6.1 outlines the duration of various stages of labor, as described in research by Emmanuel Friedman and associates. Figure 6.7 represents this graphically. New data, derived since the advent of epidural labor analgesia, suggest that the maximum slope of the normal labor curve during active phase may actually be slightly less steep.

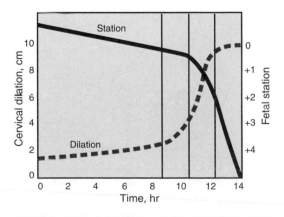

Figure 6.7. Graphic presentation of cervical dilation and station during the first and second stages of labor.

Mechanism of Labor

The mechanisms of labor (also known as the cardinal movements of labor) refers to the changes of the position of the fetus as it passes through the birth canal. The fetus usually descends in a fashion whereby the occipital portion of the fetal head is the lowermost part in the pelvis, and it rotates toward the largest pelvic segment. Because vertex presentation occurs in 95% of term labors, the cardinal movements of labor are defined relative to this presentation. To accommodate to the maternal bony pelvis, the fetal head must undergo several movements as it passes through the birth canal. These movements are accomplished by means of the forceful contractions of the uterus. *These cardinal movements of labor* do not occur as a distinct series of movements but rather as a group of movements that overlap as the fetus moves progressively through the birth canal. These movements are (1) engagement, (2) flexion, (3) descent, (4) internal rotation, (5) extension, and (6) external rotation (Figure 6.8).

Engagement is defined as descent of the biparietal diameter of the head below the pelvic inlet, suggested clinically by palpation of the presenting part below the level of ischial spines (zero station). Engagement is common days to weeks prior to labor in primigravidas, whereas in multigravidas it more commonly happens at the onset of active labor. In any event, the importance of this event is that it suggests that the bony pelvis is adequate to allow significant descent of the fetal head. *Flexion of the fetal head* allows for the smaller

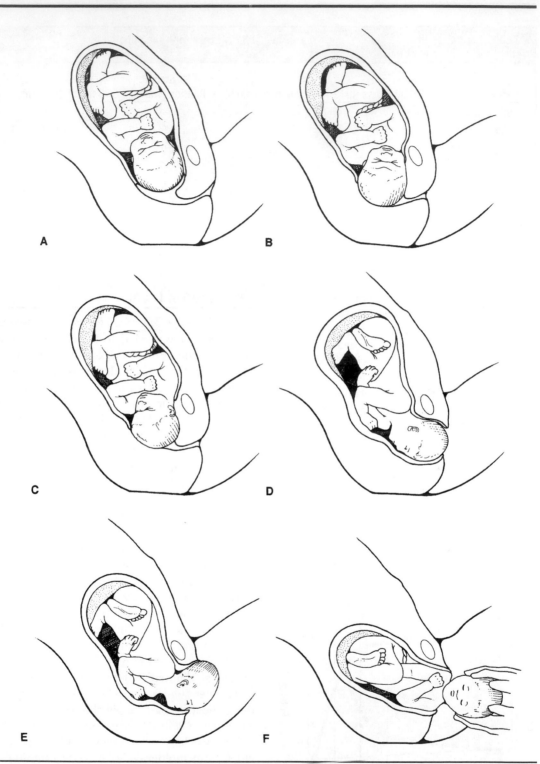

Figure 6.8. Cardinal movements of labor: engagement (**A**), flexion (**B**), descent (**C**), internal rotation (**D**), extension (**E**), and external rotation (**F**).

diameters of the fetal head to present to the maternal pelvis. *Descent of the presenting part* is a necessity for the successful completion of passage through the birth canal. The greatest rate of descent occurs during the latter portions of the first stage of labor and during the second stage of labor. Figure 6.7 is a graphic demonstration of fetal descent and dilation of the cervix. *Internal rotation,* like flexion, facilitates presentation of the optimal diameters of the fetal head to the bony pelvis, most commonly from transverse to either anterior or posterior. *Extension of the fetal head* occurs as it reaches the introitus. To accommodate the upward curve of the birth canal, the flexed head now extends. *External rotation* occurs after delivery of the head as the head rotates to "face forward" relative to its shoulders. This is known as *restitution.*

The type of pelvis may alter the presentation of the fetal vertex (see Figure 3.6). A gynecoid pelvis is most common with a wide arch, nonprominent ischial spines, and a sacral promontory that cannot be reached on digital examination. An android pelvis is most unfavorable for delivery with a narrow pubic arch, prominent spines, and sacrum. Occiput posterior presentations are common, with an anthropoid pelvis characterized by an inlet anteroposterior diameter greater than the transverse, a narrow arch, and prominent spines. Occiput transverse presentations are seen more frequently in a platypelloid pelvis, with a wide arch, nonprominent spines, and reachable promontory. Platypelloid is the least common type of pelvis.

Management of Labor

Education regarding labor pain management should occur during antepartum visits. Although the patient may have undergone some education regarding the labor and delivery process, it is important to realize that the patient has significant fears that remain. The patient should not be left unattended for any significant length of time, and a support person may be allowed to remain with the patient throughout the labor and delivery process in most cases. Maternal vital signs should be taken at least every 30 minutes during the first stage of labor. The patient should be given nothing by mouth except small sips of water, ice chips, clear liquids, or hard candies. Laboratory information, including hematocrit, type and screen, platelet count, and urinalysis for glucose and protein, are obtained when the patient is admitted to the hospital. An intravenous line (16- to 18-gauge) is frequently inserted during the active phase of labor to provide hydration and immediate access to the intravascular space should medications be necessary. As the gastrointestinal tract significantly slows in its function during labor, hydration by means of the intravenous line rather than by mouth is optimal, although allowing ice chips or even limited clear fluids poses little risk in most situations.

During the course of labor, descent of the fetus causes the bladder to be elevated relative to the lower uterine segment and cervix. This often results in the patient having difficulty voiding. The patient should, therefore, be encouraged to void frequently. Catheterization may become necessary if the bladder becomes distended.

The *position* in which a woman labors depends on her wishes, the status of her pregnancy, and the plan for labor and delivery that she and her physician have developed. Laboring in a sitting or reclining position at bed rest is common, with the lateral recumbent position often chosen to enhance uterine blood flow by taking the gravid uterus off the inferior vena cava. Other laboring positions such as sitting in a rocking chair or walking are often beneficially employed. At all times, there should be appropriate monitoring of the fetal heart rate and uterine contractions.

Electronic fetal monitoring is very common and often routine, but it is not necessary for the low-risk term pregnancy. If routine electronic monitoring is not undertaken, auscultation of the fetal heart rate should be performed at least every 15 minutes, immediately after a uterine contraction. During the second stage of labor, fetal heart rate auscultation should be performed after each uterine contraction. If electronic fetal monitoring is used, an external tocodynamometer is initially used to assess uterine activity, providing information regarding the frequency and duration of contractions, but not their intensity. Internal pressure monitoring, using an intrauterine catheter, can be performed to measure intensity more accurately by directly measuring intrauterine pressure. This internal form of fetal monitoring requires rupture of the membranes and, therefore, usually cannot be accomplished until the cervix is at least 1 to 2 cm dilated.

Fetal heart rate can be monitored externally by Doppler ultrasound, or internally by using a direct fetal electrocardiogram, which is obtained by applying a scalp electrode. The latter technique allows for more detailed evaluation of subtle changes in fetal heart rate pattern (see Chapter 8).

Whenever artificial rupture of the membranes is to be performed, the presenting part must be well applied to the cervix. This minimizes the risk of iatrogenic umbilical cord prolapse.

Monitoring of maternal conditions, including pulse, blood pressure, respiratory rate, temperature, urine output, and fluid intake, should be performed periodically throughout the course of labor. Because *analgesic and anesthetic agents* may affect the latent phase of labor, they are not used by some clinicians until the active phase of labor. Prepared childbirth classes are used to teach patients various relaxation techniques to deal with the pain of labor contractions. For some, the use of analgesics is a helpful adjunct. In the doses typically given during labor, neonatal depression is not a major concern. Commonly used medications include the narcotic meperidine (5 to 20 mg slow intravenous push every 2 to 3 hours, or 25 to 75 mg intramuscularly every 3 to 4 hours) and the synthetic opioid agonist–antagonist butorphanol tartrate (1 to 2 mg slow intravenous push every 3 to 4 hours). Any analgesic or anesthetic technique used during the labor and delivery process should take into account those sensory pathways involved and the points at which they may be affected. During the first stage of labor, pain results from the contraction of the uterus and dilation of the cervix. This pain travels along the visceral afferents, which accompany sympathetic nerves entering the spinal cord at T10, T11, T12, and L1. As the head descends, there is also distension of the lower birth canal and perineum. This pain is transmitted along somatic afferents that comprise portions of the pudendal nerves that enter the spinal cord at S2, S3, and S4.

The anesthetic technique that provides pain relief during labor is the *epidural block*. The advantage of this technique is its ability to provide analgesia during labor as well as excellent anesthesia for delivery, yet maintain the patient's sense of touch, facilitating participation in the birth process. It can also be used in either vaginal or abdominal deliveries and in postpartum procedures such as tubal ligation. *Spinal anesthetic* is usually for abdominal delivery, although on occasion it is performed for a difficult forceps delivery. A *pudendal block* with local anesthesia can be administered easily at the time of delivery to provide perineal anesthesia for a vaginal delivery (Figure 6.9). A *local block* (i.e., local injection of anesthetic) may be used at the time of an episiotomy or tear.

Epidural anesthesia is superior to spinal anesthesia in that it can be left as a continuous source of analgesia and anesthesia during both the labor and delivery process. It avoids the risk of spinal headache in the mother and reduces the risk of sympathetic blockade, which could lead to hypotension. There is also less motor blockade than with spinal anesthesia. Although the pudendal block is easy to perform and also has the least potential risk to the mother and fetus, its use is also the most limited. *General anesthesia* is reserved only for cesarean sections in selected cases. The potential risk of complications such as maternal aspiration and neonatal depression reduces its more widespread use.

Evaluation of the patient's progress of labor is accomplished by means of a series of pelvic examinations. The number of examinations should be minimized to avoid the risk of chorioamnionitis. At the time of each vaginal examination, a sterile lubricant is used. Each examination should identify cervical dilation, effacement, station, position of the presenting part, and the status of the membranes. These findings should be noted graphically on the hospital record so that abnormalities of labor may be identified. During the latter portions of the first stage of labor, patients may report the urge to push. This may signify significant descent of the fetal

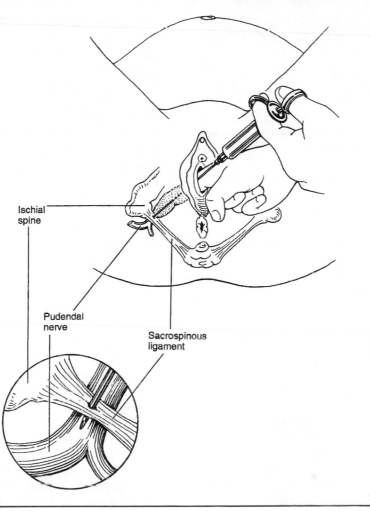

Ischial
spine

Pudendal
nerve

Sacrospinous
ligament

Figure 6.9. Pudendal block.

head with pressure on the perineum. More frequent vaginal examinations during this time may be necessary. Similarly, in the case of significant fetal heart rate decelerations, more frequent examinations may be necessary to determine whether or not the umbilical cord is prolapsed or if delivery is imminent.

In addition to rupturing the membranes to insert an intrauterine pressure catheter or a fetal scalp monitor, *artificial rupture of membranes* many be beneficial in other ways. The presence or absence of meconium (fetal stool) can be identified. Blood in the amniotic fluid may also have significance (see Chapter 20). However, rupture of the membranes does carry some risk because the incidence of infection may be increased if labor is prolonged, or umbilical

cord prolapse may occur if rupture of the membranes is undertaken before engagement of the presenting fetal part. *Spontaneous rupture of membranes* has similar risks. The fluid should be observed for meconium and blood. Fetal heart tones should be assessed after membranes spontaneously rupture.

Once the *second stage of labor* has been reached (i.e., complete, or 10 cm, of cervical dilation), voluntary maternal effort (pushing) can be added to the involuntary contractile forces of the uterus to facilitate delivery of the fetus. With the onset of each contraction, the mother is encouraged to inhale, hold her breath, and perform an extended Valsalva maneuver. This increase in intra-abdominal pressure aids in fetal descent through the birth canal.

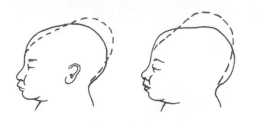

Figure 6.10. Molding of head.

It is during the second stage of labor that the fetal head may undergo further alterations. *Molding* is an alteration in the relation of the fetal cranial bones, even resulting in partial bone overlap (Figure 6.10). Some minor degree is common as the fetal head adjusts to the bony pelvis. The greater the disparity between the fetal head and the bony pelvis, the greater the amount of molding. *Caput succedaneum* is the edema of the fetal scalp caused by pressure on the fetal head by the cervix. An extended second stage may last as long as 2 to 3 hours, and the prolonged resistance encountered by the fetal vertex may prevent appropriate identification of fontanels and sutures. Both caput and molding resolve in the first few days of life. If identified before the second stage of labor, these changes should be noted on the pelvic examination and may indicate a potential problem in negotiation of the birth canal.

Delivery

The patient should be prepared for a well-controlled delivery of the fetal head. In general, nulliparous patients have a longer second stage than do parous patients. The *dorsal lithotomy position (supine on back, legs bent at knees and elevated)* is a common position for vaginal delivery in the United States, both because of custom and preference of physicians who are commonly trained in delivery technique in this position. The position offers clear advance for operative (forceps, breech) delivery and for the repair of more than minor obstetric lacerations. Other delivery positions, e.g., lateral, knee–chest, sitting, may also be used for the normal spontaneous vaginal delivery, if agreed to by patient and physician. Various delivery devices, such as a birthing chair or ball, may

also be used to advantage. With each successive contraction, the maternal force as well as uterine contractions cause more of the fetal scalp to be visible at the introitus, with progressive thinning of the perineum and distension of the vaginal canal. With slow progressive labor and good control of the fetal head and body at delivery, the risk of obstetric laceration with a normal-sized infant is low so that the need for episiotomy is minimal. If an episiotomy is needed, it should be performed only after the perineum has been thinned considerably by the descending fetal head (Figure 6.11). By enlarging the vaginal outlet, an episiotomy facilitates delivery and may be indicated in cases of instrumental delivery and/or protracted or arrested descent. Routine episiotomy is not part of modern obstetric practice. If needed, episiotomies are usually cut midline, or occasionally in a mediolateral direction. Advantages of the midline episiotomy include less pain, ease of repair, and less blood loss. The primary disadvantage is a greater risk of extension into a third- or fourth-degree laceration, involving the rectal sphincter and rectal mucosa, respectively. Performing a mediolateral episiotomy is now relatively uncommon in the United States.

As the fetal head crowns, i.e., distends the vaginal opening, it is delivered by extension to allow the smallest diameter of the fetal head to pass over the perineum. This decreases the likelihood of laceration or extension of episiotomy. To facilitate this, the physician provides support to the perineal tissues and performs a modified *Ritgen maneuver* (Figure 6.12) in which one hand is placed over the vertex as the other exerts pressure through the perineum onto the fetal chin. A sterile towel is used to avoid contamination of this hand by contact with the anus. The chin can then be delivered slowly, with control applied by both hands.

After the head is delivered, nasal and oral suction is performed with a bulb syringe. If meconium has been present, suctioning of the pharynx is accomplished using a DeLee suction catheter. The presence of a nuchal cord should be looked for, and if found, reduced over the fetal head, if possible. If the cord is tight, it may be doubly clamped and cut prior to delivery.

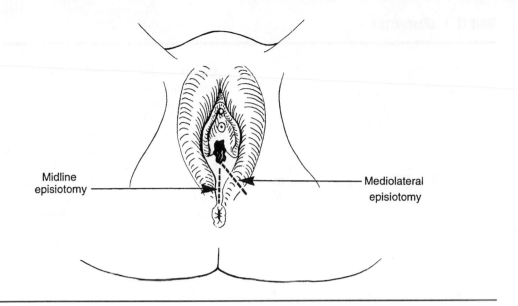

Midline episiotomy — Mediolateral episiotomy

Figure 6.11. Episiotomy.

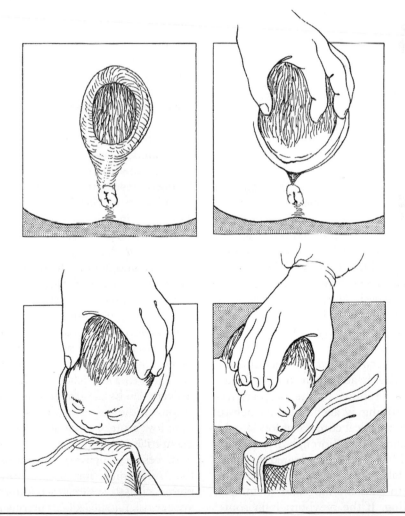

Figure 6.12. Vaginal delivery with midline episiotomy assisted by modified Ritgen maneuver.

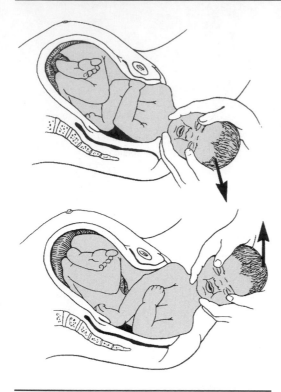

Figure 6.13. Delivery of anterior and posterior shoulders.

After delivery of the head, the shoulders descend and rotate to a position in the anteroposterior diameter of the pelvis. The attendant's hands are placed on the chin and vertex, applying gentle downward pressure, thus delivering the anterior shoulder. To avoid injury to the brachial plexus, care is taken not to put excessive force on the neck. The posterior shoulder is then delivered by upward traction on the fetal head (Figure 6.13). Delivery of the body now occurs easily.

The fetus is then cradled in the attendant's arms, with the head down to maximize drainage of secretions to the oropharynx. Further suctioning is accomplished before clamping the umbilical cord. Heat loss should be minimized by rapid, thorough drying, then wrapping with warmed crib blankets. If the newborn is stable, he or she may remain with the mother to start bonding and/or initiate breast nippling. If the newborn is in some

manner unstable, transfer to a radiant warmer and further pediatric care is indicated. Cesarean delivery now accounts for more than 30% of births in some obstetrical units. It is the most frequent operation performed in the United States. The rate of cesarean delivery was stable at <5% until 1965. Among the reasons for this increase in cesarean sections are the ready availability of neonatal intensive care units in which infants have a significantly greater survival rate than in the past, use in the delivery of fetuses in breech presentations, and greater use in cases in which more sophisticated fetal surveillance is nonreassuring. Cesarean sections are also performed as a repeat procedure. Prior to the mid-1980s, it was believed that a previous cesarean delivery mandated that all subsequent deliveries should be abdominal. Publication of data suggesting the safety of vaginal birth after cesarean (VBAC) led to a decade-long clinical trend away from the adage: "Once a cesarean, always a cesarean." Success rates of VBAC were found to be 60% to 80%. More recently, the pendulum has again swung, resulting in an increasing trend for patients and their physicians to opt for scheduled elective repeat cesarean delivery.

The American College of Obstetricians and Gynecologists' guidelines for trial of VBAC include the availability of a 24-hour blood bank, continuous electronic fetal heart rate monitoring, a physician capable of performing a cesarean delivery, in-house anesthesia services, and ability to meet a 30-minute "decision-to-incision" time frame if cesarean delivery becomes necessary.

Deciding on cesarean delivery has important ramifications because the maternal mortality rate associated with cesarean delivery is two to four times that of a vaginal birth, i.e., 1 per 2,500 to 1 per 5,000 operations. Cesarean delivery can be performed through various incisions in the uterus. An incision through the thin, lower uterine segment allows for subsequent trials of VBAC if the patient has had one prior cesarean delivery. An incision through the thick, muscular upper portion of the uterus, a classic cesarean section, carries such a greater risk for subsequent uterine rupture that repeat cesarean delivery for these patients is still recommended.

Third Stage of Labor

Immediately after delivery of the infant, the uterus significantly decreases in size. Blood from the umbilical cord should be obtained and sent for type and Rh testing. Cord blood may also be obtained for arterial blood gas determination, which should be considered if there is any concern about compromised fetal well-being or the presence of a known fetal condition that could lead to difficulties in the immediate newborn period. Any data obtained is shared with the nursery staff to assist in management of the newborn.

Delivery of the placenta is imminent when the uterus rises in the abdomen, becoming globular in configuration, indicating that the placenta has separated and has entered the lower uterine segment; a gush of blood and/or "lengthening" of the umbilical cord also occurs. These are the three classic *signs of placental separation*. Pulling the placenta from the uterus by excess traction on the cord should be avoided. Inappropriate application of force may result in *inversion of the uterus,* an obstetric emergency associated with profound blood loss and shock. Instead, it is appropriate to wait for spontaneous extrusion of the placenta, sometimes up to 30 minutes. As the placenta passes into the lower uterine segment, gentle downward pressure is applied to the fundus of the uterus, and the placenta is guided by very gentle traction on the umbilical cord (Figure 6.14).

If necessary, the placenta may be removed manually. This is accomplished by passing a hand into the uterine cavity and using the side of the hand to develop a cleavage plane between the placenta and the uterine wall. Sufficient analgesia should be employed for this maneuver; anesthesia may be required on occasion. The umbilical cord should be evaluated for the presence of the expected two umbilical arteries and one umbilical vein.

After the placenta has been removed, the uterus should be palpated to ensure that it has reduced in size and become firmly contracted. Excessive blood loss at this or any

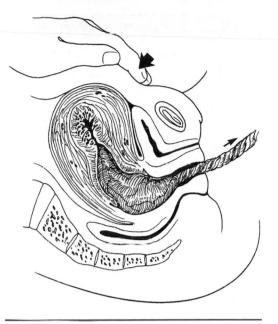

Figure 6.14. Delivery of the placenta.

subsequent time should suggest the possibility of uterine atony. The use of uterine massage as well as oxytocic agents such as oxytocin, Methergine (methylergonovine maleate), or prostaglandins (carboprost or misoprostol) may be used routinely.

Inspection of the birth canal should be accomplished in a systematic fashion. The introitus and vulvar areas, including the periurethral area, should be evaluated for lacerations. Ring forceps are commonly used to hold and evaluate the cervix. Lacerations, if present, are most commonly found at the 3 o'clock and 9 o'clock positions of the cervix. Lacerations of the vagina and/or perineum and extensions of the episiotomy are also evaluated. Repair is accomplished with an absorbable suture. Obstetric lacerations are classified in Table 6.2.

Fourth Stage of Labor

For the first hour or so after delivery, the likelihood of serious postpartum complications is at its greatest. Postpartum uterine hemorrhage occurs in approximately 1% of

Table 6.2. Classification of Obstetric Lacerations

Degree of Laceration	Description
First degree	Involves the vaginal mucosa or perineal skin, but not the underlying tissue
Second degree	Involves the underlying subcutaneous tissue, but not the rectal sphincter or rectal mucosa
Third degree	Extends through the rectal sphincter, but not into the rectal mucosa
Fourth degree	Extends into the rectal mucosa

patients. It is more likely to occur in cases of rapid labor, protracted labor, uterine enlargement (large fetus, polyhydramnios, multiple gestation), or intrapartum chorioamnionitis. Immediately after the delivery of the placenta, the uterus is palpated to determine that it is firm. Uterine palpation through the abdominal wall is repeated at frequent intervals during the immediate postpartum period to ascertain uterine tone. Perineal pads are applied and the amount of blood on these pads as well as pulse and blood pressure are monitored closely for the first several hours after delivery to identify excessive blood loss.

CHAPTER 7

ABNORMAL LABOR

This chapter deals primarily with APGO Educational Topic:

Topic 22: Abnormal Labor

The student should understand that early recognition and appropriate management of abnormalities of labor can optimize outcomes.

Abnormal labor, or *labor dystocia* (literally, "difficult labor or childbirth") results when anatomic or functional abnormalities of the fetus, the maternal bony pelvis, the uterus and cervix, and/or a combination of these interfere with the normal course of labor and delivery. The diagnosis and management of labor dystocia is a major health care issue because nearly one-third of all cesarean deliveries are performed for this indication.

Abnormal labor describes complications of the normal labor process: *slower-than-normal progress (protraction disorder)* or a *cessation of progress (arrest disorder)*. The patterns of abnormal labor are summarized in Table 7.1. Less-specific terms have also been applied to abnormal labor patterns and remain in common usage. *"Failure to progress"* describes lack of progressive cervical dilation and/or descent of the fetus, and is similar to both protraction and arrest disorders. *"Cephalopelvic disproportion"* is a disparity between the size or shape of the maternal pelvis and the fetal head, preventing vaginal delivery, and is similar to an arrest disorder. This may be caused by the size or shape of the pelvis and/or the fetal head, or a relative disparity as a result of malpresentation of the fetal head.

Causes of Abnormal Labor

Correct diagnosis and management of abnormal labor requires evaluation of the mechanisms of labor; in classic terms, the "power," the "passenger," and the "passage," otherwise referred to as the uterine contractions, fetal factors, e.g., presentation and size, and the dimensions of the maternal pelvis, respectively.

Evaluation of the "Power"

The power, or *strength, duration, and frequency of uterine contractions,* may be evaluated both qualitatively and quantitatively. Frequency and duration of contractions can be subjectively evaluated by *manual palpation of the maternal abdomen during a contraction.* Strength of uterine contractions is often judged by how much the uterine wall can be "indented" by an examiner's finger during a contraction: strong contraction, no indentation; moderate contraction, some indentation; mild contraction, considerable indentation. Although subjective, such determinations by an experienced examiner are of some value. The frequency and duration of uterine contractions may be measured more accurately by using a *tocodynamometer* while performing external electronic fetal monitor-

---

Table 7.1. Abnormal Labor Patterns

Prolonged latent phase
- No progress from latent to active phase of labor
  >20 hr for nulliparas
  >14 hr for multiparas

Protraction disorders
- Prolonged active phase of labor such that cervical dilation proceeds at
  <1.2 cm/hr for nulliparas
  <1.5 cm/hr for multiparas
- Descent of the presenting part proceeds at
  <1 cm/hr for nulliparas
  <2.0 cm/hr for multiparas

Arrest disorders
- Secondary arrest of dilation: no cervical dilation for >2 hr for nullipara or multipara in the active phase of labor
- Arrest of descent: no descent of the presenting part in >1 hr in second stage of labor

ing. A tocodynamometer is an external strain gauge that is placed on the maternal abdomen; it records when the uterus tightens and relaxes, and for how long, but does not directly measure how much force the uterus is generating, i.e., strength, for a given contraction.

The actual pressure generated within the uterus cannot be directly measured without the use of an *internal* or *intrauterine pressure catheter* (IUPC). To use an IUPC, the physician introduces into the uterine cavity a narrow flexible tube that is attached to a strain gauge. The actual intrauterine pressure is transmitted through the tubing to the strain gauge, which then records the duration and frequency, as well as the strength, of the contractions in millimeters of mercury (mm Hg) (Figure 7.1).

For cervical dilation to occur, each contraction must generate at least 25 mm Hg of peak pressure, with 50 to 60 mm Hg considered as the optimal intrauterine contractile pressure. The frequency of contractions is also important in generating a normal labor pattern; a minimum of three contractions in a 10-minute period is usually considered adequate. The expression "Montivideo units" refers to the product of the number of contractions per 10 minutes times the average intensity (above baseline) of contractions as measured by the IUPC. Normal progress of labor is usually associated with 200 or more Montivideo units. During the first stage of labor, arrest of labor should not be diagnosed until the cervix is at least 4 cm dilated; i.e., the latent phase of labor has been completed, and a pattern of uterine contractions has been established that is adequate both in frequency and intensity.

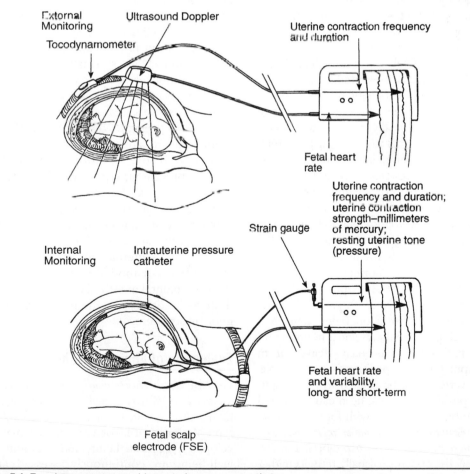

Figure 7.1. Tocodynamometers and intrauterine pressure catheters.

During the *second stage of labor,* the "powers" include both the uterine contractile forces and the voluntary maternal expulsive efforts (pushing). Maternal exhaustion, excessive pain or excessive anesthesia, or other conditions such as cardiac disease or neuromuscular disease may affect these combined forces so that they are insufficient to result in unassisted vaginal delivery. Forceps or vacuum-assisted vaginal delivery or cesarean delivery may then be required.

Evaluation of the "Passenger"

Evaluation of the passenger includes *clinical estimation of fetal weight and clinical evaluation of fetal lie, presentation, position, and attitude* (degree of flexion of the fetal head). If a fetus has an estimated weight >4,000 to 4,500 g, the incidence of dystocia, including shoulder dystocia or fetopelvic disproportion, is greater. Because ultrasound estimations of fetal weight are often inaccurate by as much as 500 to 1,000 g near term, care must be taken to use such information in conjunction with the entire clinical assessment. If the fetal head is asynclitic (turned to one side) or if the fetal head is extended, a larger cephalic diameter is presented to the pelvis, thereby increasing the possibility of dystocia. A *brow presentation* (which occurs in about 1 in 3,000 deliveries) typically converts to either a vertex or face presentation but, if persistent, causes dystocia and requires cesarean delivery. Likewise, a *face presentation* (about 1 in 600 to 1,000 deliveries) requires cesarean delivery in most cases, although a mentum anterior presentation (chin toward mother's abdomen) may be delivered vaginally. In such cases with the chin beneath the pubis, the head may undergo flexion, rather than the normal extension, with subsequent delivery of the occiput over the perineum. *Persistent occiput posterior positions* are also associated with longer labors (approximately 1 hour in multiparous patients and 2 hours in nulliparous patients). Occasionally, delivery from the occiput posterior position is not possible, and the vertex must be rotated to the occiput anterior position. The fetal head can be rotated manually or, if necessary, with forceps. In *compound presentations, when one or more limbs prolapse alongside the presenting part* (about 1 in 700 deliveries), the extremity usually retracts (either spontaneously or with manual assistance) as labor continues. When it does not, or in the 15% to 20% of compound presentations associated with umbilical cord prolapse, cesarean delivery is required. When dystocia caused by the fetal position cannot be corrected either manually or with instruments, cesarean delivery is appropriate (Figure 7.2).

Fetal anomalies, including hydrocephaly and soft tissue tumors, may also cause dystocia. The use of prenatal ultrasound significantly reduces the incidence of unexpected dystocia for these reasons.

Evaluation of the "Passage"

Unfortunately, measurements of the bony pelvis are relatively poor predictors of successful vaginal delivery. This is because of the inaccuracy of measurements, as well as case-by-case differences in fetal accommodation and mechanisms of labor. *Clinical pelvimetry,* i.e., manual evaluation of the diameters of the pelvis, cannot predict whether a fetus can successfully negotiate the birth canal, except in rare circumstances when the pelvic diameters are so small as to render the pelvis "completely contracted." Radiographic or computed tomographic pelvimetry can be helpful in some cases, although the progress (or lack of progress) of descent of the presenting part in labor is the best test of pelvic adequacy. Before assuming that the bony pelvis is preventing vaginal delivery, adequate contractions must be ensured (see Table 3.1 and Figure 3.5). In addition to the bony pelvis, there are soft tissue causes of dystocia, such as a distended bladder or colon, an adnexal mass, a uterine fibroid, an accessory uterine horn, or morbid obesity. In some instances, epidural anesthesia may contribute to dystocia by decreasing the tone of the pelvic floor musculature.

Evaluation of Abnormal Labor

Graphic documentation of progressive cervical dilation and effacement facilitates assessing a patient's progress in labor and identifying any type of abnormal labor pattern that may develop. Throughout labor, maternal and fetal well-being are continuously assessed, along with the progress in labor. The mother, and all

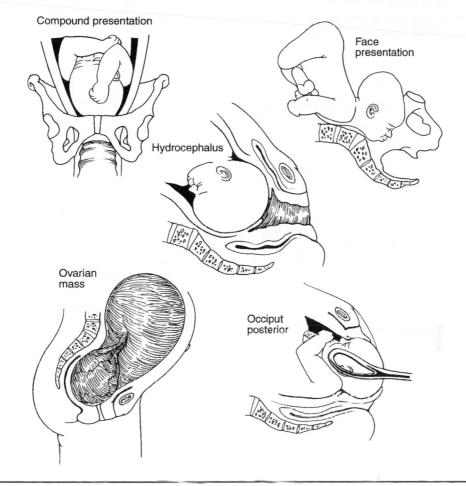

Figure 7.2. Situations associated with labor dystocia.

others present, should be provided emotional support and encouragement as the possibility of prolonged labor is faced and the various interventions are considered. Keeping the patient and support person fully apprised of the situation is an important aspect of the management of potentially abnormal labor.

Each *pelvic examination* should provide the following information: dilation of the cervix in centimeters, percentage effacement of cervix, station of the presenting part, presence or absence of caput (molding of the fetal head), and position of the presenting part. The results of each examination are compared with previous examinations and any changes are noted. In cases of failure of descent of the fetus, clinical reevaluation of the bony pelvis and its relationships to the fetus helps to identify the potential need for operative vaginal or cesarean delivery.

Uterine contractions can be assessed by manual palpation or by tocodynamometer, as previously discussed. The uterine contraction pattern and/or the force of the contractions may be inadequate, either causing the abnormal labor pattern or resulting from a mechanical disorder.

Patterns of Abnormal Labor

Abnormal labor, or dystocia, is divided into prolongation disorders and arrest disorders. These abnormal labor patterns are demonstrated graphically in Figure 7.3.

A latent phase of labor exceeding 20 hours in a nulliparous patient or 14 hours in a multiparous patient is abnormal. The causes of such a *prolonged latent phase* of labor include abnormal fetal position, "unripe" cervix when labor

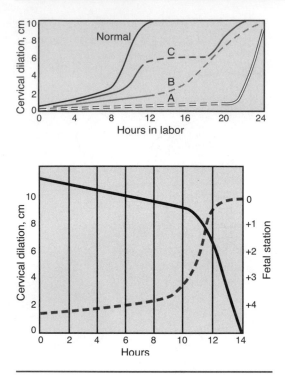

Figure 7.3. Abnormal labor. **Top.** Examples of labor patterns: A, prolonged latent phase; B, prolonged active phase; C, arrest of active phase. **Bottom.** Relation between descent of presenting part of fetus (solid line) and progressive dilation of cervix (broken line).

commences, administration of excessive anesthesia, fetopelvic disproportion, and dysfunctional/ineffective uterine contractions. The presence of a prolonged latent phase does not necessarily herald an abnormal active phase of labor. In addition, some patients who are initially thought to have a prolonged latent phase turn out only to have false labor. Although certainly of concern, particularly to the patient, a prolonged latent phase does not in itself pose a danger to the mother or fetus.

A *prolonged active phase* in the primigravid patient lasts longer than 12 hours or has a rate of cervical dilation of less than 1.2 cm/hr, and for a multipara, 1.5 cm/hr. Causes of prolonged active phase include fetal malposition, fetopelvic disproportion, excess use of sedation, inadequate contractions, and rupture of the fetal membranes before the onset of active labor. Risks associated with a prolonged active phase include an increase in operative vaginal

deliveries or cesarean delivery, intrauterine infection, and fetal compromise. In the absence of nonreassuring fetal status, slow cervical dilation poses no threat to mother or fetus and can be allowed to progress. On the other hand, secondary arrest of dilation should be assessed promptly and acted on appropriately.

In the multiparous patient, a prolonged active phase is defined as lasting more than 6 hours. Cervical dilation should occur at a rate of at least 1.5 cm/hr. Although a prolonged active phase is much less common in multiparous patients, the physician cannot be lulled into a false sense of security by the history of previous successful vaginal birth. Careful evaluation of all the factors is no less important in the multiparous patient than in the nulliparous patient.

Secondary arrest of dilation occurs when cervical dilation during the active phase of labor stops for 2 hours or more, and is demonstrated by a flattening of the labor curve. Either dilation ceases because uterine contractions are no longer sufficient to maintain the progress of labor or labor arrests in spite of adequate uterine contractions, usually associated with too large a fetus, a fetal lie/position/attitude that prevents progress in labor, or a pelvis that is too small or abnormally shaped. Because ineffective contractions can be associated with mechanical factors such as disproportion and malpresentation, careful evaluation of all factors is necessary.

Management of Abnormal Labor

Induction of labor is the stimulation of uterine contractions before the spontaneous onset of labor, with the goal of achieving delivery. *Augmentation of labor* is the stimulation of uterine contractions that began spontaneously but are either too infrequent or too weak, or both. Stimulation of labor is usually carried out with intravenous oxytocin (Pitocin) administered as an intravenous piggyback solution by means of a metered pump. In this way, exact amounts of oxytocin may be given per minute. There are several regimens for oxytocin administration; two examples, a regular-dose oxytocin program and a low-dose oxytocin program, are presented in Table 7.2.

Table 7.2. Oxytocin Administration for Induction and Augmentation of Labor

Infusion	Low Dose	Regular Dose
Initial IV infusion	1,000 mL D$_5$LR	1,000 mL D$_5$LR
Piggyback infusion	30 U oxytocin in 500 mL 0.9 N/S	20 U oxytocin in 1,000mL 0.9 N/S
Initial infusion rate	1 mU/min	1 mU/min
Interval and increment for increasing infusion rate	1 mU q 30 min	1–2 mU q 15–30 min
Maximum infusion rate	15–20 mU/min	Three contractions/10 min; 30 mU/min

N/S, normal saline.

The use of an IUPC to document actual strength as well as frequency and duration of uterine contractions stimulated by oxytocin is often recommended once a regular contraction pattern has been established, particularly if protracted labor is suspected.

Prolongation of the first stage of labor can be minimized by avoiding unnecessary intervention; i.e., labor should not be induced when the cervix is not well prepared or "ripe" (softened, anteriorly rotated, partially effaced). The degree of cervical ripening or readiness for labor is estimated by digital examination of the cervix. The Bishop score has been used to try to quantify this determination (Table 7.3). Although not especially precise, it provides an excellent schema for cervical evaluation and a rough approximation of the likelihood of successful induction of labor and vaginal delivery.

Induction of labor is indicated if the anticipated benefits of delivery exceed the risks of allowing the pregnancy to continue. There-fore, careful evaluation of both mother and fetus is needed to make this decision. Currently, "elective" induction solely for convenience is controversial. Table 7.4 summarizes commonly cited indications and contraindications to labor induction.

When a cervix is not favorable, intravaginal *prostaglandin E$_2$ gel (dinoprostone)* is often used to "ripen" the cervix and, indeed, labor often ensues without the need of oxytocin stimulation. Dinoprostone is available in a retrievable polyester tape (Cervidil) or as a gel (Prepidil) with an insertion applicator. The former contains 10 mg dinoprostone, designed to release approximately 0.3 mg/hr over a 12-hour application. The tape can be removed if active labor ensues or if nonreassuring fetal or maternal events occur. The latter is designed for a 0.5-mg dose of gel that is given in shorter intervals, usually 4 to 6 hours. The main concern in the use of prostaglandin is uterine hyperstimulation, which, in turn, may cause uteroplacental insufficiency and, rarely, uterine rupture.

Table 7.3. The Bishop Score for Cervical Status[a]

	Points			
Factor	0	1	2	3
Dilation (cm)	Closed	1–2	3–4	5+
Effacement (%)	0–30	40–50	60–70	80+
Station	−3	−2, −1	0	+1, +2
Consistency	Firm	Medium	Soft	
Position	Posterior	Mid	Anterior	

[a]A score of 0 to 4 points is associated with the highest likelihood of failed induction; a score of 9 to 13 points is associated with the highest likelihood of successful induction.

Table 7.4. Induction of Labor: Common Indications and Contraindications	
Indications	**Contraindications**
Postterm pregnancy	Placenta or vasa previa
Major maternal medical illnesses	Cord presentation
Fetal demise	Abnormal/unstable fetal lie
Suspected fetal compromise	Presenting part above inlet
Severe pregnancy-induced hypertension	Prior classic uterine incision
Premature rupture of membranes (at term)	Prior uterine incision of unknown type
Chorioamnionitis	Active genital herpes

Table 7.5. Differentiating Contractions of True and False Labor (Braxton Hicks Contractions)	
True Labor	**False Labor**
Regular intervals, gradually increasing in frequency	Irregular intervals and duration
Increasing intensity	Intensity unchanged
Cervical dilation occurs	No cervical dilation
Back and abdominal discomfort	Lower abdominal discomfort
No relief from sedation	Relief from sedation

Prostaglandins are relatively contraindicated in patients with concurrent asthma. Misoprostol is another prostaglandin cervical ripening agent. Because the risk of uterine rupture during VBAC attempts is increased when prostaglandin cervical ripening agents are used, they should be used very cautiously, if at all.

Insertion of *laminaria* is also used for cervical ripening. Laminaria, made from the stems of the seaweed *Laminaria japonica,* are hygroscopic rods that are inserted into the internal cervical os. As the rods absorb moisture and expand, the cervix is slowly dilated (Figure 7.4). The risks associated with laminaria use include failure to dilate the cervix, cervical laceration, inadvertent rupture of the membranes, and infection. A synthetic form is also available. Alternatively, insertion into the cervix of a Foley catheter has been described for this purpose.

A prolonged first stage of labor can be correctly diagnosed by accurately differentiating true labor from *false labor,* the latter being best treated with rest and sedation (Table 7.5).

A *prolonged latent phase* can be managed by either *rest* or *augmentation of labor* with intravenous oxytocin in a term pregnancy once mechanical factors have been ruled out. If the patient is allowed to rest, at times, with the addition of intramuscular morphine sulfate, one of the following will occur: she will cease having contractions, in which case she is not in labor; she will go into active labor; or she will continue as before, in which case oxytocin may be administered to augment the uterine contractions. The use of *amniotomy,* or *artificial*

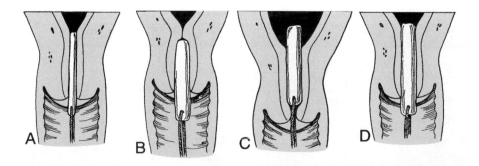

Figure 7.4. Use of laminaria. Laminaria inserted properly just beyond the internal os (**A**). Laminaria improperly inserted not far enough (**B**) and too far (**C**), increasing the risk, respectively, of failure to dilate the cervix and inadvertent rupture of the membranes. Properly placed laminaria that has expanded, causing cervical dilation (**D**).

rupture of membranes, is also advocated for patients with a prolonged latent phase. It is believed that, after amniotomy, the fetal head will provide a better dilating force than would the intact bag of water. In addition, there may be a release of prostaglandins, which could aid in augmenting the force of contractions. Before amniotomy is performed, the presenting part should generally be firmly applied to the cervix to minimize the risk of causing an umbilical cord prolapse. Amniotomy is usually performed with a thin, plastic rod with a sharp hook on the end. The end is guided to the open cervical os with the examiner's fingers, and the hook is used to snag and disrupt the amniotic sac. The clarity of the fluid should be noted and recorded, as well as the presence of meconium. The fetal heart rate should be evaluated both before and immediately after rupture of the membranes.

During the *active phase of labor,* mechanical factors such as fetal malposition and malpresentation as well as fetopelvic disproportion must be considered before augmentation of uterine contractions with oxytocin. In cases in which the fetus fails to descend with adequate contractions, disproportion is likely and cesarean delivery warranted. If no disproportion is present, oxytocin can be used if uterine contractions are judged to be inadequate. In cases of maternal exhaustion resulting in secondary arrest of dilation, rest followed by augmentation with oxytocin is often effective. If not already ruptured, artificial rupture of the membranes is also recommended.

If nonreassuring fetal or maternal status occurs, prompt intervention is warranted. If this happens during the second stage of labor with the vertex low in the pelvis, forceps or a vacuum extractor can be used to effect a prompt vaginal delivery. In all other cases, cesarean delivery may be necessary. True nonreassuring status of either mother or fetus in the first stage of labor usually mandates cesarean delivery.

Management of Prolonged Second Stage

In the past, a 2-hour second stage was considered an indication for cesarean delivery or operative vaginal delivery. Data now show that if the fetal heart rate is reassuring, it is safe to allow the mother to continue labor with the goal of vaginal delivery. As long as both mother and fetus are doing well, the second stage of labor does not have to be concluded in any specific time frame. Should disproportion exist, no amount of extra time allotted to the second stage will allow vaginal delivery, and cesarean delivery is necessary. If this is not the case, oxytocin may be used to improve the frequency and/or strength of contraction, especially if they are documented by intrauterine pressure catheter as being inadequate.

Bearing-down efforts by the patient in conjunction with the uterine contractions help bring about delivery. Because this is the one phase of labor over which the patient has some control, emotional support and encouragement are of great importance. Labor positions other than the dorsal lithotomy, where the mother is, to some extent, pushing against gravity, may facilitate delivery. In addition, alternate positions may allow subtle changes in fetal presentation relative to the birth canal and bony pelvis, facilitating better accommodation to the birth canal and, thereby, vaginal delivery. The use of such positions, e.g., knee-chest, sitting, squatting, or birth-chair, requires the ability to continue needed monitoring of fetal and maternal well-being, and the guidance of a physician or other clinician well versed in their use. Fetal accommodation within the pelvis may also be facilitated by allowing an epidural analgesia to "wear off," presumably associated with an increased tone of the pelvic floor muscles or an increased desire of the mother to push. Forceps or vacuum extraction may be used to assist the necessary descent and rotation of the fetus, resulting in vaginal delivery.

Risks of Prolonged Labor

Prolonged labor can have deleterious effects on both fetus and mother. Maternal risks include infection, maternal exhaustion, lacerations, and uterine atony with possible hemorrhage. In addition, there are the attendant risks of any operative delivery, most especially maternal soft tissue injury to the lower genital tract and fetal trauma. Fetal risks of prolonged labor include asphyxia, trauma from difficult deliveries, and infection.

Prolonged labor (along with postdatism, growth restriction, and other situations associated with decreased amniotic fluid volume) is associated with the passage of meconium into the amniotic fluid and, subsequently, the risk of *meconium aspiration syndrome*. Fetuses who inhale meconium-stained fluid during labor or from the nasopharynx just after birth may suffer this syndrome, which includes both mechanical obstruction and chemical pneumonitis from the meconium material. Pathologic factors include atelectasis, consolidation, and barotrauma as well as some degree of direct removal of pulmonary surfactant by free fatty acids in meconium. In utero aspiration of meconium can also occur.

Intrapartum management of a patient with meconium-stained amniotic fluid may include *amnioinfusion,* by which a normal saline solution is slowly infused through a tube inserted into the uterine cavity, washing meconium-stained fluid out and replacing it with the saline solution. As the head is delivered, but before delivery of the fetal chest, careful suctioning of the nasopharynx and oropharynx should be performed. Postpartum examination of the area below the vocal cords of the neonate with a laryngoscope and suctioning out of meconium below the newborn's vocal cords, using an endotracheal tube, are also recommended procedures.

Breech Presentation

Breech presentation occurs in about 2% of singleton deliveries at term, and more frequently in the early third and second trimesters. In addition to prematurity, other conditions associated with breech presentation include multiple pregnancy, polyhydramnios, hydrocephaly, anencephaly, aneuploidy, uterine anomalies, and uterine tumors. The three kinds of breech presentation–*frank, complete,* and *incomplete breech* (Figure 7.5)–are diagnosed by a combination of Leopold maneuvers, pelvic examination, ultrasonography, and at times, other imaging techniques.

The morbidity and mortality rates for mother and fetus, regardless of gestational age or mode of delivery, are higher in the breech

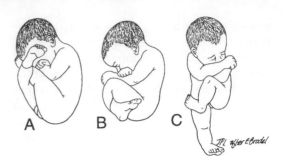

Figure 7.5. Breech presentations. (**A**) Frank breech. (**B**) Complete breech. (**C**) Incomplete breech, single footling.

than in the cephalic presentation. This increased risk to the fetus comes from associated factors such as fetal anomalies, prematurity, and umbilical cord prolapse, as well as birth trauma.

Vaginal delivery of the preterm breech fetus weighing <2,000 g is avoided by many obstetricians because of concern about an increased risk of birth injury. The practice of cesarean delivery for these smaller breech infants is common. At the other end of the spectrum, vaginal delivery of the term breech infant weighing >4,000 g is usually avoided, primarily because of concern about entrapment of the head after the vaginal delivery of the smaller body. Because of the wide margin of error in the estimated fetal weight, both by clinical estimation and by obstetrical ultrasonography, a cesarean delivery is recommended by many if the estimated fetal weight is >3,800 g.

To avoid the risks of both vaginal delivery of the breech infant at term or elective cesarean delivery for the breech infant, some clinicians attempt external cephalic version (Figure 7.6). This maneuver is successful in approximately half of properly selected cases. Selection criteria include a normal fetus with reassuring fetal heart tracing, adequate amniotic fluid, presenting part not in the pelvis, no uterine operative scars, and no labor. The risks include premature rupture of membranes, placental abruption, cord accident, and uterine rupture. External version is more often successful in parous women. Whether to use tocolytics at the time of attempted version is controversial, but the use of anti-D immune globulin in Rh-negative women is recommended.

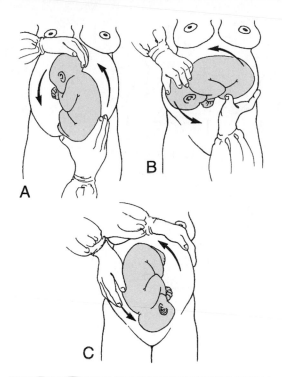

Figure 7.6. External cephalic version. Fetus is converted from breech to vertex presentation in (**A–C**).

There are three types of vaginal delivery of the breech infant (Table 7.6). The keys to successful planned vaginal delivery of the term breech infant are appropriate selection of cases and patience during the delivery, allowing as much of the delivery as possible to be spontaneous.

The suggested criteria for a vaginal breech delivery include (1) a normal labor curve, (2) an estimated fetal weight between 2,000 and 3,800 g in the frank breech presentation, (3) a reassuring fetal heart tracing, (4) an adequate

Table 7.6. Types of Vaginal Breech Deliveries
Total breech extraction
Entire body extracted
Partial breech extraction
Spontaneous delivery to umbilicus, remainder of body extracted
Spontaneous breech delivery
No traction or manipulation of the fetus, which delivers spontaneously

maternal pelvis by clinical pelvimetry (computed tomographic pelvimetry may also be employed), and (5) a normally flexed fetal head. Availability of anesthesia and neonatal support are also recommended. Hyperextension of the fetal head occurs in about 5% of term breech fetuses, requiring cesarean delivery to avoid head entrapment. Because of the risk of umbilical cord prolapse, vaginal delivery of the footling breech infant is avoided. In the event of *cord prolapse,* the following steps should be taken: place the mother in Trendelenburg position (head down); relieve pressure on the cord by pushing the fetal presenting part off of the umbilical cord; commence immediate plans for cesarean delivery.

The delivery of the aftercoming fetal head assisted with Piper forceps is shown in Figure 7.7, and the technique of breech extraction is presented in Figure 7.8.

Vaginal breech delivery is still appropriate in certain circumstances, e.g., a patient with a fetus in frank breech presentation who is ready for imminent delivery; or delivery of a second twin; however, given the increased fetal risks in all situations of vaginal breech delivery, planned vaginal breech delivery is becoming increasingly uncommon.

Indications of Operative Delivery

Techniques of operative delivery include obstetric forceps and vacuum extraction-assisted vaginal delivery, and cesarean delivery.

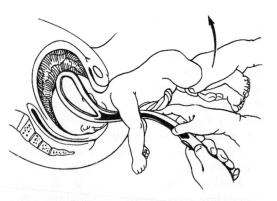

Figure 7.7. Application of Piper forceps to the aftercoming head.

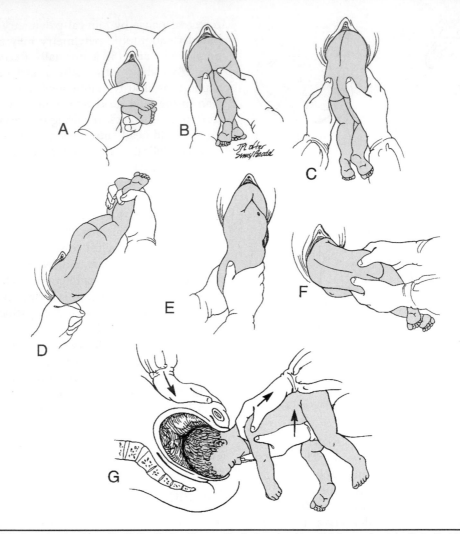

Figure 7.8. Breech extraction. (**A–C**) Gentle traction on the feet and ankles, thighs, and pelvis. Note that traction is not applied above the pelvis. (**D**) Gentle traction and rotation as the scapulae become visible, sweeping the posterior and then anterior arm free in the process. (**E–G**) Mauriceau maneuver to deliver the head.

Forceps are primarily used to supply traction to the fetal head to augment the forces expelling the fetus when the mother's voluntary efforts in conjunction with uterine contractions are insufficient to deliver the infant. Occasionally, forceps are used to rotate the fetal head before traction to complete the vaginal delivery. Forceps may also be used to control delivery of the fetal head, thereby avoiding any potentially precipitous delivery of the fetal head. Proper application of obstetric forceps by an experienced clinician is necessary to avoid the potential risk of trauma to both the maternal birth canal and the fetal head. Table 7.7 is a list of

Table 7.7. Conditions for Operative Application

Criterion	Condition
Cervix	Fully dilated
Membranes	Ruptured
Position and station of fetal head	Known and engaged
Anesthesia	Adequate for maternal comfort
Maternal pelvis	Evaluated and found adequate

Table 7.8. Forceps Classification[a]

Forceps Classification	Fetal Head Condition
Outlet forceps	The fetal skull has reached the perineal floor, the scalp is visible between contractions, the sagittal suture is in the anteroposterior diameter or in the right or left occiput anterior or posterior position, but not more than 45° from the midline
Low forceps	The leading edge of the skull is +2 station or more, rotation ≤45°
Midforceps	The head is engaged (0 station) but the leading edge of the skull is above +2 station

[a]The main controversy that has surrounded forceps delivery classification has been the definition of station used. Recently, the American College of Obstetricians and Gynecologists redefined station for the purpose of forceps delivery classification, describing the leading bony point of the fetal head in centimeters at or below the level of the maternal ischial spines (0 − +5) rather than the previously used system of thirds (0 − +3).

conditions necessary to apply forceps, and Table 7.8 is a classification of different types of forceps deliveries. Different types of forceps are available for different degrees of molding of the fetal head.

Vacuum cups applied to the fetal head are sometimes used instead of forceps. The conditions necessary to use vacuum extraction are the same as forceps. Because traction is applied only to the instrument, it is believed by some to be more physiologic than forceps, with less potential trauma to mother, although bruising or trauma to the fetal scalp may occur.

CHAPTER 8

INTRAPARTUM FETAL SURVEILLANCE

This chapter deals primarily with APGO Educational Topic:

Topic 26: Intrapartum Fetal Surveillance

The student should understand how evaluation of the fetal status during labor can detect potential abnormalities.

Evidence suggesting a *nonreassuring fetal status* during labor occurs in 5% to 10% of pregnancies. The indirect measurements of fetal status in labor can detect alterations in uteroplacental function as well as fetal and/or maternal status, which can, in some cases, result in fetal compromise with short and/or long-term sequelae. The term *fetal distress* is often used, but is now considered obsolete because it is less precise, having a low positive predictive value even in high-risk situations, and often being associated with a neonate that shows no evidence of intrauterine compromise as measured by Apgar scores and blood gas studies. An important role of the obstetric team is to identify and manage conditions that could compromise the fetus. This is often difficult because indirect measures such as fetal heart rate (FHR) monitoring, fetal acid-base measurement, amniotic fluid volume, fetal stimulation responses, and others are imprecise and difficult to interpret.

To help interpret these measurements of fetal status, the obstetric team correlates the intrapartum status with the patient's antepartum information, including historical risk factors (e.g., hypertension, maternal smoking), physical examination information (e.g., hypertension, fetal size), laboratory information (e.g., glucose tolerance data, ultrasound examinations), and dynamic testing information (e.g., biophysical profile determinations, nonstress test/oxytocin challenge testing). When interpreting this information, the obstetric team is especially alert for conditions that are known to be associated with *categories of causes of nonreassuring fetal status:* uteroplacental insufficiency, umbilical cord compression, and fetal conditions/anomalies (Table 8.1).

The *uteroplacental unit* provides oxygen and nutrients to the fetus while receiving carbon dioxide and wastes, the products of the normal aerobic fetal and placental metabolisms. *Uteroplacental insufficiency* occurs when the

Table 8.1. Causes of Nonreassuring Fetal Status

Uteroplacental insufficiency	Placental edema
	Maternal diabetes
	Hydrops fetalis
	Rh Isoimmunization
	Placental "accidents"
	Abruptio placentae
	Placenta previa ± accreta
	Postdatism
	Intrauterine growth restriction
	Uterine hyperstimulation
Umbilical cord compression	Umbilical cord accidents
	Umbilical cord prolapse or entanglement (gross, occult)
	Umbilical cord knot
	Abnormal umbilical cord insertion
	Anomalous umbilical cord
	Oligohydramnios (from any cause) with cord compression
Fetal conditions/anomalies	Sepsis (maternal/fetal; chorioamnionitis)
	Fetal congenital anomalies
	Intrauterine growth restriction
	Prematurity
	Postdatism

uteroplacental unit starts to fail at this task. Initial fetal responses include fetal hypoxia; shunting of blood flow to the fetal brain, heart, and adrenal glands; and transient, repetitive late decelerations of the FHR. *If the cause of the fetal hypoxia is progressive and is not recognized and corrected, fetal respiratory and then metabolic acidosis can ensue.* These patterns of nonreassuring fetal status are usually reversible either by altering the conditions of uteroplacental function or by rapid delivery of the infant.

Devised in 1952 by Dr. Virginia Apgar, an anesthesiologist, Apgar scores are a widely used measure of fetal status immediately after delivery *to determine the need for resuscitation of the newborn.* Five factors are rated on a three-point scale and the scores added, producing a final "Apgar" of 0 to 10 (see Table 9.1). If delivery occurs *promptly* in the face of a nonreassuring fetal status, the 1-minute Apgar score may be low, but the 5-minute score is usually high. If, however, the fetus continues to experience hypoxia, the time will come when the fetus will progressively switch over to anaerobic glycolysis, shunt more blood flow to vital organs, and progressively develop a metabolic acidosis superimposed on the respiratory one. Lactic acid accumulates as this process continues and progressive damage to vital organs occurs, especially the fetal brain and myocardium. At delivery, both the 1- and 5-minute Apgar scores are often depressed, and if the intervention was not timely, serious and possibly permanent damage (and sometimes even death) results. Apgar scores are often used incorrectly as predictors of future fetal status; the score was not designed for this purpose and does not provide such prediction.

Indeed, the correlation between such measures and neonatal encephalopathy and cerebral palsy has been and remains an important issue and area of continuous inquiry. Recently, the American College of Obstetricians and Gynecologists and the American Academy of Pediatrics released a comprehensive monograph (*Neonatal Encephalopathy and Cerebral Palsy, Defining the Pathogenesis and Pathophysiology,* January 2003) presenting current information about and understandings of these issues. *Neonatal encephalopathy (including "hypoxic-ischemic encephalopathy")* is not always as-

sociated with permanent neonatal neurologic impairment (*cerebral palsy*), although it is certain that the route from an intrapartum hypoxic-ischemic injury to cerebral palsy always involves a neonatal encephalopathy.

Cerebral palsy is a chronic central nervous system dysfunction characterized by aberrant control of movement and body posture. *Spastic quadriplegia (especially with an associated movement disorder)* is the only cerebral palsy that is associated with acute intrapartum blood flow disruption. Disorders not associated with intrapartum or peripartum asphyxia include dyskinetic or ataxic cerebral palsy (which commonly has a genetic origin) and epilepsy, mental retardation, or attention-deficit hyperactivity disorders.

It is estimated that the incidence of neonatal encephalopathy caused by intrapartum hypoxia is approximately 1.6/10,000, absent other coincident preconceptual or antepartum abnormalities. Thus, hypoxic-ischemic encephalopathy is one item in the larger category of encephalopathies that may result from conditions such as prenatal stroke, prenatal infection, genetic abnormalities, and neonatal cerebral malformation. The criteria sufficient to suggest an encephalopathy is associated with an acute intrapartum event are presented in Table 8.2.

Intrapartum Monitoring

Fetal Heart Rate Monitoring

Methods of Fetal Heart Rate Evaluation
Before the popular use of electronic fetal monitoring (EFM), intermittent auscultation of the FHR after contractions was the technique used to assess intrapartum fetal well-being. Eighty percent to 90% of births in the United States involve EFM. The idea was that the various FHR patterns that have been identified using EFM could be associated with intrauterine fetal status and, in turn, to specific situations in which interventions might result in healthier newborns. In the last few years, the now-generalized use of these monitors has undergone reevaluation. Continuous EFM of "high-risk patients" who have a predictable increased risk of intrapartum nonreassuring fe-

Table 8.2. Criteria to Define an Acute Intrapartum Hypoxic Event as Sufficient to Cause Cerebral Palsy

I. Essential criteria (must meet all four)

  a. Fetal metabolic acidosis demonstrated from umbilical cord arterial blood gas measurement (pH <7 and base deficit ≥12 mmol/liter)

  b. Early onset severe or moderate neonatal encephalopathy in newborn of ≥34 weeks of gestational age

  c. Spastic or, less commonly, dyskinetic cerebral palsy

  d. Exclusion of other identifiable causes (trauma, coagulopathy, infection, or genetic anomaly)

II. Criteria nonspecific to asphyxial insult but suggestive of intrapartum timing (close proximity to labor and delivery, within 48 hours)

  a. Sentinel hypoxic event immediately before or during labor

  b. Sudden nonreassuring fetal heart rate pattern (e.g., sudden, sustained fetal bradycardia or absent variability in the presence of persistent late or variable decelerations)

  c. Apgar scores of 0–3 beyond 5 minutes

  d. Onset of multisystem illness (e.g., acute bowel injury, renal failure, hepatic failure, cardiac damage, hematologic abnormalities) within 72 hours of birth

  e. Early cerebral imaging with evidence of acute nonfocal cerebral abnormality.

Neonatal Encephalopathy and Cerebral Palsy, Defining the Pathogenesis and Pathophysiology, January 2003, p.74.

tal status is usually not questioned. The value of EFM is questioned in "low-risk patients" whose risk of intrapartum nonreassuring fetal status is known to be small. *Intermittent FHR auscultation,* according to established guidelines for frequency of auscultation, is considered equally effective for these patients; although it is interesting that, in this group of patients, the risk of unexpected nonreassuring fetal status is highest. These intermittent auscultation guidelines suggest that the FHR in the low-risk patient should be evaluated at least every 15 minutes after a uterine contraction in the active phase and after every contraction in the second stage.

Fetal Heart Rate

Fetal heart rates by EFM are described by rate and by pattern. *The baseline FHR is the mean FHR during a 10-minute segment (rounded in 5 bpm).* A "normal FHR" at term is defined as 120 to 160 bpm, with slightly higher rates in preterm fetuses.

Fetal tachycardia is defined as >160 bpm for 10 or more minutes, and may be classified as mild if the baseline is between 161 and 180 bpm, and severe if >180 bpm. Fetal tachycardia may be transient (usually <10 minutes) and without significance, although it is sometimes associated

with situations that may require various interventions to avoid permanent fetal damage. The most common cause of fetal tachycardia is elevated maternal temperature; it is sometimes the first evidence of developing chorioamnionitis before other signs and symptoms are apparent. Because the fetal oxygen-hemoglobin dissociation curve is adversely affected by increased temperature, a fetal tachycardia coupled with increased maternal temperature should prompt administration of antipyretics to the mother. If there is evidence of chorioamnionitis, antibiotic therapy is indicated.

Fetal bradycardia is defined as <120 bpm for 10 or more minutes, and may be classified as moderate between 80 and 100 bpm and severe at <80 bpm. Heart rates between 100 and 119 bpm, although classified as a bradycardia, are rarely associated with fetal compromise unless accompanied by other evidence of nonreassuring fetal status. Fetal bradycardias may be associated with congenital heart block and with situations associated with severe fetal compromise, such as placental abruption (Figure 8.1; Table 8-3).

A *sinusoidal heart rate pattern* is seen when the rate is 120 to 160 bpm, but there is a smooth, undulating pattern of 5 to 10 bpm in amplitude (reminiscent of a sine wave) and de-

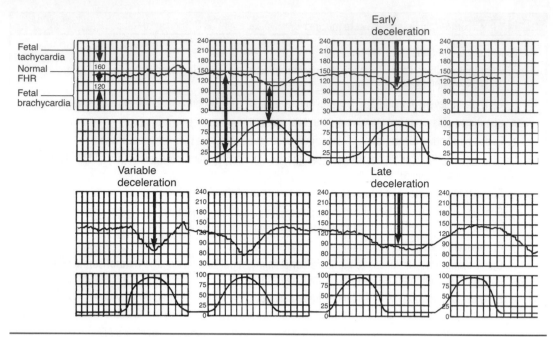

Figure 8.1. Fetal heart rate (FHR) patterns.

creased short-term variability (Figure 8.2). The cause of this pattern is unknown but it has been associated with fetal anemia, Rh isoimmunization, and newborns with significant compromise. Sinusoidal-like patterns are sometimes seen after analgesic administration, so the evaluation and treatment of this pattern are difficult. *Fetal arrhythmias* are seen in <1% of monitored labors; they are usually transient and are diagnosed by fetal electrocardiography

Table 8.3. Baseline Fetal Heart Rates		
Fetal Heart Rate (bpm)	**Description**	**Associated Causes**
>160 for >10 min	Fetal tachycardia	Maternal fever and infection
		Fetal infection
		Fetal anemia
		Maternal thyrotoxicosis
		Fetal tachyarrhythmias
		Maternal treatment with sympathomimetic or parasympatholytic (e.g., atropine) drugs
		Fetal immaturity
		Fetal hypoxia
120–160	Normal FHR	Normal function of maternal–fetal unit
<120 for >10 min	Fetal bradycardia	Maternal treatment with β-blockers (e.g., propranolol)
		Fetal congenital heart block (as in systemic lupus erythematosus where an antibody may be produced that crosses the placenta and damages the conduction system of the fetus)
		Fetal anoxia

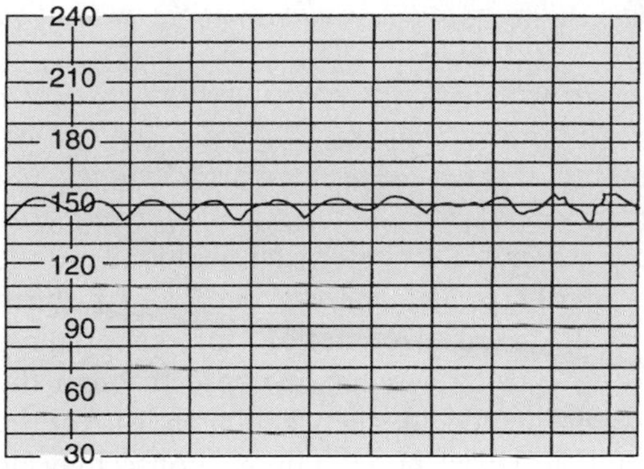

Figure 8.2. Sinusoidal fetal heart rate pattern associated with a fetal–maternal hemorrhage and severe fetal anemia.

(ECG). If they persist, evaluation of the fetus for inherent abnormalities (especially hydrops and congenital anomalies) is indicated because some treatment may be needed with delivery or during the intrapartum period.

Fetal Heart Rate Variability

Fetal heart rate variability is fluctuations in the FHR of two cycles or more, visually quantified as the amplitude of peak to trough in beats per minute. The FHR variability in general is graded according to the amplitude range (Figure 8.3):

- *Absent:* amplitude range undetectable
- *Minimal:* amplitude range detectable but at 5 bpm or less

- *Moderate:* amplitude range 6 to 25 bpm
- *Marked:* amplitude range >25 bpm.

Fetal heart rate variability is the single most reliable EFM indicator of fetal status (fetal well-being). The FHR variability results from a complex interplay of cardioinhibitory and cardioaccelerator centers in the fetal brain, which, in turn, are extremely sensitive to the fetal biochemical status (oxygenation and acid-base status). *The presence of good variability is highly suggestive of adequate fetal central nervous system (CNS) oxygenation.* Two types of variability have been described and used in clinical care for many years, and although they are the most current terminology, their continued use is anticipated and thus they are described. *Short-term variability* has been described as the variation in amplitude seen on a beat-to-beat basis, normally 3 to 8 bpm, measured from R wave to R wave by direct fetal scalp electrode. *Long-term variability* has been described as an irregular, crude, wavelike pattern with a period of 3 to 5 cycles per minute and an amplitude of 5 to 15 bpm.

Decreased variability is associated with fetal hypoxia and/or acidemia, drugs that may depress the fetal CNS (e.g., maternal narcotic analgesia), fetal tachycardia, fetal CNS and cardiac anomalies, prolonged uterine contractions (uterine hypertonus), prematurity, and fetal sleep. Care must be taken in the interpretation of decreased variability when a transient cause such as fetal sleep may be involved, lest an unnecessary intervention be considered.

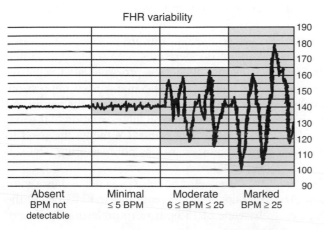

Figure 8.3. Fetal heart rate variability.

Periodic Fetal Heart Rate Changes

The FHR may vary with uterine contractions by slowing or accelerating in periodic patterns. These changes in FHR are in response to two mechanisms: (1) intrinsic reflex FHR control, especially responses to hypoxia and acidemia as well as normal reflex responses, and (2) fetal myocardial hypoxia. Periodic FHR changes are classified into patterns based on their shape, magnitude (in beats per minute), and relationship to the same parameters of the uterine contractions with which they are associated. As indirect measures of fetal well-being, these patterns have some prognostic value in the antepartum and intrapartum evaluation of the fetus and in developing management plans (Figure 8.1).

Accelerations of the FHR are defined as apparent increases (onset to peak in less than 30 seconds) in the FHR from the recent baseline FHR, with its duration defined as the time from the initial change in FHR to the return to the baseline FHR. Accelerations are considered to be present at or after 32 weeks of gestation when an acceleration has an acme of 15 bpm or more above the baseline with a duration of more than 15 seconds but less than 2 minutes. Before 32 weeks of gestational age, the acme of the acceleration is changed to 10 bpm or more. If an acceleration lasts >2 minutes but <10 minutes, it is defined as a *prolonged* acceleration. An acceleration of 10 minutes or more is a *baseline change*. Accelerations are generally considered to be associated with an intact fetal mechanism unstressed by hypoxia and academia and are therefore *considered reassuring and usually indicative of fetal well-being*. Stimulation of the fetal scalp by digital examination usually engenders a heart rate acceleration in the uncompromised, nonacidotic fetus and is used by some obstetricians as a test of fetal well-being. This is based on data that suggest that such accelerations may be associated with an arterial fetal pH of >7.20 if delivery were to occur at the time of measurement. External sound/vibration stimulation, also termed *acoustic stimulation*, elicits the same response and is also used for this purpose.

Fetal heart rate decelerations are defined as visually apparent and gradual (onset to nadir 30 seconds or more) decreases in FHR from the base- *line, returning to the baseline from the nadir of the deceleration.*

An early FHR deceleration is associated with a uterine contraction such that the nadir of the deceleration occurs at the same time as the peak of the uterine contraction (a "mirror image" of the uterine contraction). These early decelerations are the result of *pressure on the fetal head* (from the birth canal, digital examination, forceps application), causing a reflex response through the –vagus nerve with acetylcholine release at the fetal sinoatrial node. This response may be blocked with vagolytics such as atropine. *Early FHR decelerations are considered physiologic and are not a cause of concern.*

Late FHR decelerations are defined as visually apparent decreases in the FHR from the baseline FHR, associated with a uterine contraction such that the onset, nadir, and recovery of the deceleration occurs after the beginning, peak, and end of the contraction, respectively. These late decelerations are viewed as significantly nonreassuring, especially if repetitive, and most especially if associated with decreased variability. *Late decelerations are sometimes associated with uteroplacental insufficiency,* as a result of either decreased uterine perfusion or decreased placental function, and thus with decreased intervillous exchange of oxygen and carbon dioxide and *progressive fetal hypoxia and acidemia.* Therefore, they are associated with causes of uteroplacental insufficiency, including postdatism, placental abruption, maternal hypertension, maternal diabetes, maternal anemia, maternal sepsis, and problems with uterine contractions such as hyperstimulation or hypertonia, which decrease the intervals available for maximal uteroplacental blood flow.

Two mechanisms are postulated to associate late decelerations with fetal hypoxia and acidemia: chemoreceptor-mediated vagal reflex and/or hypoxic myocardial depression. Intervention is usually required, the nature and timing depending on full evaluation of the maternal and fetal status. Certainly, the need to intervene increases as nonreassuring fetal status progresses.

A *prolonged deceleration* is defined as a visually apparent decrease in the FHR below the baseline of 15 bpm or more lasting 2 minutes or more but less than 10 minutes from the onset to return to baseline.

Variable FHR decelerations are defined as abrupt (onset to nadir less than 30 seconds), visually apparent decreases in the FHR (of 15 bpm or more and a duration of 15 seconds or more but less than 2 minutes) below the baseline FHR. These variable decelerations may start before, during, or after uterine contraction starts; hence, the term "variable." Variable decelerations are also reflex-mediated, usually associated with *umbilical cord compression* and mediated through the vagus nerve with sudden and often erratic release of acetylcholine at the fetal sinoatrial node, resulting in the characteristic sharp deceleration slope of these decelerations. Umbilical cord compression may result from wrapping of the cord around parts of the fetus, fetal anomalies, or even knots in the umbilical cord, and is especially associated with oligohydramnios, in which the buffering space for the umbilical cord created by the amniotic fluid is lost. These variable decelerations are the most common periodic FHR pattern. They are often correctable by changes in the maternal position to relieve pressure on the umbilical cord. Infusion of fluid into the amniotic cavity (amnioinfusion) has also been used effectively to relieve pressure on the umbilical cord in cases of oligohydramnios or when rupture of membranes has occurred, decreasing the frequency of these decelerations, although the value with respect to improving intrapartum and immediate postpartum status is not as well established.

If the FHR falls and is sustained below 100 bpm, a vaginal examination is indicated to check for a prolapsed umbilical cord, a rare but emergent cause of the sudden development of this usually benign periodic FHR pattern. If the FHR falls below 60 to 70 bpm for more than 30 seconds, repetitive variable decelerations will often have a cumulative effect on fetal well-being, with the development of hypoxia, acidemia, and distress. If the FHR falls below 60 bpm, transient loss of fetal sinoatrial node function has been noted with transient "fetal cardiac arrest." These decelerations below 60 to 70 bpm require careful evaluation of cause.

Measurement of Fetal Acid-Base Status

Fetal acid-base balance is easily maintained despite the transient decrease in placental intervillous perfusion associated with uterine contractions when the uteroplacental unit is functioning normally. *Normal fetal acid-base status* is mirrored in the normal umbilical cord blood gas values at term (see Table 9.2). When there is *uteroplacental insufficiency,* inadequate fetal oxygenation causes a switch from fetal aerobic to fetal anaerobic metabolism, resulting in the production of lactate and progressive fetal acidosis, compounding the deleterious effects of fetal hypoxia. Initially, the fetus responds by shunting blood flow to the brain and heart from other organs. With progressive hypoxia, late decelerations develop and, with the addition of acidosis, there is loss of beat-to-beat variability. Brain and myocardial damage follow, with subsequent high risk of other end organ damage. When there are indicators of such an ominous situation (e.g., persistent late decelerations on EFM and decreased beat-to-beat variability), direct measurement of the fetal acid-base status is an option. The most common method is fetal scalp capillary blood gas or blood pH measurement.

Fetal Scalp pH/Blood Gas Evaluation

The chorioamnion must be ruptured and the presenting part descended to allow access to the presenting fetal part through the cervical os, which must be dilated at least 2 to 3 cm. Given access to the fetal part, either head or breech, a plastic or metallic cone is inserted through the os and pressed against the fetal scalp. The scalp surface is thoroughly cleaned and the cone held with enough pressure to avoid dilution of the blood with amniotic fluid. A thin layer of silicone gel is often applied to the surface, serving to provide a smooth, uniform surface on which the blood droplet may form. A small incision is then made in the fetal scalp with a specialized lancet, and the drops of blood that form are collected in a heparinized capillary tube and analyzed. Pressure is applied to the incision site through one or two uterine contractions, until bleeding stops. Care must be taken not to make the incision

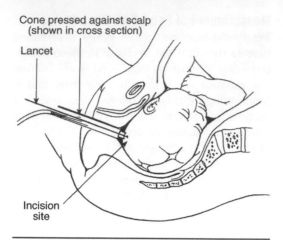

Cone pressed against scalp
(shown in cross section)

Lancet

Incision
site

Figure 8.4. Fetal scalp blood sampling.

over a fontanel or suture line. A fetal caput does not alter the pH information obtained (Figure 8.4).

Management

Interpretation of intrapartum fetal well-being measurements are made within the context of the entire obstetric situation, including maternal and fetal factors and the course and anticipated duration and outcome of labor. The number of variables to consider and the often imprecise nature of the information make these among the most difficult of medical decisions. In-depth training and experience in obstetrics (which, in modern training, includes not only classic obstetrics but also critical care medicine and components of anesthetic management) are required to perform these complex tasks adequately. Sometimes the FHR pattern demonstrates a single pattern; if it is reassuring, no intervention is usually needed; if it is not reassuring, the appropriate intervention may seem, or even be, clear. More often, however, the observed FHR strip reflects a mixture of two or more patterns with alterations in baseline rates, resulting in challenging and complex interpretations. This difficulty is underscored with the understanding that the interobserver and intraobserver variability in the interpretation of EFM shows wide variation, but is generally low, although higher if the tracing is adjudged reassuring rather than nonreassuring. Nonetheless, as a general rule, it is usually prudent to manage

the obstetric situation, factoring in both maternal and fetal status, and based on the most substantially nonreassuring of the patterns present.

In general, the efficacy of intrapartum EFM is judged by ability to minimize the need for operative vaginal delivery or cesarean section while simultaneously decreasing the incidence of intrapartum fetal death and neonatal complications such as seizures and cerebral palsy. Extant data suggest that EFM use has resulted in a decrease in perinatal mortality caused by fetal hypoxia but not by other causes, but has increased the overall cesarean delivery rate and rate of the use of vacuum and forceps-assisted vaginal delivery.

Finally, nonreassuring EFM tracings are not predictive of cerebral palsy. The positive predictive value of a nonreassuring FHR pattern to predict cerebral palsy is 0.14% in singleton pregnancies with birth weights of more than 2.5 kg. Further, the increasing use of EFM has not been chronologically associated with a decrease in the rate of cerebral palsy, which has been stable over time. Nonetheless, despite the evident limited advantages, EFM use continues to rise, from an estimated 40% of parturients in 1980 to approximately 85% in 2002. This is certainly partly related to the beneficial effects that have been demonstrated, although the increasing lack of staffing and subsequent inability to adequately perform intermittent FHR auscultation also plays a part in the decision and trend.

If there is evidence of progressive fetal hypoxia and acidosis in a situation in which the time of vaginal delivery is remote, operative delivery by cesarean section is indicated for fetal reasons. Awaiting vaginal delivery is appropriate if it is believed that delivery will occur soon enough to avoid fetal compromise, or even death. This decision could be affected by a combination of a variety of findings. For example, a scalp pH greater than 7.24 is reassuring; good variability on EFM is a reassuring factor; the presence of meconium in the amniotic fluid is associated with perinatal morbidity, which is increased by 5% to 10%, thereby serving as a nonreassuring factor.

While awaiting vaginal delivery or while preparing for cesarean delivery, one or more of the following steps is appropriate to attempt "intrauterine resuscitation": (1) discontinue oxytocin infusion that may have been started for induction or augmentation; (2) administer oxygen to the mother, usually 5 to 6 liter/min by face mask; (3) check the maternal blood pressure, treating any hypotension with intravenous fluids and, if needed, pressors such as ephedrine; (4) change the maternal position to left lateral position to decrease uterine pressure on the great vessels and thereby increase blood return to the heart, cardiac output, and utero-placental blood flow; and (5) consider using an intravenous tocolytic (such as the β-2-sympathomimetic terbutaline, 0.25 mg intravenous push or subcutaneously) to relax the uterine tone and slow the contraction rate, thereby increasing uteroplacental blood flow. Umbilical arterial and venous blood gases should be drawn immediately after the delivery from the cord attached to the placenta before placental separation. The data will help in the management of the newborn, and in some instances may help interpret intrapartum events.

CHAPTER 9

IMMEDIATE CARE OF THE NEWBORN

This chapter deals primarily with APGO Educational Topic:

Topic 12: Immediate Care of the Newborn

Newborns require immediate care that includes their assessment for problems requiring immedite care. Students should be able to explain the assessment of newborns, including situations requiring immediate intervention as well as routine care, including the elective procedure of circumcision.

Not all deliveries occur in a setting with immediate pediatric care; therefore, delivering physicians should be familiar with the initial assessment and immediate care of the newborn. Resuscitative efforts may be necessary in up to 5% of all cases of cesarean delivery and 2% of vaginal deliveries. The frequency of the need for these efforts increases in circumstances such as low birth-weight infants, prolonged labor, and nonreassuring measures of fetal well-being. It is optimal to have highly trained personnel available in circumstances in which neonatal resuscitation is anticipated. Other options include the transport of the newborn in utero to a facility with greater capacity to provide care for a potentially ill newborn, or sending a special team to the primary care site to provide immediate newborn care.

Initial Assessment

Once the newborn has been delivered, the infant is transported to a warming unit where it is thoroughly dried to minimize evaporation and a drop in core temperature. Drying the infant and removing any wet towels or wraps is critical because newborns are susceptible to rapid drops in core body temperature. The nose and oropharynx are suctioned once again as the infant is placed in the supine position with the head lowered and turned to one side. The newborn is expected to both breathe and cry within the first 30 seconds of life. Suctioning, as well as mild stimulation of the infant by rubbing the back or rubbing the sole of the feet, help to stimulate the infant and are commonly employed and beneficial.

The initial evaluation of the infant is carried out at 1 and 5 minutes, using the Apgar scoring system (Table 9.1). The Apgar score is designed as a quick assessment of the newborn to determine the need for resuscitation. The Apgar score should not be used to define birth asphyxia because it is not designed to do so and, indeed, does not provide such information. Likewise, these scores cannot be used to identify the causes of the newborn illness. In general, a low 1-minute Apgar score identifies the newborn that requires particular attention. The 5-minute Apgar score can be used to evaluate the effectiveness of any resuscitative efforts that have been undertaken, or to identify an infant needing more evaluation and management. Apgar scores at 10, 15, and multiples thereof in minutes are also often recorded. The Neonatal Resuscitation Program of the American Academy of Pediatrics and the American Heart Association recommend the assignment of Apgar scores every 5 minutes until 20 minutes, or until two scores of 8 or greater are obtained. Although not part of the original Apgar scoring system, many clinicians find these continued assessments of the newborn to be of value in ongoing clinical management.

Apgar scores of 7 to 10 are indicative of an infant who requires no active resuscitative intervention; scores of 4 to 7 are considered indicators of mildly to moderately depressed infants. Severely depressed infants with Apgar scores of less than 4 rarely require a full evaluation using

Table 9.1. Apgar Scoring System			
	Score		
Sign	**0**	**1**	**2**
Heart rate	Absent	<100	>100
Muscle tone	Limp	Some flexion of extremities	Active motion
Respiratory effort	Absent	Slow, irregular	Good cry
Reflex activity response to stimulation	No response	Grimace	Cough, sneeze, or crying
Color	Blue or pale	Body pink and extremities blue	Completely pink

Table 9.2. Normal Umbilical Cord Blood Gas Values

Blood Gas	Arterial	Venous
pH	7.25–7.30	7.30–7.40
P_{CO_2} mm Hg	50	40
P_{O_2} mm Hg	20	30
Bicarbonate mEq/hr	25	20

the Apgar score. Instead, immediate resuscitative efforts are started, which may include endotracheal intubation and suctioning, with the possible use of positive pressure oxygen.

The assessment of newborn metabolic well-being may also be done by an analysis of the umbilical cord blood gases. A 10- to 15-cm segment of umbilical cord is doubly clamped and cut so that it may be taken for assessment of pH, P_{O_2}, P_{CO_2}, and bicarbonate. It should be remembered that, in the fetus, freshly oxygenated blood from the placenta travels to the fetus through the umbilical vein, and blood metabolized by the fetus travels back to the placenta through two umbilical arteries. Accordingly, the most meaningful assessment of metabolic status of the baby at the time of delivery is through analysis of umbilical artery blood gases. Normal values for umbilical arterial and venous samples are given in Table 9.2.

Acidemia is generally accepted as an increase in hydrogen ion concentration in an umbilical arterial sample resulting in a pH of less than 7.20. Further, asphyxia is usually defined as a combination of hypoxia and/or hypercarbia of a level sufficient to produce metabolic acidosis. The terms *acidemia, acidosis,* and *asphyxia* should be used carefully when applied to the newborn condition because each term defines a series of changes that may or may not represent true metabolic compromise.

Meconium Staining of the Amniotic Fluid

Ten percent to 15% of all fetuses and over 25% of postterm fetuses pass meconium (fecal material) in utero, in some cases in association with fetal stress, albeit in others as simply a natural process. The amniotic fluid is then termed "meconium-stained," and is often graded from thin to thick and particulate. About one-third of infants born with meconium in the amniotic fluid will have meconium in the lungs, about half will have abnormal chest radiographs, and about one-tenth will develop significant respiratory distress. The latter situation is called *meconium aspiration syndrome.* Meconium aspiration syndrome may include mechanical obstruction and/or severe chemical pneumonitis associated with atelectasis, consolidation, and barotrauma, some degree of direct removal of pulmonary surfactant by free fatty acids in meconium, and/or persistent pulmonary hypertension. Ventilatory support and intensive medical management are often required, and the syndrome is associated with significant morbidity and mortality, the latter approaching 10% to 20% in some series.

Meconium aspiration syndrome was thought to be caused primarily by the aspiration of meconium material, especially when the meconium was of the thick, particulate variety. Two kinds of intervention are commonly used in an attempt to prevent meconium aspiration. The first is *amnioinfusion,* the slow infusion of normal saline into the uterus through a tube inserted through the open cervix during labor. The basic idea of the procedure is to "wash out" meconium from the amniotic fluid, replacing it with the saline fluid to decrease the amount and quality of meconium available for in utero and/or newborn aspiration. In many situations, the presence of meconium is associated with oligohydramnios, which is, in turn, associated with intermittent umbilical cord compression, decreased uteroplacental perfusion and progressive hypoxia, and fetal gasping in utero. Amnioinfusion may reverse this series of events.

The second intervention involves management of the airway immediately after birth, including immediate examination of the area below the vocal cords after birth and aspiration of any meconium material with an endotracheal tube. This procedure is generally recommended when the meconium is thick and particulate, or in any situation in which the infant is depressed, requiring positive pressure ventilation. In cases where the meconium is thin and light, clinical judgment is required, but many clinicians limit intervention to careful suctioning of the oropharynx.

Further, DeLee suctioning of the newborn's nose and mouth is often performed immediately following expulsion of the head and prior to delivery of the body. To help prevent aspiration, minimal stimulation of the newborn is done as the DeLee suctioning is performed rapidly while the head is at the level of the perineum.

Neonatal Asphyxia

The neonate for whom the diagnosis of neonatal asphyxia applies is characterized by significant neuromuscular and metabolic abnormalities (see Chapter 8).

Routine Care of the Newborn

Estimation of Gestational Age

A rapid overview of the gestational age of the newborn helps facilitate more highly skilled care if the newborn is believed to be premature. Table 9.3 provides guidelines for a rapid assessment of gestational age using five measurements.

Umbilical Cord

The umbilical cord loses its bluish-white appearance within the first 24 hours after delivery. After clamping, the cord is normally not covered, so it may be exposed to air, and thereby drying and separating more quickly. After a few days, the blackened, dried stump sloughs, leaving the granulating wound.

Urine and Stool

Over 90% of newborns pass a stool within the first 24 hours. A congenital abnormality such as imperforate anus may be suspected if a stool has not been passed during the first 36 hours of life. Voiding typically occurs shortly after birth. Concern about a congenital defect of the urinary tract is appropriate if voiding has not occurred within the first day of life.

For the first 2 or 3 days of life, the stool is greenish-brown. Initially, the stools are sterile, but after the first few hours of life, bacteria can be found. With the ingestion of milk, the stool becomes more light yellow and semisolid.

Nutrition

It is recommended for nursing to begin within the first 12 hours of delivery. Although growth-restricted or preterm infants require more frequent feedings, most term infants do well with feedings at 4-hour intervals. It is recommended that the infant be allowed to attempt to breast-feed at least 5 to 10 minutes initially, with more time required, depending on various circumstances. Encouraging breast-feeding should be one of the focuses of prenatal education because of the biologic and emotional benefits that may be derived for both mother and newborn. Support for breast-feeding can be provided both through health clinicians in the hospital and outpatient facilities as well as support groups.

As a result of the newborn's initial loss of urine, feces, and sweat, and because of the relative lack of nutrition in the first few days of life, newborn weight loss of up to approximately 10% of birth weight should be anticipated. Of note, preterm newborns lose relatively more weight and regain it at a slower rate than their term counterparts. Weight loss is usually regained in the first 1 to 2 weeks of life.

Table 9.3. Estimation of Newborn Gestational Age			
	Estimated Gestational Age (weeks)		
Anatomic Site	**<36**	**37–38**	**≥39**
Scalp hair	Fine/fuzzy	Fine/fuzzy	Coarse
Ear lobe	No cartilage	Some cartilage	Thick cartilage
Breast nodule (mm)	2	4	6
Sole creases	Anterior transverse crease	Creases across anterior two-thirds	Extensive creases covering the sole
Scrotum	Few rugae	Intermediate rugae	Extensive rugae

Circumcision

Circumcision is the surgical removal of a distal portion of the foreskin. It is usually performed in the first 2 days of life and, in modern practice, always involves the administration of anesthetic, most commonly a dorsal nerve block. For practical purposes, the procedure is entirely elective, a decision of the parents that may be made for religious reasons or simply for personal choice.

Conjunctivitis

Organisms such as *Neisseria gonorrhoeae*, *Chlamydia*, and other bacteria may cause conjunctivitis in the newborn. In most states,

application of silver nitrate as a prophylactic measure is required. In addition, various antibiotics have been used to manage the emerging resistant bacterial strains that are encountered.

Jaundice

Physiologic jaundice of the newborn (icterus neonatorum) occurs in up to one-third of all newborns. Bilirubin levels of term infants may double to 5 mg/dL by the third or fourth day of life. It is at this level that jaundice becomes clinically apparent. Expectant management is appropriate in these cases. An evaluation of the cause of jaundice, as well as treatment thereof, is needed when the cause is not apparent.

CHAPTER 10

POSTPARTUM CARE

This chapter deals primarily with APGO Educational Topics:

Topic 13: Postpartum Care
Topic 14: Lactation
Topic 21: Fetal Death
Topic 29: Anxiety and Depression

The student should be familiar with normal events to provide optimal clinical care as well as be able to identify abnormal events.

The *puerperium* is the 6- to 8-week-period following birth during which the reproductive tract, as well as the rest of the body, returns to the nonpregnant state. Some of the physiologic changes of pregnancy have returned to normal within 1 to 2 weeks postpartum. The initial postpartum examination was traditionally scheduled at 6 weeks, but is now often performed sooner as patients often return to full nonpregnant activity much sooner.

Physiology of the Puerperium

Involution of the Uterus

The *uterus* weighs approximately 1,000 g and has a volume of 5,000 mL immediately after delivery, compared with its nonpregnant weight of approximately 70 g and capacity of 5 mL. Immediately after delivery, the fundus of the uterus is easily palpable halfway between the pubic symphysis and the umbilicus. The immediate reduction in uterine size is a result of delivery of the fetus, placenta, and amniotic fluid as well as the loss of hormonal stimulation. Further uterine involution is caused by autolysis of intracellular myometrial protein, resulting in a decrease in cell size but not cell number. Through these changes, the uterus returns to the pelvis by 2 weeks postpartum, and is at its normal size by 6 weeks postpartum. Immediately after birth, uterine hemostasis is maintained by contraction of the smooth muscle of the arterial walls and compression of the vasculature by the uterine musculature.

Lochia

As the myometrial fibers contract, the blood clots from the uterus are expelled and the thrombi in the large vessels of the placental bed undergo organization. Within the first 3 days, the remaining decidua differentiates into a superficial layer, which becomes necrotic and sloughs, and a basal layer adjacent to the myometrium, which contained the fundi of the endometrial glands and is the source of the new endometrium.

This discharge is fairly heavy at first and rapidly decreases in amount over the first 2 to 3 days postpartum, although it may last for several weeks. In women who breast feed, the lochia seems to resolve more rapidly, possibly because of a more rapid involution of the uterus caused by uterine contractions associated with breast feeding. In some patients, there is an increased amount of lochia 1 to 2 weeks after delivery because the eschar that developed over the site of placental attachment has been sloughed. By the end of the third week postpartum, the endometrium is reestablished in most patients.

Cervix and Vagina

Within several hours of delivery, the cervix has reformed, and by 1 week, it usually admits only one finger (i.e., it is approximately 1 cm in diameter). The round shape of the nulliparous cervix is usually permanently replaced by a transverse, fish–mouth-shaped external os, the result of laceration during delivery. *Vulvar* and *vaginal tissues* return to normal over the first several days, although the *vaginal mucosa* reflects a hypoestrogenic state if the woman breast feeds because ovarian function is suppressed during breast feeding. The muscles of the pelvic floor gradually regain their tone. This may be aided by the use of Kegel exercises, consisting of repetitive contractions of these muscles. The hymen is now represented by several tags of tissue, the *myrtiform caruncles.*

Return of Ovarian Function

Ovulation can occur as early as 4 to 5 weeks postpartum if the woman chooses not to breast feed. The mean time to ovulation in nonlactating women is approximately 10 weeks, with 50% of women ovulating by 90 days postpartum. Among breast-feeding women, the time to first ovulation depends on how long the woman breast feeds, and can take up to 2 to 18 months. Ovulation is suppressed in the lactating woman in association with elevated prolactin levels. In these patients, prolactin remains elevated for 6 weeks, whereas in nonlactating women, prolactin levels return to normal by 3 weeks postpartum. Estrogen levels fall immediately after delivery in all patients, but begin to rise approximately 2 weeks after delivery if breast feeding is not undertaken.

Abdominal Wall

Return of the elastic fibers of the skin and the stretched rectus muscles to normal configuration occurs slowly and is aided by exercise. The silvery *striae* seen on the skin usually lighten in time. *Diastasis recti,* separation of the rectus muscles and fascia, also usually resolves over time.

Cardiovascular System

Pregnancy-related cardiovascular changes return to normal 2 to 3 weeks after delivery. Immediately postpartum, plasma volume is reduced by approximately 1,000 mL, caused primarily by blood loss at the time of delivery. During the immediate postpartum period, there is also a significant shift of extracellular fluid into the intravascular space. The increased cardiac output seen during pregnancy also persists into the first several hours of the postpartum period. The elevated pulse rate seen during pregnancy persists for approximately 1 hour after delivery, but then decreases. These conditions may contribute to decompensation sometimes seen in the early postpartum period in patients with heart disease. Immediately after delivery, approximately 5 kg of weight are lost as a result of diuresis and the loss of extravascular fluid. Further weight loss varies in rate and amount from patient to patient.

Hematopoietic System

The leukocytosis seen during labor persists into the early puerperium for several days, thus minimizing the usefulness of identifying early postpartum infection by laboratory evidence of a mild-to-moderate elevation in the white cell count. There is some degree of autotransfusion of red cells to the intravascular space after delivery as the uterus contracts.

Renal System

Glomerular filtration rate represents renal function and remains elevated in the first few weeks postpartum, then returns to normal. Therefore, drugs with renal excretion should be given in decreased doses during this time. Ureter and renal pelvis dilation regress by 6 to 8 weeks. There may be considerable edema around the urethra after vaginal delivery, resulting in transitory urinary retention.

About 7% of women experience urinary stress incontinence, which usually regresses by 3 months.

Management of the Immediate Postpartum Period

Hospital Stay

The amount of time a patient remains in the hospital after delivery continues to decrease. In the past, patients were kept in the hospital for several days. Currently, it is common for patients to be discharged 24 hours after a vaginal delivery and 48 hours after a cesarean section. The period of hospitalization has been significantly reduced primarily as a result of financial issues involving third-party payers. Concerns in these regards include the preparation of the mother for newborn care, infant feeding including the special issues involved with breast feeding, and required newborn laboratory testing. Mandatory early discharge is considered inappropriate.

Maternal–Infant Bonding

It is recognized that, shortly after delivery, the parents become totally engrossed in the events surrounding the newborn infant. Any significant separation of the mother from her infant that reduces activity such as cuddling, fondling, kissing, or gazing at the infant may have a negative impact on the involvement of maternal behaviors on a long-term basis. Contemporary obstetric units have enhanced these interactions by minimizing unnecessary medical interventions while increasing participation by the father and other family members. Rooming-in (in which mother and newborn are cared for in the same room, rather than the newborn being taken to a nursery) and an environment that facilitates breast feeding also contribute to this atmosphere. Interaction between the infant and the new parents is also observed by the nursing staff, with the resultant ability to identify any problems such as negative or even abusive actions toward the newborn.

Uterine Complications

The likelihood of serious *postpartum complications* is greatest immediately after delivery. Significant immediate postpartum hemorrhage occurs in approximately 1% of patients (see Chapter 12); infection is seen in approximately 5% of patients. Immediately after the delivery of the placenta, the uterus is palpated bimanually to ascertain that it is firm. Uterine palpation through the abdominal wall is repeated at frequent intervals during the immediate postpartum period to prevent and/or identify uterine atony. Perineal pads are applied, and the amount of blood on these pads as well as pulse and pressure are monitored closely for the first several hours after delivery to identify excessive blood loss.

Some patients will experience an episode of increased, "heavy," vaginal bleeding between days 8 and 14 postpartum, most likely associated with the separation and passage of the placental eschar. This is self-limited and needs no therapy other than reassurance. In approximately 1% of cases, this bleeding persists or is excessive, *delayed postpartum hemorrhage,* in which case oxytocic therapy and/or suction evacuation of the uterus should be considered. Suction is successful in most cases, whether or not there is retained placental tissue, as is found in one-third of cases.

Analgesia

Postpartum analgesia is primarily indicated for perineal discomfort resulting from lacerations, episiotomy, and hemorrhoids, or for postoperative pain from cesarean delivery or postpartum tubal ligation. Patients may also require pain medication for "afterbirth pains," the painful uterine contractions after delivery. This degree of discomfort from postpartum uterine contractions is seen more prominently in breast-feeding women because of the increased release of oxytocin during suckling. Common medications for this include acetaminophen (in cases of severe pain, combined with codeine), aspirin, and nonsteroidal anti-inflammatory drugs. Because hemorrhoids are varicosities of the hemorrhoidal veins, surgical treatment should not be considered for at least 6 months postpartum to allow for natural involution. Sitz baths, stool softeners, and local preparations are useful, combined with reassurance that resolution is the most common outcome.

Ambulation

Postpartum patients should be encouraged to begin ambulation as soon as possible after delivery. They should be offered assistance initially especially for patients who have delivered by cesarean section. Early ambulation helps avoid urinary retention and prevents puerperal venous thromboses and pulmonary emboli.

Breast Care

Breast engorgement in women who are not breast feeding typically occurs 3 days postpartum and may be treated with techniques such as breast binders, ice packs, and avoidance of nipple stimulation. *Bromocriptine* (Parlodel), a dopamine receptor agonist that acts to suppress prolactin release by the anterior pituitary, was previously used for lactation suppression, but is no longer recommended. Oral analgesics, such as codeine, are also useful adjuncts.

Occasionally, the breast-feeding mother may contract a *postpartum mastitis* manifest by high fever and usually chills, pain, and localized erythema and firmness of the breast. This is usually caused by infection with *Staphylococcus aureus* arising from the nursing infant's throat and nose and transmitted during nursing. Treatment includes penicillin G or a penicillinase-resistant drug such as dicloxacillin for penicillinase-producing strains. For patients who are allergic to penicillin, erythromycin would be an appropriate alternative. Nursing from the affected side may be continued without danger to the infant. If an abscess develops, surgical drainage of the abscess in addition to antibiotic therapy is necessary.

Immunizations

Women who do not have antirubella antibody should be immunized for *rubella* during the immediate postpartum period. Breast feeding is not a contraindication to this immunization. In some locations, a *tetanus toxoid booster* injection is also given at this time, if needed. If the woman is D−, is not isoimmunized, and has given birth to a D+ infant, 300 mg of anti-D immune globulin (RhoGAM) should be administered before discharge. If the mother is positive for the *hepatitis B* surface antigen

(HbSAg+), the newborn must be immunized before discharge.

Bowel Movement and Urination

It is common for a patient not to have a *bowel movement* for the first 1 to 2 days after delivery because patients have often not eaten for a long period of time. Stool softener (e.g., Colace, 100 mg orally twice daily, or Peri-Colace, 100 mg orally twice daily) is routinely prescribed in many institutions, especially if the patient has had a fourth-degree episiotomy repair or a laceration involving the rectal mucosa. Periurethral edema after vaginal delivery may cause *transitory urinary retention*. Patients should be monitored for urination after delivery, and if catheterization is required more than twice in the first 24 hours, placement of an indwelling catheter for 1 to 2 days is advisable, as is prophylactic administration of an antibiotic such as ampicillin.

Care of the Perineum

Perineal pain is minimized using oral analgesics, the application of an ice bag to minimize swelling, and/or a local anesthetic spray. Severe perineal pain unresponsive to the usual analgesics may signify the development of a hematoma, which requires evacuation if it continues to grow in size or becomes infected. *Infection of the episiotomy* is rare (<0.1%) and usually is limited to the skin and responsive to broad-spectrum antibiotics. *Necrotizing fasciitis* is a rare but extremely serious infection requiring extensive resection and debridement of the perineum, cardiovascular support, and broad-spectrum antibiotic therapy. *Dehiscence*, like infection, is uncommon, with repair individualized on the basis of the nature and extent of the wound.

Contraception

Postpartum care in the hospital should always include discussion of *contraception*. Approximately 15% of nonnursing women are fertile at 6 weeks postpartum. All forms of contraception should be considered, although natural family planning methods (basal body temperature and cervical mucus evaluation) are not reliable until regular menses have been reestablished. Combined estrogen–progestin oral contraceptive preparations are not contraindicated by breast feeding, although they may inhibit lactation slightly. Progestin preparations (oral northindrone or depo medroxyprogesterone acetate) have no effect or may slightly facilitate lactation. Once lactation is established, neither the volume nor the composition of breast milk is adversely affected by the administration of hormonal contraceptives, and there is no effect on the growth of breast-fed infants. Intrauterine device insertion in the immediate postpartum interval is acceptable in the appropriately selected patient, but it must be remembered that the expulsion rate rises in this group to 10% to 20% compared with an expulsion rate of 1% to 2% in the first year in the gynecologic patient (see Chapter 25). If a patient desires an intrauterine device for contraception, it is best to insert it at her initial postpartum visit.

Postpartum sterilization by tubal ligation is a popular method of permanent contraception, but usually the decision for this procedure should be made during the antepartum period and well documented in the chart. Then, if after delivery the patient still wishes sterilization, it may be performed without concern about the decision process (see Chapter 26). Because postpartum sterilization is associated with an increased incidence of guilt and regret when compared with "interval sterilization," consideration may be given to the advantages of laparoscopic sterilization 6 to 12 weeks postpartum, allowing time for further consideration of the permanence of the procedure in a time removed from childbirth, and allowing time to ensure that the newborn is healthy. Finally, vasectomy should be considered as an alternative method of family planning for the couple.

Sexual Activity

Coitus may be resumed when the patient is comfortable. She should be counseled, especially if breast feeding, that coitus may initially be uncomfortable because of a lack of lubrication because of low estrogen levels, and that the use of exogenous, water-soluble lubrication is helpful. The female superior position may be recommended, as the woman is thereby able to control the depth of penile penetration. The lactating patient may also be counseled to apply topical estrogen or a lubricant to the vaginal mucosa to minimize the dyspareunia caused by coital trauma to the hypoestrogenic tissue.

Patient Education

Patient education at the time of discharge should not be solely focused on postpartum and contraceptive issues. This is a good opportunity to reinforce the value and need for preventive health care and health care maintenance for both mother and infant. This should include a review of follow-up that has been arranged for the newborn and frequency and scope of health care for the new mother. Previously identified high-risk behaviors such as alcohol, tobacco, and drug abuse should once again be addressed. Infant safety concerns (e.g., automobile child restraints) are also appropriate topics of discussion. Postpartum follow-up of any preexisting medical conditions should also be reviewed.

Weight Loss

Postpartum patients typically experience about 5 to 6 kg weight loss immediately after delivery, then about 2 to 3 kg per week. Most patients should return to their nonpregnancy weight by 6 months postpartum.

Lactation and Breast Feeding

An increasing belief in the advantages of breast feeding has led many physicians to recommend this form of infant nutrition. As a result, more patients breast feed and do so for a longer period of time. Benefits of breast feeding include increased convenience for some mothers, decreased cost, improved infant nutrition for a variable period of time, and some protection against infection and allergic reaction. Successful breast feeding depends on several factors, particularly the motivation of the mother and her ability to include breast feeding in her daily activities. For some women, breast feeding may be impossible, even if desired, because of restrictions on time caused by work. *Support by family and health care providers for the decision that best fits the total needs of the mother and baby is very important.* If breast feed-

ing is chosen, rooming-in during the hospital stay allows the mother to begin the process in a less pressured setting while allowing the hospital staff to provide helpful recommendations and support. *The decision to breast feed or bottle feed is best made before delivery, and is facilitated by balanced discussion during the antepartum visits.*

At the time of delivery, the drop of estrogen and other placental hormones is a major factor in removing the inhibition of the action of prolactin. Also, suckling by the infant stimulates release of oxytocin from the neurohypophysis. The increased levels of oxytocin in the blood result in contraction of the myoepithelial cells and emptying of the alveolar lumen of the breast. The oxytocin also increases uterine contractions, thereby accelerating involution of the postpartum uterus. Prolactin release is also stimulated by suckling, with resultant secretion of fatty acids, lactose, and casein. *Colostrum* is produced in the first 5 days postpartum and is slowly replaced by maternal milk. Colostrum contains more minerals and protein but less fat and sugar than maternal milk, although it does contain large fat globules, the so-called colostrum corpuscles, which are probably epithelial cells that have undergone fatty degeneration. Colostrum also contains immunoglobulin A, which may offer the newborn some protection from enteric pathogens. Subsequently, on approximately the third to sixth day postpartum, milk is produced.

For milk to be produced on an ongoing basis, there must be adequate insulin, cortisol, and thyroid hormone, and adequate nutrients and fluids in the diet. Nutrients and fluids are especially important because maternal fat stores deposited during pregnancy provide only one-third of the fat and calories needed to produce 850 mL of milk each day. The remainder must be supplied by an appropriate diet and fluid intake. All vitamins except K are found in human milk, but because they are present in varying amounts, maternal vitamin supplementation is recommended. Vitamin K may be administered to the infant to prevent hemorrhagic disease of the newborn. To maintain breast feeding, the alveolar lumen must be emptied on a regular basis.

Nipple care is also important during breast feeding. The nipples should be washed with water and exposed to the air for 15 to 20 minutes after each feeding. A water-based cream such as lanolin or A and D ointment may be applied if the nipples are tender. Fissuring of the nipple may make breast feeding extremely difficult. Temporary cessation of breast feeding, manual expression of milk, and use of a nipple shield will aid in recovery.

Engorgement, mastitis, and plugged duct (galactocele) are the three causes of an enlarged, tender breast postpartum. They may be differentiated according to their signs and symptoms, presented in Table 10.1. Engorgement is treated by continued nursing or expression of milk by breast pump as well as application of heat and oral analgesics. It usually resolves spontaneously in 72 hours if the patient is not breast feeding. Mastitis is associated with infection by *S. aureus*, β-*hemolytic streptococci*, and *Haemophilus influenzae* and is treated with antibiotics (dicloxacillin, 500 mg orally four times a day) for at least 1 week. Nursing may be continued during treatment. A plugged duct is treated with warm packs and a breast pump. Rarely, incision and drainage may be required.

Drugs in the breast milk are a common concern for the breast-feeding mother. Less than 1% of the total dosage of any medication is seen in breast milk. This should be considered when any medication is prescribed by a physician or when any over-the-counter medications are contemplated by the patient (Table 10.2). Specific medications that would contraindicate breast feeding include lithium carbonate, tetracycline, bromocriptine, methotrexate, and any radioactive substance, as well as all substances of abuse such as amphetamine, cocaine, heroin, marijuana, nicotine, and phencyclidine (PCP).

Anxiety, Depression, and the Postpartum Period

Although pregnancy and childbirth are usually joyous times, for some patients the experience is followed by significant emotional distress. Identification of specific risk factors for postpartum and antepartum anxiety and depression is an important first step in identifying and dealing with these problems. Approximately 25% of patients with previous postpartum mental disease have a recurrence after their next pregnancy. One-third of patients with psychiatric illness during the postpartum period have a history of psychiatric disease. The exact cause of most of the postpartum emotional changes is unknown, although suggested causes include changing hormone levels (as is seen with premenstrual changes), difficulty adjusting to a new lifestyle, and the stresses of parenthood.

There is a wide spectrum of response to pregnancy and delivery, ranging from mild depression ("maternity blues") to postpartum depression to the extreme response of postpartum psychosis (Table 10.3). The overall incidence of depression during the postpartum period does not appear to be significantly greater than at other times of a woman's life. Early symptoms of depression include sleeplessness, loss of self esteem, irritability, and mood swings. More serious symptoms include

Table 10.1. Differential Diagnosis of an Enlarged, Tender Breast Postpartum

Finding	Engorgement	Mastitis	Plugged Duct
Onset	Gradual	Sudden	Gradual
Location	Bilateral	Unilateral	Unilateral
Swelling	Generalized	Localized	Localized
Pain	Generalized	Intense, localized	Localized
Systemic symptoms	Feels well	Feels ill	Feels well
Fever	No	Yes	No

Table 10.2. Medications and Breast Feeding

Medication or Substance	Reason for Concern/Effect on Lactation
Contraindicated During Breast Feeding	
Bromocriptine (Parlodel)	Suppresses lactation
Cyclophosphamide (Cytoxan)	Possible immune suppression; neutropenia; unknown effect on growth
Cyclosporine	Possible immune suppression; unknown effect on growth
Doxorubicin (Adriamycin)	Concentrated in milk; possible immune suppression; unknown effect on growth
Ergotamine (Ergotrate)	In dosages for migraine, emesis, diarrhea, convulsions
Lithium	50% therapeutic level in infant
Methotrexate	Possible immune suppression; unknown effect on growth
Substances of abuse	Growth restriction; neurologic damage; obstetric accidents (amphetamines, cocaine, heroin, marijuana, nicotine, and phencyclidine)
Uncertain Effects but of Concern when Breast Feeding	
Antianxiety medications	No reported effects, but may be of special concern to nursing mothers taking antidepressants, and because of primary drug effect when given to nursing mothers taking antipsychotics for long periods of time
Chloramphenicol	Idiosyncratic bone marrow suppressions
Metoclopramide (Reglan)	Concentrated in milk; dopaminergic blockade
Metronidazole (Flagyl)	In vitro mutagen; consider discontinuing breast feeding for 12–14 hr to allow secretion of single-dose regimens

anorexia, obsessive behavior, panic, and delusions. A most disturbing symptom is the patient's estrangement from the newborn.

Both internal and external forces may result in postpartum psychiatric illness. A patient who does not cope well with stress is particularly susceptible to such potentially traumatic stimuli as previous infertility, complications of the antepartum, intrapartum, or postpartum course, or conflicts in the roles of

Table 10.3. Three Categories of Postpartum Mood Disorders

	Postpartum Psychosis	Postpartum Depression	Maternity Blues
Incidence (%)	0.1–0.2	≥10	50–80
Average time	2–3 days PP	2 weeks to 12 months PP	1–5 days PP
Average duration	Variable	3–14 months	2–3 days, resolution within 10 days
Symptoms	Similar to organic brain syndrome: confusion, attention deficit, distractibility, clouded sensorium	Irritability, labile mood, difficulty falling asleep, phobias, anxiety; symptoms worsen in evening	Mild insomnia, tearfulness, fatigue, irritability, poor concentration, depressed affect
Treatment	Apsychotic pharmacotherapy, antidepressant, 50% of patients also meet depression criteria	Antidepressant, pharmacotherapy, psychotherapy	Time, reassurance, watchful waiting; leads to PPD in 20% of patients

PP, postpartum; PPD, postpartum depression.

mother and wife. A supportive spouse and family can minimize the severity of any symptom complex.

Anxiety is common during the antepartum and intrapartum periods, but can be minimized by having the patient as an active participant in the planning of and carrying out of the birthing process plan. Prepared childbirth and the rational use of minimal anesthesia at the patient's discretion may help the patient feel a sense of control. Active involvement of nursing personnel in the identification of significant anxiety and depression is also critical because they observe the patient on a more ongoing basis than do physicians.

Treatment must be tailored to the patient's individual situation, with most cases of mild postpartum depression being managed by the attending physician in conjunction with the support of hospital staff such as nursing personnel and social workers. The mother who is fearful of, or is averse to, contact with the newborn should not be forced into contact. Both psychotherapy and medication such as antidepressants or lithium carbonate may be provided, usually in consultation with a clinical psychologist or psychiatrist. If conditions worsen despite outpatient efforts, inpatient therapy is warranted.

Whether during the antepartum, intra partum, or postpartum period, depression and anxiety should be viewed as significant problems. It should be noted, however, that they are not necessarily solely related to pregnancy or its complications. Specifically, women are clinically depressed twice as frequently as men. Anxiety accompanies depression in three-fourths of cases. The earliest clinical clue to the diagnosis of depression may be the inability to experience pleasure or happiness (anhedonia). Women particularly susceptible to depression are those with young children, those who are living in poverty, those who are abused, and those who have professional careers.

There appears to be some evidence for a hereditary factor that predisposes some patients to the development of anxiety disorders. This may occur in as many as 10% to 15% of the population. Because every patient is subjected to some degree of stress, anxiety is usually seen in all patients, resulting in some shifts

in mood as part of the normal life experience. As with depression, however, anxiety can become dysfunctional, with the patient seeing the world as a hostile or unsafe environment. Nonspecific nervousness, panic, irritability, and fear of losing control suggest significant anxiety disorder and require treatment.

Perinatal Grief

The loss of a child results in grief in the patient and the family. Grief occurs as the result of any significant loss, whether it is the death of an infant, the loss of the fetus before birth, or the loss of the "ideal child," as in the case of the birth of a disabled infant. Perinatal grief is typically more severe the closer the loss is to term (i.e., third-trimester loss brings about a more extensive grief reaction than a first-trimester pregnancy loss). Health care providers should be sensitive to the patient's sense of guilt and failure in these circumstances. Postpartum depression is both more common and more severe in cases of perinatal loss.

Management of grief must occur not only in the postpartum period, but also during the prenatal period in the case of fetal death or diagnosis of abnormality before birth. Management of perinatal grief includes:

1. Anticipate the grief response.
2. Provide accurate information.
3. Encourage open expression of feelings.
4. Encourage photographing of the newborn and/or seeing and touching the infant.
5. Encourage active participation of the support person.
6. Assist the patient in disseminating information to family and friends.
7. Provide information regarding future pregnancies.
8. Arrange for appropriate consultations.

The Postpartum Visit

At the time of the first postpartum visit, inquiries should be made into the following: status of breast feeding, return of menstruation, resumption of coital activity, use of contraception, interaction of the newborn with the family, and resumption of other physical activities such as return to work. Involutional changes will have occurred in most instances. Inflammatory changes because of the healing of the cervix may result in minor atypia on a Pap smear performed at this time. Unless there is a past history of significant cervical dysplasia, repeating the Pap smear in 3 months is appropriate.

CHAPTER 11

ISOIMMUNIZATION

This chapter deals primarily with APGO Educational Topic:

Topic 19: Isoimmunization

Problems involving the red cell antigen–antibody system may result in
hemolysis and severe newborn illness. Students should be able to describe the
circumstances leading to isoimmunization (including specifically D isoimmunization), its pathophysiology, and the techniques used to determine its presence and severity in mother and newborn, as well as the appropriate use of
immunoglobulin prophylaxis.

Isoimmunization refers to the development of antibodies to red blood cell antigens following exposure to such antigens from another individual. Transfusion is a source of such antigens, and in pregnancy, the "other individual" may be the fetus, 50% of whose genetic makeup is derived from the father. If the mother is exposed to fetal red cells during pregnancy or at delivery, she may develop antibodies to fetal cell antigens. Later in that pregnancy, or more commonly with a subsequent pregnancy, the antibodies can cross the placenta and hemolyze fetal red cells, leading to fetal anemia. In a pregnancy complicated by isoimmunization, the manufacture of maternal antibody that destroys fetal red cells is countered by the ability of the fetus to manufacture sufficient red cells to permit survival and growth.

Natural History

Isoimmunization can involve many of the *several hundred blood group systems.* This disorder is frequently referred to as Rh isoimmunization, because the Rhesus (Rh) system that comprises the CcD–Ee antigens is most frequently involved, although it should be remembered that isoimmunization can and does develop with many other blood systems such as Kell, Duffy, Kidd, and others.

Within the Rh system, there are several specific antigens, the one most commonly associated with hemolytic disease being the D antigen. If a fetus is Rh+, having received the genes for the Rh D antigen from its father, and the mother lacks the Rh antigen (i.e., she is Rh−, there is no "small d" antigen), the conditions exist for the development of isoimmunization. In the woman's first such pregnancy, the infant typically has no complications. If, however, the mother's blood is exposed to fetal red cells, even minuscule amounts, the woman can develop antibodies to the Rh D antigen. This can occur at the time of childbirth or in other situations where fetomaternal hemorrhage may occur. These situations include amniocentesis; threatened, spontaneous, or elective/therapeutic abortion; ectopic pregnancy; bleeding associated with placenta previa and placental abruption; abdominal trauma; and external version. Antibody development occurs in approximately 15% of index pregnancies involving an Rh− mother and Rh+ fetus. In a subsequent pregnancy, passage of minute amounts of fetal blood across the placenta, which occurs quite frequently, can lead to an *anamnestic response* of maternal antibody production. If the mother produces immunoglobulin M (IgM)-type antibodies, the molecules do not cross the placenta because they are too large. In the case of Rh factor, however, the maternal antibody is predominantly the smaller IgG-type, which can freely cross the placenta and enter the fetal circulation. Once in the fetal vascular system, the antibody attaches to the Rh+ red blood cells and hemolyzes them. The bilirubin produced in this hemolytic process is transferred back across the placenta to the mother and metabolized. *The condition of the fetus is determined by the amount of maternal antibody transferred across the placenta and the ability of the fetus to replace the red blood cells that have been destroyed.*

In the first affected pregnancy, the infant may be anemic at delivery and may soon develop elevated levels of bilirubin because hemolysis continues after birth and the newborn must now rely on its own, somewhat immature, liver to metabolize the bilirubin. *In subsequent pregnancies,* with an Rh+ fetus, the process of antibody production and transfer may be accelerated, leading to the development of more significant anemia. In such cases, the fetal liver can manufacture additional red cells. However, this activity reduces the amount of proteins manufactured by the fetal liver. In turn, the reduced protein production can lead to a decreased oncotic pressure within the fetal vascular system, resulting in fetal ascites and subcutaneous edema. At the same time, the severe fetal anemia can lead to high-output cardiac failure. This combination of findings is referred to as *hydrops fetalis.*

The tendency is for each subsequent baby to be more severely affected, but this is not always the case. The level of fetal disturbance may remain the same or, occasionally, may even be less than in the previous pregnancy. If subsequent fetuses are Rh−, which is commonly the case if the father is a heterozygote for the D antigen, the fetus is not affected at all (Table 11.1).

Table 11.1. Risk of Rh Sensitization

Obstetric/Medical Event	Chance of Sensitization (%)
Ectopic pregnancy	<1
Full-term pregnancy	1–2
Amniocentesis	1–3
Spontaneous abortion	3–4
Induced abortion	5–6
Full-term delivery, ABO compatible or incompatible	14–17
Mismatched blood transfusion	90–95

Diagnosis

Although previous pregnancy history can increase the suspicion for the diagnosis of isoimmunization, the gold standard for diagnosis is the indirect antibody screen. As part of routine antenatal *laboratory evaluation,* maternal blood is tested for the presence of a variety of antibodies that may cause significant disturbances in the fetus. Any significant antibodies are further evaluated for the strength of antibody response, which is reported in a titer format (1:4, 1:16, and so on). During this testing process, other antibodies may be discovered that do not cause significant fetal/neonatal problems. The two most common of these are the anti-Lewis and anti-I. When these antibodies are found, titers are not reported because of their lack of clinical importance.

Determination of the genetic father's Rh status is helpful. If he is Rh−, the fetus is not affected. If he is Rh+, genotype testing can determine whether he is homozygous or heterozygous. Recently, direct Rh testing of the fetus has become possible using cultured fetal cells obtained by amniocentesis. In limited clinical settings, fetal DNA extracted from the maternal circulation can be used to determine the fetal blood type.

Management

Antibody titers would seem to be good markers of maternal antibody production, but in fact,

such titers are of limited usefulness. In the first sensitized pregnancy, titers do seem to be helpful, but thereafter they are of virtually no value because they do not reflect the current fetal condition. Even in the initial sensitized pregnancy, the greatest value is in distinguishing those pregnancies for which antibody production is so low that it is nonthreatening to the fetus from those for which there are likely to be significant consequence. *A titer of 1:16 or greater is generally considered the critical point* at which there is sufficient risk of fetal jeopardy to warrant additional evaluation.

Amniotic fluid assessment is of value as the *level of bilirubin in the amniotic fluid accurately reflects the condition of the fetus.* In the second half of normal pregnancy, the level of bilirubin normally decreases progressively, whereas the level of bilirubin in an affected, isoimmunized patient can be evaluated in relation to natural decline. The level of bilirubin in the amniotic fluid is determined using a spectrophotometer. Normal amniotic fluid subjected to spectrophotometric analysis has a characteristic optical density curve that may be compared with that found in an affected pregnancy. The relative degree of elevation of bilirubin optical density at the 450-nm wavelength correlates with the severity of fetal disease and may be used to determine the timing of intrauterine transfusion or of delivery.

The peak velocity of middle cerebral artery blood flow as determined by ultrasonography provides a noninvasive way to follow fetuses at risk for developing severe anemia. Gestational age-specific peak velocity norms have been determined and correlated with fetal hematocrit at the time of periumbilical blood sampling (PUBS). The degree of peak velocity elevation beyond the mean has correlates with fetal hematocrit, and therefore the degree of anemia. The sensitivity of an increased peak systolic velocity in the middle cerebral artery (MCA) for prediction of moderate-to-severe anemia is 100% with a false–positive rate of 12%.

Periodic anatomic assessment by ultrasonography can also be very helpful in detecting severe signs of the hemolytic process, namely subcutaneous edema, pericardial and pleural effusions, and ascites. These findings are referred to as fetal hydrops (hydrops fetalis) and are indicative of a fetal hematocrit of <12% to 15%. Under ultrasound guidance, the umbilical cord can be sampled directly (by PUBS) and fetal blood can be taken for hematocrit determination to assess the severity of anemia. Later in pregnancy, general tests of fetal well-being are used in the isoimmunized patient because the ability of an affected fetus to withstand the stresses of pregnancy and labor may be compromised.

Transfusions

Transfusion of Rh− red blood cells to the fetus is indicated when, on the basis of the previous assessment, it is determined that the fetus is at risk for developing clinically significant anemia, defined as a hematocrit of <30%. Traditionally, blood was transfused into the fetal abdominal cavity where absorption of the transfused cells takes place over subsequent days. Recently, direct fetal transfusions into the umbilical cord (PUBS) under ultrasonography guidance are being used more frequently, with positive results. Specialized physicians trained specifically in the assessment of fetal anemia and the procedure of PUBS are critical to its success. The procedure carries with it a risk of fetal death of 1% to 3%, a risk that must be weighed against the predicted future course for the fetus in utero and the potential adverse consequences of preterm delivery. The quantity of red blood cells to be transferred can be calculated using the gestational age and size of the fetus and the current and desired fetal hematocrit. Because the transferred cells are Rh−, they are not affected by the transplacental maternal antibody. Timing of subsequent transfusions can be determined based on the severity of disease and the predicted life span of the transfused cells.

Prevention

Maternal exposure and subsequent sensitization to fetal blood usually occur at delivery and much less commonly during pregnancy. In the late 1960s, it was determined that the antibody to the D antigen of the Rh system could be prepared from donors previously sensitized to the antigen. Subsequently, it was found that *administration of this antibody (Rh immune globulin) soon after delivery could, by passive immunization, prevent an active antibody response by the mother in most cases.* Rh immune globulin is effective only for the D antigen of the Rh system. No similar preparations are available for patients sensitized with the many other possible antigens. It is now standard practice for Rh− patients who deliver Rh+ infants to receive an intramuscular dose of 300 mg of Rh immune globulin (i.e., RhoGAM) within 72 hours of delivery. With this practice, the risk of subsequent sensitization decreases from approximately 15% to approximately 2%. This residual 2% was determined to be the result of sensitization occurring *during the course of pregnancy* (as opposed to occurring at delivery), usually in the third trimester. Administration of a 300-mg dose of Rh immune globulin to Rh− patients at 28 weeks was found to reduce the risk of sensitization to approximately 0.2%.

Prophylaxis with Rh immune globulin in Rh− women is not necessary if the father of the pregnancy is *known with certainty* to be Rh−. Although testing of the father can be done, *if there is any question as to the paternity, prophylactic administration of Rh immune globulin should be given as described* because the risk is negligible and the potential benefits are considerable.

In summary, Rh− pregnant patients who have no antibody on initial screening are retested at 28 weeks to detect the rare patient who was sensitized earlier in pregnancy. If no sensitization has occurred, the patients are given Rh immune globulin to protect them from antibody formation for the remainder of the pregnancy. If the father is known to be Rh−, this practice is not necessary. After delivery, the child's blood type and Rh status are determined, and if the child is Rh+, a second dose of Rh immune globulin is given to the new mother.

There are other situations when Rh immune globulin should be administered (Table 11.2). Because the amount of fetal red cells required to elicit an antibody response is minute, approximately 0.01 mL, *any circumstance in pregnancy in which fetomaternal hemorrhage can occur warrants Rh immune globulin administration.* Furthermore, because fetal red cell production begins within 6 weeks of conception, sensitization can occur in patients who have a spontaneous

Table 11.2. Indications for Rh Immune Globulin Administration in an Unsensitized Rh-negative Patient[a]

At approximately 28 weeks' pregnancy

Within 3 days of delivery of an Rh-positive infant

At the time of amniocentesis

After positive Kleihauer-Betke test

After an ectopic pregnancy

After a spontaneous or induced abortion

[a]Unless the father of the infant is known to be Rh negative.

or scheduled pregnancy termination. Because the dose of antigen in such situations is low, a reduced dose of 50 mg of Rh immune globulin can be used to prevent sensitization. Amniocentesis and other trauma (e.g., from an auto accident) during pregnancy are also indications for the standard 300-mg dose of Rh immune globulin. In cases of trauma or bleeding during pregnancy, the extent to which fetomaternal hemorrhage has occurred, if any, can be evaluated using the Kleihauer–Betke test or a similar test that allows for the identification of fetal cells in maternal circulation. In the test, a sample of maternal blood is subjected to a strong base such as potassium hydroxide (KOH). Maternal cells are sensitive to changes in pH and, therefore, promptly lyse and become "ghost" cells. Fetal cells are much more resistant to such agents and remain intact. The ratio of fetal to maternal cells can be assessed by counting 1,000 or more total cells under the microscope and determining how many cells retain the dark appearance (representing fetal cells). Then the maternal blood volume is calculated and, using the ratio just described, the total amount of fetomaternal hemorrhage is derived. Because a standard 300-mg dose of Rh immune globulin effectively neutralizes 15 mL of fetal red blood cells, the appropriate dose can then be administered.

Management of Other Irregular Antibodies

As the scheduled use of Rh immune globulin has become routine, an increasing number of isoimmunization cases are associated with other irregular antibodies. Differences in the frequencies of these antibodies and the likelihood that their presence will cause hemolytic disease of the newborn depends on several factors, including the size and frequency of the antigenic stimulus, the relative potency of the antigen, and the type of antibody response (IgG or IgM).

Both Rh+ and Rh− mothers can produce these antibodies. When at risk for fetomaternal or exogenous antibody exposure, a positive antibody screen should be managed (Figure 11.1). Anti-Kell is the most important non-Rh cause of hemolytic diseases of the newborn and is usually associated with previous blood transfusion. When the mother is anti-Kell antibody positive, paternal Kell genotyping should be carried out. Ninety percent of fathers and their fetuses are Kell negative, and no further workup is required as long as paternity is certain.

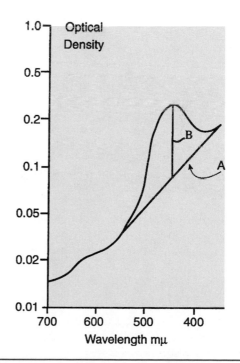

Figure 11.1. Management of other irregular antibodies. The more common irregular antibodies may be managed according to this flow sheet. It is important to determine paternity and paternal genotype before deciding against amniocentesis.

Anemia resulting from Kell isoimmunization, unlike that from the other red cell antigens, is not the result of a hemolytic process, but rather fetal bone marrow suppression. Therefore, infants experiencing Kell isoimmunization require longer follow-up and often require serial transfusions until their hematopoietic system functions normally.

ABO hemolytic disease is associated with milder fetal kernicterus and, rarely, hydrops, probably because of the relatively smaller number of A and B antigenic sites on fetal red blood cells and because anti-A and anti-B are IgM and thus do not traverse the placenta well; those that do cross have a high propensity for other binding sites besides fetal red blood cells. This disease usually occurs in the first pregnancy, and amniocentesis and early delivery are rarely indicated. Non-Rh D/non-ABO hemolytic disease is frequently associated with blood transfusion because "compatible blood" is matched only to the ABO and DD antigens.

CHAPTER 12

POSTPARTUM HEMORRHAGE

This chapter deals primarily with Educational Topic:

Topic 27: Postpartum Hemorrhage

The prevention or management of postpartum hemorrhage is important, as it remains a major cause of maternal morbidity and mortality. Students should be able to explain the risk factors, differential diagnosis, and management of postpartum hemorrhage.

Excessive bleeding after delivery is a serious and potentially fatal complication. Hemorrhage can be sudden and profuse, or blood loss can occur more slowly but be prolonged and persistent. Postpartum hemorrhage is usually defined as a delivery-associated blood loss in excess of 500 mL. Many patients lose considerably more blood than this; the figure of 500 mL may actually represent the average amount of blood loss after vaginal delivery, with twice this amount lost at cesarean delivery

General Management of Patients With Postpartum Hemorrhage

Once excessive blood loss is identified, prompt assessment is mandatory. A general approach to management is outlined in Table 12.1. Because most cases of postpartum hemorrhage are caused by uterine atony, the uterus should be palpated abdominally, seeking the soft, boggy consistency of the relaxed uterus. If this is found, oxytocin infusion should be increased and either Methergine or prostaglandins administered if the excessive bleeding continues.

There are other questions that may help direct assessment:

- Was expulsion of the placenta spontaneous and apparently complete?
- Were forceps or other instrumentation used in delivery?
- Was the baby large or the delivery difficult or precipitous?
- Were the cervix and vagina inspected for lacerations?
- Is the blood clotting?

As the cause of the hemorrhage is being identified, general supportive measures for patients with hemorrhage of any cause are initiated. Such measures as large-bore intravenous access; crystalloid infusions; type, cross match, and administration of blood or blood components as needed; periodic assessment of hematocrit and coagulation profile; and monitoring of urinary output are all important.

The management of postpartum hemorrhage is greatly facilitated if patients at high risk are identified and preliminary preparations are made before the bleeding episode. Table 12.2 reviews such precautionary measures.

Major Causes of Postpartum Hemorrhage

Uterine Atony

Uterine atony is by far the most common cause of postpartum hemorrhage. Ordinarily, the uterine corpus contracts promptly after delivery of the placenta, constricting the spiral arteries in the newly created placental bed, and preventing excessive bleeding from them. This muscular contraction, rather than coagulation, prevents excessive bleeding from the placental implantation site. When contraction does not occur as expected, the resulting uterine atony gives rise to postpartum hemorrhage.

A number of *factors predispose to uterine atony* (Table 12.3). These include conditions in which there is extraordinary enlargement of the uterus, such as hydramnios or twins, abnormal labor (both precipitous, prolonged, or augmented by oxytocin), and conditions that interfere with contraction of the uterus, such as uterine leiomyomas or use of magnesium sulfate. The clinical diagnosis of atony is based largely on the tone of the uterine muscle on palpation. Instead of the normally firm, contracted uterine corpus, a softer, more pliable–often called "boggy"–uterus is found. The cervix is usually open. Frequently, the uterus contracts briefly when massaged, only to become relaxed again when the manipulation ceases.

Management of uterine atony is both preventive and therapeutic. In the management of a normal delivery, it is customary to infuse oxytocin diluted in intravenous fluids (usually 20 units in 1 liter of fluid infused at 200 to 500 mL/hr) starting soon after the placenta has been delivered. Oxytocin promotes contraction of the uterine corpus and decreases the likelihood of uterine atony. Gentle bimanual massage of the uterus is also commonly performed in the belief that this will hasten uterine contraction. Immediate breast feeding also causes uterine contractions.

Once uterine atony occurs and is diagnosed, management can be categorized as manipulative, medical, and surgical. Management must be individualized in cases of severe uterine atony, taking into account the degree of hemorrhage, the overall status of the patient, and her future childbearing desires (Table 12.1). When hem-

Table 12.1. Management of the Patient With Postpartum Hemorrhage

Evaluate promptly once excessive bleeding is detected.

Notify other members of obstetrics team (i.e., obtain help!)

Review clinical course for probable cause.

    Any difficulty removing placenta?

    Were forceps used?

    Other predisposing factors?

Perform bimanual examination in recovery area/delivery room.

Uterus boggy? Massage. Initiate or increase oxytocin; give Methergine, 0.2 mg IM if not hypertension (HTN). Other uterotonics (prostaglandins) if no response.

Placental fragments within uterus on exploration or on ultrasound examination? If so, return to delivery room for curettage.

Laceration or hematoma? Repair in delivery room.

Monitor and maintain circulation. This should be done while performing above.

    Large-bore intravenous catheters: one or two well-functioning lines.

    Type and cross match blood.

    Check hematocrit and coagulation profile with platelet count for baseline.

Notify obstetric physicians, nurses, and anesthesia and operating room personnel of potential need for surgical intervention.

Visualize cervix and vagina in search of lacerations.

    Repair if present.

    Remember that postpartum hemorrhage may be from multiple causes (e.g., atony plus lacerations).

Observe patient constantly. Repeat bimanual examination. If bleeding persists, is the blood clotting? If not, consider disseminated intravascular coagulopathy.

Inform patient of the problem and what measures are being taken to correct it.

    Get an appreciation of her desires regarding further childbearing and hysterectomy.

Operative measures

    Ligation of vessels:

        Uterine artery ligation—bilateral (O'Leary stitch).

        B-Lynch suture.

        Hypogastric artery ligation.

    Selective arterial embolization. Move to preoperative management options above.

    Hysterectomy is treatment of last resort in patient who wants to retain her uterus.

Intensive care measures.

    Hemodynamic, renal, and coagulation surveillance measures.

orrhage does occur, multiple large-bore intravenous access sites should be obtained, and blood should be typed and cross matched for possible transfusion.

Uterine massage alone is often successful in causing uterine contraction, and this should be done while preparations for other treatments are underway (Figure 12.1). Medical treatments include oxytocin, *Methergine* (methylergonovine maleate), and several prostaglandin preparations, administered separately or in combination. Methergine is a potent constrictor that can cause uterine contractions within several minutes. It is always given intramuscularly because rapid intravenous administration can lead to dangerous hypertension. Prostaglandin

Table 12.2. Precautionary Measures to Prevent or Minimize Postpartum Hemorrhage

Before delivery	Determine baseline hematocrit
	Send blood specimen to blood bank for group and screen
	Establish well-functioning intravenous line with large-bore catheter
	Obtain baseline coagulation studies and platelet count if indicated
	Identify any predisposing factors
In delivery room	Avoid excessive traction on umbilical cord
	Inspect placenta for complete removal
	Perform digital exploration of uterus (if indicated)
	Massage uterus
	Visualize cervix and vagina
	Remove all clots in uterus and vagina before transfer to recovery area
In recovery area	Closely observe patient for excessive bleeding
	Frequently palpate uterus with massage
	Determine vital signs frequently

F_{2a} may be given intramuscularly or directly into the myometrium, and prostaglandin E_2 may be given by vaginal suppository. Both of these prostoglandins result in strong uterine contractions. Prostaglandin E_1 (misoprostil), administered rectally, also causes strong uterine contractions, and has recently begun to be used for treatment of postpartum hemorrhage. Typically, oxytocin is given prophylactically, as noted previously; if uterine atony occurs, the infusion rate is increased, and Methergine or prostaglandin, or both, are given sequentially.

Occasionally, uterine massage and oxytocics are unsuccessful in bringing about appropriate uterine contraction, and surgical measures must

Table 12.3. Factors Predisposing to Uterine Atony

Precipitous labor
General anesthesia
Prolonged labor
Uterine leiomyomas
Macrosomia
Chorioamnionitis
Multiparity
Oxytocin use in labor
History of postpartum hemorrhage
Amniotic fluid embolus
Polyhydramnios
Magnesium sulfate in laboring patient
Multiple gestation
Hypotension

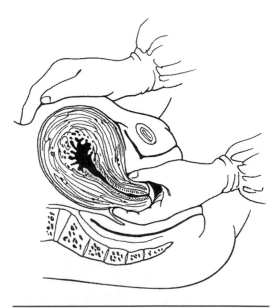

Figure 12.1. Management of uterine atony with manual massage. One hand gently massages the uterus from the abdomen while the other is inserted so that the cervix is cradled in the fingers and thumb to allow for maximal compression and massage.

be used. Surgical management of uterine atony may include ligation of the uterine arteries or hypogastric arteries, selective arterial embolization, and hysterectomy (Figure 12.2). At times, these procedures may be lifesaving.

Lacerations of the Lower Genital Tract

Lacerations of the lower genital tract are far less common than uterine atony as a cause of postpartum hemorrhage, but they can be serious and require prompt surgical repair. *Predisposing factors* include an instrumented delivery with forceps, a manipulative delivery such as a breech extraction, a precipitous labor, presentations other than occiput anterior, and a macrosomic infant.

Although minor lacerations to the cervix in the process of cervical dilation and delivery are routinely found, lacerations >2 cm in length and those that are actively bleeding usually require repair. To minimize blood loss caused by significant cervical and vaginal lacerations, all patients with any predisposing factors, or any patient in whom blood loss soon after delivery appears to be excessive despite a firm and contracted uterus, should have a careful repeat inspection of the lower genital tract. This vaginal examination may require assistance to allow adequate visualization. As a rule, repair of these lacerations is usually not difficult if adequate exposure is provided (Figure 12.3).

Lacerations of the vagina and perineum (first- through fourth-degree vaginal and periurethral lacerations) are not commonly causes of substantial blood loss, although the steady loss of blood, which may come from deeper lacerations, may be so significant that their repair when bleeding is requisite. Periurethral lacerations may be associated with sufficient edema to occlude the urethra causing urinary retention; a Foley catheter for 12 to 24 hours usually alleviates this problem.

Retained Placenta

Separation of the placenta from the uterus occurs because of cleavage between the *zona basalis* and the *zona spongiosa*. Once separation occurs, expulsion is caused by strong uterine contractions. Retained placenta can occur when either the process of separation or the process of expulsion is incomplete. Predisposing factors to retained placenta

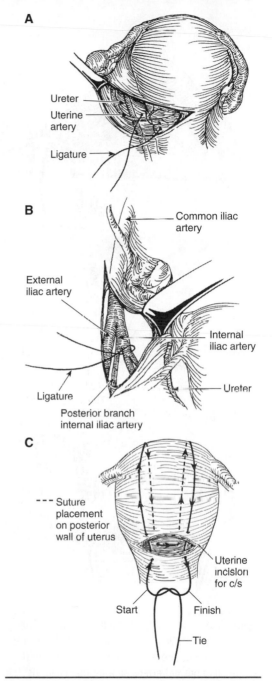

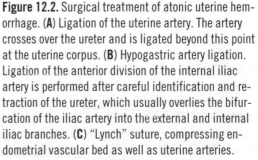

Figure 12.2. Surgical treatment of atonic uterine hemorrhage. (**A**) Ligation of the uterine artery. The artery crosses over the ureter and is ligated beyond this point at the uterine corpus. (**B**) Hypogastric artery ligation. Ligation of the anterior division of the internal iliac artery is performed after careful identification and retraction of the ureter, which usually overlies the bifurcation of the iliac artery into the external and internal iliac branches. (**C**) "Lynch" suture, compressing endometrial vascular bed as well as uterine arteries.

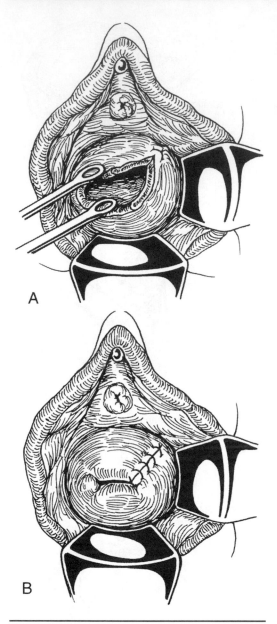

Figure 12.3. Repair of a cervical laceration. (**A**) After careful demonstration of the entire extent of the laceration, the first suture is placed above the apex of the laceration to prevent extension after the repair. (**B**) The laceration is then repaired, whether with interrupted sutures, as shown, or with figure-of-eight or running sutures.

include a previous cesarean delivery, uterine leiomyomas, prior uterine curettage, and succenturiate placental lobe.

Placental tissue remaining in the uterus can prevent adequate contractions and predispose to excessive bleeding. After expulsion, every placenta should be inspected to detect missing cotyledons, which may remain in the uterus. If retained placenta is suspected, either because of apparent absent cotyledons or because of excessive bleeding, it can often be removed by inserting two fingers through the cervix into the uterus and manipulating the retained tissue downward into the vagina. If this is unsuccessful, or if there is uncertainty regarding the cause of hemorrhage, an ultrasound examination of the uterus is helpful. Curettage with a suction apparatus and/or a large, sharp curette may be used to remove the retained tissue. Care must be exercised to avoid perforation through the uterine fundus.

Placental tissue may also remain in the uterus because separation of the placenta from the uterus may not occur normally. At times, placental villi penetrate the uterine wall to form what is generally called *placenta accreta*. More specifically, abnormal adherence of the placenta to the superficial lining of the uterus is termed "placenta accreta"; penetration into the uterine muscle itself is called *placenta increta,* and complete invasion through the thickness of the uterine muscle is termed *placenta percreta*. If this abnormal attachment involves the entire placenta, no part of the placenta separates. Much more commonly, however, attachment is not complete and a portion of the placenta separates and the remainder remains attached. Major, life-threatening hemorrhage can ensue. Hysterectomy is often required; however an attempt to separate the placenta by curettage or other means of controlling the bleeding (such as uterine artery ligation or hypogastric artery ligation) is usually appropriate in trying to avoid a hysterectomy in a woman who desires more children.

Other Causes of Postpartum Hemorrhage

Hematomas

Hematomas can occur anywhere from the vulva to the upper vagina as a result of delivery trauma. Hematomas may also develop at the site of episiotomy or perineal laceration. Hematomas may occur without disruption of the vaginal mucosa, when the fetus or forceps causes shearing of the submucosal tissues without mucosal tearing.

Vulvar or vaginal hematomas are characterized by exquisite pain with or without signs of shock. Hematomas that are <5 cm in diameter and are not enlarging can usually be managed expectantly by frequent evaluation of the size of the hematoma and close monitoring of vital signs and urinary output. Application of ice packs can also be helpful. Larger and enlarging hematomas must be managed surgically. If the hematoma is at the site of episiotomy, the sutures should be removed and a search made for the actual bleeding site, which is then ligated. If not at the episiotomy site, the hematoma should be opened at its most dependent portion and drained, the bleeding site identified, if possible, and the site closed with interlocking hemostatic sutures. Drains and vaginal packs are often used to prevent reaccumulation of blood.

Coagulation Defects

Virtually any congenital or acquired abnormality in blood clotting can lead to postpartum hemorrhage. Abruptio placentae, amniotic fluid embolism, and severe preeclampsia are obstetric conditions commonly associated with disseminated intravascular coagulopathy. The treatment of coagulation defects is aimed at correcting the coagulation defect. When assessing a patient with postpartum hemorrhage, it should always be noted whether the blood that is passing from the genital tract is clotting. It also should be recalled that profuse hemorrhage itself can lead to coagulopathy.

Amniotic Fluid Embolism

Amniotic fluid embolism is a rare, sudden, and often fatal obstetric complication presumably caused primarily by entry of amniotic fluid into the maternal circulation, although there are probably significant biochemical as well as physical mediators of the syndrome. The diagnosis is classically based on the identification of fetal squames and lanugo in the maternal pulmonary system on autopsy, although these findings are absent in perhaps one-third of cases. The clinical diagnosis is based on five findings that occur in sequence: respiratory distress, cyanosis, cardiovascular collapse, hemorrhage, and coma. The syndrome also of-

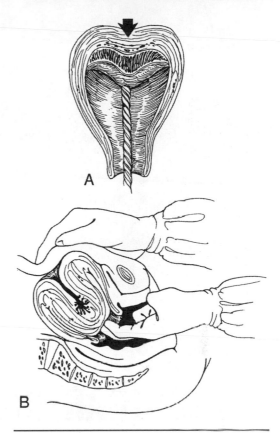

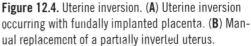

Figure 12.4. Uterine inversion. (**A**) Uterine inversion occurring with fundally implanted placenta. (**B**) Manual replacement of a partially inverted uterus.

ten results in severe coagulopathy. Treatment is directed toward total support of the cardiovascular and coagulation systems, although maternal mortality still approaches 30% to 50% in most series.

Uterine Inversion

Uterine inversion is a rare condition; the uterus literally turns inside out, with the top of the uterine fundus extending through the cervix into the vagina and sometimes even past the introitus (Figure 12.4). Hemorrhage with uterine inversion is characteristically severe and sudden. Treatment includes administration of an anesthetic that causes uterine relaxation (such as halothane) or another agent with uterus-relaxing properties (such as terbutaline or nitroglycerine), followed by replacement of the uterine corpus. If this fails, surgical treatment, possibly including hysterectomy, may be needed.

CHAPTER 13

POSTPARTUM INFECTION

This chapter pertains primarily to Educational Topic:

Topic 28: Postpartum Infection

Postpartum infection engenders substantial risk for maternal morbidity and mortality. Students should be able to identify the risk factors for postpartum infection as well as the common organisms involved, their pathophysiology, and the evaluation and management of postpartum infection.

Infections occurring during the puerperium are a relatively frequent cause of morbidity and, rarely, even mortality. Many factors predispose to postpartum infection, including general health and concurrent medical problems, immune status, and concurrent infections (Table 13.1). Even the mode of delivery is itself a determinant of infection. After vaginal delivery, infection occurs much less frequently than after cesarean birth. The incidence of infection varies from 10% to as high as 50% in some populations (see Table 13.1).

Puerperal Febrile Morbidity

The definition of puerperal febrile morbidity is a *temperature of 38.0°C (100.4°F) or higher, the temperature to occur on any 2 of the first 10 days postpartum, exclusive of the first 24 hours.* This guideline was written with the intent to help distinguish true infection from minor temperature elevations commonly seen in the early puerperium, and presumed to be the result of breast engorgement. *Practically speaking, significant elevations in maternal temperature even within the first 24 hours postpartum, especially when accompanied by other evidence of infection, are usually* thought to represent frank infection, and treatment is often instituted. However, this "official" definition of puerperal morbidity does serve as a reminder that *not every postpartum temperature elevation reflects infection, and that, in borderline cases, expectant management is warranted.*

Evaluation of the Febrile Postpartum Patient

Persistent fever greater than 38°C in the postpartum patient requires evaluation for extrapelvic as well as pelvic sources of infection. *The most common cause of persistent fever following delivery is genital tract infection.* The most common infection is endomyometritis (infection of the uterine cavity and adjacent tissue), which is usually associated with the development of fever on the first or second day postpartum. The "sequence" of other infection sites is somewhat predictable after vaginal or surgical delivery. On the first postoperative day, the lungs are the common cause of fever (atelectasis, pneumonia); on the second day, the urinary tract (cystitis, pyelonephritis); on the third day, the wound (superficial infection, necrotizing fasciitis); and on the fourth day, the extremities (thrombophlebitis). The common mnemonic phrase is *Wind, Water, Wound, and Walking.* Finally, infection of the breast (mastitis) is seen in the first few weeks postpartum, usually in patients who are breast feeding.

When evaluating a febrile patient, a *history* of the labor and delivery can be helpful. If, for example, the patient had amnionitis and was febrile through labor, one would suspect endomyometritis as the cause of fever. *In addition, the mode of delivery is the single most important risk factor for postpartum uterine infection, and women delivered by cesarean section are at greatest risk.* A careful history regarding pulmonary symptoms, urinary tract disturbance, and abdominopelvic pain and tenderness is important. Pertinent information from the prenatal course of care is also often useful, such as medical problems that predispose to infection, a history of sexually transmitted diseases, or bacterial vaginosis. *Examination* should include the lungs, the back (for costovertebral tenderness), palpation of the abdomen, careful inspection of the incision site, a check for the presence of bowel sounds,

Table 13.1. Factors That Predispose to Postpartum Infections
Maternal
Obesity
Low socioeconomic status
Anemia
Immunosuppression
Chronic disease (e.g., diabetes mellitus)
Vaginal infection, especially bacterial vaginosis
Associated with labor and delivery
Cesarean birth
Rupture of fetal membranes
Intra-amniotic infection
Prolonged labor
Multiple pelvic examinations during labor
Internal electronic fetal monitoring, fetal scalp electrode, and/or intrauterine pressure catheter

examination of the perineum (if an episiotomy was performed or if a laceration occurred), a pelvic examination, assessment for calf tenderness, and inspection of any intravenous site. Although a pelvic examination may not elicit any findings other than uterine tenderness, one can confirm that lochia drainage is, in fact, occurring, and baseline information can be obtained concerning adnexal masses that may be important if the fever persists and an abscess develops. Blood cultures are not usually obtained as they are of little value in management unless the infection appears severe, sepsis is suspected, fever is especially high, or the response to limited therapy is delayed.

Endomyometritis

The most common infection after cesarean delivery is infection of the uterus. These infections usually extend well beyond the thin endometrial lining into the adjacent myometrium, the loose fibroareolar tissues within the parametrium, and sometimes beyond, with pelvic abscess formation (Figure 13.1). Various terms have been used to describe postpartum uterine infection,

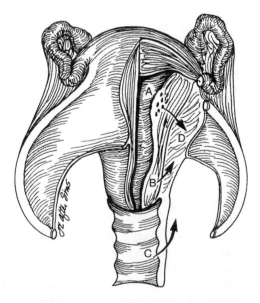

Figure 13.1. Endomyometritis may result from the spread of infection from the placental site, (**A**) cervical or vaginal lacerations or infections, (**C**) or vagina, and may spread to and through the myometrium (**B**) & (**D**), at times into the loose parametrial tissues.

including endomyometritis, endometritis, metritis, and metritis with pelvic cellulitis. Although endomyometritis is the more comprehensive term, the abbreviated term "metritis" is common and will be used for the remainder of this discussion. The route of delivery, duration of labor, duration of rupture of membranes, and the presence of amnionitis during labor are the major factors leading to the development of metritis.

Fever is the characteristic feature in the diagnosis of metritis, and it may be accompanied by cervical motion and especially *uterine tenderness.* If the infection has spread to the parametrium and adnexa, tenderness may be present there as well. Signs of peritoneal irritation and diminished or absent bowel sounds, especially associated with ileus, indicate more serious infection, including the possibility of abscess formation. A leukocytosis in the range of 15,000 to 30,000 cells/mL^3 is common but difficult to interpret in the presence of the normal, early puerperium leukocytosis.

As with virtually all pelvic infections, metritis is polymicrobial in origin. Both aerobic and anaerobic organisms are commonly isolated, with anaerobic organisms predominating. The most common of these organisms are listed in Table 13.2. Because bacteria are normally found in the vagina and endocervix, it is difficult to culture the endometrial cavity properly because sampling devices are contaminated on transcervical sampling. Furthermore, the organisms involved in metritis are those commonly found in the lower genital tract and rectum, and can usually be predicted without the need for endometrial cultures. On a practical basis, treatment using broad antibiotic coverage against a variety of common microorganisms is usually prescribed without cultures.

Various choices of *initial antibiotic therapy* are used, most of which are successful (Table 13.3). Single-agent therapy has the benefit of ease of administration and is often cost saving; cephalosporins such as cefotetan and cefoxitin are commonly used. A combination of ampicillin and an aminoglycoside is also popular, as is the combination of clindamycin with gentamicin. Adequate anaerobic coverage is especially important following cesarean delivery. Many initial therapies have "gaps" in their total

Table 13.2. Common Organisms Associated with Pelvic Infections

Aerobes		Anaerobes	
Gram-positive	**Gram-negative**	**Gram-positive**	**Gram-negative**
Staphylococcus	*Escherichia coli*	*Peptococcus*	*Bacteroides*
Streptococcus (A,B)	*Proteus*	*Peptostreptococcus*	
Enterococci (group D)	*Klebsiella*	*Clostridium Streptococcus*	

coverage, that is, one or more major pathogens are not sensitive to the antibiotic treatment. Therefore, *it is customary to provide additional antibiotic coverage if there has been no response within 48 to 72 hours.* Intravenous antibiotic administration while the patient is hospitalized is preferred for initial treatment. *Intravenous antibiotic therapy is continued until the patient is asymptomatic, has normal bowel function, and has been afebrile for at least 24 hours.* Subsequent outpatient oral antibiotic treatment is usually unnecessary.

Occasionally a *pelvic abscess* further complicates the patient's recovery. Evidence that suggests abscess formation includes persistent fever despite antibiotic therapy, protracted malaise, delayed return of gastrointestinal function, localization of pain and/or tenderness in the abdominal cavity, and detection of a mass on pelvic/abdominal examination.

Table 13.3. Antibiotic Therapy for Metritis

Drug	Dosage
Single-drug regimens	
Cefazolin (Ancef)	1 g IV q 8 hr
Cefotetan (Cefotan)	2 g IV q 12 hr
Cefoxitin (Mefoxin)	1–2 g q 8 hr
Ampicillin w/sulbactam (Unasyn)	1.5–3.0 g q 6 hr
Ticarcillin w/clavulanic acid (Timentin)	3.1 g q 6 hr
Multiple-drug regimens	
Clindamycin–gentamicin	
Clindamycin (Cleocin)	900 mg IV q 8 hr
Gentamicin (Garamycin)	70–100 mg IV q 8 hr[a]
Clindamycin–aztreonam	
Clindamycin (Cleocin)	900 mg IV q 8 hr
Aztreonam (Azactam)	2 g IV q 8 hr
Cefoxitin–doxycycline	
Cefoxitin (Mefoxin)	1–2 g q 8 hr
Doxycycline	100 mg IV q 8 hr
Ampicillin–gentamicin–clindamycin	
Ampicillin	2 g q 6 hr
Gentamicin (Garamycin)	
Clindamycin (Cleocin)	

[a]Adjust for impaired renal function; check serum levels for therapeutic range on first day.

Ultrasonography, computed tomography, or magnetic resonance imaging may be helpful in diagnosing a pelvic abscess. Management of a persistent pelvic abscess includes drainage either by percutaneous techniques, colpotomy, or laparotomy. Intra-abdominal rupture of a pelvic abscess is a surgical emergency. Sepsis may occur in association with pelvic infection, with or without frank abscess formation.

Prophylactic antibiotic therapy at the time of cesarean delivery has been shown to significantly reduce the likelihood of postpartum infection. A single dose of a broad-spectrum antibiotic (for example, 1 g cefazolin sodium [Ancef]) is usually given at the time of clamping of the umbilical cord, a practice designed to avoid confounding of subsequent bacterial cultures of the infant, should they be necessary. Additional doses of antibiotics given after surgery do not provide added protection against infection.

Wound Infections, Separations, and Dehiscence

Infection of the *incision site* after cesarean delivery can occur, but is uncommon (3% to 8% of cases in most series, reduced by 50% with prophylactic antibiotic use). Risk factors include obesity, diabetes, corticosteroid therapy, immunosuppression, anemia, and poor hemostasis from any cause, with subsequent hematoma formation. Fever accompanied by pain, tenderness, and erythema around the incision are seen most frequently on the third and fourth days after delivery. Induration and drainage from the incision site may also be noted. Cesarean wound infections are often preceded by metritis, and fever persists despite apparently adequate antibiotic coverage. As with any wound infection, the cesarean incision site must be opened to determine the extent of infection, to ensure that the fascia is intact, and to permit adequate drainage of purulent or serosanguineous material. A culture of the site should be obtained, after which broad-spectrum antibiotic treatment is often initiated, although drainage alone may be adequate. Meticulous care of the open wound is also vital. If the infection disrupts the closure of the fascia, the patient must be returned to the operating room for debridement and reapproximation of the wound, with

delayed closure of the skin being the usual management.

Infections of the episiotomy site are uncommon (probably less than one-fourth of 1% of cases), which is somewhat surprising, given the bacterial milieu in that area. Infected episiotomy sites are tender and swollen. Poor tissue turgor often leads to breakdown of the sutures used in the initial repair. The sutures should be removed and drainage permitted, both to limit further spread of infection and to promote healing. Sitz baths also help in healing. Subsequent repair of the episiotomy site, if necessary, can be accomplished soon after the infection has cleared.

Necrotizing fasciitis is a rare infection that may be seen on the perineum or with abdominal incisions. Risk factors include obesity, diabetes, and hypertension. Necrotizing fasciitis is caused by gas-forming organisms, including *Clostridium.* This especially virulent and frequently fatal infectious process involves necrosis of the subcutaneous tissue, muscle, and fascia. Early in the process, the skin may be normal or relatively benign in appearance, despite extensive underlying necrosis. The necrosis may spread downward along the thighs or upward onto the abdomen and chest. This necrotic tissue must be debrided immediately until healthy tissue is reached. Antibiotics, cardiovascular system support, and subsequent skin grafting comprise the overall treatment. Without such vigorous care, fatality is virtually ensured; even with treatment, approximately 50% of the patients with necrotizing fasciitis do not survive. The key factor is early recognition of the possibility that a wound infection, whether perineal or abdominal, may represent this overwhelming infection.

Septic Pelvic Thrombophlebitis

Septic pelvic thrombophlebitis is an uncommon infection and is a sequela of pelvic infection. The venous drainage of the pelvic organs tends to flow in a left-to-right fashion through the right ovarian vein. Venous stasis in these widely dilated veins, along with the presence of multiple bacteria if infection is present, can lead to septic thrombosis in these vessels; subsequent *microembolization* of the lungs or other organs by way of the inferior vena cava is possible.

Clinically, this infection manifests as *residual fever and tachycardia* after several days of antibiotic treatment for presumed metritis. Usually the patient is asymptomatic with respect to uterine tenderness and bowel function. Although it is possible to diagnose this condition with computed tomographic scanning or other such imaging, a negative study does not rule it out. Treatment in most cases is empiric. Addition of heparin therapy may result in prompt resolution of the fever and tachycardia, usually within 24 hours. Anticoagulation therapy is recommended for at least 7, and up to 30, days. Clinical resolution of fever can also occur with continued parenteral antibiotics and no heparin therapy.

Respiratory Complications/Infection

Respiratory complications are especially common in the first 24 hours after delivery, particularly if general anesthesia with endotracheal intubation was used. *Atelectasis* is also common if general anesthesia was used. Preoperative training in the use of an inspiratory inhaler and its postoperative use under supervision significantly reduce the incidence and severity of this complication. Atelectasis is arguably a cause of postoperative fever, but it is certainly associated with it, and its resolution often coincides with clinical defervescence. *Postoperative pneumonia* is uncommon and is usually seen in those patients with predelivery respiratory disease. *Aspiration pneumonia* is a feared, although uncommon, complication.

Urinary Tract Infections

Urinary tract infections are also commonly seen after cesarean delivery but also may occur after vaginal delivery. Bladder catheterization, a practice common with both cesarean deliveries and epidural anesthesia, introduces bacteria into the lower urinary tract, which can lead to infection.

Dysuria (painful urination) is not as common in the puerperium as at other times because of a relative insensitivity of the bladder after delivery. *Frequency* of urination is also a normal occurrence postpartum, minimizing the value of this symptom during the postpartum period.

Costovertebral tenderness may suggest an upper urinary tract infection. When a urinary tract infection is suspected, a clean-catch or catheterized urine sample should be obtained for urinalysis and for culture. Antibiotic treatment is begun with one of a variety of broad-spectrum agents, and if the patient is especially uncomfortable, urinary analgesia may be provided (200 mg phenazopyridine, three times a day). The antibiotic can be changed if the culture results (usually available 24 to 48 hours later) indicate resistance of the bacteria to the initial antibiotic, especially if symptoms persist.

Mastitis

In the lactating woman, breast infection occurs most commonly several weeks postpartum, but it can occur much later. Initially, symptoms can be misleading. Patients often complain of significant *fever* (often 103°F or more), *chills, malaise,* and *general body aching.* Breast symptoms may be somewhat vague, although breast tenderness is described if patients are asked specifically about this. Commonly, patients think they have a generalized viral infection and call their physician seeking information regarding medications to take for the flu while lactating.

After the onset of these signs and symptoms, evidence of infection becomes more localized to the breasts over the following days. Erythema and tenderness are present, often with a brawny and indurated area to palpation, which may be segmented in orientation. The infection is virtually always unilateral. Once the infection has progressed to produce fever and clinical findings, it may proceed to generalized sepsis quickly, often in a matter of just a few hours. *Staphylococcus aureus* is cultured from the breast milk in about 50% of cases; no single predominant organism is identified in other cases. The origin of the infection is, in fact, the infant's pharynx; accordingly, there should be no concern on the part of the mother with respect to transmitting the infection to the infant.

It is no longer common practice to culture the breast milk. However, because of the prevalence of the *S. aureus* as the offender, an antibiotic that is penicillinase-resistant, such as *dicloxacillin* (500 mg orally every 6 hours) is recommended. Resolution of symptoms is usually prompt, with marked improvement within 24 to 36 hours. Persistent fever or the development of a mass may indicate a breast abscess. Patients should be cautioned to complete the full antibiotic course to prevent recurrence of mastitis. It is *not necessary to withhold nursing* on the infected breast, although some patients benefit greatly from uninterrupted rest for the first day or two of therapy. If nursing is discontinued, pumping of the breast is necessary to optimize response to therapy and prevent abscess formation.

Mastitis is usually distinguished from a blocked (inspissated) duct (see Chapter 10) on the basis of fever. At times, however, it may be difficult to distinguish these two entities, and antibiotic treatment is usually begun empirically. *Breast engorgement* may occur in the first 24 hours following initial milk production and is characterized by transient low-grade fever and bilaterally distended, firm, and nodular breasts. Treatment is supportive and includes breast binders (if not breast feeding), pumping of the breasts, and nonsteroidal anti-inflammatory agents.

CHAPTER 14

ABORTION

This chapter deals primarily with Educational Topics:

Topic 16: Spontaneous Abortion
Topic 21: Fetal Death
Topic 34: Abortion

Students should be able to define the types of spontaneous abortion (spontaneous, recurrent, incomplete, septic) and explain their diagnosis and management, including the differential diagnosis of bleeding in the first trimester. Students should also be able to explain the indications, risks and benefits, and means for elective and therapeutic abortion. Students should be able to evaluate and manage fetal death in each trimester, including appropriate counseling for the parents.

Abortion is the loss (or termination or end) of a pregnancy before viability, typically defined as 20 weeks from the first day of the last normal menstrual period, or a fetus weighing <500 g. Whether spontaneous or induced, there are profound medical as well as emotional implications associated with abortion. Because the lay expression for spontaneous abortion is "miscarriage," care should be taken to be certain that communications between patient and physician are clear.

Spontaneous Abortion

The *incidence of spontaneous abortion* is estimated at 50% of all pregnancies, based on the understanding that many pregnancies spontaneously terminate without clinical recognition. An incidence of recognized spontaneous abortion of 15% to 25% is commonly cited, with approximately 80% occurring during the first 12 weeks of pregnancy.

Approximately 50% of early spontaneous abortions are attributed to chromosomal abnormalities, of which trisomy accounts for 40% to 50%, monosomy X for 15% to 25%, triploidy

for approximately 15%, and tetraploidy for approximately 5%. Risk factors associated with spontaneous abortion include increasing parity, increasing maternal age, increasing paternal age, and conception within 3 months of a live birth. Abnormal development of the early pregnancy (including the zygote, embryo, fetus, or placenta) is a common pathologic finding in spontaneous abortion. Expulsion of the pregnancy is typically preceded by death of the embryo or fetus.

The further that a pregnancy progresses before undergoing spontaneous abortion, the less likely that the fetus is chromosomally abnormal compared with first-trimester abortions. Second-trimester abortions are more likely to be caused by maternal systemic disease, abnormal placentation, or other anatomic considerations. This difference is of great clinical significance because these conditions associated with later abortions can often be treated, and recurrent abortions can thereby potentially be prevented.

Table 14.1 lists the causes of spontaneous abortion, which will be discussed in the following sections.

Table 14.1. Causes of Spontaneous Abortion

Genetic factors (10%–50%)	*Ureaplasma urealyticum*
Advaned maternal or paternal age	Toxoplasmosis
Balanced translocation/carrier state	Syphilis
Endocrine abnormalities (25%–50%)	Systemic disease
Luteal-phase defect	Diabetes mellitus
Thyroid disease	Chronic renal disease
Hyperandrogenism	Chronic cardiovascular disease
Reproductive tract abnormalities (6%–12%)	Systemic lupus/lupus anticoagulant
Leiomyomata uteri (submucous)	Antiphospholipid antibody syndrome
Septate uterus	Inherited thrombophias
Bicornuate or unicornuate uterus	Environmental factors
In utero exposure to diethylstilbestrol	Toxins
Incompetent cervix	Radiation
Intrauterine adhesions	Smoking
Abnormality of placentation	Alcohol
Infection	Heavy caffeine intake
Listeria monocytogenes	
Mycoplasma hominis	

Maternal Factors

Infectious Factors

Maternal systemic conditions that have been associated with spontaneous abortion include infections such as *Listeria monocytogenes, Mycoplasma hominis, Ureaplasma urealyticum,* and toxoplasmosis as well as viral infections, including rubella and cytomegalic inclusion disease. However, these are uncommon causes of spontaneous abortion.

Systemic Factors

Insufficient secretion of progesterone by the corpus luteum or the placenta may be associated with spontaneous abortion. *Luteal-phase inadequacy* occurs in 3% of the general population, but more frequently in those suffering spontaneous pregnancy loss. Luteal-phase defect is diagnosed by appropriately timed endometrial biopsy, not serum progesterone assay. Treatment may include clomiphene, which acts by increasing follicle-stimulating hormone, and human chorionic gonadotropin (hCG), which is the physiologic luteotropic stimulus, or progesterone vaginal suppositories. Although uncommon, untreated medical conditions such as *hypothyroidism, systemic lupus erythematosus,* antiphospholipid antibody syndrome, inherited thrombophilias, and *diabetes mellitus* are also associated with an increased incidence of spontaneous abortion.

Environmental Factors

Spontaneous abortion has also been related to environmental toxins and radiation. *Smoking, heavy caffeine intake, and alcohol consumption* have been linked to miscarriages. Women who smoke more than one pack of cigarettes per day have an almost twofold increase in their rate of spontaneous abortion. Consumption of more than four to five cups of coffee per day (500 mg or more of caffeine per day) has been associated with a doubling of the risk of miscarriage. Women who drink alcohol more than 2 days per week experience twice the abortion rate of those who do not.

Uterine Factors

Submucous leiomyomata uteri have been associated with spontaneous abortion. Removal of the leiomyomata (myomectomy) is recommended only if it is determined that pregnancy wastage has been caused by this anatomic distortion.

Twenty percent to 30% of women with a unicornuate or septate uterus have reproductive difficulties; the most frequent difficulty is recurrent spontaneous abortion. In utero exposure to *diethylstilbestrol (DES)* has been associated with abnormally shaped uteri as well as cervical incompetence and spontaneous abortion.

Intrauterine synechiae (Asherman syndrome) has been linked to spontaneous abortion, caused by an inadequate amount of endometrium to support implantation. This condition is typically a sequela of uterine curettage with subsequent destruction and scarring of the endometrium.

Paternal Factors

Occasionally, a chromosomal abnormality in either parent may be a cause of spontaneous abortion. As a result, couples suffering recurrent abortions should have karyotyping of both parents. In addition, as with eggs, advanced paternal age may also increase the rate of spontaneous abortion.

Fetal Factors

Genetic abnormalities of the conceptus are the most common cause of spontaneous abortion. More than 50% of abortions in the first trimester are caused by chromosomal anomalies, approximately half of which are autosomal trisomies. Whereas chromosomally abnormal pregnancies tend to terminate early, chromosomally normal pregnancies are usually lost later in gestation.

Differential Diagnosis of Abortion

Because the differential diagnosis of bleeding in the first trimester of pregnancy includes a wide range of possibilities, such as ectopic pregnancy, hydatidiform mole, cervical polyps, and cervicitis, the patient should be examined whenever there is bleeding in early pregnancy. Any vaginal bleeding in the first half of an intrauterine pregnancy is presumptively called a *threatened abortion,* unless another specific diagnosis can be made.

Threatened Abortion

Threatened abortion occurs in up to 25% of pregnancies, with approximately half of these patients proceeding to spontaneous abortion. This condition is characterized by bleeding in the first trimester without loss of fluid or tissue. Those who carry a pregnancy complicated by threatened abortion to viability are at greater risk for preterm delivery, an infant of low birth weight, and a higher incidence of perinatal mortality. There does not, however, appear to be a higher incidence of congenital malformations in these newborns. Some patients describe bleeding at the time of their expected menses, sometimes referred to as the *placental sign or implantation bleeding,* which may be the result of ruptured blood vessels in the endometrium. Low abdominal pain may accompany the bleeding. On examination, the cervix is usually closed. Ultrasonography is especially useful to determine if an early pregnancy is intact. Lack of a gestational sac does not, however, rule out an early viable pregnancy. Ultrasonography, in conjunction with quantitative hCG, has been used to identify viable pregnancies at various stages of gestation. Transabdominal ultrasonography can identify an intact gestation if the quantitative β-hCG exceeds 5,000 to 6,000 mIU/mL, whereas transvaginal ultrasonography can typically identify an early intact pregnancy when the β-hCG level exceeds 1,500 mIU/mL.

Inevitable Abortion

An *inevitable abortion* is defined as rupture of the membranes and/or cervical dilation during the first half of pregnancy so that pregnancy loss is unavoidable. It is unusual for a pregnancy to successfully reach viability in this circumstance. Uterine contractions typically follow, and the products of conception are expelled. Conservative management of these patients significantly increases the risk of maternal infection.

Complete Abortion

Complete abortion refers to a documented pregnancy that spontaneously passes all of the products of conception. Early in pregnancy, the fetus and placenta are often expelled in toto.

Incomplete Abortion

In those cases of spontaneous abortion in which partial expulsion of pregnancy tissue has occurred, bleeding and pain result. Suction curettage of the uterus is usually necessary to remove the remaining products of conception and prevent further bleeding and infection (see Chapter 24). Postevacuation treatment with an ergot derivative (Methergine [methylergonovine maleate], 0.2 mg orally every 4 hours for 24 hours) and an antibiotic (doxycycline, 100 mg orally, twice daily for 3 days) reduces the risk of postabortal syndrome, further bleeding, and infection. Medical evacuation, primarily using prostaglandins, is also effective and avoids some risks of operative procedures.

Missed Abortion

A *missed abortion* is the retention of a failed intrauterine pregnancy for an extended period, usually defined as more than two menstrual cycles. These patients have an absence of uterine growth and may have lost some of the early symptoms of pregnancy. Although unusual, disseminated intravascular coagulopathy can occur when an intrauterine fetal demise in the second trimester has been retained beyond 6 weeks after the death of the fetus. Evacuation of the uterus with suction curettage is recommended for pregnancy in the first trimester, whereas dilation and evacuation, or prostaglandins, are used for evacuation in pregnancies that have advanced to the second trimester.

Recurrent Abortion

Recurrent abortion is a term used when a patient has had more than two consecutive, or a total of three spontaneous, abortions. In early abortions, there is a great likelihood of a chromosomal abnormality, whereas in later abortions, a maternal cause is more likely. Karyotyping is recommended for both parents when recurrent early abortion occurs because there is a 3% chance that one parent is a symptomless carrier of a chromosomal abnormality after two fetal losses. The possibility of immunologic factors should also be explored. Correction of maternal medical conditions and/or anatomic deformities should be pursued for those patients with recurrent late abortions.

These include surgical correction of uterine abnormalities, cerclage of the incompetent cervix, or lysis of intrauterine synechiae.

Recurrent abortion can be the result of *uterine anomalies,* such as septate uterus, with only approximately 25% of patients with septate uteri having problems with fetal wastage. Getting pregnant is usually not a problem, but maintaining pregnancy may require surgical management. Such management may include hysterography, operative hysteroscopy, and laparoscopy.

The *incompetent cervix* is diagnosed mainly by its classic history of sudden expulsion of a normal sac and fetus between the eighteenth and thirty-second week of pregnancy without prior pain or bleeding. Diagnosis is by history and observation of a lax, open cervical os. Increasingly, ultrasound visualization of shortening and funneling of the cervical canal during pregnancy is being used to make this diagnosis. Treatment is surgical by the *cerclage procedures,* which involve the placement of a purse-string suture about the cervix to close the incompetent cervix (Figure 14.1). Such sutures are commonly placed during pregnancy when the cervix is found to be dilating asymptomatically. The suture must be

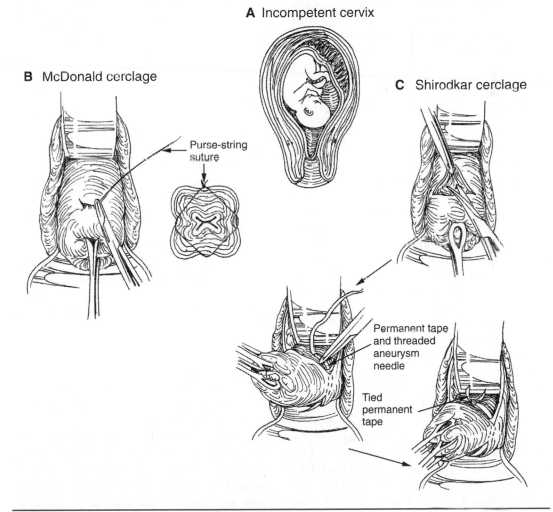

A Incompetent cervix

B McDonald cerclage

Purse-string suture

C Shirodkar cerclage

Permanent tape and threaded aneurysm needle

Tied permanent tape

Figure 14.1. Cerclage for the treatment of incompetent cervix. (**A**) Incompetent cervix. (**B**) McDonald cerclage: purse-string, through-and-through suture about the cervical canal. (**C**) Shirodkar cerclage: purse-string submucosal suture, facilitated by an aneurysm needle threaded below the mucosae and used to pull the suture through, beneath the mucosae.

removed when labor ensues or the patient must be delivered by cesarean birth. Allowing a patient who has been treated with cerclage to undergo labor risks extensive laceration of the cervix and/or uterine rupture.

Intrauterine synechiae associated with *Asherman syndrome* may occur after a vigorous curettage has denuded the endometrium past the layer of the basalis so that webs of myometrium develop across the uterine cavity (the synechiae). Asherman syndrome is associated with amenorrhea or irregular menses, infertility, and recurrent pregnancy loss. The diagnosis is confirmed by a hysterogram that shows the characteristic webbed pattern or by hysteroscopy. Treatment involves lysis of the synechiae and postoperative treatment with high doses of estrogen to facilitate endometrial proliferation, leading to the reestablishment of a normal endometrial layer.

Treatment of Spontaneous Abortion

No intervention is necessary for patients with threatened abortion even if the bleeding is accompanied by low abdominal pain and cramping. If there is no evidence of significant abnormality on ultrasound evaluation, and if the pregnancy is found to be intact, the patient can be reassured and allowed to continue normal activities. Intercourse is usually proscribed for 2 to 3 weeks or longer, depending on the cause of bleeding. Although commonly recommended, a short period of bed rest has no documented benefit.

If pain and bleeding persist, especially with significant hemodynamic alterations, or if ultrasound and hormonal evaluation identify a nonviable pregnancy, evacuation of the uterus should be carried out. Immediate considerations include control of bleeding, prevention of infection, pain relief, and emotional support.

Bleeding is controlled by ensuring that the products of conception have been expelled or removed from the uterus. In cases of complete abortion, the uterus is small and firm, the cervix is closed, and ultrasound identifies an empty uterus. Evacuation of the uterus is accomplished by curettage in cases of incomplete, inevitable, missed, or septic abortions. Hemostasis is enhanced through uterine con-

traction stimulated by Methergine. Removal of the products of conception also decreases the risk of infection, and this, combined with vaginal rest (no tampons, douches, or intercourse), provides adequate protection against infection in most cases.

A mild analgesic may be required and should be offered. Rh-negative mothers should receive Rh immune globulin (RhoGAM). Chromosomal evaluation of spontaneous abortions is not recommended unless there is a history of recurrent abortion.

Emotional support is important for both the short- and long-term well-being of the patient as well as her partner. No matter how well prepared a couple is for the possibility of pregnancy loss, the event is a significant disappointment and cause of stress. When appropriate, the couple should be reassured that the loss was not precipitated by anything that they did or did not do, and that there was nothing that they could have done to prevent the loss.

A follow-up office visit is generally scheduled for 2 to 6 weeks after the loss of a pregnancy. This is an appropriate time to evaluate uterine involution, assess the return of menses, and discuss reproductive plans. The causes (or lack of causes) of the pregnancy loss should also be reiterated. The impact of this loss on future childbearing should be discussed. A single pregnancy loss does not significantly increase the risk of future losses. Multiple pregnancy losses carry an increased risk for future pregnancies, partly on the basis of the higher likelihood of a continuing causative condition such as fibroids, immune diseases, or genetic disorders.

Induced Abortion

Termination of an intact pregnancy before the time of viability can be done to safeguard the health of the mother, because of severe fetal abnormality, or on an elective (i.e., voluntary) basis. Elective abortion has been legal since the 1973 Supreme Court decision of *Roe v. Wade*. Since that time, various local and state laws have been proposed to significantly limit access to elective abortion. These laws will continue to undergo many court challenges as our society struggles to define a consistent national policy.

Before undergoing an elective abortion, patients must be aware that choices are available. These include continuation of pregnancy with subsequent adoption, continuation of pregnancy and keeping the child, and elective abortion during either the first or second trimester. First-trimester pregnancies are typically terminated by means of suction curettage (i.e., vacuum aspiration performed through the cervix). Second-trimester abortions are most commonly performed through the cervix, using suction or destructive forceps, or by the use of prostaglandins, as in the form of intra-amniotic injections or vaginal suppositories. Early first-trimester medical abortion can be performed by the administration of misoprostil and mifepristone (RU486).

Medical and/or surgical complications are associated with all choices, with the fewest complications related to elective abortion in the first trimester. Although there are complications associated with pregnancy termination, they are significantly fewer complications than those associated with carrying a pregnancy.

The most common complication following an induced abortion is infection. The patient usually presents with fever, pain, a tender uterus, and mild bleeding. Oral antibiotics and antipyretics are usually sufficient to manage these mild infections. If tissue remains in the uterus (incomplete abortion), suction curettage is also necessary. The second most common complication following induced abortion is bleeding. Risk of death from abortion during the first 2 months of pregnancy is less than 1 per 100,000 procedures, with increasing rates as pregnancy progresses (versus 7.7 maternal deaths per 100,000 live births). There is no apparent risk to future pregnancies if the first- or second-trimester abortion has been free of complications. There appears to be a slightly increased risk of premature delivery if more than three first-trimester pregnancies are terminated by elective abortion.

Medical (i.e., nonsurgical) methods to induce first-trimester abortion include the antiprogesterone medication RU486 (mifepristone), which is used in conjunction with a prostaglandin analog and methotrexate. Abortion is not always complete with this medical method, and suction and curettage to remove retained products of conception may be required.

Septic Abortion

Occasionally, patients may present with a *septic abortion,* an infected complete or incomplete abortion in which the patient has sepsis, shock, hemorrhage, and possibly renal failure. It rarely occurs as a complication of a legal abortion but is more commonly associated with criminal abortions (i.e., those done illegally, under unsterile conditions, by persons who may have little or no knowledge of medicine or anatomy). Broad-spectrum parenteral antibiotics, fluid therapy, and prompt evacuation of the uterus are indicated. A careful evaluation for trauma, including perforation of the uterus or vagina, should also be carried out.

Postabortal Syndrome

Postabortal syndrome develops when the uterus fails to remain contracted after spontaneous abortion (with or without suction curettage) or elective/therapeutic abortion. The patient presents with cramping pain and/or bleeding, and is found to have an open cervix, bleeding, and a large, "softer-than-expected" uterus. The clinical situation is often indistinguishable from incomplete abortion, and the question is resolved only on receipt of a pathology report of the tissue/material removed at suction curettage, which is the treatment for the condition. Treatment is completed by oxytocic and antibiotic therapy as in the treatment of incomplete abortion.

CHAPTER 15

ECTOPIC PREGNANCY

This chapter deals primarily with APGO Educational Topic:

Topic 15: Ectopic Pregnancy

The student should understand that ectopic pregnancy is a leading cause of maternal morbidity and mortality, and that early diagnosis and intervention can preserve fertility and save lives.

Incidence

Implantation outside the uterine cavity is termed *ectopic pregnancy,* a condition that significantly jeopardizes the mother and is incompatible with continuing the pregnancy. Catastrophic bleeding may occur when the implanting pregnancy erodes into blood vessels or ruptures through structures not suited to accommodate the growing conceptus (typically the fallopian tubes). The effect of the ectopic pregnancy reaches beyond the incident pregnancy, reflected in decreased fertility and increased risk of recurrent ectopic pregnancy, depending on the amount of damage caused by the ectopic pregnancy, the treatment(s) used, and underlying causes.

Primarily because of an increasing prevalence of pelvic inflammatory disease, the incidence of ectopic pregnancy has been increasing in the United States, from 4.5 per 1,000 pregnancies in 1970 to an estimated 19.7 per 1,000 pregnancies in 1992. Despite this nearly 2% incidence of ectopic pregnancy, maternal mortality rates have decreased markedly. In the 1970s, there were 3.5 maternal deaths per 1,000 cases

of ectopic pregnancy; today the rate is <1 per 1,000. This improvement is primarily the result of earlier detection, which allows intervention before massive bleeding occurs and, in some cases, even prior to the development of any symptoms.

Pregnancies may implant in many locations in the genital tract and pelvis (Figure 15.1). Most ectopic gestations (95%) occur in the fallopian tube (*tubal pregnancy*). Four of five tubal pregnancies occur in the ampullary portion of the fallopian tube. Infrequent locations include the cervix, ovary, and peritoneal cavity (termed *cervical, ovarian, and abdominal pregnancy,* respectively). For women who have used assisted reproductive technology to achieve pregnancy, there is a significant increase in the incidence of nontubal ectopic pregnancies, especially the heretofore rare combined (or heterotopic) pregnancy, in which one pregnancy is intrauterine and a second one is ectopic.

Tubal pregnancy may result in any of three clinical scenarios: (1) tubal rupture with intraperitoneal hemorrhage, (2) tubal abortion (i.e., expulsion of the pregnancy out the fimbriated end with or without hemorrhage), or

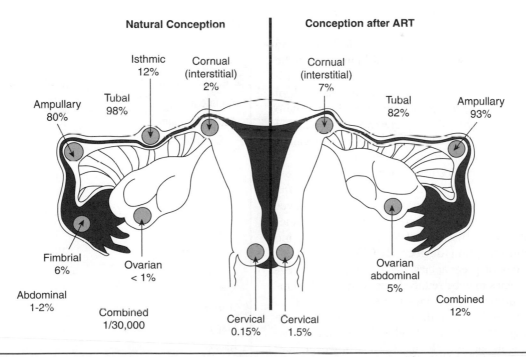

Figure 15.1. Incidence of types of ectopic pregnancy by location, after natural cycles and for women who have used assisted reproductive technology (ART).

rarely (3) tubal abortion with subsequent implantation on an intraperitoneal structure.

Patients with ectopic pregnancy are at risk for immediate morbidity and mortality from acute blood loss and risk of anatomic damage, and they also have a significantly reduced fertility rate, with fewer than half of the patients subsequently having a live full-term birth. As the *second leading cause of maternal mortality in the United States, ectopic pregnancy should be high in the differential diagnosis for any woman of reproductive age with acute pelvic or lower abdominal pain, with or without abnormal vaginal bleeding, and with a positive pregnancy test.*

Causes of Ectopic Pregnancy

Knowing which patients are at higher risk can aid the physician in making an early diagnosis. The primary risk factor for ectopic pregnancy is a prior history of *salpingitis.* Damage from such infection may retard the passage of the fertilized ovum through the tube to the endometrial cavity, facilitating extrauterine implantation. Women with a history of salpingitis have a sixfold increase in their risk of ectopic pregnancy. *A previous ectopic pregnancy also increases the risk of future ectopic implantations by approximately 10-fold.*

Age is an important risk factor. Women 35 to 44 years old have a threefold increase in the rate of ectopic pregnancy compared with women 15 to 24 years old. More than half of all ectopic pregnancies occur in women who have had *three or more pregnancies.* Finally, *Black and Hispanic women* also have a significantly higher risk of ectopic pregnancy.

Contrary to some reports, *sterilization, contraception, and abortion do not increase the frequency of ectopic pregnancy.* Oral contraceptives prevent ovulation, thereby significantly reducing pregnancies in all locations. Intrauterine contraception devices (IUCDs) prevent all types of pregnancies, although ectopic pregnancies may be reduced relatively less than intrauterine pregnancies, thereby giving the false impression that they are a risk factor. The higher prevalence of pelvic inflammatory disease in patients who use IUCDs, however, may increase the patient's risk even after the removal of the device.

In patients with previous sterilization, the chance of ectopic pregnancy is increased, but because sterilization failures are so uncommon, the net effect of sterilization is to protect against ectopic pregnancies. Although 85% of sterilization failures are associated with intrauterine pregnancies, the possibility of an ectopic pregnancy should always be considered in patients with sterilization failures. Abortion itself does not predispose to ectopic pregnancy, although associated infection may do so. There has been a reported effect of ovulation induction in increasing the risk of ectopic pregnancy. This has been difficult to determine because there is the potential for subclinical tubal disease in some infertile patients, which may itself be the primary cause of the ectopic pregnancy.

Clinical Evaluation of Possible Ectopic Pregnancy

Symptoms of Tubal Pregnancy

The classic presentation of a patient with an ectopic pregnancy includes *abdominal pain, amenorrhea, and vaginal bleeding.* The frequency of symptoms in patients with ectopic pregnancy is presented in Table 15.1.

Table 15.1. Symptoms of Ectopic Pregnancy	
Symptom	**Prevalence (%)**
Abdominal pain	95–100
Generalized	50
Unilateral	35
Shoulder	20
Back	5–10
Abnormal uterine bleeding	65–85
Amenorrhea	75–95
<2 weeks	45
<6 weeks	35
Syncope	10–18
Dizziness	20–35
Pregnancy symptoms	10–20
Nausea	15
Urge to defecate	5–15

Early ectopic pregnancies are asymptomatic. As the pregnancy grows, the most common symptom is abdominal or pelvic pain, which is present in nearly all patients. Pain is a result of the distended fallopian tube and/or irritation of the peritoneum by blood. The pain is generally described as colicky in character and may be unilateral (not necessarily on the same side as the ectopic) or bilateral, intermittent or constant, and located in the lower or even upper abdomen. The proximal portions of the fallopian tube are not as able to adapt to the growing pregnancy, so an ectopic pregnancy in this area is likely to become symptomatic earlier in gestation.

In up to one-fifth of patients with extensive intra-abdominal bleeding, irritation of the diaphragm causes referred pain to the shoulder. Irritation of the posterior cul-de-sac may cause an urge to defecate. Patients may present with a history of feeling faint or passing out while they are straining to have a bowel movement. Syncope occurs in one-third of patients with ruptured tubal pregnancies, and less frequently in unruptured cases.

Although patients with ectopic pregnancy typically have missed their normal menses, this history often is not given. By the time symptoms have developed, it has usually been 6 weeks since the last normal menstrual period. At this early stage, symptoms of pregnancy are not always present and cannot be used to rule in or rule out ectopic pregnancy.

As long as placental hormones are produced, there is usually no vaginal bleeding.

Irregular vaginal bleeding results from the sloughing of the decidua from the endometrial lining. Vaginal bleeding in patients with an ectopic gestation may range from little or none to heavy, menstrual-like flow. In some patients, the entire "decidual cast" is passed intact, simulating a spontaneous abortion (Figure 15.2). Histologic evaluation of this tissue confirms whether placental villi are present. In any patient with a positive pregnancy test, whenever evaluation of tissue passed spontaneously or obtained by curettage does not demonstrate villi, an ectopic implantation should be assumed to be present until proved otherwise.

Physical Findings in Tubal Pregnancy

Physical examination findings range from a totally normal examination in early, unruptured ectopic pregnancy to hypovolemic shock and an acute abdomen in cases of ruptured ectopic pregnancy. Most healthy reproductive-age women are able to compensate for mild-to-moderate degrees of blood loss so that extensive blood loss is usually required to cause a decrease in blood pressure and an increase in pulse. Five percent of patients with ectopic pregnancies present in hypovolemic shock, although blood loss is the major factor in 85% of ectopic pregnancy deaths. A summary of physical examination findings is presented in Table 15.2.

Fever is not expected, although a mild elevation in temperature in response to intraperitoneal blood may occur. A temperature of >38°C may suggest an infectious cause to a patient's symptoms. Abdominal distension and

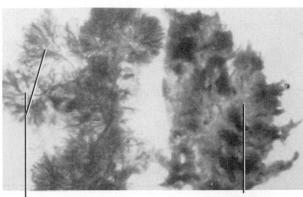

Villi

Shaggy decidua

Figure 15.2. Left. Typical fluffy villi of placenta. Right. Shaggy decidua. (From Munsick RA. Clinical test for placenta in 300 consecutive menstrual aspirations. *Obstet Gynecol* 1982;60:738.)

Table 15.2. Physical Examination in Ectopic Pregnancy

Finding	Prevalence (%)
Abdominal tenderness	80–90
Peritoneal signs	
Ruptured ectopic pregnancy cases	50
Unruptured ectopic pregnancy cases	5
Adnexal tenderness	75–90
Unilateral	40–75
Bilateral	50–75
Cervical motion tenderness	50–75
Adnexal mass	30–50
Contralateral	20
Uterus	
Normal size	70
Enlarged	15–30
Orthostatic changes	10–15
Temperature >37°C	5–10
Vomiting	15

tenderness, with or without rebound, rigidity, or decreased bowel sounds, may be seen in cases of intra-abdominal bleeding. Abdominal tenderness is variable; it is present in 50% to 90% of patients with ectopic pregnancies. Cervical motion tenderness, caused by intraperitoneal irritation, and adnexal tenderness are commonly found. An adnexal mass is present in roughly one-third of cases, but its absence does not rule out the possibility of an ectopic implantation. The uterus may enlarge and soften throughout the first trimester, thus simulating an intrauterine pregnancy. A slightly open cervix with blood or decidual tissue may be found and mistaken for a threatened and/or spontaneous abortion.

Differential Diagnosis

The rapid and accurate diagnosis of ectopic pregnancy is imperative to reduce the risk of serious complications or death. Up to half of ectopic pregnancy-related maternal deaths have had a lag in treatment because of delayed or inaccurate diagnoses. *Any sexually active woman in the reproductive age group who presents with pain, irregular bleeding, and/or amenorrhea should have ectopic pregnancy as a part of the initial differential diagnosis.* Other elements of the differential diagnosis include complications of an intrauterine pregnancy (threatened, missed, completed, or incomplete abortion), nonpregnancy-related gynecologic conditions (acute and chronic salpingitis, follicular or corpus luteum cyst rupture, endometriosis, or adnexal torsion), and nongynecologic conditions (e.g., gastroenteritis and appendicitis).

Diagnostic Procedures

The initial assessment in the otherwise hemodynamically stable patient must include a *pregnancy test.* With the sensitive assays available today, a negative pregnancy test excludes the possibility of ectopic pregnancy. Urinary pregnancy tests, which detect human chorionic gonadotropin (hCG) levels to 50 mIU/mL, are now commonly available. These tests detect hCG as early as 14 days after conception and are positive in more than 90% of cases of ectopic pregnancy. Serum assays can detect the presence of hCG as early as 5 days after conception (i.e., before the missed menstrual cycle). However, because they require additional time and expertise to perform, they are often not used in a potentially emergent clinical setting.

If a positive pregnancy test is found when ectopic pregnancy is suspected, the remainder of the workup should focus on evaluation of the viability and location of the pregnancy. *Quantitative β-hCG levels* can be followed at 2-day intervals. Early in pregnancy, these levels should increase by at least 66% in 48 hours. Failure to meet this criterion suggests that a pregnancy is not growing appropriately, thus increasing the suspicion of ectopic pregnancy. An inappropriate increase in hCG identifies a potentially abnormal pregnancy but does not identify its location. No single hCG result can be used to rule in or rule out ectopic pregnancy, unless it is negative.

A useful adjunct to serial quantitative levels of hCG is pelvic *ultrasonography* (Figure 15.3). Ultrasonography cannot be relied on to routinely image a pregnancy outside the uterine cavity, but it can identify an intrauterine

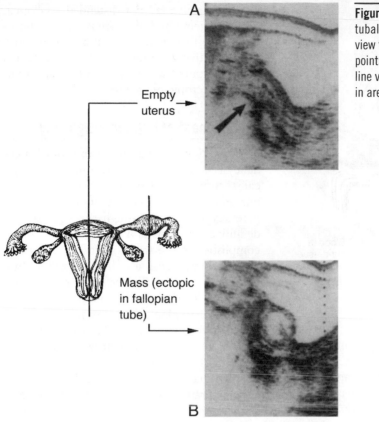

Figure 15.3. Sonographic findings in tubal ectopic pregnancy. (**A**) Midline view through empty uterus (arrow points to empty uterus). (**B**) Paramidline view (arrow points to cystic mass in area of fallopian tube).

Empty uterus

Mass (ectopic in fallopian tube)

A

B

pregnancy with considerable accuracy, thus effectively ruling out ectopic pregnancy, with the exception of the rare possibility of coexistent intrauterine and extrauterine gestations (heterotopic pregnancy). Transabdominal ultrasonography should be able to identify an intrauterine gestation by the time the hCG level reaches 5,000 to 6,000 mIU/mL. The more sensitive transvaginal ultrasonography should show the pregnancy by the time the hCG level is 1,500 mIU/mL. Failure to do so should further increase the suspicion that an ectopic pregnancy exists.

Although a low hematocrit is unusual, a complete blood count can document possible blood loss anemia and identify leukocytosis. If the white blood cell (WBC) count is >20,000 (WBC/dL), it is more likely that there is infection rather than an ectopic pregnancy.

Serum progesterone concentration has also been used as a screening test for ectopic pregnancy. A progesterone of less than 5.0 ng/mL strongly suggests a nonviable pregnancy, either intrauterine or extrauterine. Serum progesterone levels >25 ng/mL help in cases of suspected ectopic gestation because only 2.5% of all abnormal pregnancies (ectopic or intrauterine) have serum progesterone levels above this level.

Curettage of the uterine cavity can also help rule out ectopic pregnancy, but should only be undertaken after the possibility of interrupting an intact pregnancy has been considered. Although intrauterine and ectopic pregnancy can exist simultaneously in rare cases, identification of chorionic villi in curettings identifies an intrauterine location of the pregnancy and essentially rules out ectopic pregnancy. The Arias-Stella reaction, a hypersecretory endometrium of pregnancy seen on histologic examination, is compatible not only with ectopic pregnancy but also with intrauterine pregnancy and therefore is not useful in identifying an ectopic pregnancy.

Culdocentesis can identify hemoperitoneum, which may indicate a ruptured ectopic pregnancy, although it is also consistent with other

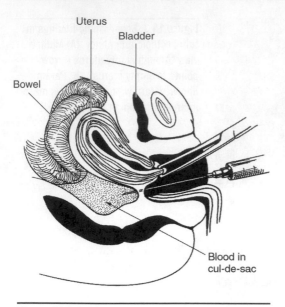

Figure 15.4. Culdocentesis.

causes such as a ruptured corpus luteum cyst. An 18-gauge needle is inserted posterior to the cervix, between the uterosacral ligaments, and into the cul-de-sac of the peritoneal cavity (Figure 15.4). Aspiration of clear peritoneal fluid (*negative culdocentesis*) indicates no hemorrhage into the abdominal cavity, but does not rule out an unruptured ectopic pregnancy. Aspiration of blood that clots can indicate either penetration of a vessel or such rapid blood loss into the peritoneal cavity that the blood clot has not had time to undergo fibrinolysis. Nonclotting blood is evidence of hemoperitoneum (*positive culdocentesis*) in which the blood clot has undergone fibrinolysis. If nothing is aspirated (*equivocal or nondiagnostic culdocentesis*), no information is obtained. Because no finding on culdocentesis can definitively rule in or rule out ectopic pregnancy, its use in clinical practice has declined. When used, the primary utility of culdocentesis is that a positive culdocentesis identifies blood in the peritoneal cavity and confirms the need for further evaluation to identify the source of the bleeding.

The most accurate technique of identifying an ectopic pregnancy is by direct visualization, which is done most commonly via laparoscopy. Even laparoscopy, however, has a 2% to 5% misdiagnosis rate. For example, an extremely early tubal gestation may not be

identified as it may not distend the fallopian tube sufficiently to be recognized as an abnormality (false–negative). On the other hand a false–positive diagnosis may result from a hematosalpinx being misinterpreted as an unruptured ectopic pregnancy.

Management of Ectopic Pregnancy

The traditional management of a tubal pregnancy is surgical removal. Conservative surgical techniques have been developed that maximize preservation of reproductive organs. If removal is done through the laparoscopy, definitive diagnosis and treatment can be accomplished at the same operation with minimal morbidity, cost, and hospitalization. In a *linear salpingostomy* (Figure 15.5), the surgeon makes an incision on the fallopian tube over the site of implantation, removes the pregnancy, and allows the incision to heal by secondary intention. A *segmental resection* is the removal of a portion of the affected tube with the potential of reanastomosing the tube at the initial operation or at a later time (Figure 15.6). *Salpingectomy* is removal of the entire tube, a procedure reserved for those cases in which little or no normal tube remains.

Nonsurgical therapy for the early, unruptured ectopic pregnancy includes expectant management and methotrexate. Expectant management involves no surgery and no medical therapy but allows the pregnancy to

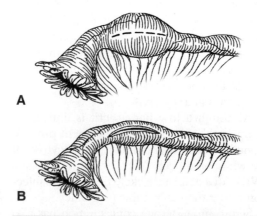

Figure 15.5. Surgical management of ectopic pregnancy: linear salpingostomy. (**A**) Site of linear incision. (**B**) Linear incision.

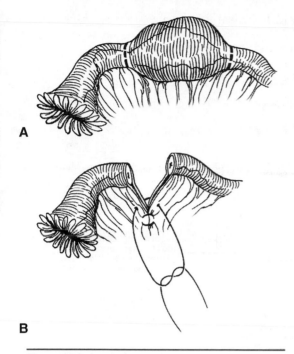

Figure 15.6. Surgical management of ectopic pregnancy: segmental resection (**A**) and tubal reanastomosis (**B**).

spontaneously regress as documented by serial hCG levels. *Methotrexate,* a folic acid antagonist, may be given via the oral or intramuscular routes, as well as by direct injection into the ectopic gestational sac. Table 15.3 shows a management protocol using methotrexate as a

Table 15.3.	Single-Dose Methotrexate Protocol for Ectopic Pregnancy Treatment	

Day	Therapy
0	hCG, D&C, CBC, SGOT, BUN, creatinine, blood type + Rh
1	MTX, hCG[a]
4	hCG[b]
7	hCG

[a]In those patients not requiring D&C before MTX initiation (hCG <2,000 mIU/mL and no gestational sac on transvaginal ultrasound), days 0 and 1 are combined.
[b]With a 15% decline in hCG titer between days 4 and 7, follow weekly until hCG is <10 mIU/mL.
BUN, blood urea nitrogen; CBC, complete blood count; D&C, dilation and curettage; hCG = quantitative β-human chorionic gonadotropin; MTX, intramuscular methotrexate, 50 mg/m²; SGOT, serum glutamic oxaloacetic transaminase.

single-dose intramuscular treatment for unruptured ectopic gestations. This therapy is usually reserved for cases in which the ectopic gestation is less than 3.5 cm in diameter and there is no cardiac activity in the pregnancy as seen on ultrasound.

When conservative surgery or nonsurgical treatment is used, the patient must be followed posttherapy with serial quantitative β-hCG levels to monitor regression of the pregnancy. Subsequent surgery or methotrexate therapy is needed if trophoblastic function persists as evidenced by persistent or rising levels of hCG.

Rh-negative mothers with ectopic pregnancy should receive *Rh immune globulin* (Rho-GAM) to prevent Rh sensitization.

Although traditionally diagnosed at the time of surgery, ectopic pregnancies are increasingly suspected and treated without either laparoscopy or laparotomy, thereby avoiding the inherent morbidity and cost of surgery. The algorithm shown in Figure 15.7 is an example of the nonsurgical diagnosis and treatment of ectopic pregnancy. Figure 15.8 demonstrates how this may be accomplished with minimal use of surgery.

Cornual Pregnancy

A pregnancy that implants in the cornual segment of the tube tends to present several weeks later than a tubal pregnancy because the muscular cornu of the uterus is better able to expand and accommodate an enlarging pregnancy. As a result, rupture of a *cornual (isthmic) pregnancy* typically occurs between the eighth and sixteenth gestational weeks, and is often associated with massive hemorrhage, frequently requiring hysterectomy.

Combined Pregnancy

Combined pregnancy (coincident or heterotopic pregnancy) occurs in approximately 1 in 30,000 pregnancies with simultaneous intrauterine and extrauterine gestations. Associated with abnormal development of one twin or superfetation, the treatment of the intrauterine pregnancy is individualized depending on the maternal status and wishes, as well as the gestational age and clinical status of the pregnancy. Management of the extrauterine pregnancy

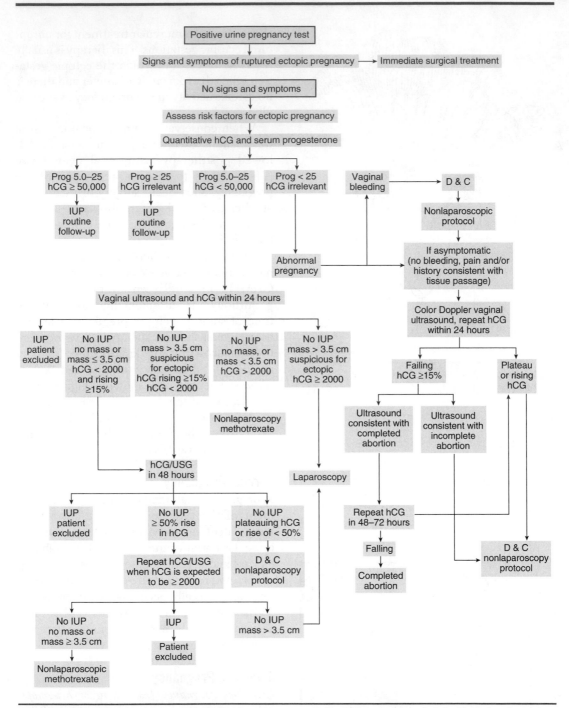

Figure 15.7. Algorithm for nonsurgical diagnosis and treatment of ectopic pregnancy. D & C, dilation and currettage; IUP, intrauterine pregnancy.

must account for the possible effect on the intrauterine gestation. Of the limited number of cases reported, approximately one in three of the intrauterine pregnancies is reported as surviving.

Nontubal Ectopic Pregnancy

Ectopic implantations outside the fallopian tube may present in a variety of ways and at different times in gestation, primarily related to the site of implantation. All are uncommon, deriving part

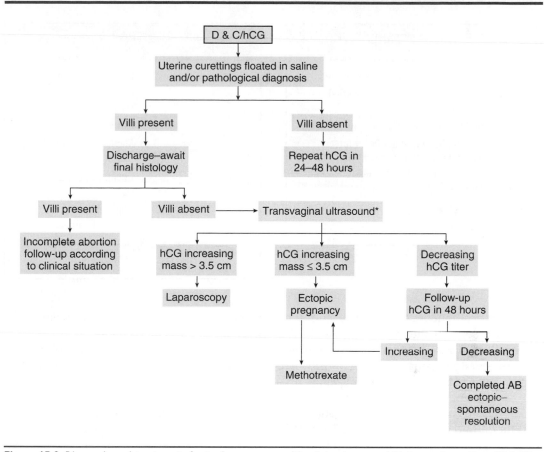

Figure 15.8. Diagnosis and treatment of ectopic pregnancy with minimal surgery (dilation and curettage [D & C]). *Repeat transvaginal ultrasound if performed >48 hours earlier. AB, abortion.

of their morbidity from their locations and the remainder from delayed diagnosis.

Abdominal pregnancy occurs in 1 in 3,000 to 4,000 pregnancies and more frequently occurs after assisted reproductive technology. In *primary abdominal pregnancy*, the fertilized ovum implants on peritoneal surfaces–in order of frequency, on the adnexae, broad ligaments, sigmoid colon, uterine fundus, and elsewhere in the abdominopelvic cavity. It occurs in association with müllerian tract anomalies, delayed ovulation, endometriosis, pelvic inflammatory disease, and fallopian tube dysfunction. *Secondary abdominal pregnancy* is more common and involves reimplantation in the abdominal cavity after the pregnancy has been separated from its primary site of implantation, such as in tubal abortion (expulsion of a tubal pregnancy out the fimbriated end), tubal pregnancy rupture, or uterine rupture. Physical findings

and symptoms are widely variable, depending on gestational age and site of implantation. Diagnosis is confirmed primarily by ultrasonography.

Abdominal pregnancy is usually discovered long before fetal viability; treatment is removal of the pregnancy. Survival of the fetus occurs in only 10% to 20% of cases, with up to one-half having significant deformity. The patient is given the option of continuing the pregnancy to fetal viability with operative delivery, or operative termination of the pregnancy at the time of diagnosis. In either case, removal of the placenta is usually not attempted because of the risk of uncontrollable hemorrhage. Treatment with methotrexate is commonly used to induce regression of the retained placenta.

Cervical pregnancy occurs in 1 in 10,000 to 20,000 pregnancies, when the ovum implants

Table 15.4. Rubin's Criteria for Cervical Pregnancy

- Cervical glands opposite placental attachment, chorionic villi in cervical canal, no chorionic villi in corpus
- Intimate attachment of placenta to cervix
- All or part of placenta must be situated below entrance of uterine vessels and anterior/posterior uteroperitoneal reflections
- No fetal elements in corpus uteri
- Internal cervical os closed, external cervical os open or closed

Table 15.5. Spiegelberg's Criteria for Ovarian Pregnancy

Fallopian tube	1. Intact, including fimbria
	2. Clearly separate from ovary
	3. Microscopically free of gestational tissue
Ovary	1. Occupies normal position
	2. Connected to uterus by ovarian ligament
	3. Ovarian tissue in wall of gestational sac

in the cervical mucosa below the level of the histologic cervical internal os (Table 15.4). Cervical pregnancy presents as an incomplete or threatened abortion, with uncontrollable hemorrhage as removal of the pregnancy tissue is attempted. Surgical treatment that avoids hysterectomy, i.e., conization, and arterial embolization have successfully treated cervical pregnancy; however, hysterectomy is often needed to control the bleeding that ensues when the cervical pregnancy is disrupted. Hysterectomy is especially common when the pregnancy is 12 weeks or more of gestational age. Methotrexate has been used when the

diagnosis is made earlier, thereby avoiding the need for surgical intervention.

Ovarian pregnancy occurs uncommonly, with an incidence estimated from 1 in 7,000 to 1 in 50,000 pregnancies. The types of ovarian pregnancy are primary and reimplantation, or secondary, as with abdominal pregnancy. The criteria of Spiegelberg define the requirements for ovarian pregnancy (Table 15.5), which has a low morbidity rate because it is often diagnosed as a tubal pregnancy and successfully treated by surgery, either wedge resection of the pregnancy or oophorectomy, depending on the extent of ovarian damage.

CHAPTER 16

MEDICAL AND SURGICAL CONDITIONS OF PREGNANCY

This chapter deals primarily with APGO Educational Topic:

Topic 17: Medical and Surgical Conditions of Pregnancy

Students should be able to discuss the diagnosis of each of the listed problems during pregnancy, the impact of pregnancy on the condition and the condition on the pregnancy (mother and fetus), and the initial management during pregnancy.

A. Anemia
B. Diabetes mellitus
C. Urinary tract disorders
D. Infectious diseases, including
   1. Herpes
   2. Rubella
   3. Group B Streptococcus
   4. Hepatitis
   5. HIV, human papillomavirus, and other sexually transmitted infections
   6. Cytomegalovirus
   7. Toxoplasmosis
   8. Varicella and parvovirus

E. Cardiac disease
F. Asthma
G. Alcohol, tobacco and substance abuse
H. The "surgical" abdomen during pregnancy.

Maternal medical or surgical condition can complicate the course of a pregnancy and/or be affected by pregnancy. Physicians providing obstetric care must have a thorough understanding of the effect of pregnancy on the natural course of a disorder, the effect of the disorder on a pregnancy, and the change in management of the pregnancy and/or disorder caused by their coincidence. In this chapter, a small portion of possible medical and surgical disorders are discussed, with more detailed coverage the province of textbooks of maternal–fetal medicine, internal medicine, and surgery.

Anemia

The plasma and cellular composition of blood changes significantly during pregnancy because of an expansion of plasma volume proportionally greater than that of the red blood cell mass. On average, there is a 1,000 mL increase in plasma volume and a 300 mL increase in red cell volume (a 3:1 ratio). Because the hematocrit (Hct) reflects the proportion of blood made up primarily of red blood cells, Hct demonstrates a "physiologic" decrease during pregnancy; therefore this decrease is not actually an anemia. *Anemia in pregnancy is generally defined as an Hct less than 30% or a hemoglobin of <10 g/dL.* Because of monthly blood loss with menstrual flow and contemporary dietary practices that may lack sufficient iron and protein, women often enter pregnancy with a lowered store of iron and sometimes a lowered Hct. When faced with the expansion of the maternal red cell mass and fetal iron needs, additional demands on the mother for iron outstrip the stores that are available; the result is iron deficiency anemia. It is for these reasons that supplemental iron is appropriately prescribed for pregnant women. Iron deficiency anemia is by far the most frequent type of anemia seen in pregnancy, accounting for more than 90% of cases.

Iron Deficiency Anemia

Because *iron deficiency is the most common form of anemia in pregnancy*, extensive evaluation of anemic pregnant patients should usually be delayed until an empiric trial of iron therapy is given and the effect observed. If the presumed iron deficiency anemia is severe, the classic findings are small, pale erythrocytes manifest on peripheral blood smears (microcytic, hypochromic anemia) and red cell indices that indicate a low mean corpuscular volume and low mean corpuscular hemoglobin concentration. Further laboratory studies usually demonstrate a decreased serum iron, an increased total iron-binding capacity, and a decrease in serum ferritin. A recent dietary history is obviously important, especially if pica exists (the consumption of non-nutrient substances such as starch, ice, or dirt). Such dietary compulsions may contribute to iron deficiency by decreasing the amount of nutritious food and iron consumed.

For patients with iron deficiency anemia, iron therapy is generally given in the form of ferrous sulfate, a 325-mg tablet taken twice daily. Each tablet contains approximately 60 mg of elemental iron, as do most standard prenatal vitamin/mineral supplements, thus a total elemental iron supplementation of about 120 mg/day. The response to therapy is first seen as an increase in the reticulocyte count approximately 1 week after the institution of iron therapy. Because of the plasma expansion associated with pregnancy, the Hct may not increase significantly, but rather stabilizes or increases only slightly.

Folate Deficiency Anemia

The second most common form of anemia seen in pregnancy is folate deficiency. Folate is found in green leafy vegetables and is now an added supplement in cereal, bread, and grain products. The demands of fetal and maternal growth during pregnancy (800 mcg/day) exceed the usual adult intake of 50 to 100 mcg/day, requiring folate supplementation. Folate deficiency is especially likely in multiple gestations or when patients are taking medications such as phenytoin (Dilantin), nitrofurantoin, or trimethoprim. Treatment of folate deficiency anemia is 1 mg of folate orally on a daily basis, the amount generally found in most prenatal vitamin supplements.

Other Anemias

The hereditary hemolytic anemias are also rare causes of anemia in pregnancy. Some examples are hereditary spherocytosis, an autosomal dominant defect of the erythrocyte membrane; glucose 6-phosphate dehydrogenase deficiency; and pyruvate kinase deficiency.

Thalassemia trait may also present as microcytic, hypochromic anemia, but unlike iron deficiency anemia, the serum iron and total iron-binding capacity are normal and the hemoglobin A_2 (HbA$_2$) is elevated.

Fetal Consequences of Maternal Anemia

The direct fetal consequences of anemia are minimal, although infants born to mothers with iron deficiency may have diminished iron stores as neonates. The maternal consequences of anemia are those associated with any adult anemia. If anemia is corrected, the woman with an adequate red cell mass enters the labor and delivery better able to respond to acute peripartum blood loss and to avoid the risks of blood or blood product transfusion.

The Hemoglobinopathies

The *hemoglobinopathies*, including the sickle cell diseases and the thalassemias, are disorders of polypeptide chains that comprise the oxygen-carrying hemoglobin molecule found in the blood cells (Table 16.1). These disorders usually involve abnormalities of the β-globulins; the oxygen-carrying capacity of the hemoglobin molecule, including its structural integrity under conditions of low oxygen tension, is impaired. When this results in deformity of the normal spheroid shape of the red blood cell, vaso-occlusive "crisis" ensues.

Besides the genetic implications, patients with the sickle cell trait (HbSA) have an increased risk of urinary infections, but experience no other pregnancy complications. Although the course of pregnancy can vary according to the type of hemoglobinopathy, there is individual variation among patients with the same type of disorder. Pregnancies in patients with HbS-β-thal are generally unaffected. Patients who are HbSS or HbSC, in contrast, may suffer vaso-occlusive episodes (crises), although infections are more common and should be ruled out before attributing any pain to a crisis. Although prophylactic maternal red cell transfusions have been popular in the past, the risks of multiple blood transfusions and the general improvement in outcome in patients with hemoglobinopathies without transfusion have shifted the therapeutic emphasis to conservative management. Transfusions are, for the most part, reserved for complications of hemoglobinopathies such as congestive heart failure, sickle cell disease crises unresponsive to hydration and analgesics, and severely low levels of hemoglobin. Antenatal assessment of fetal well-being and growth is an important part of managing patients with hemoglobinopathies.

Diabetes Mellitus

Approximately 2% of pregnancies are complicated by diabetes that either develops during pregnancy or was antecedent to pregnancy. In either case, diabetes has significant implications for mother and fetus during pregnancy, and conversely, pregnancy significantly affects diabetes.

Classification of Diabetes in Pregnancy

The White classification was used for many years to group cases of diabetes during pregnancy on the basis of age at onset of diabetes, duration of diabetes, and complications such as vascular disease. In recent years, the simpler classification of the American Diabetic Association (ADA) has become more commonly used. Three forms of glucose intolerance are identified in the ADA classification. *Type I diabetes* refers to diabetes diagnosed in childhood and is often brittle and difficult to control. It is thought to result from an immunologic destruction of cells of the pancreas. Diabetic

Table 16.1. The Hemoglobinopathies

Characteristic	Sickle Cell	HbSC Disease	Sickle Cell β-Thalassemia	α-Thalassemia	β-Thalassemia
Globin abnormality	HbS (valine substituted for glutamic acid at the sixth position) in one or both chains	One globin is HbS and the other is HbC (lysine substituted for valine at the position)	One globin is HbS and one globin allele codes for β-thalassemia; decreased synthesis of HbA	Normal hemoglobins; decreased production of globin chains	Normal hemoglobin; decreased production of β-globin chains
Genetics	Autosomal recessive sickle cell trait: heterozygous (one chain affected); <40% HbS; 1 in 12 Black Americans sickle cell disease: homozygous (both chains affected); 1 in 500 pregnancies in Black Americans	Autosomal recessive; 1 in 700 patients at risk	Autosomal recessive; 1 in 1,700 pregnancies; severity of disease depends on β-allele— from no HbA production (severe disease) to moderate production (milder disease)	Autosomal recessive; severity of disease (microcytic, hypochromic anemia) depends on expression and amount of globin produced— from none (homozygous) to 25%–75% (heterozygous)	Autosomal recessive; point mutations cause decreased β-chain synthesis Homozygous: β-thalassemia major (Cooley's anemia); no HbA produced; most is HbF or HbA_2; severe disease Heterozygous: β-thalassemia or β-thalassemia minor; one normal and one abnormal β-globin allele; usually mild-to-moderate disease
Risk groups	African, Mediterranean, Turkish, Arabian, and East Indian heritage			Asian, African, East Indian, and Mediterranean heritage	Mediterranean, Middle Eastern, African, East Indian, and Asian heritage

ketoacidosis (DKA) is common in patients with this type of diabetes.

Type II diabetes refers to the patient who has adult-onset glucose intolerance. These patients are frequently overweight and the disease can often be controlled with a carefully followed diet. This type of diabetes is thought to result from exhaustion of the cells rather than their destruction. *Gestational diabetes* refers to a new glucose intolerance identified during pregnancy. In most patients, it subsides postpartum, although glucose intolerance in subsequent years occurs more frequently in this group of patients.

Diabetes in Pregnancy: Physiology and Pathophysiology

Dietary habits are frequently changed during pregnancy, most notably with a decrease in food intake early in pregnancy because of nausea and vomiting and altered food choices. Several pregnancy-associated hormones also have a major effect on glucose metabolism. Most notable of these is human placental lactogen (hPL), which is produced in abundance by the enlarging placenta. The hPL affects both fatty acid and glucose metabolism. It promotes lipolysis with increased levels of circulating free fatty acids and causes a decrease in glucose uptake. In this manner, hPL can be thought of as an anti-insulin. The increasing production of this hormone as pregnancy advances generally requires ongoing changes in insulin therapy to adjust for this effect.

Other hormones that have demonstrated lesser effects include estrogen and progesterone, which interfere with the insulin-glucose relation, and insulinase, which is produced by the placenta and degrades insulin to a limited extent. These effects of pregnancy on glucose metabolism make the management of pregnancy-associated diabetes difficult. Diabetic ketoacidosis, for example, is more common in pregnant patients.

With increased renal blood flow, the simple diffusion of glucose in the glomerulus increases beyond the ability of tubular reabsorption, resulting in the *normal glucosuria of pregnancy*, commonly of approximately 300 mg/day. In patients with diabetes, this glucosuria may be much greater, but because of the poor correlation of pregnancy glucosuria values and simultaneous blood glucose concentrations, using urinary glucose is of little value in glucose management during pregnancy. This glucose-rich urine is also an excellent environment for bacterial growth so that pregnant women with diabetes have twice the incidence of urinary tract infection than pregnant women without diabetes experience.

In addition to the added difficulties of glucose management and the increased risk of DKA during pregnancy, mothers with diabetes have a twofold increase in the incidence of pregnancy-induced hypertension, or preeclampsia, compared with patients without diabetes. Diabetic retinopathy worsens in approximately 15% of pregnant patients with diabetes, some proceeding to proliferative retinopathy and loss of vision if the process remains untreated by laser coagulation.

Infants of mothers with diabetes are at a threefold increased risk of congenital anomalies over the 1% to 2% baseline risk of all patients. The most commonly encountered anomalies are cardiac and limb deformities. Sacral agenesis is a unique but rare anomaly for this group. Excessive fetal growth, or macrosomia (usually defined as a fetal weight in excess of either 4,000 or 4,500 g), is more common in pregnant patients with diabetes because of the fetal metabolic effects of increased glucose transfer across the placenta. This excessive neonatal size can lead to problems with fetopelvic disproportion during labor, requiring cesarean section or causing shoulder dystocia at the time of attempted vaginal delivery.

The neonatal hypoglycemia often encountered in these infants results from the sudden change in the steady-state arrangement, wherein increased glucose crossing the placenta was countered in the fetus by an increase in insulin levels. Once separated from the maternal supply of glucose, the higher level of insulin can cause a significant neonatal hypoglycemia. In addition, these newborns are subject to an increased incidence of neonatal hyperbilirubinemia, hypocalcemia, and polycythemia.

Another complication of pregnancy in patients with diabetes is an increase in amniotic fluid volume above 2,000 mL, a condition known as hydramnios, or polyhydramnios. Encountered in approximately 10% of mothers with diabetes, the increases in amniotic fluid volume and uterine size are associated with an increased risk of abruptio placentae and preterm labor as well as postpartum uterine atony.

The risk of spontaneous abortion is similar in patients with well-controlled diabetes and in patients without diabetes, but the risk is significantly increased for the patients with diabetes if glucose control is poor. There is also an increased risk of intrauterine fetal demise and stillbirth, especially when diabetic control is inadequate.

Infants of mothers with diabetes also tend to have an increased frequency of respiratory distress syndrome. The usual tests of lung maturity may be less predictive for these infants.

Laboratory Diagnosis of Glucose Intolerance/Diabetes in Pregnancy

Approximately 1% of all pregnant patients are diabetic before pregnancy. For these patients, management ideally begins before conception with the goal of optimal glucose control before and during pregnancy.

Gestational diabetes is usually identified by prenatal screening of all pregnancy patients, although it may be suspected in patients with known risk factors for gestational diabetes, including a history of giving birth to an infant weighing >4,000 g, a history of repeated spontaneous abortions, a history of unexplained stillbirth, a strong family history of diabetes, obesity, and/or persistent glucosuria. However, 50% of patients identified as having gestational diabetes do not have such risk factors, and this is the rationale for universal glucose screening in pregnancy.

The most commonly used screening test for glucose intolerance during pregnancy does not require the patient to be in a fasting state: 1 hour after consuming 50 g of glucose solution, blood is drawn for plasma glucose determination. Patients whose glucose value exceeds 140 mg/dL require a standard 3-hour glucose tolerance test using 100 g of glucose. (Some tests use 135 mg/dL as the upper limit of normal for the 1-hour screen, increasing the number of patients with diabetes discovered at the expense of an increase in the number of women screened.) Two or more abnormal values on the 3-hour test make the diagnosis of gestational diabetes.

In patients lacking any risk factors, the 1-hour glucose screening is usually performed between 24 and 28 weeks of gestation because glucose intolerance is generally manifest by that time. In patients with factors suggesting possible glucose intolerance, the testing is performed at the onset of prenatal care and, if normal then, repeated as the third trimester commences. Using this screening method, approximately 15% of patients have an abnormal screening test. Of those patients who then proceed to have the standard 3-hour oral glucose tolerance test, approximately 15% are diagnosed as having gestational diabetes.

Management of Diabetes During Pregnancy

Often overlooked or underemphasized in the overall management of a patient whose pregnancy is complicated by diabetes mellitus is the importance of patient education. The patient with long-standing diabetes should realize that much tighter control of her glucose levels is advised during pregnancy, with greater attention to, and more frequent monitoring of, glucose values. The impact of pregnancy on diabetes, and vice versa, must also be emphasized to the pregnant patient with diabetes. The patient with newly diagnosed diabetes should receive general diabetic counseling, along with information about the unique features of the combination of diabetes and pregnancy. Home glucose monitoring is the norm, and instruction in technique should be provided. Whether diabetes is newly diagnosed or long-standing, intense management may be stressful, and all those involved with obstetric care should be mindful of the extra emotional attention many of these patients need.

The overall goal of management is to control glucose values within fairly circumscribed limits, to serially evaluate fetal well-being, and to time delivery to maximize outcome for both mother and fetus/neonate. The mainstay of diabetes management is nutritional counseling about an appropriate diet. The recommended diet is about 35 Kcal/kg of ideal body weight, composed of approximately 45% complex carbohydrates, 35% fat, and 20% protein. With careful attention to diet, most gestational mothers with diabetes do not require insulin.

Patients are instructed to obtain a morning fasting glucose, along with periodic glucose values throughout the day and evening. The precise goals for glucose control vary, but in general the fasting plasma glucose should be maintained in the 90 to 100 mg/100 mL range, and the values obtained throughout the day at less than 120 to 140 mg/100 mL.

For patients who do not need exogenous insulin, the perinatal outcome is good. Pregnancy is allowed to continue to term, with delivery planned at that time.

For patients unable to achieve the goals for glucose as stated, exogenous insulin is prescribed. Frequently a combination of NPH (neutral protamine Hagedorn) and regular insulin is used, based on the time of day or night when glucose values are high. Insulin does not cross the placenta and, therefore, does not directly affect the fetus. However, glucose does cross the placenta (by facilitated diffusion) and, at high levels, can affect the infant soon after delivery, as previously noted. Also, the increased insulin production converts glucose to fat, resulting in the heavier infants (macrosomia) often noted in patients with diabetes.

Patients with diabetes are followed closely through pregnancy, usually at 1- to 2-week intervals. Insulin adjustments are made on the basis of the glucose logs maintained by the patient. Also, as previously described, insulin requirements of a pregnant patient are expected to increase as pregnancy advances because of the rising production of hPL by the placenta, with its insulin-resistant effect.

A fraction of hemoglobin known as hemoglobin A_{1c} reflects glucose values over the preceding 6 to 8 weeks. This test has been used to monitor glucose control and to predict the likelihood of congenital anomalies in patients with diabetes early in pregnancy. Pregnant patients with diabetes, especially type I diabetes, are prone to DKA. This serious complication can usually be avoided with frequent monitoring of blood glucose levels, attention to diet, careful insulin administration, and the avoidance of infections. Management of DKA is not different from management of DKA in nonpregnant patients, and consists of adequate fluids, insulin, glucose, and electrolyte stabilization. Fetal death can accompany DKA, so electronic fetal monitoring of the fetus is essential until the maternal metabolic status is stabilized. At the other end of the spectrum, hypoglycemia is encountered at times, especially early in pregnancy, when nausea and vomiting interfere with caloric intake. Although hypoglycemia does not have untoward effects on the fetus, the symptoms and potential trauma that the patient may experience should be avoided.

Infections are more frequently encountered in mothers with diabetes, especially urinary tract infections because the risk of urinary tract infection and pyelonephritis is increased.

Patients should also be told to promptly report any other symptoms that suggest infection so identification and treatment can be initiated.

Because of the risk of progressive retinopathy, patients with diabetes should have an ophthalmologic evaluation. Also, because of the risk of renal disease and the higher likelihood of developing preeclampsia later in pregnancy, 24-hour urine collections to determine the level of proteinuria and creatinine clearance are often used.

Beginning at approximately 30 to 32 weeks of gestation, various measures to evaluate the fetal growth and well-being are undertaken. Daily fetal kick counts are an inexpensive and reliable screening test for fetal well-being. Serial nonstress testing and/or biophysical profile measurements are also initiated, usually on a once or twice weekly schedule, but more frequently if clinical indicators warrant. Serial ultrasonography is performed to detect fetal anomalies and developing polyhydramnios and to follow fetal growth. Fetuses of mothers with diabetes are more prone to cardiac defects, so specialized fetal cardiac ultrasounds are often recommended. Both intrauterine growth restriction and macrosomia are seen in infants of mothers with diabetes. When the estimated fetal weight by ultrasound late in pregnancy is >4,000 g, cesarean section is often recommended to avoid the risk of shoulder dystocia and other birth trauma.

With respect to delivery, the usual goal is for the patient with diabetes to deliver a healthy child vaginally. The adequacy of glucose control, the well-being of the infant, estimated fetal weight by ultrasound, the presence of hypertension or other complications of pregnancy, the gestational age, the presentation of the fetus, and the status of the cervix are all factors involved in decisions regarding delivery. *In the well-controlled patient with diabetes who has no complications, induction at term (38 to 39 weeks) is often undertaken.* If an earlier delivery is deemed necessary for either fetal or maternal indications, fetal maturity studies may be performed on amniotic fluid obtained by amniocentesis.

Whether the patient's labor begins spontaneously or is induced, intrapartum glucose control may be managed by a constant glucose infusion of a 5% dextrose solution at 100 mL/hr with frequent plasma glucose assessments. Short-acting insulin may be administered if needed, usually by constant intravenous infusion. Somewhat surprisingly, patients whose glucose has been difficult to control through pregnancy often have satisfactory levels of glucose in labor when so managed.

With delivery of the placenta, the source of the "anti-insulin" factors, hPL, is removed. With its short half-life, its effect on plasma glucose is evident within hours. Many patients do not require any insulin whatsoever in the first several postpartum days, and routine management generally consists of frequent glucose determinations using a sliding scale approach with minimal insulin injections. The goals for optimal glucose values are less stringent in the puerperium than during pregnancy. For patients with gestational diabetes, no further insulin is required postpartum. In patients with preexisting diabetes, insulin is generally resumed at 50% of the prepregnant dose once a patient is consuming a normal diet. Thereafter, insulin can be adjusted over the ensuing weeks, with requirements usually reaching the prepregnancy level.

Over 95% of mothers with gestational diabetes return to a completely normal glucose status postpartum. Glucose tolerance screening is advocated 2 to 4 months postpartum for these patients to detect the 3% to 5% who remain diabetic and require treatment. A fasting plasma glucose of >140 mg/dL or a 2-hour post-75 g glucose load of >200 mg/dL requires close follow-up.

For contraception, barrier methods or intrauterine devices are often chosen; patients who choose oral contraceptives should monitor their glucose values to identify an increase that is sometimes seen with this method.

Urinary Tract Disorders

Urinary tract infections are common in pregnancy. Approximately 8% of all women (pregnant and nonpregnant) have >10^5 colonies of a single bacterial species on a midstream culture. Approximately 25% of the pregnant portion of this group develop an acute, symptomatic urinary tract infection. Compared with non-pregnant women with similar colony counts on urine culture, asymptomatic bacteriuria in pregnancy is more likely to lead to cystitis and pyelonephritis. The increased incidence of symptomatic infection during pregnancy is thought to be caused by pregnancy-associated urinary stasis and glucosuria. This relative urinary stasis in pregnancy is a result of progesterone-induced decreased ureteral tone and motility, mechanical compression of the ureters at the pelvic brim, and compression of the bladder and ureteral orifices. In addition, the pH of the urine is increased because of increased bicarbonate excretion, which also enhances bacterial growth.

It is standard to obtain a urine culture at the onset of prenatal care and to treat patients with *asymptomatic bacteriuria*. Ampicillin (500 mg orally four times a day), sulfisoxazole (Gantrisin; 1 g orally four times a day), or nitrofurantoin (Macrodantin; 50 mg orally four times a day) for 7 to 10 days is usually effective. The most common organism identified is *Escherichia coli*. Approximately 25% to 30% of patients not treated for asymptomatic bacteriuria proceed to symptomatic urinary tract infection; hence, this treatment should prevent approximately 70% of symptomatic urinary tract infections in pregnancy. However, 1.5% of patients with initial negative cultures also develop symptomatic urinary tract infections in pregnancy. Suppressive antimicrobial therapy (nitrofurantoin, 50 to 100 mg orally four times a day) is indicated if there are repetitive urinary tract infections during pregnancy or following pyelonephritis during pregnancy. Consideration should be given to postpartum radiographic evaluation of these patients to identify renal parenchymal and urinary-collecting duct abnormalities.

Acute cystitis occurs in approximately 1% of pregnancies, and the treatment is the same as for asymptomatic bacteriuria.

Patients with *pyelonephritis* are acutely ill, with fever, costovertebral tenderness, general malaise, and often dehydration. Approximately 20% of these ill patients demonstrate increased uterine activity and preterm labor, and approximately 10% have positive blood cultures if they are obtained in the acute febrile phase of the disease. Pyelonephritis occurs in 2% of all pregnant patients and is one of the most common medical complications of pregnancy requiring hospitalization, especially in its context as a major cause of maternal mortality (septic shock). After a urinalysis and urine culture are obtained, patients are treated with intravenous hydration and antibiotics, commonly cephalosporin or ampicillin and gentamicin. Uterine contractions may accompany these symptoms, and specific tocolytic therapy may be required if preterm labor ensues. It is known that *E. coli* can produce phospholipase A, which in turn can promote prostaglandin synthesis, resulting in an increase in uterine activity. Fever is also known to induce contractions, so antipyretics are required for a temperature >100°F. Attention must be paid to the patient's response to therapy and her general condition; sepsis occurs in 2% to 3% of patients with pyelonephritis, and adult respiratory distress syndrome can be seen. If improvement does not occur within 48 to 72 hours, urinary tract obstruction or urinary calculus should be considered along with a reevaluation of antibiotic coverage. An ultrasound or other imaging study will sometimes identify a calculus or abscess. The organisms most commonly cultured from the urine of symptomatic pregnant patients are *E. coli* and other Gram-negative aerobes. Follow-up can be with either frequent urine cultures and/or empiric antibiotic suppression with an agent such as nitrofurantoin.

Recurrent symptoms or failure to respond to usual therapy suggests another cause for the findings. In these patients, a complete urologic evaluation 6 weeks after pregnancy may be warranted.

Urinary calculi are identified in approximately 1 in 1,500 patients during pregnancy, although pregnancy per se does not promote stone development. Symptoms similar to those of pyelonephritis but without fever suggest urinary calculi. Microhematuria is more common with this condition than in uncomplicated urinary tract infection. Although renal colic pain may be found typically, it is seen less frequently in pregnancy than in the nonpregnant state because of the hormone-induced relaxation of ureteral tone. Usually, hydration and expectant management, along with straining of urine in search of stones, suffice as management.

Occasionally, however, the presence of a stone can lead to infection and/or complete obstruction, which may require drainage by either ureteral stent or percutaneous nephrostomy.

Pregnancy in patients with preexisting renal disease is encountered frequently because treatments such as dialysis and transplantation allow these patients to have health sufficient to support ovulation and pregnancy. During preconception counseling, these patients should be advised of the significant risks involved in a pregnancy, and that pregnancy outcome is related to the degree of serum creatinine elevation and the presence of hypertension.

Overall, pregnancy does not seem to have a negative impact on chronic renal diseases. In general, patients with mild renal impairment (serum creatinine <1.5 mg/dL) have relatively uneventful pregnancies, provided other complications are absent. Patients with moderate renal impairment (serum creatinine 1.5 to 3.0 mg/dL) have a more guarded prognosis with an increased incidence of deterioration of renal function. Patients with severe renal impairment have the worst outcome. In approximately 50% of patients with renal disease, proteinuria is noted. An increase in proteinuria during pregnancy is not, by itself, a serious consequence. The presence of hypertension before pregnancy or the development of hypertension during pregnancy is a more worrisome finding with respect to both the course of the patient's renal disease and the pregnancy.

In addition to hypertension, there is an increased incidence of *intrauterine growth restriction in patients with chronic renal disease*. Serial assessments of fetal well-being and growth are frequently performed. Pregnancy following renal transplantation is generally associated with a good prognosis if at least 2 years have elapsed since the transplant was performed, and thorough renal assessment reveals no evidence of active disease or rejection. Drug therapy should be minimal.

Infectious Diseases in Pregnancy

Herpes

Herpes simplex virus (HSV) is a DNA virus that poses significant risk to the fetus/neonate. There are two types of HSV: HSV-1, which is usually involved in oral lesions, and HSV-2, which is primarily responsible for genital infections. However, up to 15% of genital herpes cases are caused by HSV-1. Herpes infections are categorized as first episode primary (no HSV-1 or HSV-2 antibodies), first episode nonprimary (with circulating antibodies, usually to HSV-1), or recurrent disease. It is the primary form that poses the greatest risk to the fetus. The fetus/neonate is infected either from ascending infection following spontaneous rupture of membrane, or from passage through an infected lower genital tract at delivery. With a primary infection, the neonatal risk approaches 50%; it is far lower with recurrent infection, as the size of the inoculum is much decreased. Most infants with localized herpes ultimately do well; as a rule, those infants with disseminated infection do very poorly.

The diagnosis of HSV infection is suspected when clinical examination shows the characteristic tender vesicles with ulceration followed by crusting. Confirmation is by cell culture, with most positive results reported within 72 hours. Multinucleated giant cells can be seen on Pap smears or with the use of a Tzanck test in approximately 50% of cases.

If infection with herpes virus is suspected during the course of pregnancy, a culture from a lesion is generally obtained to confirm the diagnosis. In such patients, or any patient with a history of herpes virus infection, careful visualization of the lower genital tract is important at the onset of labor or when rupture of membranes occurs. If no lesions are identified, vaginal delivery is deemed safe. Cesarean delivery is recommended if herpes lesions are identified on the cervix, in the vagina, or on the vulva at the time of labor or spontaneous rupture of membrane. This is true whether or not the lesions are associated with primary or recurrent infection. Acyclovir or related compounds are used if symptoms are serious, and also may be, and often are, used as prophylaxis against outbreaks near term.

Rubella

Rubella (German or 3-day measles) is an RNA virus with important perinatal impact if infection occurs during pregnancy. Widespread immunization programs in the last 30 years have prevented periodic epidemics of rubella, but about 15% of reproductive-age women lack immunity to this virus and are, therefore, susceptible to infection. A history of prior infection is unreliable in 50% of cases. Once infection occurs, immunity is lifelong.

If a woman develops rubella infection in the first trimester of pregnancy, there is an increased risk of both spontaneous abortion and congenital rubella syndrome. Although 50% to 70% of infants with congenital rubella appear normal at birth, many subsequently develop signs of infection. Common defects associated with the syndrome include congenital heart disease (e.g., patent ductus arteriosus), mental retardation, deafness, and cataracts. The risk of congenital rubella is related to the gestational age at the time of infection, from about 50% if acquired in the first month of pregnancy, decreasing to about 5% if acquired midpregnancy. Primary infection can be diagnosed using acute and convalescent sera for IgM and IgG antibodies.

Because of the serious fetal implications, prenatal screening for IgG rubella antibody is routine. Young women should be vaccinated when they are not pregnant if they are *susceptible*. The vaccine uses a live attenuated rubella virus that induces antibodies in more than 95% of vaccinations. It is recommended that pregnancy be delayed 3 months following immunization, although congenital rubella syndrome following vaccination during an undiagnosed pregnancy has not been reported. In women whose prenatal screen identifies a lack of rubella antibody, vaccination at the time of hospital discharge postpartum is recommended. Such management poses no risk to the newborn or other children; breast feeding is not contraindicated.

Because there is no effective treatment for a pregnant patient infected with rubella, patients who do not have immunity are advised to avoid potential exposure. Human immune g-globulin does not prevent or lessen the effect of infection; no antiviral therapy is available. Maternal treatment is supportive.

Group B Streptococcus

The group B β-hemolytic streptococcus (GBS) is an important cause of perinatal infections.

Asymptomatic cervical colonization occurs in up to 30% of pregnant women, but cultures may be positive only intermittently, even in the same patient. Approximately 50% of infants exposed to the organism in the lower genital tract will become colonized. For most of these infants, such colonization is of no consequence, but for approximately 2 to 3 infants per 1,000 live births, significant clinical infection occurs.

There are two manifestations of clinical infection of the newborn, termed early-onset (2 to 3 per 1,000 neonates) and late-onset (1/1,000 neonates). Early-onset infection is manifest as septicemia and septic shock, pneumonia, and/or meningitis. Such an infection is much more likely in premature infants than in term gestations. Late-onset infection occurs up to 4 weeks after delivery. Meningitis is the most common specific infection, but bone and joint infections can occur. Prematurity is not a factor for late-onset infection.

Recommendations regarding GBS management during pregnancy have evolved. To avoid serious infections in a few neonates (2 to 3 per 1,000), what should be done to the many pregnant patients (up to 30%) who harbor the organism at various times during the course of pregnancy? Currently, mothers with a high risk for perinatal infection (e.g., preterm labor, ruptured membranes) are treated empirically when the factor is identified, and all patients are screened with cultures of the vagina/rectum late in pregnancy; those patients with positive cultures are treated in labor. Patients with negative cultures are treated in labor if the duration of rupture of membranes exceeds 18 hours. Other indications for empiric treatment include a history of a previous infant with GBS infection, an intrapartum fever, or a history of maternal urinary tract infection with GBS (denotes high inoculum of the organism).

In the mother, postpartum endometritis may be caused by infection with GBS. The onset is often sudden and within 24 hours of delivery. Significant fever and tachycardia are present; sepsis may follow.

Hepatitis

Hepatitis A has no specific effects on pregnancy or the fetus. Immunoglobulin administration to exposed patients is safe.

Hepatitis B is a much more serious infection, regardless of pregnancy status. The carrier rate for hepatitis B is 1/1,000 adults in the United States, and much higher in some other countries. Testing for hepatitis B surface antigen (HBsAg) during pregnancy is routine, as about half of pregnant women infected lack traditional high-risk factors. Vertical transmission of hepatitis occurs to a significant, but variable, extent. It is related to the presence or absence of maternal HBeAg: if the patient is positive for the "e" antigen, her fetus has up to a 90% risk of becoming infected, and most will become chronic carriers. If negative for this "e" antigen, transmission may be as low as 10%, and far fewer of those infected remain carriers. Fetal/neonatal infection is more common if maternal infection occurs in the third trimester or the several months following delivery; neonatal infection can also be via breast milk. In utero, transplacental infection is unusual.

All infants now receive vaccination against hepatitis B, with the initial injection given within 2 two days of delivery. Infants of mothers with evidence of hepatitis B are also given hepatitis B immune globulin (HBIG) very soon after delivery.

Hepatitis C is a growing problem with obstetric implications. Similar to hepatitis B in transmission, it is often asymptomatic. Screening for evidence of infection is not routine. The presence of hepatitis C antibody does not prevent transmission of infection. Vertical transmission occurs in about 5% of cases, with the risk of fetal infection directly related to the hepatitis C RNA virus load.

HIV/AIDS Syndrome

Worldwide, women account for nearly 50% of those infected with HIV. The U.S. Centers for Disease Control and Prevention (CDC) estimates that 22% of those living with AIDS in America were women. Of these women, 61% were exposed through heterosexual contact and 36% through injection drug use. One percent of those living with AIDS were children under the age of 13, most of whom acquired the infection perinatally

The HIV is a single-strand, RNA-enveloped human retrovirus that has the ability to become incorporated into cellular DNA. The virus attaches to cells with high CD4 surface receptor concentrations such as lymphocytes, monocytes, and some neural cells. Once infected, seroconversion usually occurs from 3 to 12 weeks, but may take up to 12 months. Based on an antigen-antibody reaction, the HIV enzyme-linked immunosorbent assay (ELISA) generally becomes positive at a mean of about 4 months' time. The Western blot test, which identifies antibodies to specific portions of the virus, is performed to confirm the diagnosis. A serologic test is reported as positive if both the ELISA and the Western blot analyses are positive. If the Western blot test is negative, the test is reported as negative.

The sensitivity and specificity of HIV serologic testing is >99%. The usual estimated latency period from untreated HIV to AIDS is about 11 years. The HIV infection becomes AIDS as the helper (CD4) lymphocyte count decreases and the host becomes more susceptible. With the availability of increasingly effective antiretroviral drugs, life span and quality of life are improving.

Rapid HIV testing is a valuable alternative to the conventional testing previously discussed. Results can be available as soon as 1 to 2 hours after the blood sample is obtained, and thus is especially useful when a patient of unknown HIV status presents in labor.

Universal, voluntary HIV screening for pregnant women is standard and should be included in the prenatal laboratory "package" unless a patient states that she does not want HIV testing.

The HIV infection appears to have no direct effect on pregnancy course or outcome. Likewise, pregnancy does seem to affect the course of HIV. Both HIV and pregnancy may affect the natural history, presentation, treatment, or significance of certain infections, and these, in turn, may be associated with pregnancy complications or perinatal infection. These infections include vulvovaginal candidiasis, bacterial vaginosis, genital herpes simplex, human papilloma virus, syphilis, cytomegalovirus, toxoplasmosis, and hepatitis B and C. In both HIV-positive and HIV-negative women there is a decline in absolute CD4 cell counts in pregnancy, which is thought to be secondary to hemodilution. On the other hand, the percentage of CD4 cells remains relatively stable. Therefore, percentage, rather than absolute number, may be a more accurate measure of immune function for HIV-infected women.

The baseline rate of perinatal HIV transmission without prophylactic therapy is approximately 25%, and is generally related to higher viral loads and lower CD4 counts. With zidovudine monotherapy, perinatal transmission was reduced to ~8%. Finally, with vigorous antiretroviral therapy and a viral load of <1,000 copies, perinatal transmission is reduced to 1% to 2%. There is evidence that transmission can occur vertically, intrapartum, or postpartum through breast-feeding; however, 66% to 75% of transmission appears to occur during or close to the intrapartum period, particularly in non breast-feeding populations.

In regard to duration of rupture of membranes, the likelihood of transmission increased linearly with increasing duration or rupture of membranes, with a 2% increase in risk for each hourly increment. Women with clinical AIDS have the most pronounced risk, with a 31% probability of transmission after 24 hours of ruptured membranes. The use of fetal scalp electrodes or fetal scalp sampling increases exposure of the fetus to maternal blood and genital secretions, and may increase the risk of vertical transmission, depending on the serum and genital HIV viral load. Use of episiotomy or vacuum extraction or forceps may potentially increase risk of transmission by increasing exposure to maternal blood and genital secretions. However, judicious use of these techniques to shorten duration of labor or rupture of membranes with vaginal delivery may decrease the likelihood of transmission. Antiretroviral therapy in pregnancy is a key component to reduction of perinatal transmission to as low as 1.1%. Finally, cesarean delivery performed before the onset of labor and rupture of membrane significantly reduces the risk of perinatal HIV transmission, from 8% to 2%.

Breast feeding plays a significant role in perinatal HIV transmission; it is estimated to have accounted for up to 50% of newly infected children globally. Breast feeding in the setting of established maternal infection has an estimated additional risk of 14% transmission.

Human Papillomavirus

More than one-third of sexually active females have been exposed to human papillomavirus. The lesions (condyloma acuminate) increase in size and area during pregnancy, and, if extensive, may require cesarean delivery to avoid excessive trauma to the lower genital tract. Human papillomavirus is discussed elsewhere in the text (see Chapter 28).

Syphilis

Syphilis is caused by the motile spirochete pallidum, which survives only in vivo. The spirochete is transmitted by direct contact, invading intact mucous membranes or areas of abraded skin. A painless ulcer at the site of inoculation follows, usually within 6 weeks following exposure. The ulcer is firm, with elevated edges; it lasts for several weeks. One to 3 months later, a skin rash occurs, or, in some patients, raised lesions (condyloma lata) appear on the genitalia.

Treponema pallidum is generally considered to cross the placenta to the fetus after 16 weeks of gestation, although transmission has been documented at as early as 6 weeks of gestation.

Abortion, stillbirth, and neonatal death are more frequent in any untreated patient, whereas neonatal infection is more likely in primary or secondary rather than latent syphilis. Infants with congenital syphilis may be asymptomatic or have the classic stigmata of the syndrome, although most infants do not develop evidence of disease for 10 to 14 days after delivery. Early evidence of disease includes a maculopapular rash, "snuffles," mucous patches on the oropharynx, hepatosplenomegaly, jaundice, lymphadenopathy, and chorioretinitis. Later signs include Hutchinson teeth, mulberry molars, saddle nose, and saber shins.

Screening in pregnancy is mandatory. Serologic testing is the mainstay of diagnosis. Nontreponemal tests (Venereal Disease Research Laboratory [VDRL], rapid plasma reagin) are sometimes falsely positive; treponemal-specific tests (fluorescent treponemal antibody absorption) are used to confirm infection and identify antibody specific against *T. pallidum*. Importantly, a positive result indicates either active disease or previous exposure, i.e., the test remains positive.

Treatment consists of a single 2.4 MIU intramuscular benzathine penicillin injection for primary and secondary infection, or latent disease of a duration <1 year. For latent disease of a duration >1 year, three injections are given at weekly intervals. Patients with known penicillin sensitivity generally require desensitization because penicillin is the only antibiotic that can cross the placenta in adequate amounts to treat the fetus. Posttreatment titers should be followed serially for 2 years. A fourfold increase in serologic titer or persistent or recurrent signs or symptoms indicates inadequate treatment or reinfection, and re-treatment is indicated in either case. Response to therapy is again evaluated by following serologic titers.

Gonorrhea

Routine antepartum screening for *Neisseria gonorrhoeae* is universal, with recovery rates of 1% to 7%, depending on the population. Treatment is with ceftriaxone or any of several other alternative regimens. Infection above the cervix (i.e., of the uterus, including the fetus, and the fallopian tubes) is rare after the first weeks of pregnancy. At delivery, however, infected mothers may transmit the organism, causing gonococcal ophthalmia in the neonate. In the past, such infection was a prominent cause of blindness, but currently used routine prophylactic treatment of the newborn's eyes with silver nitrate, erythromycin, or tetracycline is generally effective in preventing neonatal gonorrhea.

Cytomegalovirus

Cytomegalovirus (CMV) infection affects 1% of births in the United States, and it is the most common congenital infection. A DNA virus, it may be transmitted in saliva, semen, cervical secretions, breast milk, blood, or urine. A CMV infection is often asymptomatic, although it can cause a short febrile illness. Similar to the herpes virus to which it is related, CMV may have dormant periods, only to reactivate at a later time. The prevalence of antibodies to CMV is inversely proportional to socioeconomic status.

Primary maternal infection, which occurs in 1% to 2% of pregnancies, is associated with a 50% risk of intrauterine infection, whereas the risk of intrauterine infection with recurrent infection is much lower, 2.0% or less. Intrauterine growth restriction is sometimes noted. Many infants are asymptomatic, but petechiae, hepatosplenomegaly, and thrombocytopenia may be seen. Microcephaly, chorioretinitis, hearing loss, and mental retardation may also be identified. The virus can be cultured, and IgM and IgG serology testing is available.

There is no treatment of maternal infection. Acyclovir treatment of newborn infection has been used, but remains experimental.

Toxoplasmosis

Infection with the intracellular parasite *Toxoplasma gondii* occurs primarily through ingestion of the infectious tissue cysts in raw or poorly cooked meat or through contact with feces from infected cats, which contain infectious sporulated oocytes. The latter may remain infectious in moist soil for more than 1 year. Only cats that hunt and kill their prey are reservoirs for infection; those that eat prepared cat food are not. In humans, asymptomatic infection is common. Approximately one-third of reproductive-age women have antibodies to toxoplasmosis.

Risk of congenital infection is limited to pregnant women with primary infection. Infection in the first trimester causes more severe fetal disease than infection in the third trimester, but, conversely, the risk of infection declines as pregnancy advances.

Over half of infants whose mothers are infected during the last trimester of pregnancy have serologic evidence of infection, but three-fourths of these show no gross evidence of infection at birth. However, congenital disease can cause severe mental retardation with chorioretinitis, blindness, epilepsy, intracranial calcifications, and hydrocephalus.

Because infection is usually asymptomatic, diagnosis depends on serologic testing. Unfortunately, these tests cannot predict the time of infection with accuracy, so the routine screening of patients is not recommended. Furthermore, such testing is of limited value in specific clinical situations. Fetal blood testing is possible, and is sometimes used if infection is likely to have occurred in the first half of pregnancy.

Treatment of toxoplasmosis with pyrimethamine and sulfadiazine may decrease the risk of congenital infection and/or the severity of manifestations.

Prevention of infection should be an important part of prenatal care, including the strong suggestion that all meats are to be thoroughly cooked and that cats are to be kept indoors and fed only processed foods. If a cat is kept outside, someone other than a pregnant woman should feed and care for the cat and its wastes.

Varicella

Congenital varicella (chicken pox) infection can be serious, but this is very unusual. It almost always occurs when maternal infection occurs in the first half of pregnancy. Most patients are immune, even if they or their families do not recall their having been infected. A pregnant patient who is thought to be susceptible can have serologic testing (IgM and IgG) within 4 days of exposure, and, if truly susceptible, be given varicella zoster immune globulin. It is unclear whether varicella zoster immune globulin reduces the risk of, and severity of, maternal and fetal infection.

If clinical infection occurs in a patient between 5 days prior to delivery and 2 days after delivery, neonatal infection can be severe, even deadly. Varicella zoster immune globulin is given to infants in such situations, though protection is not complete.

Varicella pneumonia is much more common in adults than in children, and can be serious. It seems to occur more frequently during pregnancy. Treatment is with acyclovir.

Parvovirus

Parvovirus (fifth disease) has particular ramifications during pregnancy because maternal infection can lead to abortion, fetal nonimmune hydrops fetalis, and even death. Maternal immune status can be determined by antibody determination; IgM reflects recent infection and IgG indicates infection in the past. Exposed mothers should have testing for B19-specific IgG; if negative, testing for IgM follows. If positive, weekly ultrasound testing to look for evidence of fetal hydrops (ascites, edema) is performed. Intrauterine transfusions may be necessary if hydrops develops. There is no specific treatment for parvovirus infection.

Cardiac Disease

Modern treatment of congenital and acquired heart disease allows many patients to reach their reproductive years and become pregnant. As a result, patients with rheumatic heart disease and acquired infectious valvular heart disease (often associated with drug use) comprise only 50% of pregnant cardiac patients, the remainder consist of other lesions previously less commonly encountered in pregnancy. Considering that pregnancy is associated with a cardiac output increase of 40%, the risks to mother and fetus are often profound for patients with preexisting cardiac disease. Ideally, cardiac patients should have preconceptional care directed at maximizing cardiac function. They should also be counseled about the risks their particular heart disease poses in pregnancy.

Classification of Heart Disease in Pregnancy

The classification of heart disease of the New York Heart Association is useful to evaluate all types of cardiac patients with respect to pregnancy (Table 16.2). It is a functional classification, and is independent of the type of heart disease. Patients with septal defects, patent ductus arteriosus, and mild mitral and aortic valvular disorders often are in classes I or II and do well throughout pregnancy. Primary pulmonary hypertension, uncorrected tetralogy of Fallot, Eisenmenger syndrome, and certain other conditions are associated with a much worse prognosis (frequently death) through the course of pregnancy. For this reason, patients with such disorders are strongly advised not to become pregnant.

Management of Cardiac Disease in Pregnancy

General management of the pregnant cardiac patient consists of avoiding conditions that add additional stress to the workload of the heart beyond that already imposed by pregnancy, including prevention and/or correction of anemia, prompt recognition and treatment of any infections, a decrease in physical activity and strenuous work, and proper weight gain. Adequate rest is essential. For patients with class I or II heart disease, increased rest at home is advised, and in cases of higher class levels, hospitalization and treatment of cardiac failure may be required. Coordinated management between obstetrician, cardiologist, and anesthesiologist is especially important for patients with significant cardiac dysfunction.

The fetuses of patients with functionally significant cardiac disease are at increased risk for low birth weight and prematurity. A patient with congenital heart disease is 1% to 5% more likely to have a fetus with congenital heart disease; antepartum fetal cardiac assessment using ultrasound is recommended.

The antepartum management of pregnant cardiac patients includes serial evaluation of maternal cardiac status as well as fetal well-being and growth. Anticoagulation, antibiotic prophylaxis for subacute bacterial endocarditis, invasive cardiac monitoring, and even surgical correction of certain cardiac lesions during pregnancy can be all accomplished if necessary. The intrapartum and postpartum management of pregnant cardiac patients includes consideration of the increased stress of delivery and postpartum physiologic adjustment. Labor in the lateral position to facilitate cardiac function is often desirable. Every attempt is made to facilitate vaginal delivery because of the increased cardiac stress of cesarean section. Because cardiac output increases by 40% to 50% during the second

Table 16.2.	New York Heart Association Functional Classification of Heart Disease		
Class	**Description**
I	No cardiac decompensation
II	No symptoms of cardiac decompensation at rest; minor limitations of physical activity
III	No symptoms of cardiac decompensation at rest; marked limitations of physical activity
IV	Symptoms of cardiac decompensation at rest; increased discomfort with any physical activity

stage of labor, shortening this stage by the use of forceps is often advisable. Epidural anesthesia to reduce the stress of labor is also recommended. Even with patients who are stable at the time of delivery, it must be remembered that an additional increase in cardiac output is manifest in the puerperium because of the additional 500 mL added to the maternal blood volume as the uterus contracts. Indeed, the majority of obstetric patients who die with cardiac disease do so following delivery.

Rheumatic heart disease remains a common cardiac disease in pregnancy. As the severity of the associated valvular lesion increases, these patients are at higher risk for thromboembolic disease, subacute bacterial endocarditis, cardiac failure, and pulmonary edema. A high rate of fetal loss is also seen in women with rheumatic heart disease. Approximately 90% of these patients have mitral stenosis, whose associated mechanical obstruction worsens as cardiac output increases during pregnancy. Mitral stenosis associated with atrial fibrillation has an especially high likelihood of congestive failure.

Maternal cardiac arrhythmias are occasionally encountered during pregnancy. Paroxysmal atrial tachycardia is the most commonly encountered maternal arrhythmia and is usually associated with overly strenuous exercise. Underlying cardiac disease such as mitral stenosis should be suspected when atrial fibrillation and flutter are encountered.

Peripartum cardiomyopathy is an unusual but especially severe cardiac condition identified in the last month of pregnancy or the first 6 months following delivery. It is difficult to distinguish from other cardiomyopathies (e.g., myocarditis) except for its association with pregnancy. In many cases, no apparent cause can be determined. Treatment is generally unchanged from cardiac failure unassociated with pregnancy, except the angiotensin-converting enzyme inhibitors are avoided if the patient is pregnant. Management includes bed rest, digoxin, diuretics, and in some cases, anticoagulation. The mortality rate is high and is related to cardiac size 6 to 12 months later. If cardiac size returns to normal, prognosis is improved, although it remains guarded. Steriliza-tion counseling is warranted for patients with cardiomyopathy.

Asthma

Bronchial asthma is encountered in approximately 2% to 3% of pregnant patients, about 15% of whom have one or more severe asthma attacks during pregnancy. The overall course of asthma tends to be the same from pregnancy to pregnancy with about one-third of patients noting improvement in their asthma symptoms, one-third worsening, and one-third remaining the same. In addition to pulmonary complications, hypertension, gestational diabetes, preterm labor and low birth weight infants occur more frequently in asthmatic patients. Management is similar to that provided to nonpregnant patients, with emphasis on avoiding exciting allergens and other causes of acute asthmatic exacerbation.

Surgical Abdomen

Obviously, patients who are pregnant can experience the same surgical conditions as those who are not pregnant, such as appendicitis, cholecystitis, and bowel injury. In early gestation, ectopic pregnancy and torsion of the adnexa should be considered. Later in pregnancy, placental abruption and uterine rupture can cause an acute abdomen.

The management of patients with surgical conditions should provide optimal care for the mother and consideration for optimal perinatal outcome. Any pregnant patient presenting with a potential surgical condition should be fully evaluated regardless of her pregnant status (i.e., necessary radiographic or other studies should not be avoided just because the patient is pregnant). For procedures such as radiographs of the chest, an abdominal shield may be used to avoid unnecessary exposure to the fetus. Exposure to low doses of radiation is safe for the fetus when considered against failure to treat or misdiagnosis of a serious surgical condition.

The fetus should be monitored as thoroughly as possible, consistent with the stage of gestation and need for intervention. For a viable pregnancy, this means electronic fetal monitoring for fetal heart tones and for preterm labor.

The supine position should be avoided, if possible, to prevent the supine hypotensive syndrome. Oxygen administration may be helpful. In general, those caring for these patients should be constantly aware of both maternal and fetal considerations. For example, the residual lung volume is diminished in pregnancy, which provides less reserve for respiratory function. Delayed gastric emptying makes aspiration of stomach contents more likely. The appendix may be displaced upward as pregnancy advances.

CHAPTER 17

HYPERTENSION IN PREGNANCY

This chapter deals primarily with APGO Educational Topic:

Topic 18: Preeclampsia-Eclampsia Syndrome

Students should be able to define and classify hypertensive disease in pregnancy, including preeclampsia and its associated syndromes; to discuss the pathophysiology of preeclampsia and its diagnosis, evaluation, and initial management, including labor management and the appropriate use of magnesium sulfate; understand and be able to discuss the effects of preeclampsia on pregnancy (mother and fetus) and the converse.

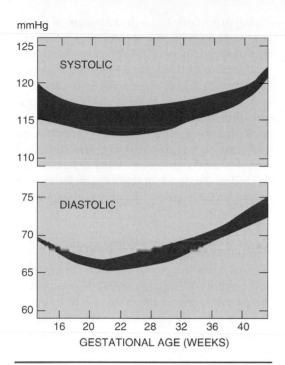

Figure 17.1. Range of blood pressures in normotensive pregnancy. Note the decrease in blood pressure in the second trimester.

Hypertensive disorders are among the most common, and yet serious, conditions seen in obstetrics, causing substantial morbidity and mortality for both mother and fetus. The cause of hypertension unique to pregnancy remains unknown.

Hypertension in pregnancy is generally defined as a sustained systolic blood pressure at or above 140 mm Hg, or a diastolic blood pressure of 90 mm Hg or greater. This definition requires that the increased blood pressures be present on at least two separate occasions, 6 hours or more apart. Although this definition seems clear, its use in clinical practice is difficult because of various problems in obtaining a reliable assessment of blood pressure.

The position of the patient influences blood pressure. It is lowest with the patient lying in the lateral position, highest when the patient is standing, and at an intermediate level when she is sitting (Figure 17.1). The choice of the correct size blood pressure cuff also influences blood pressure readings, with falsely high measurements noted when normal-sized cuffs are used on large patients. Also, during the course of pregnancy, blood pressure typically declines slightly in the second trimester, increasing to prepregnant levels as gestation nears term. If a patient has not been seen previously, there is no baseline blood pressure against which to compare new blood pressure determinations, thereby making the diagnosis of pregnancy-related hypertension more difficult.

Pregnancy-induced hypertension develops in 5% to 10% of pregnancies that proceed beyond the first trimester, with a 30% incidence in multiple gestation, regardless of parity. Maternal morbidity is directly related to the severity and duration of hypertension, although maternal mortality is rare, even when associated with such complications as abruptio placentae, hepatic rupture, or preeclampsia and eclampsia. Primarily because of the association with increased uteroplacental insufficiency and abruptio placentae, perinatal mortality increases progressively with increasing mean arterial pressure

Hypertensive Disease in Pregnancy

Classification

Various classifications of hypertensive disorders in pregnancy have been proposed. Table 17.1 presents a commonly used classification. Because hypertensive disorders in pregnancy

Table 17.1. Hypertensive Disorders in Pregnancy
Pregnancy-induced hypertension
Transient hypertension
Preeclampsia
Mild
Severe
Eclampsia
Chronic hypertension preceding pregnancy (any cause)
Chronic hypertension (any cause) with superimposed pregnancy-induced hypertension
Superimposed preeclampsia
Superimposed eclampsia

Classification of the American College of Obstetricians and Gynecologists.

represent a spectrum of disease, classification systems should not be considered as rigid markers on which all management decisions are made.

Hypertension in late pregnancy in the absence of other findings that are suggestive of preeclampsia has been termed *transient hypertension of pregnancy* or *gestational hypertension*. Although isolated hypertension is certainly seen in late pregnancy and in the first few days postpartum, caution should be taken in assuming that these patients have hypertension alone.

Preeclampsia is defined as *the development of hypertension with proteinuria induced by pregnancy, generally in the second half of gestation*. The high prevalence of edema in pregnancy has led to this clinical finding being dropped from the classic diagnostic criteria. Preeclampsia is more common in women who have not carried a previous pregnancy beyond 20 weeks, and is more frequent at the extremes of the reproductive years. Preeclampsia is classified as severe if there is a blood pressure ≥ 160 mm Hg systolic or 110 mm Hg diastolic, marked proteinuria (generally >1 g per 24-hour urine collection, or 2+ or more on dipstick of a random urine), oliguria, cerebral or visual disturbances such as headache and scotomata (spots before the eyes), pulmonary edema or cyanosis, epigastric or right upper quadrant pain (probably caused by subcapsular hepatic hemorrhage or stretching of Glisson capsule), evidence of hepatic dysfunction, thrombocytopenia, or oligohydramnios/fetal growth restriction. These myriad changes illustrate the multisystem alterations associated with preeclampsia.

Eclampsia is the additional presence of convulsions in a woman with preeclampsia, and is not a neurologic disorder. Eclampsia occurs in 0.5% to 4% of deliveries. Most cases of eclampsia occur within 24 hours of delivery, but approximately 3% of cases are diagnosed between 2 and 10 days postpartum.

Chronic hypertension is defined as hypertension present before the twentieth week of gestation or beyond 6 weeks postpartum. Chronic hypertension can be the result of a variety of causes, although the majority of cases are deemed essential hypertension. The greatest risk to a woman with chronic hypertension during pregnancy is the development of superimposed preeclampsia or eclampsia, which occurs in approximately 25% of cases. At times, it is difficult to distinguish between preeclampsia and chronic hypertension when a patient is seen late in pregnancy with an elevated blood pressure. In such cases, it is always wise to assume that the findings represent preeclampsia and treat accordingly. Finally, *preeclampsia or eclampsia superimposed on chronic hypertension* is defined as the development of preeclampsia or eclampsia in a patient with preexisting chronic hypertension.

Pathophysiology

Hypertension in pregnancy affects the mother and newborn to widely varying degrees. Given the characteristic multisystem effects, it is clear that several pathophysiologic mechanisms are involved. The one common pathophysiologic finding in hypertension in pregnancy, especially when there is progression to preeclampsia, is maternal *vasospasm*. Several potential causes for maternal vasospasm have been postulated:

1. *Uterine vascular changes:* Instead of noting the physiologic trophoblast-mediated vascular changes in the uterine vessels (decreased musculature in the spiral arterioles leads to the development of a low resistance, low pressure, high-flow system), inadequate maternal vascular response is seen in cases of preeclampsia and/or intrauterine fetal growth restriction. Endothelial damage is also noted within the vessels.

2. *Hemostatic changes:* Increased platelet activation with increased consumption in the microvasculature is noted during the course of preeclampsia. Endothelial fibronectin levels are elevated and antithrombin III and α-2-antiplasmin levels are decreased, reflecting endothelial damage. Low antithrombin III levels are permissive for microthrombi. Endothelial damage is then thought to promote further vasospasm.

3. *Changes in prostanoids:* Prostacyclin (PGI_2) and thromboxane (TXA_2) are increased during pregnancy, with the balance in favor of PGI_2. In patients who

develop preeclampsia, the balance shifts to favor TXA_2. Again, PGI_2 functions to promote vasodilatation and decrease platelet aggregation, and TXA_2 promotes vasoconstriction and platelet aggregation. Because of this imbalance, vessel constriction occurs.

4. *Changes in endothelium-derived factors*: Nitric oxide, a potent vasodilator is decreased in patients with preeclampsia and may explain the evolution of vasoconstriction in these patients.

5. *Lipid peroxide, free radicals, and antioxidant release*: Lipid peroxides and free radicals have been implicated in vascular injury and are increased in pregnancies complicated by preeclampsia. Decreased antioxidant levels are also noted.

These five mechanisms, in any combination or permutation, are thought to lead to the following common pathophysiologic changes seen in patients with preeclampsia:

1. *Cardiovascular effects*: Elevated blood pressure is seen as the result of potential vasoconstriction (persistent angiotensin II sensitivity) as well as an increase in cardiac output.

2. *Hematologic effects*: Plasma volume contraction may develop, with risk of rapid onset hypovolemic shock, if hemorrhage occurs. Plasma volume contraction is demonstrated by increased hematocrit. Thrombocytopenia/disseminated intravascular coagulation may also develop from microangiopathic hemolytic anemia. Involvement of the liver may lead to hepatocellular dysfunction and further evolution of coagulopathy. Third spacing of fluid may be noted because of increased blood pressure and decreased plasma oncotic pressure.

3. *Renal effects*: Decreased glomerular filtration rate and proteinuria (urine protein >300 mg per 24 hours) develop secondary to atheroscleroticlike changes in the renal vessels (glomerular endotheliosis). Uric acid filtration is decreased; therefore, elevated maternal serum uric acid levels may be an indication for evolving disease.

4. *Neurologic effects*: Hyperreflexia/hypersensitivity may develop, although it does not correlate with the severity of the disease. In severe cases, grand mal seizures may develop.

5. *Pulmonary effects*: Pulmonary edema may occur and can be related to decreased colloid oncotic pressure, pulmonary capillary leak, left heart failure, iatrogenic fluid overload, or a combination of these factors.

6. *Fetal effects*: Decreased intermittent placental perfusion secondary to vasospasm is the potential cause for the increased incidence of intrauterine growth restriction, oligohydramnios, low birth weight infants, and increased perinatal mortality of infants born to mothers with preeclampsia. An increased incidence of placental abruption is also seen. With the stress of uterine contractions during labor, the placenta is often incapable of supporting the fetus, resulting in intrapartum uteroplacental insufficiency with progressive fetal hypoxia and acidosis.

Presumably because of vasospastic changes, placental size and function are decreased. The results are progressive fetal hypoxia and malnutrition as well as an increase in the incidence of intrauterine growth restriction, oligohydramnios, and dysmaturity.

Evaluation

The history and physical examination are directed toward detection of pregnancy-associated hypertensive disease and its stigmata. A review of current obstetric records, if available, is especially helpful to ascertain changes or progression in findings. *Visual disturbances,* especially scotomata, or unusually severe or persistent *headaches* are indicative of vasospasm. *Right upper quadrant pain* may indicate liver involvement, presumably involving distention of the liver capsule. Any history of *loss of consciousness or seizures,* even in the patient with a known seizure disorder, may be significant.

The patient's weight is compared with her pregravid weight and with previous weights during this pregnancy, with special attention to excessive or too-rapid weight gain. Peripheral edema is common in pregnancy, especially in the lower extremities; however, persistent edema unresponsive to resting in the supine position is not normal, especially when it also involves the upper extremities, sacral region, and face. Indeed, the puffy-faced, edematous, hypertensive pregnant woman is the classic picture of severe preeclampsia. Careful blood pressure determination in the sitting and supine positions is necessary. Funduscopic examination may detect vasoconstriction of retinal blood vessels, presumably indicative of similar vasoconstriction of other small vessels. Tenderness over the liver, attributed partly to hepatic capsule distension, may be associated with complaints of right upper quadrant pain. The patellar and Achilles' deep tendon reflexes should be carefully elicited, and hyperreflexia noted. The demonstration of clonus at the ankle is especially worrisome.

The maternal and fetal laboratory evaluations for pregnancy complicated by hypertension are presented in Table 17.2 and demonstrate, by the wide range of tests, the multi-system effects of hypertension in pregnancy. Maternal liver dysfunction, renal insufficiency, and coagulopathy are significant concerns and require serial evaluation. Evaluation of fetal well-being with ultrasonography, nonstress test/oxytocin challenge test, and/or biophysical profile is crucial.

Management

The goal of management of hypertension in pregnancy is to balance the management of both fetus and mother and to optimize the outcome for each. Maternal blood pressure should be monitored and the mother should be observed for the sequelae of the hypertensive disease. Intervention for maternal indica-

Table 17.2. Laboratory Assessment of Pregnant Hypertensive Patients

Test or Procedure	Rationale
Maternal studies	
Complete blood count	Increasing hematocrit may signify worsening vasoconstriction and decreased intravascular volume
Platelet count	Thrombocytopenia and coagulopathy are associated with worsening PIH
Coagulation profile (PT, PTT)	Hepatocellular dysfunction is associated with worsening PIH
Fibrin split products	
Liver function studies	
Serum creatinine	Decreased renal function is associated with worsening PIH
24-hour urine for creatinine clearance	
Total urinary protein	
Uric acid	
Fetal studies: To assess for pregnancy-associated hypertension effects on the fetus	
Ultrasound examination	IUGR
Fetal weight and growth	Oligohydramnios
Amniotic fluid volume	Chronic fetal stress/distress
Placental status	
NST/OCT	
Biophysical profile	

IUGR, intrauterine growth restriction; NST/OCT, nonstress test/oxytocin challenge test; PIH, pregnancy-induced hypertension; PT, prothrombin time; PTT, partial thromboplastin time.

tions should occur when the risk of permanent disability or death for the mother without intervention outweighs the risks to the fetus caused by intervention. For the fetus, there should be regular evaluation of fetal well-being and fetal growth, with intervention becoming necessary if the intrauterine environment provides more risks to the fetus than delivery with subsequent care in the newborn nursery.

Management of Preeclampsia

The severity of the preeclampsia and the maturity of the fetus are the primary considerations in the management of preeclampsia. Care must be individualized, but there are well-accepted general guidelines.

The mainstay of management for patients with *mild preeclampsia* and an immature fetus is *bed rest*, preferably with as much time as possible spent in a lateral decubitus position. In this position, cardiac function and uterine blood flow are maximized and maternal blood pressures in most cases are normalized. This improves uteroplacental function, allowing normal fetal growth and metabolism. For a patient with mild preeclampsia who has access to medical care and is motivated to care for herself, bed rest at home with daily weighing (if possible), fetal movement count records, and home blood pressure determinations (if available) usually suffice. The patient is instructed to recognize the signs and symptoms that indicate worsening of the preeclampsia and to notify her physician in such an event. In the absence of significant changes in her condition, such care allows the fetus to grow and become more functionally mature. In addition, induction of labor, if needed, is more likely to be successful as gestational age approaches term.

Hospitalization is recommended if the patient lacks either transportation for frequent prenatal visits or motivation to maintain bed rest, or for the patient in whom expectant management at home does not result in normalization of blood pressure. The same regimen is used in the hospital, but better compliance is ensured in this more controlled environment.

For the patient with *worsening preeclampsia* or the patient who has *severe preeclampsia*

Table 17.3. Criteria for Diagnosis of Severe Preeclampsia
BP >160–180 mm Hg systolic or >110 mm Hg diastolic
Proteinuria >5g/24 hr
Elevated serum creatinine
Grand mal seizures (eclampsia)
Pulmonary edema
Oliguria (<500 mL/24 hr)
Microangiopathic hemolysis
Thrombocytopenia
Hepatocellular dysfunction
IUGR or oligohydramnios
Symptoms suggesting significant end organ involvement (headache, visual disturbances, or epigastirc/RUQ pain)

BP, blood pressure; IUGR, intrauterine growth restriction; RUQ, right upper quadrant.

(Table 17.3), stabilization with magnesium sulfate, antihypertensive therapy (as indicated), monitoring for maternal and fetal well-being, and delivery by either induction or cesarean delivery are required. A 48-hour delay in delivery to allow for steroid administration to enhance fetal pulmonary maturity may be indicated in some cases, depending on gestational age.

For more than half a century, *magnesium sulfate* has been used to prevent eclamptic convulsions. It has virtually no effect on blood pressure. In the event of *eclampsia*, other anticonvulsants such as diazepam and phenytoin are infrequently used. Magnesium sulfate, when used as a seizure prophylactic for patients with the diagnosis of preeclampsia or as an anticonvulsant in the patients with eclampsia, may be administered by intramuscular or intravenous routes, although the latter is far more common. An initial 4-g loading dose is given intravenously over 20 to 30 minutes, followed by a constant infusion of 1 to 3 g/hr. In 98% of cases, convulsions will be prevented. Therapeutic levels are 4 to 7 mEq/L, with toxic concentrations having predictable consequences (Table 17.4). Frequent evaluations of the patient's patellar reflex and respirations are

Table 17.4. Magnesium Toxicity

Serum Concentration (mg/dL)	Manifestation
1.5–3	Normal concentration
4–7	Therapeutic levels
5–10	ECG changes
8–12	Loss of patellar reflex
9–12	Feeling of warmth, flushing
10–12	Somnolence; slurred speech
15–17	Muscle paralysis; respiratory difficulty
>30	Cardiac arrest

necessary to monitor for manifestations of rising serum magnesium concentrations. In addition, because magnesium sulfate is excreted solely from the kidney, maintenance of urine output of at least 25 mL/hr will help avoid accumulation of the drug. Reversal of the effects of excessive magnesium concentrations is accomplished by the slow intravenous administration of 10% calcium gluconate, along with

oxygen supplementation and cardiorespiratory support, if needed.

Antihypertensive therapy is indicated if the diastolic blood pressure is repeatedly above 110 mm Hg. Hydralazine (Apresoline) is often the initial antihypertensive medication of choice, given in 5-mg increments intravenously until an acceptable blood pressure response is obtained. A 10- to 15-minute response time is usual. The goal of such therapy is to reduce the diastolic pressure to the 90 to 100 mm Hg range. Further reduction of the blood pressure may impair uterine blood flow to rates that are dangerous to the fetus. Other antihypertensive agents may be used (Tables 17.5 and 17.6).

Once anticonvulsant and antihypertensive therapies are established in patients with severe preeclampsia or elcampsia, attention is directed toward *delivery*. Induction of labor is often attempted, although cesarean delivery may be needed either if induction is unsuccessful or not possible, or if maternal or fetal status is worsening. At delivery, blood loss must be closely monitored because patients with preeclampsia or eclampsia have significantly reduced blood volumes. *After delivery*, patients are kept in the labor and delivery area

Table 17.5. Antihypertensive Medications Used in Pregnancy

Medication	Mechanism of Action	Effects
Thiazide	Decreased plasma volume and CO	CO decreased; RBF decreased; maternal electrolyte depletion; neonatal thrombocytopenia
Methyldopa	False neurotransmission, CNS effect	CO unchanged; RBF unchanged; maternal lethargy, fever, hepatitis, and hemolytic anemia
Hydralazine	Direct peripheral vasodilation	CO increased; RBF unchanged or increased; maternal flushing, headache, tachycardia, lupuslike syndrome
Propranolol	β-adrenergic blocker	CO decreased; RBF decreased; maternal increased uterine tone with possible decrease in placental perfusion; neonatal depressed respirations
Labetalol	α- and β-adrenergic blocker	CO unchanged; RBF unchanged; maternal tremulousness, flushing, headache; neonatal depressed respirations
Nifedipine	Calcium-channel blocker	CO unchanged; RBF unchanged; maternal orthostatic hypotension and headache (also a tocolytic); no neonatal effects known

CNS, central nervous system; CO, cardiac output; RBF, renal blood flow.

Table 17.6. Drug Therapy for Hypertensive Emergencies in Pregnancy

Drug	Regimen	Course of Action
Hydralazine (Apresoline)	10–50 mg IM q 3–6 hr; 5–25 mg IV q 3–6 hr	Onset, 10–20 min; maximum effect, 20–40 min; duration, 3–8 hr
Nifedipine	10 mg po q 4–8 hr	Onset, 5–10 min; maximum effect, 10–20 min; duration, 4–8 hr
Labetalol	20–50 mg IV q 3–6 hr	Onset, 1–2 min; maximum effect, 10 min; duration, 6–16 hr

for 24 hours, or longer if the clinical situation warrants, for close observation of their clinical progress and further administration of magnesium sulfate to prevent postpartum eclamptic seizures. Approximately 25% of all patients with preeclampsia who have eclamptic seizures have them before labor, approximately 50% have them during labor, and approximately 25% have them after delivery. Usually, the vasospastic process begins to reverse itself in the first 24 to 48 hours after delivery, as manifest by a brisk diuresis.

The management of patients with *chronic hypertension in pregnancy* involves closely monitoring maternal blood pressure and watching for the superimposition of preeclampsia or eclampsia, and following the fetus for appropriate growth and fetal well-being. Also, the patient should be encouraged to increase the amount of time she rests. Medical treatment of milder forms of chronic hypertension has been disappointing in that no significant improvement in pregnancy outcome has been demonstrated.

Antihypertensive medication is generally not given unless the diastolic blood pressure exceeds 110 mm Hg; the purpose of such medications is to reduce the likelihood of maternal stroke. Methyldopa has been and is a commonly used antihypertensive medication for this purpose, although beta blockers such as labetolol and calcium channel blockers such as amlodipine are also commonly used today. It was formerly taught that diuretics were contraindicated during pregnancy, but diuretic therapy is no longer discontinued in, and indeed is usually continued in, the patient who was already on such therapy before becoming pregnant.

Management of the Eclamptic Seizure

The eclamptic seizure is life threatening for mother and fetus. Maternal risks include musculoskeletal injury (including biting the tongue), hypoxia, and aspiration. Maternal therapy consists of inserting a padded tongue blade, restraining gently as needed, providing oxygen, assuring maintenance of an adequate airway, and gaining an intravenous access. Eclamptic seizures are usually self-limited, so medical therapy should be directed to the initiation of magnesium therapy (4 g slowly, intravenously) to prevent further seizures, rather than to anticonvulsant therapy with diazepam or similar drugs. Transient uterine hyperactivity for up to 15 minutes is associated with fetal heart rate changes, including bradycardia or compensatory tachycardia, decreased beat-to-beat activity, and late decelerations. These are self-limited and are not dangerous to the fetus unless they continue for 20 minutes or more. Delivery during this time imposes unnecessary risk for mother and fetus and should be avoided. Arterial blood gases should be obtained, any metabolic disturbance should be corrected, and a Foley catheter should be placed to monitor urinary output. If the maternal blood pressure is high, if maternal urinary output is low, or if there is evidence of cardiac disturbance, consideration of a central venous catheter and, perhaps, continuous electrocardiogram monitoring is appropriate.

The HELLP Syndrome

The acronym HELLP is for a specific set of hypertensive patients who have *hemolysis (H), elevated liver (EL) enzymes, and low platelet (LP) count.* This syndrome is now appreciated as a distinct clinical entity, occurring in 4% to 12% of patients with severe preeclampsia or eclampsia. Patients with HELLP syndrome are often multiparous, somewhat older than the average obstetric patient, and somewhat less hypertensive than many preeclamptic patients. The liver dysfunction may be manifest as right upper quadrant pain and is all too commonly misdiagnosed as gallbladder disease or indigestion. Major morbidity and mortality with unrecognized HELLP make accurate diagnosis imperative. Unfortunately, the first symptoms are often rather vague, including nausea and emesis and a nonspecific viral-like syndrome.

Treatment of these gravely ill patients is best done in a high-risk obstetric center and consists of cardiovascular stabilization, correction of coagulation abnormalities, and delivery. Platelet transfusion before or after delivery is indicated if the platelet count is fewer than 20,000/mm^3, and it may be advisable to transfuse patients with a platelet count below 50,000/mm^3 before proceeding with a cesarean birth. In cases in which HELLP syndrome develops before 32 weeks estimated gestational age, and in the setting of reassuring fetal status and absent maternal end organ symptoms, stabilization of maternal platelet count may result from intravenous treatment with steroids.

CHAPTER 18

MULTIFETAL GESTATION

This chapter addresses APGO Educational Topic:

Topic 20: Multifetal Gestation

The student should understand that a multifetal gestation requires modifications in antepartum, intrapartum, and postpartum care.

Incidence of Multiple Gestation

The overall incidence of recognized twins in the United States is almost 3%, with the rate rising as a result of an increase in older gravidas and the more frequent use of assisted reproductive technologies. The natural rate of twinning is approximately 1 in 90 and is slightly higher in Blacks than in Whites. Twin gestations can be characterized as dizygotic (fraternal) or monozygotic (identical).

Dizygotic twins occur when two separate ova are fertilized by two separate sperm and, in fact, represent two siblings who happen to be born at approximately the same time. *Monozygotic twins* represent division of the fertilized ovum at various times after conception. There is a marked difference in the incidence of twinning in various populations, almost exclusively the result of the incidence of dizygotic twinning. The *incidence of monozygotic twinning* is fairly constant around the world at *approximately 1 in 250 pregnancies,* whereas *dizygotic twinning* occurs as frequently as *1 in 20 pregnancies* in certain African countries. Increasing age and increasing parity are independent factors for dizygotic twinning. A familial factor is present in twinning that follows the maternal lineage.

Serial ultrasound assessments have shown that only 50% of twin pregnancies detected in the first trimester result in the delivery of viable twins. The other 50% of cases deliver a single fetus because of the intrauterine demise and ultimate resorption of one embryo/fetus *(vanishing twin syndrome)*. During the first ultrasonographic examination that confirms a twin gestation, chorionicity should be determined because the potential morbidity and mortality associated with a monochorionic gestation is different from that of a dichorionic gestation. Chorionicity can be determined with almost 100% certainty as early as 9 to 10 weeks of gestational age.

The likelihood of twinning is increased significantly if *fertility agents or other assisted reproductive technologies* are used. With clomiphene citrate induction of ovulation, the twinning rate is approximately 6% to 8%. With the use of exogenous gonadotropin therapy, the rate increases to approximately 25% to 35%. Because in vitro fertilization programs typically insert several fertilized ova into the uterine cavity, multiple fetuses would be expected to occur in some instances; in fact, the rate of two or more fetuses is approximately 35% to 40%. Although the exact mechanism is not known, monozygotic twinning is also increased in pregnancies that conceived by using artificial reproductive techniques.

The natural incidence of three or more fetuses may be approximated by 90 raised to the power of the number of fetuses minus one. Thus, triplets are 1 in 90^2, or 1 in 8,100; quadruplets are 1 in 90^3, or 1 in 729,000, and so forth.

Natural History

As the number of fetuses increases, the expected gestational age at delivery decreases. Compared with singleton pregnancies, which deliver at 40 weeks, twins deliver at an average of 37 weeks, triplets at 33 weeks, and quadruplets at an average of 29 weeks. Thus, with each additional fetus, the length of gestation is decreased by approximately 4 weeks. Although all twins face certain risks, *monozygotic twins face additional risks related to the time when twinning occurs.* The developmental sequence associated with the separation of the conceptus into twins explains the basis for these problems as well as the configuration of the fetal membranes at delivery. If division of the conceptus occurs within 3 days of fertilization, each fetus will be surrounded by an amnion and chorion, and the membranes are termed *dichorionic diamniotic* (approximately 20% to 30% of all monozygotic gestations). If division occurs between the fourth and eighth day following fertilization, the chorion has already begun to develop, whereas the amnion has not. Therefore, each fetus will be surrounded by an amnion, but a single chorion will surround both twins, a condition termed *monochorionic diamniotic* (approximately 70% to 80% of monozygotic gestations). In 1% of monozygotic gestations, division occurs between days 9 and 12, after development of both the amnion and the chorion, and the twins will share a common sac, a condition termed *monochorionic/monoamniotic* (approximately 1% of monozygotic gestations). This carries a mortality rate of up to 50%, usually before 32 weeks. Division thereafter is incomplete, resulting in the development of conjoined twins, which may be fused in any of a multitude of ways, but usually at the chest and/or abdomen. This rare condition is seen in approximately 1 in 70,000 deliveries. Figure 18.1 illustrates these twin conditions.

As development of a monochorionic gestation progresses, various vascular anastomoses between the fetuses can develop that, in turn, can lead to a condition known as *twin–twin transfusion syndrome*. In this circumstance, blood flow of the fetuses mixes so there is net flow from one twin to another, at times with disastrous consequences. The so-called donor twin can have impaired growth, anemia, hypovolemia, and other problems. On the other hand, the recipient twin can develop hypervolemia, hypertension, polycythemia, and congestive heart failure as a result of this abnormal transfusion. A secondary manifestation involves the amniotic fluid dynamics. Because of transudate across the skin or, probably more importantly, increased urinary output owing to its hypervolemia, the recipient produces abundant amniotic fluid, whereas the donor twin may have oligohydramnios. The hydramnios in one twin further compounds the risk of

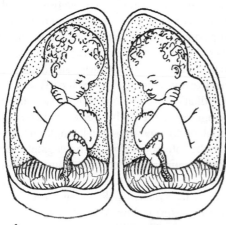

A Two placentas, two amnions, two chorions — dichorionic diamniotic

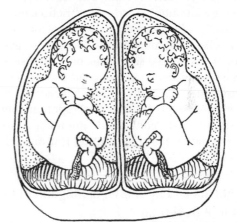

B One placenta, two amnions, two chorions — dichorionic diamniotic

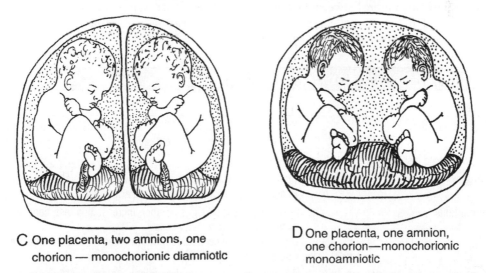

C One placenta, two amnions, one chorion — monochorionic diamniotic

D One placenta, one amnion, one chorion—monochorionic monoamniotic

Figure 18.1. Development of the amnion and chorion in twin pregnancies. **A–D** on the figure describe the resultant conditions.

preterm labor in multifetal pregnancies. Recently, intrauterine laser ablation of the vascular anastomoses has met with some success in treating this difficult problem. Other vascular abnormalities include absence of an umbilical artery, which may be associated in 30% of cases with other congenital problems, especially renal agenesis. A single umbilical artery is seen in approximately 3% to 4% of twins, compared with 0.5% to 1% of singletons.

Multifetal pregnancy is associated with *increased perinatal morbidity,* 3 to 4 times that for a comparable singleton pregnancy in the case of twin gestation. The most significant cause of morbidity is preterm labor and delivery, followed by intrauterine growth restriction, polyhydramnios (in approximately 10% of multiple gestations, predominantly monochorionic gestations), maternal disease (e.g., preeclampsia is 3 times more frequent), congenital anomalies, postpartum hemorrhage, and placental and umbilical cord accidents. Both spontaneous abortions and congenital anomalies are approximately twice as common in multiple gestation.

Diagnosis and Antenatal Management of Multiple Gestation

Twin pregnancy is usually *suspected when the uterine size is large for the calculated gestational age.* A difference of 4 cm or more between the weeks of gestation and the measured fundal height should prompt evaluation with ultrasound to detect the cause; e.g., inaccurate gestational age, multiple gestation, hydramnios, gestational trophoblastic disease, or pelvic tumor.

Once the diagnosis of twin pregnancy has been made and chorionicity has been assigned, subsequent antenatal care addresses each of the *potential concerns* for mother and fetus, as listed in Table 18.1. Although the maternal blood volume is greater with a twin gestation than with singleton pregnancy, the anticipated blood loss at delivery is also greater. Anemia is more common in these patients, and a balanced diet with iron, folate, and possibly other micronutrients is important. Because of the increased risk for preterm labor in multiple gestations, careful attention to detection of uterine contractions is important, and the patient should be cautioned about signs of preterm labor, such as low back pain, a thin vaginal discharge, and diarrhea. Cervical examinations to detect early effacement and dilation are usually done every 1 to 2 weeks beginning in the midtrimester. When available, serial endovaginal cervical length ultrasounds may be interspersed with the vaginal examinations. Adjunctive to cervical length assessment, a cervical swab for fetal fibronectin may aid in predicting preterm delivery in women experiencing preterm labor. A negative screen predicts with almost 1 in 125 certainty that the patient will not deliver within the next 2 weeks. At each visit, evidence suggesting pregnancy-induced hypertension is also gathered, which includes

Table 18.1. Antenatal Management of Twin Pregnancies	
Concern	**Action**
Adequate nutrition	Balanced diet; additional 300 kcal in daily intake; multivitamin, and mineral supplements (e.g., folate)
Increased blood loss at delivery	Prevent anemia (iron)
Fetal growth	Increasing rest beginning at 24–26 weeks; the value of this is unclear, but also may decrease preterm labor
Preterm labor	Educate patient on signs of labor; increase bed rest; cervical examinations every 1–2 weeks alternating with cervical length ultrasounds; fetal fibronectin assessment
Pregnancy-induced hypertension	Frequent blood pressure determinations; frequent urinary protein assessment
Fetal growth, discordant growth	Periodic ultrasonographic examinations

careful measurement of blood pressure and testing for protein in the urine. Beginning at 30 to 32 weeks, daily fetal kick counts are usually begun to help assess *fetal well-being*. Although somewhat surprising, patients can almost always distinguish movements of different fetuses. Nonstress tests or other fetal monitor testing is begun as the pregnancy approaches term.

The chief antenatal assessment in twin pregnancy remains the periodic ultrasonographic examination, which is done approximately every 4 weeks after 20 weeks of gestation. At each examination, growth of each fetus is assessed and an estimate of amniotic fluid volume is made. If growth is discordant, usually defined as a 20% to 25% difference in weight (the difference in weight divided by the weight of the larger fetus is 20% to 25% or more), or if either fetus has an estimated fetal weight of less than the tenth percentile, ultrasonography should be performed more often. Other criteria used to define discordant growth include a 20-mm difference in abdominal circumference, a 5% difference in head circumference, or a 5-mm difference in biparietal diameter.

Intrapartum Management

Intrapartum management is largely *determined by the presentation of the twins*. In general, if the first (presenting) twin is in the cephalic (vertex) presentation, labor is allowed to progress to vaginal delivery, whereas if the presenting twin is in a position other than cephalic, cesarean delivery is often performed. During labor, the heart rate of both fetuses is monitored separately. Approaches to the delivery of twins vary, depending on gestational age, presentation of the twins, and the experience of the attending physicians. Regardless of the delivery plan, access to full obstetric anesthetic and pediatric services is mandatory because cesarean delivery may be required on short notice.

If vaginal delivery of the first twin is accomplished and the second twin is also cephalic, vaginal delivery of the second twin generally proceeds smoothly (40% of all twin deliveries). With proper monitoring of the second twin, there is no urgency in accomplishing the second delivery. If the second twin is presenting in any way other than cephalic (40% of all twin deliveries), there are two primary manipulations that

may effect vaginal delivery (Figure 18.2). The first is *external cephalic version* whereby, using ultrasonographic visualization, the fetus is gently guided into the cephalic presentation by abdominal massage and pressure. The second maneuver is *breech extraction/internal podalic version,* in which the physician reaches a hand into the uterine cavity, grasps the lower extremities of the fetus, and gently delivers the infant via breech delivery. Delivering the second twin via cesarean delivery is another management option. The possibility of a prolapsed umbilical cord must always be borne in mind when delivery of twins is to be accomplished. Twin gestations in which the first twin is in the breech presentation (20% of all twin deliveries) are most often delivered via cesarean delivery. Some clinicians and their patients plan for cesarean delivery unless both fetuses are in a cephalic presentation.

Postpartum, the overdistended uterus may not contract normally, leading to uterine atony and postpartum hemorrhage.

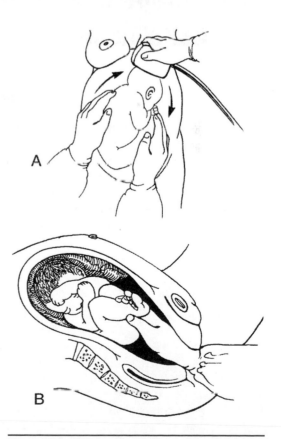

Figure 18.2. (A) External cephalic version. **(B)** Breech extraction (internal podalic version).

CHAPTER 19

FETAL GROWTH ABNORMALITIES
Intrauterine Growth Restriction and Fetal Macrosomia

Chapter 19 deals primarily with APGO Educational Topic:

Topic 31: Fetal Growth Abnormalities

Students should be able to define the two major fetal growth abnormalities, macrosomia and fetal growth restriction, as well as discuss their evaluation and management. Students should also be able to identify the major morbidities and causes of mortality for each condition.

Intrauterine Growth Restriction

Intrauterine growth restriction (IUGR) describes infants whose weights are much lower than expected for their gestational age. *A fetus or infant whose weight lies in the lowest 10% of the normal population for a specified gestational age is designated as having IUGR,* a determination based on standard weight/gestational age tables. By definition, the prevalence of IUGR will be 10%. Unlike "low birth weight," IUGR is based on weight for a *specific gestational age.* Therefore, careful assessment of gestational age is crucial to diagnosing and, therefore, managing patients with IUGR.

The fetus with IUGR should be viewed as fragile, that is, potentially lacking adequate reserves for continued intrauterine life, the stress of labor, or neonatal adaptation. Infants with IUGR are at greater risk for intrauterine fetal death, neonatal death, asphyxia, and fetal intolerance of labor. Once delivered, they are at risk for meconium aspiration, hypoglycemia, hypothermia, and respiratory distress. Perinatal morbidity and mortality is significantly increased in IUGR fetuses. *In general, the smaller the fetus with IUGR, the greater the risk.* Indeed, the perinatal mortality rate is increased sevenfold to 10-fold with IUGR–approximately 120 per 1,000 for all cases of growth restriction and approximately 100 per 1,000 if anomalous infants are excluded. About one third of stillborns are growth restricted. Thus, it is important to identify such infants in utero so that management may maximize the quality of their intrauterine environment, plan and implement their delivery using the safest means possible, and provide needed care in the neonatal period.

Cause

Intrauterine growth restriction is a descriptive term and diagnosis, but it is important to remember that it is the consequence of many possibly different maternal or fetal causes (specific diagnosis).

For a fetus to thrive in utero, an adequate number of fetal cells must be present and differentiated properly. In addition, sufficient foodstuffs, other nutrients, and oxygen must be available via an adequately functioning uteroplacental unit to allow growth in the number of cells and then in cell size. *Early in pregnancy, fetal growth is primarily by cellular hyperplasia, or cell division, so that early-onset IUGR leads to an irreversible diminution of organ size and perhaps function.* This type of IUGR is associated with heritable factors, immunologic abnormalities, chronic maternal disease, fetal infection, and multiple pregnancies. Later in pregnancy, fetal growth depends increasingly more on cellular hypertrophy rather than hyperplasia so that *delayed-onset IUGR results in decreased cell size and it is amenable to restoration of size with adequate nutrition.* The normal fetus grows throughout pregnancy, but the rate of growth falls off after 37 weeks of gestational age as the fetus begins to use energy to deposit fat in addition to cellular growth. Uteroplacental insufficiency is the primary cause of this kind of IUGR. The placenta grows early and rapidly compared with the fetus, reaching a maximum surface area of about 11 m^2 and weight of 500 g at approximately 37 weeks of gestational age. Thereafter, there is a slow but steady decline in placental surface area (and, hence, function), primarily because of microinfarctions of its vascular system. Because there is a close relationship between placental surface area and fetal weight, factors that act to decrease placental size (surface area, weight) are associated with decreased (restricted) growth.

Although a number of *causes of IUGR* have been recognized (Table 19.1), a definite cause of IUGR cannot be identified in approximately 50% of all cases. Up to 50% to 60% of all fetuses with actual IUGR are improperly thought to be simply constitutionally small but otherwise healthy. Causes of IUGR can be conveniently grouped into maternal and fetal origins. Maternal smoking has been known for many years to be associated with decreased birth weight, to a magnitude of roughly 0.5 pound at term. Because maternal habits are important causes of growth restriction, modification of such behavior can improve outcome. Certain drugs are also associated with IUGR and include, but are not limited to, drugs of abuse such as alcohol and cocaine, certain anticonvulsants, long-term steroids, and immunosuppressants.

Weight gain in pregnancy has not correlated well with IUGR except with extreme

Table 19.1. Causes and Risk Factors of Intrauterine Growth Restriction

Maternal

Cardiovascular

    Hypertension

    Cyanotic heart disease

    Cyanotic pulmonary disease

Metabolic

    Low maternal prepregnancy weight (< 90% ideal body weight)

    Poor nutrition, poor weight gain

    Diabetes

    Significant anemia; hemoglobinopathies

Behavioral

    Substance abuse (drugs, alcohol), Smoking

Obstetric

History of growth restriction in previous pregnancy

Elevated MSAFP/hCG

Antiphospholipid syndrome

Multifetal pregnancy

Abnormal placentation

Fetal

Infection: rubella, cytomegalovirus

Congenital anomalies

MSAFP/hCG, maternal serum α-fetoprotein/human chorionic gonadotropin.

nutritional deficiencies and in teens, who themselves are still growing and requiring a portion of nutritional intake. The recommended maternal *weight gain* during pregnancy is approximately 25 to 35 pounds (11.4 to 15.9 kg) in a normal-weight woman. It is difficult to define the role of less severe forms of nutritional deficiencies on fetal growth. In pregnancies with multiple fetuses, even normal food intake may not be enough to provide adequate nutrition for all fetuses, a factor that results in IUGR.

The most common known maternal factor associated with IUGR is *hypertensive disease* (either preexisting hypertension or pregnancy-associated hypertensive disease such as preeclampsia), which accounts for 25% to 30% of all cases of IUGR. Hypertension causes a decrease in placental perfusion, with subsequent growth restriction. Severe early onset hypertensive disease in pregnancy is associated with abnormal placentation in the first and early second trimester, as evidenced by placental pathologic studies. In severe preeclampsia, there is a failure of the trophoblast to invade the maternal uterine spiral arterioles with subsequent endothelial cell dysfunction, failure of maternal plasma volume expansion, and diminished uteroplacental blood flow. The overall result is, in general, a placenta that is smaller in size and surface area and with diminished function and reserve. Other maternal disorders, such as systemic lupus erythematous, antiphospholipid antibody syndrome, certain thrombophilias, *cyanotic heart disease, and the hemoglobinopathies,* may likewise interfere with fetal growth.

Fetal causes of IUGR include congenital infections and anomalies. The most clearly understood *fetal infections* that interfere with growth are rubella and cytomegalovirus infections, especially at early gestational ages. Although these infections may be manifest only as mild "flu-like" illnesses, their effects are far from mild. Damage to the fetus during organogenesis can result in a decreased cell number, which is manifest by diminished growth later in gestation, with or without multiple congenital anomalies. Five percent or fewer of all cases of IUGR are related to early infection with these or other viral agents. Bacterial infections have not been implicated in IUGR. *Congenital anomalies* account for up to 15% of all cases of IUGR. Chromosomal anomalies such as trisomy 13 and trisomy 18 syndrome, are typically associated with diminished fetal growth.

Evaluation and Management

The diagnosis of IUGR is based on a fetus whose weight falls below the tenth percentile for a given age. Unfortunately, this definition requires two data (gestational age and fetal weight) whose intrauterine measurement is both difficult and imprecise. Late prenatal care, a common problem, further exacerbates this imprecision because dating is more difficult later in pregnancy. Some elements of maternal history are associated with IUGR, and the presence of these factors alerts the clinician to a higher possibility of the development of IUGR (see Table 19.1). A patient with a history of having a child with IUGR is at increased risk for a recurrence of this problem.

Physical examination is limited in usefulness in recognizing IUGR or in making specific diagnosis, but it is an important screening test for abnormal fetal growth. Maternal size and weight gain throughout pregnancy have a limited use, but access to such information is readily available; a low maternal weight or little or no weight gain during pregnancy may suggest IUGR. Serial measurement of fundal height at every antepartum visit is perhaps the most useful screening evaluation for IUGR. Between approximately 15 and 36 weeks of gestation, *fundal height measurement* should advance in centimeter increments and in parallel with gestational age in weeks (Figure 19.1). Thus, a patient at 28 weeks of gestation would be expected to have a fundal height of 28 cm. Serial measurements, especially by the same examiner, can serve as an effective screening test for IUGR because a fundal height 3 to 4 cm less than expected suggests the diagnosis of IUGR and increases the need for an ultrasound examination. Clinical estimations of fetal weight are not very helpful in diagnosing IUGR, except when fetal size is grossly diminished.

Ultrasonography has become the standard for the recognition of IUGR and assessment for specific cause. Measurements of standard fetal biometry can be compared with standardized tables that reflect normal growth for a certain gestational age. The measurement of the biparietal diameter, head circumference, abdominal circumference, and femur length are among the most common measurements obtained. Ratios of these measurements and equations can provide useful information with respect to fetal size. The diameter of the cerebellum appears to be unaltered by a number of the factors that lead to growth restriction. Accordingly, in patients with uncertain gestational age, measurement of the diameter of the cerebellum may prove helpful.

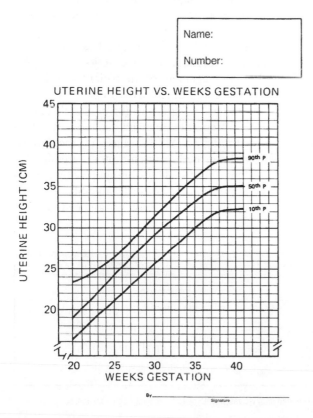

Figure 19.1. Fundal height evaluation as a screening test for intrauterine growth restriction. (Reprinted with permission from Scott JR, Di Saia PJ, Hammond CB, et al. *Danforth's Obstetrics and Gynecology.* 8th Ed. Philadelphia: Lippincott Williams & Wilkins, 1999.)

Ultrasonography, can determine whether IUGR is asymmetric or symmetric. *Asymmetric IUGR* refers to an unequal decrease in the size of structures. In asymmetric IUGR, the abdominal circumference is small, but the biparietal diameter of the head is nearly normal. Such asymmetry is seen with a primary placental cause, nutritional deficiencies, and hypertensive disease in pregnancy, when fetal access to nutrients is compromised. In *symmetric IUGR,* all structures are approximately equally diminished in size with a relative sparing of fetal brain and heart compared with asymmetric IUGR. Congenital anomalies or early intrauterine infection can alter cell number and lead to this symmetric type of IUGR. This distinction between symmetric and asymmetric IUGR is not always clear, but it does serve as a guide in seeking the cause of IUGR (Table 19.2).

In patients at increased risk for IUGR, a *baseline ultrasonographic* examination should be obtained early in prenatal care and usually repeated periodically. Because growth restriction is related to gestational age, all patients whose length of pregnancy is uncertain should be assessed with physical examination and ultrasonography to establish an accurate gestational age as early in pregnancy as possible. Ultrasonography also can identify the amount of amniotic fluid present. *The combination of oligohydramnios (diminished amniotic fluid volume) and IUGR is especially worrisome* because it is associated with severe disease and/or worsening outcome. The mechanism in this situation is thought to be decreased placental perfusion of oxygen and nutrients, with a compensatory redistribution of fetal blood favoring the brain, adrenal gland, and heart, and a

consequent decrease in fetal blood to the kidneys. This, in turn, leads to a reduction of urine output, a primary source of amniotic fluid in the second half of pregnancy.

Direct invasive studies of the fetus are useful in selected patients with IUGR. Fetal karyotyping and viral cultures and polymerase chain reaction can be accomplished by removing about 20 mL of amniotic fluid via amniocentesis (and evaluation of fetal fibroblasts floating in the amniotic fluid). Chorionic villus sampling (or biopsy of placenta) and direct blood sampling (percutaneous umbilical blood sampling, or removal of fetal plasma and cells) also permit karyotyping, immunoglobulin studies, and viral cultures. Percutaneous umbilical blood sampling and, to some extent, chorionic villus sampling are less widely available than ultrasound-directed amniocentesis.

Once IUGR, with or without specific diagnosis reflecting cause, has been diagnosed, *the goal is to deliver the healthiest possible infant at the optimal time.* This involves a balance between the degree of prematurity estimated at the time of diagnosis with the degree of suspected fetal compromise. Initial management consists of a comprehensive attempt to determine a cause for the IUGR. If a correctable cause is found, corrective action should be taken. Management of the patient with IUGR can be categorized as antepartum, intrapartum, and postpartum (or neonatal) (Table 19.3). Antepartum management consists of efforts to determine the cause of the IUGR, promote growth, and monitor carefully for fetal compromise. Ultrasonography by experienced personnel can usually identify congenital anomalies that may be associated with

Table 19.2. Symmetric and Asymmetric Intrauterine Growth Restriction		
Ultrasound Measurement	**Asymmetric**	**Symmetric**
BPD	Appropriate for dates	May be smaller than dates suggest
EFW	<10th percentile for dates	<10th percentile for dates
HC/AC ratio	>95th percentile for dates	In "normal" range for dates
AFV	Low for dates	Normal or low for dates

AFV, amniotic fluid volume; BPD, biparietal diameter; EFW, estimated fetal weight; HC/AC, head-to-abdominal circumference.

Table 19.3. Assessment and Management of Patient with Intrauterine Growth Restriction

Antepartum	Intrapartum	Postpartum (Neonatal)
Eliminate cause, if possible	Electronic fetal monitoring	Pharyngeal suction
Bed rest, frequent fetal movement counts	Preparation for cesarean delivery; amnioinfusion	Effective neonatal resuscitation as needed
Serial sonography	Oxygen therapy	Avoid hypoglycemia
NST, CST, BPP	Neonatal/anesthesia consultation	Avoid hypothermia; oxygen therapy, if needed
Amniocentesis for maturity studies		Doppler ultrasound
PUBS		Avoid hyperviscosity syndrome

BPP, biophysical profile; CST, contraction stress test; NST, nonstress test; PUBS, percutaneous umbilical blood sampling.

IUGR. Measurements of amniotic fluid volume and fetal biometry should be done on a serial basis. The degree of IUGR can then be followed in the ensuing weeks. Ultrasound evaluation every 3 or 4 weeks to follow the extent of growth restriction, and whether it is improving or worsening, is an important part of the overall management plan for IUGR. Worsening IUGR, for example, may be a key factor in the timing of delivery in combination with gestational age and measurements of fetal well-being. Bed rest, or at least limited activity, is often prescribed for patients with IUGR because limitation of activity, especially with the patient lying in the left-lateral position, maximizes uterine blood flow. This has a salutary effect on fetal growth.

Recently, Doppler velocimetric examination of certain fetal vessels, both arterial and venous, has provided much insight into the fetal response to IUGR and has become part of the standard assessment for the fetus with IUGR. Examination of blood flow through the umbilical artery was one of the first vessels to be studied with Doppler in an attempt to evaluate the fetal placental circulation. It is measured by a systolic/diastolic (S/D) ratio, which indirectly measures impedance or resistance downstream within the placental vessels. As placental resistance increases, diastolic flow decreases and the S/D ratio increases. A normal S/D ratio at term is 1.8 to 2.0. By the mid-1990s, it was well known that fetuses with IUGR who had no end diastolic flow or reversed diastolic flow had progressively worse perinatal outcomes. Doppler velocimetric examination of the fetal middle cerebral artery may also be used to measure the pathophysiologic adaptation of fetal brain sparing, and is characterized by an increase of diastolic and mean blood flow velocity in the middle cerebral artery. The fetus with IUGR seems to be at even greater risk if the ductus venosus is abnormal by Doppler examination.

Determination of fetal activity by the so called kick counts is a useful way of assessing *fetal well-being*. Various electronic fetal monitoring tests, such as the nonstress test or contraction stress test, or electronic fetal monitoring combined with ultrasound (the biophysical profile) can be used once or twice a week, or even more frequently, to assess the condition of the fetus. Although these tests can be helpful if the results are normal, the high false–positive rate must be considered in making management decisions regarding delivery. Use of these tests in combination may reduce this false–positive rate in some patients with IUGR

The decision regarding proper *time for delivery* is based on a combination of factors. Amniocentesis for tests of fetal lung maturity may provide information that is helpful in selecting the timing of delivery. Recently, several researchers have described the temporal sequence of abnormal Doppler studies, with each subsequent abnormality reflecting deterioration in the fetal status. Early abnormal Doppler examination includes studies of the umbilical artery and the fetal middle cerebral artery. Late abnormal Doppler examination includes findings in the ductus venosus and the umbilical vein.

The fetus that is thought to be in marked jeopardy may be delivered by scheduled cesarean section without a trial of labor if the ability of the fetus to withstand labor is questionable and an induced labor is likely to be lengthy. If induction of labor is undertaken, however, constant electronic fetal monitoring to detect signs that suggest fetal jeopardy is important. Recent studies suggest that fetuses with abnormal Doppler findings have a high incidence of fetal intolerance of labor. Preparations for cesarean delivery should be made because of rapid deterioration of the optimal care of the patient and her newborn. Amnioinfusion (instillation of warmed normal saline via transcervical catheter) may be helpful if fetal heart rate decelerations are thought to be caused by diminished amniotic fluid.

Common neonatal complications of IUGR and associated early delivery include respiratory distress, hyperviscosity syndrome, hypoglycemia, and hypothermia. Hyperviscosity syndrome results from the fetus' attempt to compensate for poor placental oxygen transfer by increasing the hematocrit to more than 65%. After birth, this marked polycythemia can cause multiorgan thrombosis, heart failure, and hyperbilirubinemia. Growth-restricted fetuses also have had less fat deposition in late pregnancy, so newborn euglycemia cannot be maintained by the normal mechanism of mobilization of glucose by fat metabolism. Fortunately, infants who survive the neonatal period have a generally good prognosis.

Fetal Macrosomia

Fetal macrosomia is variably defined as a fetus of 4,000 or 4,500 g, or a fetal weight greater than the ninetieth percentile for a given gestational age. Identification of these fetuses is important and, when possible, the underlying cause must be treated. The physician must anticipate the potential problems of vaginal delivery of a large infant, including a prolonged second stage of labor, shoulder dystocia, and immediate neonatal injury.

Macrosomia is associated with maternal obesity, maternal diabetes, and excessive maternal weight gain during pregnancy. Diagnosis is suspected when the fundal height is >4 cm above the expected height for a given gestational age (see Figure 19.1). The differential diagnosis includes a large but normal fetus ("constitutionally large"), multiple gestations, polyhydramnios, uterine leiomyoma or other gynecologic tumor, and early molar pregnancy. The diagnosis is confirmed by ultrasonography. It is important to understand that the precision of ultrasound in the determination of fetal weight at term is far from perfect. Nevertheless, it is the best test currently available. The American College of Obstetricians and Gynecologists suggests that a primary cesarean delivery should be offered for estimated fetal weights >5,000 g in a patient without diabetes and >4,500 g in a patient with diabetes. Macrosomia itself is not an indication for induction because it does not change perinatal outcomes.

Antepartum care focuses on management of any treatable cause of macrosomia; intrapartum management consists of choice of delivery route. Shoulder dystocia is addressed by maneuvers such as hyperflexion of the thighs (McRoberts maneuver) (see Figure 21.1) as well as suprapubic pressure (see Figure 21.2).

CHAPTER 20

THIRD-TRIMESTER BLEEDING

This chapter deals primarily with APGO Educational Topic:

Topic 23: Third-Trimester Bleeding

Students should be able to list the causes of bleeding in the third trimester, describe their evaluation and management, and discuss the maternal and fetal effects of such bleeding. Students should also be able to describe the management of acute blood loss, including the proper use of blood and blood products.

Table 20.1. Causes of Bleeding in the Second Half of Pregnancy

Vulva
    Varicose veins
    Tears or lacerations
Vagina
    Tears or lacerations
Cervix
    Polyp
    Glandular tissue (normal)
    Cervicitis
    Carcinoma
Intrauterine
    Uterine rupture
    Placenta previa
    Abruptio placentae
    Vasa previa

About 5% of women describe bleeding of some extent during pregnancy, from bleeding that is hardly more than "spotting" to profuse hemorrhage, which can lead to maternal death. Minimal spotting may occur following sexual intercourse, presumably related to trauma to the friable ectocervix. Table 20.1 lists causes of bleeding in the second half of pregnancy. A previous Pap test and examination of the lower genital tract should eliminate the likelihood of lower genital tract neoplasms in most cases. At times, patients may mistake bleeding from hemorrhoids or even hematuria for vaginal bleeding, but the difference is easily distinguished by examination.

The two causes of hemorrhage in the second half of pregnancy that require greatest attention–because of the associated maternal and fetal morbidity and mortality rates–are *placenta previa* and *abruptio placentae*. Various characteristics of these entities are compared in Table 20.2.

Placenta Previa

Placenta previa refers to an *abnormal location of the placenta over, or in close proximity to, the internal cervical os.* Placenta previa can be categorized as *complete or total* if the entire cervical os is covered; *partial,* if the margin of the placenta extends across part but not all of the internal os; *marginal,* if the edge of the placenta lies adjacent to the internal os; and *low lying,* if the placenta is located near but not directly adjacent to the internal os (Figure 20.1). The cause of placenta previa is not understood, but abnormal vascularization has long been proposed as a mechanism for this abnormal placement of the placenta. In some cases, such as in twin pregnancy or if the placenta is hydropic, the placenta may extend to the region of the

Table 20.2. Characteristics of Placenta Previa and Abruptio Placentae

Characteristic	Placenta Previa	Abruptio Placentae
Magnitude of blood loss	Variable	Variable
Duration	Often ceases within 1–2 hr	Usually continues
Abdominal discomfort	None	Can be severe
Fetal heart rate pattern on electronic monitoring	Normal	Tachycardia, then bradycardia; loss of variability; decelerations frequently present; intrauterine demise not rare
Coagulation defects	Rare	Associated, but infrequent; DIC often severe when present
Associated history	None	Cocaine use; abdominal trauma; maternal hypertension; multiple gestation; polyhydramnios

DIC, disseminated intravascular coagulation.

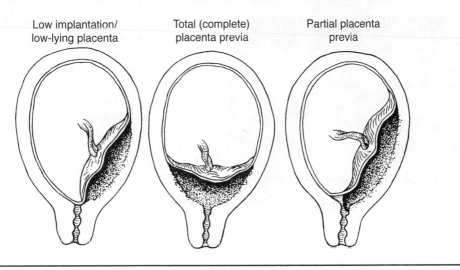

Low implantation/ low-lying placenta   Total (complete) placenta previa   Partial placenta previa

Figure 20.1. Placenta previa.

internal cervical os because of its size alone. Increasing maternal age, increasing parity, and previous cesarean delivery are factors commonly associated with placenta previa, although recent evidence suggests that age alone is not an important factor.

The incidence of placenta previa varies with gestational age. It is usually reported overall as approximately 1 in 250 pregnancies, although there is a great variation in incidence with parity. The incidence in nulliparas is only 1 in 1,000 to 1,500, whereas the incidence in grand-multiparas is as high as 1 in 20. Women with the highest risk for placenta previa are grand-multiparas, those who have had a previous placenta previa (4% to 8%), and those who have had four or more cesarean sections. With common use of ultrasonographic examinations, it has been shown repeatedly that the placenta may cover the internal cervical os in approximately 5% of pregnancies when examined at midpregnancy, a finding seen even more frequently earlier in gestation. Because of subsequent growth of both the upper and lower uterine segments, the placenta appears to "migrate" away from the internal os in the majority of cases. The likelihood of this apparent movement diminishes as the gestational age at first detection increases.

The average gestational age at the time of the first bleeding episode is 29 to 30 weeks. Although the bleeding may be substantial, it almost always ceases spontaneously, unless labor, digital examination, or other trauma occurs. The bleeding is caused by separation of part of the placenta from the lower uterine segment and cervix, possibly in response to mild uterine contractions. The blood that is lost is usually maternal in origin. The patient often describes a sudden onset of bleeding without any apparent antecedent signs. There is no pain associated with placenta previa in most cases, unless coincident with labor or with abruptio placentae (approximately 5% to 10% of cases).

Ultrasonography has been of enormous benefit in localizing the placenta, especially when the placenta is anterior or lateral. If the placenta lies in the posterior portion of the lower uterine segment, its exact relation with the internal os may be more difficult to ascertain. In most cases, though, ultrasonographic examination can accurately diagnose placenta previa (Figure 20.2) or, by illustrating the placenta location away from the cervix and lower uterine segment, exclude it as a cause for bleeding. Transvaginal ultrasonography is often used in this circumstance to complete the placental localization.

The basic management of patients with symptomatic placenta previa includes initial hospitalization with hemodynamic stabilization, followed by expectant management until fetal maturity has occurred. Ideal expectant

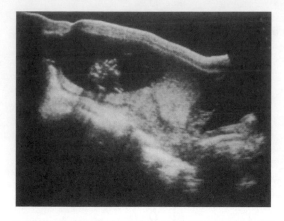

Figure 20.2. Posterior placenta previa shown on transabdominal ultrasound.

management would be continuous hospitalization with enforced bed rest and immediate access to emergency care, but this is increasingly prohibited by cost issues. After initial hospital management, care as an outpatient may be considered if certain criteria are met. These include a highly motivated patient who clearly understands and will comply with instructions concerning restrictions of activity, the constant attendance of a responsible adult to assist in the event of an emergency situation, and the presence of ready transportation to the hospital.

The number of bleeding episodes is unrelated to the degree of placenta previa or to the prognosis for fetal survival. Such expectant management combined with appropriate use of blood transfusion and cesarean birth have resulted in the lowering of the maternal mortality rate from 25% to 30% to <1%, and the perinatal mortality rate from 60% to 70% to <10%. If the fetus is thought to be mature by gestational age criteria or by amniocentesis for fetal lung maturity testing, there is little benefit to be gained by a delay in delivery. The further from term that bleeding from placenta previa occurs, the more important it is to delay delivery to allow for further fetal growth and maturation. The degree of bleeding and the maturity of the fetus must be constantly weighed in managing these patients. Fetal maturity is usually assessed at approximately 36 weeks, with cesarean delivery performed once the fetus is deemed mature.

Before the widespread use of ultrasound, a *double setup examination was frequently used to determine route of delivery for patients suspected of having placenta previa.* This procedure involves careful evaluation of the cervix in the operating room with full preparations for rapid cesarean delivery. If placental tissue is seen or palpated at the internal cervical os, prompt cesarean delivery is performed. This procedure is rarely done today, but may still be an important tool in selected cases.

An attempt at vaginal delivery of a patient with placenta previa may be indicated if the delivery can be accomplished with minimal blood loss and if the fetus is dead, has major fetal malformations, or is clearly previable. If making such an attempt is appropriate, ceasing the process and moving to cesarean delivery for a maternal indication must always be considered. Some patients with only marginal placenta previa may also be candidates for vaginal delivery under controlled circumstances. Placenta previa is associated with a nearly doubling of the rate of congenital malformations; the most serious malformations include major anomalies of the central nervous system, gastrointestinal tract, cardiovascular system, and respiratory tract. At the time of diagnosis of placenta previa, a detailed fetal survey should be performed for anomalies.

Abnormal placental location can be further complicated by abnormal growth of the placental mass into the substance of the uterus, a condition termed *placenta previa accreta.* In placenta previa accreta, the poorly formed decidua of the lower uterine segment offers little resistance to trophoblastic invasion. The incidence of this severe complication is variously reported as 5% to 10% of placenta previa cases, although the incidence is much higher in patients with multiple previous cesarean sections. At the time of delivery, sustained and significant bleeding may ensue, often requiring hysterectomy.

Abruptio Placentae

Whereas placenta previa refers to the abnormal location of the placenta, abruptio placentae, often called placental abruption, refers to the *premature separation of the normally im-*

planted placenta from the uterine wall. Although it shares some clinical features with placenta previa, particularly vaginal bleeding, other characteristics serve to distinguish abruptio placentae from placenta previa, the most important of which are abdominal discomfort and painful uterine contractions (see Table 20.2).

Placental abruption occurs when there is hemorrhage into the decidua basalis, leading to premature placental separation and further bleeding. The cause for this bleeding is often not known. Placental abruption is associated with maternal hypertension and sudden decompression of the uterus in cases of rupture of membranes in a patient with excessive amniotic fluid (hydramnios) or after delivery of the first of multiple fetuses. A more recent and serious association involves cocaine use by the mother, which leads to intense vasoconstriction and, in some cases, sudden separation of the placenta from the uterine wall. Placental abruption can also occur following trauma, even when the extent of injury is not considered serious. For example, pregnant women involved in motor vehicle accidents can sustain placental abruption even though lap belts and shoulder strap restraints are used. Moreover, direct trauma to the abdomen is not required because sudden force applied elsewhere to the body can result in coup and contrecoup injury.

The anatomic relation between vaginal bleeding and placental abruption is shown in Figure 20.3. If the bleeding and subsequent separation of a placenta permit access to the cervical os, vaginal bleeding will be apparent. If the placental location is higher in the uterus, or if the bleeding is more central and the margins of the placenta remain attached to the underlying uterus, blood may not escape into the vagina but is instead trapped under the placenta Thus, the amount of vaginal bleeding is extremely variable, from none to heavy, with even substantial placental abruptions. The bleeding into the basalis stimulates the uterine muscle to contract, and the uterus will be painful to the patient and tender to touch. Unusually painful and frequent uterine contractions may occur, or the uterus may feel constantly tense. At times, the bleeding can penetrate the uterine musculature to such an extent that, at the time of cesarean delivery, the entire uterus has a purplish or bluish appearance, owing to such extravasation of blood (*Couvelaire uterus*). Despite its unusual appearance, no treatment is required because spontaneous resolution of the condition occurs postpartum.

Because the separation of the placenta from the uterus interferes with oxygenation of the fetus, a nonreassuring fetal status is common in cases of significant placental abruption. Thus, in any patient in whom placental abruption is suspected, electronic fetal moni-

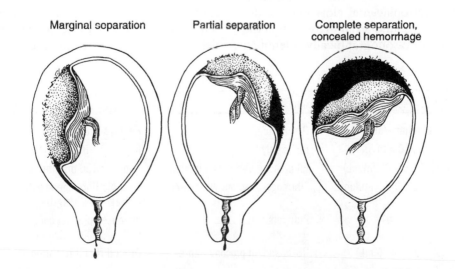

Marginal separation   Partial separation   Complete separation, concealed hemorrhage

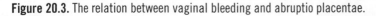

Figure 20.3. The relation between vaginal bleeding and abruptio placentae.

toring should be included in the initial management. Fetal death caused by deprivation of oxygen is, unfortunately, not rare with placental abruption.

Coagulation abnormalities may also be found, thereby compounding the patient's already compromised status. Placental abruption is the most common cause of consumptive coagulopathy in pregnancy and is manifest by hypofibrinogenemia as well as by increased levels of fibrin-degradation products. The platelet count can also be decreased, and prothrombin time and partial thromboplastin time can be increased as well. Such coagulopathy is a result of intravascular and retroplacental coagulation. The intravascular fibrinogen is converted to fibrin by way of the extrinsic clotting cascade. Thus, not only is serum fibrinogen decreased but platelets and other clotting factors are thereby also depleted. Transfusion with crystalloid, packed red blood cells and, potentially, platelets and fresh-frozen plasma should be implemented as soon as possible for those patients who require either volume replacement or oxygen-carrying capacity. Table 20.3 provides a list of blood-replacement products. The extent of placental abruption is generally categorized as the proportion of the maternal surface of the placenta on which a clot is detected at the time of delivery (e.g., 50% abruption).

Ultrasound is of little benefit in diagnosing placental abruption, except to exclude placenta previa as a cause for the hemorrhage. Relatively large retroplacental clots may be detected on ultrasound examination, but the absence of ultrasonographically identified retroplacental clots does not rule out the possibility of placental abruption, and, conversely, a retroplacental echogenic area can be seen in patients without placental abruption. The diagnosis rests on the classic clinical presentation of vaginal bleeding, a tender uterus, and frequent uterine contractions with some evidence of fetal distress. The extravasation of blood into the uterine muscle causes contractions so the resting intrauterine pressure, when measured with an intrauterine pressure catheter, is often elevated; this sign can be helpful in making the diagnosis.

Management of a patient with placental abruption when the fetus is mature is hemodynamic stabilization and delivery. Careful attention to blood component therapy is critical, and the coagulation status must be followed closely. Unless there is evidence of fetal distress or hemodynamic instability, vaginal delivery by oxytocin induction of labor is preferable to a cesarean delivery, although the maternal or fetal status may require that abdominal delivery be performed. When the fetus is not mature and the placental abruption is limited and not associated with premature labor or fetal or maternal distress, observation with close monitoring of both fetal and maternal well-being may be considered while awaiting fetal maturity.

Vasa Previa

Although rarely encountered, *vasa previa* presents significant risk to the fetus. In vasa previa, the umbilical cord inserts into the membranes

Table 20.3. Blood-Replacement Products		
Component (volume/unit)	**Discussion**	**Factors Present**
Packed RBCs (250 mL)	RBCs only	Replaces RBC cell mass only
Fresh-frozen plasma (250 mL)	All procoagulants; no platelets	Supplies 150 mg fibrinogen/unit
Cryoprecipitate (20–50 mL/unit)	Fibrinogen; factors VIII and XIII	Variable fibrinogen content; averages 0.25 mg/bag
Platelets (50 mL/unit)	Platelets only	Increases platelet count 5,000–8,000/mcL/unit
Fresh whole blood (500 mL)	RBCs and all procoagulants	Often difficult to obtain

RBCs, red blood cells.

of the placenta (rather than into the central mass of the placental tissue), and one such vessel lies below the presenting fetal part in the vicinity of the internal os. If this vessel ruptures, fetal bleeding occurs. Because of the low blood volume of the fetus, seemingly insignificant amounts of blood may place the fetus in jeopardy. A small amount of vaginal bleeding associated with fetal tachycardia may be the clinical presentation. A test to distinguish fetal blood from maternal blood, such as the Betke–Kleihauer or the Apt test, can be of value when such a condition is suspected. These tests distinguish between maternal and fetal blood on the basis of the marked resistance to pH changes in fetal red cells compared with the friable nature of adult red cells in the presence of strong bases. Immediate cesarean section is the only way to save the fetus in vasa previa.

Uterine Rupture as a Cause of Obstetric Hemorrhage

Separation of the muscular wall of the pregnant uterus occurs in a fraction of 1% of pregnancies, most commonly associated with labor in a patient who has had a cesarean section (vaginal birth after cesarean section). The incidence approaches 0.5% for patients with an uncomplicated previous lower segment transverse cesarean section, but may approach one in four to one in three patients with previous incisions of the upper uterine segment or fundus (previous classic cesarean section, previous myomectomy, or repair of congenital uterine anomaly). Other conditions associated with such intrapartum rupture include uterine hyperstimulation (either endogenous, as in chorioamnionitis, or exogenous with Pitocin induction or augmentation of labor), uterine anomalies, placenta increta or percreta, grandmultiparity, obstructed labor (fetal macrosomia, uterine myomas blocking the birth passage, fetopelvic disproportion), and previous perforation of the uterus associated with dilatation and curettage, hysteroscopy, or forceps delivery. Often such separation occurs slowly, involving only the muscular wall without breach of the overlying peritonium. In this case, *uterine scar dehiscence or uterine window formation,* bleeding is minimal, the fetus remains in utero, uterine function continues, there is no disruption of placental function if the scar is not under the placenta, and delivery is unimpeded. The rent is discovered during the postpartum examination. Uterine rupture occurs when the rent is relatively more rapid, with disruption of the peritoneum and uterine wall, bleeding, extrusion of the fetus from the uterus, separation of the placenta with nonreassuring fetal status, and/or shock, and occasionly disseminated intravascular disease.

Because uterine rupture may be difficult to recognize, close intrapartum surveillance with appreciation of the risk factors is requisite. The most common early finding is nonreassuring fetal status, with fetal heart rate decelerations, bradycardia, and/or failure to detect fetal heart activity in about one-half to three-fourths of cases. Bleeding, loss of fetal station, shock, pain, and altered uterine activity are also noted in varying numbers of patients. Management consists of immediate exploratory laparotomy, retrieval and the hopeful resuscitation of the fetus, and repair of the uterine rent. In most cases, repair is possible, although in some cases damage is sufficiently severe that hysterectomy is required. The management of women with a previous uterine rupture confined to the lower uterine segment is controversial because the repeat rupture rate is about 5%. If the uterine rupture involves the upper segment of the uterus, the repeat rate approaches 33% and cesarean delivery at 36 to 37 weeks is recommended.

Antepartum uterine rupture is rarely spontaneous, rather it is associated with trauma in most situations. Auto accidents with improper seat belt placement and assault are the two most common situations encountered.

CHAPTER 21

POSTTERM PREGNANCY

This chapter deals primarily with APGO Educational Topic:

Topic 30: Postterm Pregnancy

Students should be able to identify the normal period of gestation, and the evaluation and management in pregnancy when gestation extends beyond this normal period. Students should also be able to discuss the maternal and fetal complications of gestation extending beyond the normal period.

Normal pregnancy lasts from 38 to 42 weeks, which is considered "term." Stated another way, term is the due date or estimated date of confinement ±2 weeks. *A patient who has not delivered by the completion of the forty-second week* (294 days from the first day of the last normal menstrual period) is said to be postterm (a common synonym is *postdates*). This condition occurs in approximately 8% to 10% of pregnancies and carries with it an increased risk of adverse outcome. The increased morbidity and mortality in a small percentage of cases, however, warrants careful evaluation of all postterm pregnancies. In addition, postterm pregnancies can create significant stress for the patient, her family, and those caring for her. Therefore, the physician should reassure the patient and discuss with her the options for management.

leads to the erroneous classification of a pregnancy as postterm has two important sequelae. First, these pregnancies are labeled "high-risk," costly increased evaluations are employed, and the likelihood of intervention increases. The latter leads to the second sequela: increased intervention usually means delivery by induction or cesarean section, both of which are associated with increased maternal and fetal morbidity. Other less common causes of postterm pregnancy are listed in Table 21.1. Uterine contractility has also been shown to be diminished in some cases of postterm pregnancy, suggesting a cause intrinsic to the myometrium. Whatever the cause, there is a tendency for recurrence of postterm pregnancy. *Approximately 50% of patients having one postterm pregnancy will experience prolonged pregnancy with the next gestation.*

Cause

The most common "cause" of postterm pregnancy is inaccurate estimation of gestational age (dating). Inaccurate dating is more likely in women with irregular menses, those who seek prenatal care later in pregnancy, those with delayed ovulation (for example, a woman who has just stopped using oral contraceptives), and those who simply do not remember their last menstrual period accurately. Inaccurate dating that

Effects

The morbidity and mortality rates for the postterm fetus increase severalfold compared with term pregnancies. Stillbirth and neonatal mortality rates increase steadily after 37 weeks, approaching 1 in 300 at 42 weeks. It is impossible to discuss postterm without discussing macrosomia, diabetes mellitus, meconium aspiration syndrome, and shoulder dystocia as these co-morbidities are closely related.

Table 21.1. Factors Associated With Postterm Pregnancy	
Factor	**Discussion**
Inaccurate or unknown dates	*Most common cause;* high association with and major risk factor of late or no prenatal care
Irregular ovulation; variation in length of follicular phase	Results in overestimation of gestational age
Altered estrogen:progesterone ratio	
Anencephaly	Decreased production of 16α-hydroxydehydroepiandrosterone sulfate, a precursor of estriol
Fetal adrenal hypoplasia	Decreased fetal production precursors of estriol
Placental sulfatase deficiency	X-linked disease prevents placenta conversion of sulfated estrogen precursors
Extrauterine pregnancy	Pregnancy not in uterus, no labor (see Chapter 15)

Approximately 25% of prolonged pregnancies result in a *macrosomic infant* (i.e., birth weight >4,000 or 4,500 g, depending on the definition used) and may occur in any prolonged pregnancy, although maternal obesity or diabetes mellitus raises the risk. These infants may demonstrate altered glucose and bilirubin metabolism and are at risk for hypoglycemia and hyperbilirubinemia. They have an increased incidence of birth trauma, especially shoulder dystocia, fracture of the clavicle, and associated brachial plexus injury (Erb, or Erb–Duchenne, palsy) during vaginal delivery as well as of the need for cesarean section as a result of fetopelvic disproportion. *Brachial plexus injury* is reported in approximately 1 in 500 term deliveries and is especially likely in the delivery of macrosomic infants, breech deliveries, or in difficult deliveries, although it may occur in the seemingly uneventful, easy delivery. In the *Erb (or Erb–Duchenne) palsy,* or paralysis, stretch or tear injury to the upper roots of the brachial plexus results in paralysis of the deltoid and infraspinatus muscles and flexor muscles of the forearm, causing the limb to hang limply close to the side, forearm extended and internally rotated; finger function is usually retained. Less frequently, damage is limited to the lower nerves of the brachial plexus, causing *Klumpke paralysis,* or paralysis of the hand. Because most injuries are mild, treatment is expectant, with splints and physical therapy and the anticipation of complete or nearly complete recovery in 3 to 6 months. In fetal macrosomia, there can also be maternal trauma, with lacerations of the maternal perineum or, in the case of cesarean delivery, of the uterus and other pelvic organs.

Another special concern in postterm pregnancies is meconium passage and the *meconium aspiration syndrome*, which can lead to severe respiratory distress from mechanical obstruction of both small and large airways as well as meconium chemical pneumonitis. Meconium passage is not limited to postterm pregnancies, although postterm pregnancy, especially if there is oligohydramnios, is a substantial risk factor; it is seen in 13% to 15% of all term pregnancies. The incidence of meconium passage increases as pregnancy becomes prolonged, as does the incidence of meconium aspiration syndrome. Increasingly severe *placental dysfunction* with decreased transfer of water, electrolytes, glucose, amino acids, and oxygen can occur in postterm pregnancy. In normal pregnancy, the placenta reaches its maximum size and surface area at approximately 37 weeks of gestational age with functional peak at the same time. Thereafter, size, surface area, and function decrease. To compensate, especially in the postdates intervals, the fetus may decrease its energy requirements by decreasing growth and deposition of fat and glycogen. Second, it may slow movement. Lastly, it may experience degrees of hypoxia, during movement or with contractions, or at rest. Approximately 40% of placentas from postterm pregnancies demonstrate placental infarcts, calcification, and fibrosis consistent with decreased functional capability. Placental dysfunction is the primary mechanism that causes oligohydramnios postterm, and is the reason for close antenatal surveillance for oligohydramnios and its sequela.

Diagnosis

The diagnosis of postterm pregnancy rests on establishment of the correct gestational age. Every effort should be made to accurately assess gestational age as early as possible in pregnancy, when the parameters used for this purpose are most discriminating and reliable. With improved access to prenatal care and the greater importance placed on accurate gestational age assessment, the percentage of patients in whom postterm pregnancy is suspected but whose dates are uncertain has diminished. Nonetheless, a substantial number of patients do not seek prenatal care early in pregnancy or do not have an accurate gestational age determination. Physicians should be suspicious of the presumed due date of any patient who first appears for prenatal care late in pregnancy who might be "1 or 2 months overdue." Care should be taken to properly evaluate and monitor her fetus for these problems associated with postterm pregnancy.

Management

The first step in management of postterm pregnancy is a careful review of the information used to establish the gestational age to be as certain as possible that the estimate is correct. *Once a patient approaches 41 weeks of gestation (1 week past her due date), the management options are either to induce labor or to continue surveillance of fetal well-being until spontaneous labor occurs.*

If gestational age is believed to be firmly established, factors that influence the decision of whether or not to deliver rest with the patient's concerns and desires, the assessment of fetal well-being, and the status of the cervix. Induction of labor is appropriate if the cervix is favorable (see Chapter 7 regarding induction of labor and the Bishop score) and if the patient prefers labor induction

Several studies have shown no difference in cesarean rates comparing 41-week induction to expectant management until 42 weeks.

If the cervix is not favorable or if the patient does not wish induction of labor, fetal well-being is monitored while awaiting spontaneous labor or a change in the cervix so that induction is appropriate. A variety of management schemes have been devised for this "waiting period," none of which is clearly superior. Daily fetal movement counting is included in most management plans, with decreased perceived fetal movement an indication for further, timely evaluation of fetal well-being. Weekly monitoring of amniotic fluid volume is commonly employed, often by using an amniotic fluid index measurement in which the largest pocket of fluid is measured in each of the four quadrants of the uterus and summed; a value of more than 5 or so is considered within normal limits, and less than that it is considered as oligohydramnios. This diagnosis is usually considered a sufficient indication for delivery. Antepartum fetal heart rate monitoring is also commonly used, with the nonstress tests employed twice a week, or oxytocin challenge tests employed once or twice a week. The biophysical profile is a combination of ultrasound and fetal heart rate monitoring information, and may be used once or twice a week. Doppler flow studies of the umbilical artery are also considered useful. These studies are discussed in Chapter 5. All of these tests are most useful when the data obtained are viewed in the context of the whole pregnancy, maternal and fetal factors.

If the gestational age is not well established, the clinician uses whatever information is available to determine the best date. Amniocentesis is not especially helpful because fetal lung maturity is rarely a question in the postterm evaluation. When the best date is selected, a management plan similar to that for a postterm pregnancy with well-established dates is used.

Although there is no absolute time within which labor must be induced, most physicians believe that delivery should be effected between 41 and 42 weeks. Proponents of such cutoff dates are said to favor *"aggressive management,"* citing increased morbidity and mortality after 41 completed weeks of gestation. Modern methods for surveillance of fetal well-being make it less logical to be dogmatic about mandatory induction at a given gestational age. Proponents of *"expectant management"* allow pregnancy to continue for some time as long as there is evidence of fetal well-being. Several different agents are now available for induction of labor: intravenous oxytocin (Pitocin); intracervical or intravaginal preparation of prostaglandin; Foley bulb placed through the cervix; laminaria, a hydrophilic device that dilates the cervix; and Misoprostol (see Chapter 7). The choice will depend on the readiness of the cervix, the condition of the fetus, and the experience of the physician. Rarely, cesarean section without attempted induction may be performed.

Because of the risk of macrosomia-associated birth trauma, ultrasonographic estimation of fetal weight should be obtained before any induction of labor in a postterm pregnancy when macrosomia is suspected. If the estimated fetal weight is >5,000 g in a woman who does not have diabetes or 4,500 g in a woman with diabetes, primary cesarean delivery should be offered.

Patients with postterm pregnancies should be advised to come promptly to the hospital when labor pains commence. Once the onset of regular contractions occurs, careful electronic fetal monitoring should be used throughout labor because of the risk of fetal stress/distress. Intrapartum management includes the artificial rupture of membranes, when possible, to allow detection of meconium and to allow the placement of a fetal scalp electrode and intrauterine pressure catheter. If the decreased amniotic fluid is sufficient to permit undue pressure on

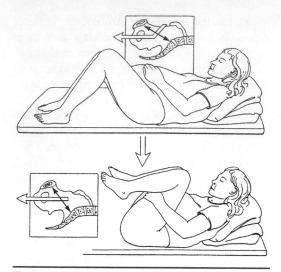

Figure 21.1. McRoberts maneuver: hyperflexion of thighs to aid in the management of shoulder dystocia.

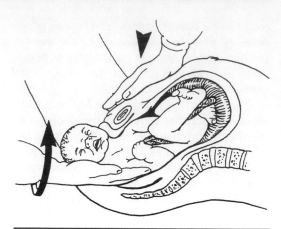

Figure 21.2. Rotation plus suprapubic pressure to aid in the management of shoulder dystocia.

the umbilical cord, deceleration of the fetal heart rate may occur. Infusion of normal saline through the intrauterine pressure catheter (amnioinfusion) may provide a buffer for the cord and eliminate these decelerations. Because of the increased risk of cesarean delivery for a nonreassuring fetal heart rate tracing and because of the potential problems associated with meconium, both anesthesia and pediatric personnel should be alerted that a postterm patient is in labor.

At the time of delivery, special precautions are taken. If meconium passage has been noted, the infant's nasopharynx and oropharynx should be suctioned before delivery of the shoulders. Pediatric support should be available in the delivery room whenever possbile, to provide prompt evaluation of the infant. In a depressed infant, aggressive suctioning of the fetus with a laryngoscope decreases, but does not eliminate, the likelihood of meconium aspiration syndrome. In a vigorous infant with meconium, laryngoscopy and aggressive suctioning is no longer indicated. Because of the risk of macrosomia in postterm pregnancy, the delivery team should be familiar with the techniques used to treat shoulder dystocia, such as exaggerated flexion of the thighs (McRoberts maneuver [Figure 21.1]) and suprapubic pressure (Figure 21.2).

CHAPTER 22

PRETERM LABOR

This chapter deals primarily with APGO Educational Topic:

Topic 24: Preterm Labor

Students should be able to list the risk factors associated with preterm labor and delivery, and discuss the evaluation and management of preterm labor, including counseling. Students should similarly be able to describe the same issues with respect to cervical incompetence.

Preterm birth is delivery that occurs prior to the completion of 37 weeks of gestation. Because *preterm birth* is the most common cause of perinatal morbidity and mortality, its prevention and treatment are major concerns in obstetric care. The *consequences of preterm birth* occur with increasing severity and frequency the earlier the gestational age of the newborn. Seventy-five percent of neonatal deaths that are not the result of congenital malformations are associated with premature labor and birth. Besides perinatal death in the very young fetus, common complications of preterm birth include respiratory distress syndrome (formerly called hyaline membrane disease), intraventricular hemorrhage, necrotizing enterocolitis, sepsis, neurologic impairment, and seizures. Long-term morbidity associated with preterm delivery includes bronchopulmonary dysplasia and developmental abnormalities, including cerebral palsy. The significant impact of preterm birth is best summarized by this fact: *The 11% to 12% of babies born prematurely account for 60% to 75% of all perinatal morbidity and mortality in the United States.*

Preterm birth may occur as the result of spontaneous preterm labor (PTL) or preterm premature rupture of membranes (PROM). These births are collectively known as spontaneous preterm births. Some preterm births (20% to 30%) are the result of deliberate intervention for a variety of pregnancy complications and have unavoidable perinatal complications (e.g., delivery of a preterm fetus because of maternal eclampsia) and are considered indicated preterm births. Preterm PROM will be considered in more depth in a subsequent chapter.

It is important to *separate the concepts of low birth weight and prematurity* when discussing preterm delivery and labor. Prematurity reflects gestational age, whereas low birth weight is based on the single parameter of weight, usually 2,500 g or less. For example, a growth-restricted fetus of a hypertensive patient may weigh well under 2,500 g at 40 weeks of gestation. Such an infant is a low birth weight infant but not preterm, and will suffer the consequences associated with low birth weight and the effects of maternal hypertension, but not of premature birth. Likewise, an

infant of a mother with diabetes may be delivered before term, weigh in excess of 2,500 g, and still have the significant perinatal morbidities of preterm birth and maternal diabetes.

Preterm labor is functionally defined as the presence of *regular uterine contractions, occurring with a frequency of every 10 minutes or less between 20 and 36 weeks of gestation, with each contraction lasting at least 30 seconds. This uterine activity is accompanied by cervical effacement, cervical dilation, and/or descent of the fetus into the pelvis.* However, variations of this definition are commonly used, and much of the criteria rest with data whose subjective measurement is difficult, so it is often difficult to know when a patient is really in PTL. This presents a problem because treatment appears to be more effective when initiated early in the course of PTL; waiting for cervical changes to occur to establish a definitive diagnosis may limit successful therapy.

Cause, Prediction, and Prevention of Preterm Labor

A number of causes and associated factors have been implicated in PTL (Table 22.1). About 10% of preterm births are in multiple gestations, although multiple gestation accounts for only about 1% of pregnancies. If a patient's first pregnancy ends in PTL and delivery, her risk in a subsequent pregnancy is increased twofold, and if she has a second PTL and delivery, her risk increases still further to threefold for the next pregnancy. However, an intervening term labor and delivery decrease the risk in similar proportion. African-American women have at least twofold increased rates of preterm birth because of PTL or preterm PROM when compared with other racial and ethnic groups. Subclinical intra-amniotic infection has also been associated with PTL and preterm PROM, especially at the earlier gestational ages. Unfortunately, in most cases, PTL is idiopathic (i.e., no cause or risk factor can be identified).

Infant morbidity and mortality following preterm birth have decreased over the last several decades as the result of several factors, and despite the identification of successful strategies to predict and prevent PTL. First, neona-

Table 22.1. Factors Associated With Preterm Labor

African-American race	Excessive uterine enlargement
Prior history of preterm birth	Polyhydramnios
Preterm uterine contractions	Multiple gestation
Premature rupture of membranes (PROM)	Uterine distortion
Incompetent cervix	Leiomyomas
Primary	Septate uterus, uterine didelphis, and other anomalies
Secondary to surgery (e.g., cone biopsy of cervix)	Placental abnormalities
Shortened cervix by TV ultrasonography	Abruptio placentae
Presence of cervicovaginal fetal fibronectin	Placenta previa
Infections	Maternal smoking (associated with PROM)
Urinary	Other substance abuse
Vaginal	Iatrogenic: induction of labor
Bacterial vaginosis	
Intra-amniotic	

tal management strategies for preterm infants have greatly improved outcome. For women in PTL presenting to hospitals without sophisticated neonatal intensive care, maternal transport to a regional tertiary care center is indicated for the neonate to receive this care. Second, the use of corticosteroids administered to a mother at immediate risk for preterm birth (such as a woman in PTL) has resulted in decreased incidence of respiratory distress syndrome and associated infant morbidity and mortality. Therapy to stop contractions in a woman in PTL (tocolytic therapy) may prolong pregnancy for up to 48 hours and allow time to administer corticosteroids. Finally, prophylaxis against perinatal infection with group B streptococcus in women with PTL or preterm PROM has also improved infant morbidity and mortality rates in the United States.

Prediction of Preterm Labor

Patient and physician education has focused on *recognition of the signs and symptoms* that suggest PTL (Table 22.2). Patients with such symptoms are counseled to seek and to receive prompt medical attention. Patient education to help recognize these signs and symptoms is an important part of care. Patients destined to develop frank PTL may have increased uterine irritability and more frequent contractions in the weeks before the PTL develops, but maternal ability to distinguish normal preterm uterine activity from PTL often lacks accuracy. *Home uterine activity monitoring* using remote tocodynamometry was hoped to be effective in the recognition of PTL, but no differences in outcome with the use of this monitoring have

Table 22.2. Symptoms and Signs of Preterm Labor

Menstrual-like cramps
Low, dull backache
Abdominal pressure
Pelvic pressure
Abdominal cramping (with or without diarrhea)
Increase or change in vaginal discharge (mucous, watery, light bloody discharge)
Uterine contractions, often painless

been demonstrated in properly designed studies, and its use is no longer recommended.

An *increase in the concentration of fetal fibronectin (fFN) in cervicovaginal secretions* is found with PTL. Fetal fibronectin is an extracellular glycoprotein normally found in the cervical mucus in early pregnancy and then again near term. A preterm rise in the concentration of fFN may be associated with the impending onset of PTL. However, *the greatest benefit of fFN appears to be its negative predictive value in that its absence from cervicovaginal secretions is uncommonly associated with a patient who delivers in the 7 days after the sample is taken.*

Bacterial vaginosis is a common alteration of the vaginal flora in up to 40% of pregnant women and has been associated with PTL and preterm PROM. Bacterial vaginosis is diagnosed using the documented presence of three of four possible clinical findings: (1) homogeneous vaginal discharge, (2) clue cells on saline microscopy, (3) amine or "fishy" odor with the addition of KOH to vaginal secretions, and (4) vaginal pH >4.5. Bacterial vaginosis diagnosed in symptomatic pregnant patients should thus be treated. Unfortunately, widespread screening and treatment for bacterial vaginosis in asymptomatic low-risk women and women with previous preterm birth has not been beneficial in decreasing the occurrence of PTL and is not recommended.

Early asymptomatic dilation and effacement of the cervix (incompetent cervix) seems to be associated with an increased likelihood of PTL and delivery. Cervical examinations can be performed periodically through the second half of gestation, although their sensitivity and specificity is low, primarily because of examiner-interrelator variability. *Transvaginal ultrasound examination of the cervix* is a reliable and reproducible method to assess cervical length when performed by trained personnel. As the cervical length decreases in midpregnancy, the risk for preterm birth increases. Unfortunately, interventions such as prophylactic cervical cerclage (see Chapter 24, "Obstetric Procedures") on sonographic recognition of a shortened cervical length (often defined as <2.5 cm against a normal value of 4) has not proved beneficial in

several studies, although the issue is highly controversial and many obstetricians disagree on its lack of usefulness and continue to use cerclage.

Thus, for the general population and for women with risk factors associated with PTL, there are currently no uniformly effective interventions to prevent PTL and preterm birth. Recently, a significant decrease in PTL has been demonstrated in women at risk with weekly intramuscular injections of the progesterone, 17-α-hydroxyprogesterone caproate. Its use is increasingly common.

Evaluation of a Patient in Suspected Preterm Labor

Once a patient describes symptoms and signs suggestive of PTL, evaluation should be prompt. Application of an *external electronic fetal monitor (tocodynamometer)* may help to quantify the frequency and duration of contractions; the intensity of which is still best evaluated by abdominal palpation by experienced personnel. The status of the cervix should be determined, either by visualization with a speculum or by gentle digital examination. Because digital examination may increase the risk of infection if there is premature rupture of membranes, speculum evaluation should be performed first if there is indication of membrane rupture. If there is membrane rupture, cervical dilation and effacement are estimated by inspection rather than by digital examination. Changes in cervical effacement and dilation on subsequent examinations are important in the evaluation of both the diagnosis of PTL and the effectiveness of management. Subtle changes are often of great clinical importance, so serial examinations by the same examiner are optimal to decrease interrater reliability error, although this is not always practical.

Because urinary infections can predispose to uterine contractions, a *urinalysis and urine culture* should be obtained. At the time of speculum examination, a cervical culture should be taken for group B streptococcus. Empiric treatment for group B streptococcus with penicillin or ampicillin is generally given until culture results are available. When indicated by history or physical examination findings, cultures for *Chlamydia* and *Neisseria gonorrhoeae* should be obtained.

Ultrasound examination is useful in assessing the gestational age of the fetus, estimation of the amniotic fluid volume (spontaneous rupture of membranes with fluid loss may precede PTL and may be unrecognized by the patient), fetal presentation, and placental location, as well as the existence of fetal congenital anomalies. Because placenta previa and abruptio placentae may lead to preterm contractions, patients should also be monitored for bleeding.

Because either clinical or subclinical infection of the amniotic cavity is thought to be associated with PTL in some cases, *amniocentesis* may be performed. The presence of bacteria in amniotic fluid is correlated not only with PTL but also with the subsequent development of infection, which is less responsive to therapy. The presence of white cells in the amniotic fluid may also indicate infection. Antibiotic therapy before delivery is instituted if infection is diagnosed or strongly suspected. If intrauterine infection on amniocentesis is confirmed, then delivery is generally indicated and clinical evidence of infection (chorioamnoinitis) should prompt delivery regardless of

Table 22.3. Agents Used in Treating Preterm Labor

Class (Example)	Action	Adverse effects	Comments
Magnesium sulfate	Competes with calcium for entry into cells	May cause flushing or headaches; at high levels may cause respiratory depression (12–15 mg/dL) or cardiac depression (>15 mg/dL)	High degree of safety; often used as first agent; contraindicated in patients with hypocalcemia or who have myasthenia gravis
β-adrenergic agents (ritodrine, terbutaline)	Increase cAMP in cell, which decreases free calcium	Hypotension, tachycardia, anxiety, chest tightening or pain, ECG changes; increased pulmonary edema occurs very infrequently but is possible, especially with fluid overload; relatively contraindicated in patients with coronary artery disease and in those with renal failure	β-receptors are of two types: $β_1$-receptors predominate in the heart and intestines and $β_2$-receptors predominate in the uterus, lungs, and blood vessels;
Prostaglandin synthetase inhibitors (indomethacin)	Decrease PG production by blocking conversion of free arachidonic acid to PG	Premature constriction of ductus arteriosus possible especially after 34 weeks; reversible impaired fetal renal function and oligohydramnios with prolonged exposure (72 hr or more)	Second line of therapy
Calcium-channel blockers (nifedipine)	Prevent calcium entry into muscle cells	Problems include possible decrease in uteroplacental blood flow, fetal hypoxia, and hypercarbia	May potentiate side effects of magnesium sulfate

cAMP, cyclic adenosine monophosphate; ECG, electrocardiogram; PG, prostaglandin.

the gestational age. At the time of amniocentesis, additional amniotic fluid may be obtained for pulmonary maturity studies, which could have bearing on subsequent management, and for glucose, a low level of which is suggestive of intrauterine infection. Tocolysis, or the suppression of uterine contractions by pharmacologic means, is not appropriate in the setting of intrauterine infection and may not be appropriate if there is indication of fetal lung maturity because lung maturity does not necessarily correlate with all aspects of fetal maturity.

Management of Preterm Labor

The purpose in treating PTL is to delay delivery, if possible, until fetal maturity is attained. Management involves *two broad goals:* (*1*) the detection and treatment of disorders associated with PTL, and (*2*) therapy for the PTL itself. Although it is fortunate that more than 50% of patients with preterm contractions have spontaneous resolution of abnormal uterine activity, this complicates the evaluation of treatment. One may not know whether there was actual PTL or simply normal preterm uterine activity. It may be difficult to know whether it was the treatment that stopped the PTL or whether it would have stopped without therapy.

Because dehydration has been known to lead to uterine irritability, *therapy often begins with intravenous hydration.* In a significant number of patients, this therapy alone causes

Table 22.5. Administration of Nifedipine for Preterm Labor

- Loading dose: 30 mg
- Immediate tocolysis: 20 mg po q 6–8 hr; may increase to q 4 hr if blood pressure remains >80/50
- Maintenance: 10–20 mg q 8 hr if necessary
- Cautions: Contraindicated in patients with myasthenia gravis, renal failure, hypoglycemia, or active hepatitis and/or hepatic failure; may potentiate the effect of magnesium sulfate, leading to hypotension and respiratory depression
- Pharmacology: Inhibits calcium transport through L-type or slow-type channels, causing significant reductions in systemic and pulmonary vascular resistance and tocolysis; specific uterine effects include inhibition of myometrial contractility and reduction of uterine vascular resistance; potentiates magnesium sulfate but may be used concurrently with β-blockers such as terbutaline
- Side effects: Flushing is common; headache in 5%–10% of patients; hypotension and tachycardia are rare; no known teratogenic effects
- Other uses: Treatment of hypertension in pregnancy

cessation of uterine contractions, although its value in patients who are already well hydrated is controversial. Furthermore, hydration does not stop PTL.

Various tocolytic therapies have been used in the management of PTL (Table 22.3); two specific regimens are detailed in Tables 22.4 and 22.5. *Unfortunately, tocolytics have not clearly shown to prolong pregnancy beyond several days.* Different treatment regimens address specific mechanisms involved in the maintenance of uterine contractions, and each, therefore, may be best suited for certain patients.

Typically, *patients with a diagnosis of PTL receive one form of therapy, with the addition or substitution of other forms if the initial treatment is considered unsuccessful.* As noted in Table 22.3, adverse side effects, at times serious and even life threatening to the mother, can occur.

Table 22.4. Administration of Magnesium Sulfate for Preterm Labor

- 6 g MgSO$_4$ are mixed in 100–150 mL of D$_5$W and infused over 15–20 min as a loading dose
- 40 g MgSO$_4$ are mixed in 1,000 mL of D$_5$W, providing an MgSO$_4$ concentration of 1 g MgSO$_4$ in 25 mL of solution
- Using a piggyback infusion via an infusion pump, the physician usually begins infusion at 2 g/hr (50 mL/hr) and increases it in 0.5-g/hr increments as needed

These possibilities must be taken into account in selecting a therapy. The maturity of the fetus is a consideration in deciding how aggressively to pursue therapy, and, in general, the vigor with which therapy is undertaken diminishes as the gestational age of the fetus increases. One might be more willing to accept potential adverse effects for a patient in PTL at 26 weeks as opposed to 33 weeks. It is customary not to initiate or to stop therapy after 35 to 36 weeks. Treatment sequences may vary from hospital to hospital, depending on the individual hospital experience and the success rate with various therapeutic regimens.

Contraindications to tocolysis include advanced labor, a mature fetus, a severely anomalous fetus, intrauterine infection, significant vaginal bleeding, conditions in which the adverse effects of tocolysis may be marked, and a variety of obstetric complications that contraindicate delay in delivery.

From 24 to 34 weeks, management generally includes administration of certain *steroids,* such as betamethasone, *to enhance pulmonary maturity*. Both the incidence and severity of respiratory distress syndrome appear to be reduced with this therapy. In addition, other sequelae of prematurity such as interventricular hemorrhage and necrotizing enterocolitis occur less frequently in infants whose mothers received betamethasone. The salutatory effect for the fetus appears to wane after 7 days; however, routine weekly courses are not recommended because of potential negative neurologic fetal effects. If there has been some time between initial treatment with corticosteroids (such as >4 weeks), though, a "rescue" course of steroids may be considered.

Because tocolytic therapy is often unsuccessful, maternal transfer of a woman in PTL (after stabilization) to a center with a neonatal intensive care unit is highly advisable.

CHAPTER 23

PREMATURE RUPTURE OF MEMBRANES

This chapter deals primarily with APGO Educational Topic:

Topic 25: Premature Rupture of Membranes

Students should be able to explain the risk factors associated with premature rupture of the membranes, its diagnosis by physical examination and laboratory study, and expectant versus immediate delivery managements. Students should also know the risks and benefits for mother and infant from both kinds of management and how to counsel patients about them.

Amniotic fluid is produced continuously as the result of passage of fluid across the fetal membranes and across the skin, fetal urine production, and fetal pulmonary effluent. It provides protection against infection, fetal trauma, and umbilical cord compression. It also allows for fetal movement and fetal breathing, which, in turn, permits full fetal respiratory development. Decreased or absent amniotic fluid can lead to compression of the umbilical cord and decreased placental blood flow. Disruption (rupture) of these fetal membranes is associated with loss of protective effects and developmental roles of amniotic fluid.

Premature rupture of membranes (PROM) is defined as rupture of the chorioamniotic membrane before the onset of labor. Premature rupture of membrane occurs in approximately 10% to 15% of all pregnancies. The PROM is associated with about 10% of term pregnancies (37 weeks or more of gestational age) and is generally followed by the onset of labor. *The primary risk of PROM at less than 37 weeks of gestation is preterm labor and delivery,* with about 75% of patients with preterm PROM delivering within 1 week of the time of membrane rupture. Preterm PROM is associated in about 30% of preterm deliveries. Premature rupture of membranes leading to preterm delivery is, in turn, associated with neonatal complications of prematurity such as respiratory distress syndrome, intraventricular hemorrhage, neonatal infection, necrotizing enterocolitis, neurologic and neuromuscular dysfunction, and sepsis. A major complication of PROM is intrauterine infection (chorioamnionitis; 30% to 50% of cases), the incidence of which increases with decreasing gestational age at PROM. The presence of lower genital tract infections such as *Neisseria gonorrhoeae,* bacterial vaginosis, and group B streptococcus increase the risk of intrauterine infection associated with PROM. Other complications include prolapsed umbilical cord and abruptio placentae.

The consequences of preterm PROM differ substantially, depending on the gestational age, increasing as gestational age decreases. Midtrimester preterm PROM (between 16 and 26 weeks of gestational age) complicates about 1% of all pregnancies. Today, survival is increasingly likely in the 24- to 26-week group, although the morbidities of extreme prematurity in this group of neonates are more substantial and frequent in inverse proportion to gestational age. Oligohydramnios at <20 to 22 weeks of gestation is associated with incomplete alveolar development and the development of pulmonary hypoplasia. Infants born with pulmonary hypoplasia cannot be adequately ventilated regardless of the gestational age at birth, and soon succumb to hypoxia and barotrauma from high-pressure ventilation.

The *cause* of PROM is not clearly understood. Sexually transmitted diseases and other lower genital tract conditions such as bacterial vaginosis may play a role, as such *infections* are more commonly found in women with PROM than in those without sexually transmitted disease or bacterial vaginosis. However, intact fetal membranes and normal amniotic fluid do not fully protect the fetus from infection because it appears that subclinical intra-amniotic infection may be responsible for PROM in certain cases. Metabolites produced by bacteria may either weaken the fetal membranes or initiate uterine contractions through stimulating prostaglandin synthesis. The risk of PROM is at least doubled in *women who smoke* during pregnancy. Other risk factors for PROM include *prior PROM* (approximately twofold), a short cervical length, prior preterm delivery, hydramnios, multiple gestation, and bleeding in early pregnancy (threatened abortion).

The relation between PROM and preterm contractions also is unclear. It is theorized that preterm contractions may cause dilation of the cervix, thereby exposing the fetal membranes to microorganisms in the vagina or cervix, which may then cause spontaneous rupture of the membranes. There is also uncertainty about the impact of gestational age and the length of time since membrane rupture on the likelihood of intrauterine infection.

Chorioamnionitis poses a major threat to the mother and fetus. Fetal sepsis is associated with an increased risk for morbidity, particularly neurologic abnormalites such as periventricular leukomalacia and cerebral palsy. Patients with intra-amniotic infection can experience significant fever (generally, 100.5°F), tachycardia (maternal and fetal), and uterine tenderness. Purulent cervical discharge is usually a very late finding. The maternal white blood cell count is generally elevated, but this finding is nonspecific in pregnancy and after corticosteroids and may be misleading. Patients with chorioamnionitis frequently enter spontaneous and often tumultuous labor. Once the diagnosis of chorioamnionitis is made, treatment consists of antibiotic therapy and prompt delivery, either by induction or augmentation of labor, if needed, or cesarean section, either for primary indication or if vaginal delivery is expected to be substantially delayed.

Diagnosis

Fluid passing through the vagina must be presumed to be amniotic fluid until proved otherwise. At times, patients describe a "gush" of fluid, whereas at other times they note a history of steady leakage of small amounts of fluid. *Intermittent urinary leakage* is common during pregnancy, especially near term, and this can be confused with PROM. Likewise, the normally increased vaginal secretions in pregnancy as well as perineal moisture (especially in hot weather) may be mistaken for amniotic fluid.

The *nitrazine test* uses pH to distinguish amniotic fluid from urine and vaginal secretions. Amniotic fluid is alkaline, having a pH above 7.0; vaginal secretions in pregnancy usually have pH values of <6.0. To perform the nitrazine test, a sample of fluid obtained from the vagina during a speculum examination is placed on a strip of nitrazine paper. The paper turns dark blue in response to amniotic fluid. Cervical mucus, blood, and semen are possible causes of false–positive results (Table 23.1).

The *"fern test"* is also used to distinguish amniotic fluid from other fluids. It is named from the pattern of arborization that occurs when amniotic fluid is placed on a slide and is allowed to dry in room air. The resultant pattern, which resembles the leaves of a fern plant, is caused by the sodium chloride content of the amniotic fluid. The ferning pattern from amniotic fluid is fine, with multiple branches, as shown in Figure 23.1; cervical mucus does not fern or, if it does, the pattern is thick with much less branching. This test is considered more indicative of ruptured membranes than

Table 23.1. Causes of False–Positive and False–Negative Nitrazine Tests	
False–positive	**False–negative**
Basic urine	Remote PROM with no residual fluid
Semen	Minimal amniotic fluid leakage
Cervical mucus	
Blood contamination	
Some antiseptic solutions	
Vaginitis (especially trichomonas)	

PROM, premature rupture of membrane.

the nitrazine test, but, as with any test, it is not 100% reliable.

Ultrasound can be helpful in evaluating the possibility of rupture of membranes. If ample amniotic fluid around the fetus is visible on ultrasound examination, the diagnosis of PROM must be questioned; however, if the amounts of amniotic fluid leakage are small, sufficient amniotic fluid will still be visible on scan. When there is less than the expected amount of fluid seen on ultrasound, the differential diagnosis of oligohydramnios must also be considered.

The differential diagnoses for PROM include urinary incontinence, increased vaginal secretions in pregnancy (physiologic), increased cervical discharge (pathologic, infection), exogenous fluids (such as semen or douche), and vesicovaginal fistula.

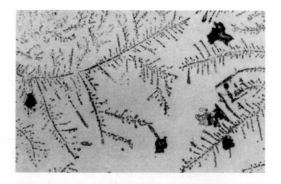

Figure 23.1. Ferning pattern from amniotic fluid.

Evaluation and Management

Patients with PROM are *hospitalized for their initial evaluation* and further management. In the hospital environment, evaluations may proceed quickly and efficiently so that delivery may be accomplished if needed. *Factors to be considered in the management of the patient with PROM include* the gestational age at the time of rupture, the presence of uterine contractions, the likelihood of chorioamnionitis, the amount of amniotic fluid around the fetus, and the degree of fetal maturity.

The patient's history as well as the management factors listed previously must be carefully evaluated for information relevant to the diagnosis. Abdominal examination includes palpation of the uterus for tenderness and fundal height measurement for evaluation of gestational age and fetal lie.

A sterile speculum examination is performed to assess the likelihood of vaginal infection and to obtain cervical or vaginal cultures for *N. gonorrhoeae,* β-hemolytic streptococcus, and possibly *Chlamydia trachomatis.* The cervix is visualized for its degree of dilation as well as for the presence of free-flowing amniotic fluid. Fluid is obtained from the vaginal vault for nitrazine and/or fern testing. If there is fluid pooled in the vaginal vault, it may be sent for *fetal maturity testing* if the gestational age warrants. The test for phosphatidylglycerol (PG) is considered the most reliable indicator of fetal lung maturity because PG is not found in vaginal secretions or blood. *Because of the risk of infection, intracervical digital examination should be avoided unless, and until, the patient is in active labor, or if there is evidence that is highly suggestive of an occult prolapsed umbilical cord.*

Ultrasound examination can be helpful in determining gestational age, verifying the fetal presentation, and assessing the amount of amniotic fluid remaining within the uterine cavity. It has been shown that labor is less likely to occur when an adequate volume of amniotic fluid remains within the uterus.

Term Premature Rupture of Membranes

If PROM occurs at term (37 weeks or more of gestational age), spontaneous labor will ensue in 90% of women within about 24 hours. Awaiting the onset of spontaneous labor for 12 to 24 hours is reasonable and has limited risk of infection, unless there are risk factors such as previous or concurrent vaginal infection or multiple digital pelvic examinations. However, induction of labor at any time after presentation of PROM is also considered appropriate, with informed consent. Information that the physician shares with the patient as this decision is made includes, in addition to the risk of infection, that immediate oxytocin administration is associated with a decreased risk of chorioamnionitis and endometritis, although there is a decrease in the incidence of cesarean section in patients managed expectantly. Serial evaluation for the development of intrauterine infection and other complications of PROM is requisite with expectant management, which, in most cases, should not extend beyond 24 hours in term pregnancy.

Preterm Premature Rupture of Membranes

The time from PROM to labor is the latency period and is inversely related to gestational age. Between term and about 28 weeks of gestational age, about 50% of patients labor within 24 hours and 80% within 1 week, and only 50% of patients whose gestational age is 24 to 28 weeks labor within 1 week of PROM.

If the gestational age is thought to be in the transitional time of fetal maturity (i.e., from 34 to 36 weeks), the management is variable, depending on the center. Immediate delivery with the low risk for morbidity at >34 weeks of gestation is reasonable, as is continued expectant management and delivery at 35 to 36 weeks. If there is clinical suspicion for the presence of uterine infection, delivery should be effected as soon as possible. Amniocentesis in the setting of PROM and oligohydramnios may be difficult. However, tests of fetal maturity can be performed and evaluation for intra-amniotic infection with the presence of bacteria on Gram's stain or a positive culture may be indicated. Fetal lung maturity may also be tested with amniotic fluid obtained from the vagina.

If the evaluation suggests *intrauterine infection,* antibiotic therapy and delivery are indicated. The antibiotic prescribed should have a broad spectrum of coverage because of the polymicrobial nature of the infection. Delivery is usually accomplished by induction of labor or, if the infant is a preterm breech, possibly by cesarean delivery. If the patient is beginning to have uterine contractions or if the cervix is dilated beyond approximately 3 cm, labor is usually allowed to proceed. As in cases of labor not related to PROM, oxytocin augmentation may be necessary. Persistent contractions after PROM may be a manifestation of infection, possibly subclinical, so most clinicians do not attempt to inhibit labor when such contractions begin spontaneously.

If the fetus is significantly preterm and in the absence of infection or other evidence of fetal compromise (such as a nonreassuring fetal heart rate), expectant management is generally chosen. Patients are assessed carefully on a daily basis for uterine tenderness as well as maternal or fetal tachycardia. White blood cell counts may be obtained and compared with baseline, although the maternal WBC count is again nonspecific. Intermittent ultrasound assessment helps to determine amniotic fluid volumes because leaking of fluid from the vagina may cease and allow amniotic fluid to reaccumulate around the fetus. Antibiotic therapy prolongs the latency period (time from PROM to delivery) after preterm PROM and improves the perinatal outcome and should be used. Daily fetal movement monitoring by the mother can also be helpful to assess fetal well-being. In the absence of sufficient amniotic fluid to buffer the umbilical cord from external pressure, compression of the cord can lead to fetal heart rate decelerations. If these are frequent and severe, there should be early and expeditious delivery to avoid fetal compromise or death. Unfortunately, such an umblical cord accident often is unrecognized for a time regardless of the monitoring regimen instituted. Electronic fetal monitoring is used frequently during the initial evaluation period to search for any fetal heart rate decelerations, although the fetal cardiac control mechanisms are often insufficiently developed to allow meaningful evaluation for fetal heart rate variability.

To enhance fetal pulmonary maturity in patients with preterm PROM, corticosteroid therapy (such as betamethasone) is generally recommended in patients whose gestational age is 32 weeks or less. Despite the immunosuppressive property of steroids, they do not seem to predispose the mother or fetus to infection. It is reasonable to consider tocolytic therapy in preterm PROM to allow time for corticosteroid therapy.

Premature rupture of membranes at very early gestational ages, such as before 20 to 22 weeks of gestation, presents additional problems. Along with the risks of prematurity and infection already discussed, the very premature fetus faces the further hazards of *pulmonary hypoplasia* and other consequences of prolonged oligohydramnios. The relation of PROM with both of these entities is both interesting and important. For normal fetal lung development to occur, it is necessary that fetal breathing movements take place. During intrauterine life, the fetus normally inhales and exhales amniotic fluid. This adds substances generated in the respiratory tree to the amniotic fluid pool, including the phospholipids that form the basis for many of the fetal maturity tests. If rupture of fetal membranes occurs before 20 to 22 weeks of gestation, the lack of amniotic fluid interferes with this normal breathing process and, therefore, with pulmonary development. The result is a failure of normal growth and differentiation of the respiratory tree. If severe, the fetus is said to have *pulmonary hypoplasia.* Neonatal death then occurs because of an inability to maintain ventilation. The development of pulmonary hypoplasia is not necessarily an all-or-none phenomenon, but rather represents a spectrum of disordered development. On the brighter side, PROM that occurs early in pregnancy following genetic amniocentesis has a greater likelihood of sealing over with reaccumulation of amniotic fluid.

CHAPTER 24

OBSTETRIC PROCEDURES

This chapter deals primarily with APGO Educational Topic:

Topic 32: Obstetric Procedures

Students should understand and be able to explain each of the procedures or assessment and evaluation topics listed in the chapter, and list their indications and complications. The list is not exhaustive and there are other important procedures included throughout this book.

Women's health care physicians must be familiar with the procedures common in obstetric and gynecologic practice. Whether the physician performs the procedure or not, he or she should understand the indications, contraindications, risks, benefits, and the appropriate language needed to inform the patient about her diagnoses and therapeutic options.

Amniocentesis

Amniocentesis is the withdrawal of fluid from the amniotic sac to obtain fluid and cells for a variety of tests (Figure 24.1). Biochemical studies can identify the presence of fetal physiologic markers (e.g., deficiency of hexosaminidase A or Tay–Sachs disease) or the presence of substances indicating fetal abnormalities (e.g., α-fetoprotein in neural tube defects or bilirubin in Rh incompatibility). Evaluation of the DNA of fetal cells grown in tissue culture allows genetic evaluation of the fetus.

In more advanced gestations, fluid obtained through amniocentesis is used to assess the degree of fetal lung maturity. This indication of fetal lung readiness is extremely valuable in the management of premature labor or the timing of delivery for patients with medical complications. Fluid obtained at amniocentesis may also be cultured and stained to evaluate for intrauterine infection (i.e., chorioamnionitis).

Amniocentesis is associated with a 0.5% risk of fetal loss because of bleeding, infection, preterm labor, or fetal injury. To reduce this risk, the procedure is usually performed using ultrasonographic guidance.

Chorionic Villus Sampling

In chorionic villus sampling, a small cannula is passed through the cervix to aspirate villus cells for genetic analysis of an early gestation (Figure 24.2). Cells may also be acquired via transabdominal aspiration. The cells that are obtained are cultured for genetic studies.

Because chorionic villus sampling carries an approximately 0.5% risk of fetal loss, it is usually reserved for patients with a >0.5% chance of an abnormality (e.g., those over the age of 35 or with a history of genetic abnormalities). Bleeding or infections are infrequent complications.

Compared with amniocentesis, chorionic villus sampling can be performed earlier in pregnancy and with a more rapid availability of results. This allows for an earlier decision regarding possible pregnancy termination in the case of significant fetal abnormality.

Periumbilical Artery Blood Sampling

In *periumbilical artery blood sampling*, a fetal blood sample is obtained via a transabdominal

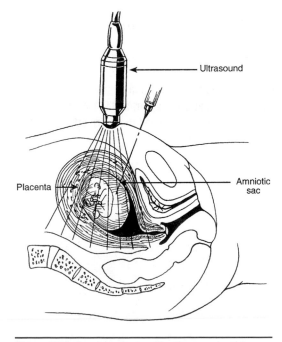

Figure 24.1. Amniocentesis with ultrasound guidance. Cross section of uterus and fetus, with the needle in a pocket of amniotic fluid.

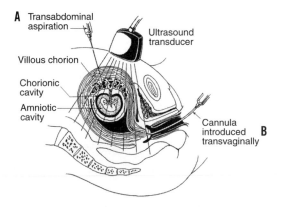

Figure 24.2. Chorionic villus sampling. (**A**) Transabdominal apporach. (**B**) Transvaginal approach.

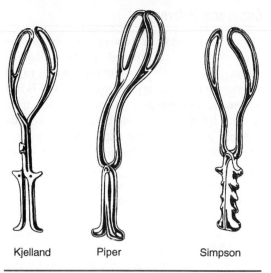

Kjelland   Piper   Simpson

Figure 24.3. Commonly used obstetric forceps.

needle aspiration of the umbilical cord under real-time ultrasonographic guidance. Various analyses may be performed on the fetal blood sample obtained, including fetal blood gas and metabolic evaluation, fetal hemogram and blood chemistries, and fetal genetics studies. The risks of this procedure are the same as those of amniocentesis plus an approximately 1% risk to the fetus from bleeding at the umbilical puncture site. This procedure is also referred to as *cordocentesis*.

Forceps Delivery and Vacuum Extraction

Operative vaginal deliveries, using either forceps (Figure 24.3) or a vacuum extractor, are designed to augment the expulsive forces during the second stage of labor, as well as to direct these forces in an optimal manner. In addition to enhancing expulsive forces, forceps can facilitate the rotation of the fetal head, facilitating the fetus' completion of the cardinal movements of labor allowing vaginal delivery (Figure 24.4).

Forceps deliveries are classified as outlet, low, or mid, based on the level of descent of the fetal head into the pelvis (station) at the time the forceps are applied. When the fetal head is not engaged (the biparietal diameter of the fetal head passing the plane of the pelvic inlet), forceps and vacuum delivery is prohibited.

A variety of types of forceps can be used to aid the expulsive forces (for example, *Simpson [or Tucker] forceps;* Figure 24.3). Some have different construction and are used to rotate the head (for example, the *Kjelland [Kielland] forceps).* Almost all forceps are designed for application to the fetal head, with one important exception. The *Piper forceps* are specially designed to facilitate the delivery of the "after-coming head" in vaginal breech deliveries (Figure 24.5).

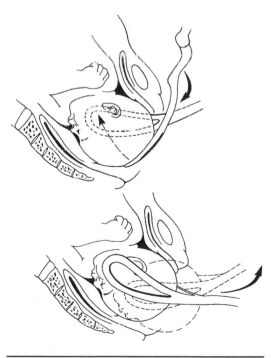

Figure 24.4. Correct biparietal, bimalar, cephalic forceps application.

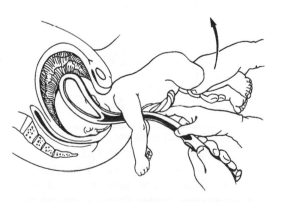

Figure 24.5. Use of Piper forceps on an after-coming head during breech delivery.

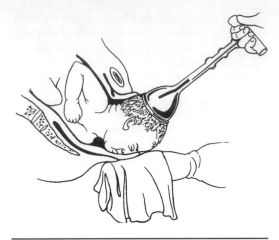

Figure 24.6. Vacuum extractor applied to head.

The *vacuum extractor* is a suction cup-like device that is applied to the fetal scalp (Figure 24.6). Traction is then used to aid maternal expulsive efforts and expedite delivery; it is not used to facilitate rotation. The indications and criteria for vacuum-assisted vaginal delivery are the same as for the use of obstetric forceps.

Cesarean Delivery

Cesarean delivery (or cesarean section) is the delivery of the fetus through an abdominal incision. This route may be chosen when rapid delivery is required and vaginal delivery is not imminent (nonreassuring fetal status at a time remote from vaginal delivery), when vaginal delivery is not advisable (e.g., placenta previa, fetal anomalies, or malpresentation), or when vaginal delivery cannot be accomplished by the normal forces of labor (e.g., cephalopelvic disproportion, macrosomia, malpresentation, or uterine dysfunction). Currently, the cesarean delivery rate in the United States is between 25% and 30%.

Cesarean sections are not classified by the kind of abdominal incision made, but rather by the type of incision made in the uterus. An incision in the lower, noncontractile portion of the uterus, whether transverse or vertical, is termed a lower uterine segment incision. Most incisions are transverse. When the incision into the uterine cavity is made in the upper, con-

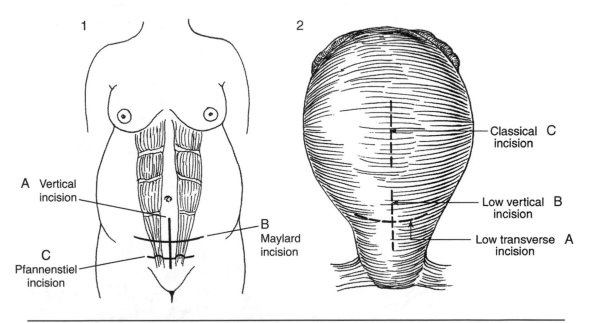

Figure 24.7. Incisions at cesarean section. **1.** *Abdominal incisions,* including the midline incision through the less-vascular midline space (**A**); the Maylard incision, which involves incision of the rectus sheath and muscles (**B**); and the Pfannenstiel incision, in which the rectus sheath and muscles are retracted away rather than incised (**C**). In general, midline incisions allow somewhat more rapid access but at the expense of a less-pleasing cosmetic effect and more postoperative discomfort than the transverse abdominal incisions. **2.** *Uterine incisions,* by which cesarean sections are classified: the lower segment transverse (lower segment transverse cesarean section) (**A**), the lower segment vertical cesarean section (**B**), and the classic cesarean section in which the incision is through the thick, contractile, upper uterine segment (**C**).

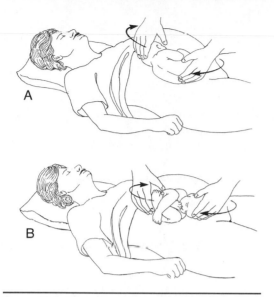

Figure 24.8. External cephalic version. Steady, gentle pressure is applied to "squeeze" the fetus from the breech to the cephalic, more often in a "forward roll" motion, as noted.

tractile portion of the uterus, it is commonly referred to as a classic incision (Figure 24.7).

The risk of uterine rupture in a subsequent pregnancy is related to the type of uterine incision performed. If a classic incision was used, the risk of rupture is about 8%, so a repeat cesarean delivery is generally recommended. Patients who have had incisions of the upper uterus for other reasons (e.g., myomectomy, cornual resection) are at greater risk of rupture of the uterine scar before or during labor and generally are not allowed to labor in subsequent pregnancies.

Because healing of the cesarean incision is stronger when it has occurred in the lower uterine segment, the risk of rupture is about 1%, usually in the process of labor. With that in mind, subsequent vaginal delivery may be possible (vaginal birth after cesarean).

External Cephalic Version

The application of gentle constant pressure to the breech fetus between 36 and 39 weeks of gestation may facilitate version to the cephalic presentation (Figure 24.8). In a woman of normal body habitus, a fetus of normal size with adequate amniotic fluid volume, and proper relaxation (which may include tocolysis), success rates of 50% to 75% may be expected, with half or more remaining in the cephalic presentation until labor ensues. The cesarean section rate for these patients is one half of that for those who do not undergo version, balanced against infrequent risks of cord compression and placental abruption. Electronic fetal monitoring and/or ultrasonographic monitoring before and after the procedure is recommended, and Rh-negative women should receive Rh-immune globulin because of the risk of feto-maternal transfusion.

Circumcision

Circumcision of the newborn male (the removal of the foreskin from the penis) has been practiced for centuries as social custom, for religious reasons, and for the belief that there are health benefits. Controversy continues over the health value of this surgical procedure. It has been argued that circumcision represents mutilation, reduces penile sensitivity, and carries a greater risk of operative complications (surgical damage, bleeding, and infection) than is warranted by its benefits. Proponents point to improved hygiene and a reduced incidence of penile cancer and phimosis, as well as social benefits. Circumcision is elective surgery and should be performed only if the newborn is stable and healthy; local anesthesia is requisite.

Female circumcision is proscribed by most of the world's health organizations and societies, viewed as having no value and serving only to mutilate.

UNIT III

GYNECOLOGY

CHAPTER 25

CONTRACEPTION

This chapter deals primarily with APGO Educational Topic:

Topic 33: Contraception

Students should be able to list the various types of contraception by type, and describe their mechanisms of action, effectiveness, risks and benefits, as well as indications and contraindications.

The ability to control fertility has had a more wide-ranging impact on society than almost any other aspect of medical practice, past or present. Because the subject of contraception has personal, religious, and political overtones, it can often lead to conflict, emotionality, and confusion. Before the physician can advise a couple on their contraceptive options, he or she must understand the physiologic or pharmacologic basis of action, the effectiveness, the indications and contraindications, complications, and advantages and disadvantages of the contraceptive methods available, as well as the cultural context of the couple.

There are many methods of contraception that are considered reliable, as well as numerous methods of dubious or no value arising from superstition or ignorance. Because no method is 100% reliable, failures are reflected in the descriptive measures of *method failure* (the failure rate inherent in the method if the patient uses it correctly 100% of the time, the *lowest expected rate*) and *patient failure* (the failure rate seen when patients actually use the method, i.e., make the mistakes in usage everyone will make from time to time, or actual noncompliance, the *typical rate*) (Table 25.1).

How Contraceptives Work

All available contraceptive methods act to prevent sperm and egg from uniting, or to prevent implantation and growth of the embryo. These goals are accomplished by (1) inhibiting the development and release of the egg (oral contraceptives, long-acting progesterone injection, contraceptive patch and ring), (2) imposing a mechanical, chemical, or temporal barrier between sperm and egg (condom, diaphragm, foam, rhythm, and intrauterine devices), or (3) altering the ability of the fertilized egg to implant and grow (intrauterine devices, diethylstilbestrol, post-coital oral contraceptives). RU 486 (mifepristone) is sometimes described as a contraceptive, and while it does have some contraceptive effect, it acts primarily by inducing menstruation or abortion by inhibiting progesterone receptors. Each approach may be used successfully, individually or in combination, to prevent pregnancy, and each method has its own unique advantages and disadvantages, risks, and benefits.

Factors Affecting Choice of Contraceptive Method

Although efficacy is important in the choice of contraceptive methods, it is not the only factor on which the final decision is based. Factors such as safety, availability, cost, degree to which the method relies on or interferes with coitus (coital dependence), and personal acceptability to patient and partner, all have a role to play in the decision. Although we tend to think of safety in terms of significant health risks, for many patients this also includes the possibilities of side effects. For a couple to use a method, it must be accessible (i.e., immediately available, especially in coitally dependent or use-oriented methods) and affordable for the patient. The effects of a method on spontaneity or modes of sexual expression may be important in some cases. The ability of a contraceptive method to provide some protection against sexually transmitted diseases may also be relevant. Furthermore, cultural, religious, or social considerations may influence a couple's choice of contraceptive method. Career or other life choices as well as plans for future fertility may influence the type and duration of the method chosen. Finally, the couple's feelings about which partner should take responsibility for contraception may be important. The clinician must be sensitive to all these factors that might influence the decision and provide factual information that fits the needs of the patient and her partner. A decision tree based on this concept is presented in Figure 25.1.

Hormonal Contraceptives

For many women, "*birth control*" is synonymous with the oral contraceptive pill, or hormonal contraception. Recently, the choices have expanded to injectable hormonal preparations (injectable medroxyprogesterone [Depo-Provera], injectable medroxyprogesterone acetate and estradiol cypionate [Lunelle]), contraceptive

242

Table 25.1. Contraceptive Technique Pregnancy Rates in the First Year of Use in the United States

Method	Percentage of Women With Pregnancy	
	Lowest Expected[a]	Typical[b]
No method of contraception	85.0%	85.0%
Hormonal contraceptives		
Combination pill	0.1	3.0
Progestin-only pill	0.5	3.0
Contraceptive patch	0.6	0.8
NuvaRing	0.65	<1.0
Depo-Provera	0.3	0.3
Implanon	0.1	0.1
Barrier contraceptives		
Spermicides	3.0	20.0
Male condom	2.0	12.0
Female condom	5.0	21.0
Cervical cap	6.0	18.0
Diaphragm and spermicide	6.0	18.0
IUDs		3.0
Progesterone IUD (Mirena)	0.2	0.2
Copper T 380A	0.8	<1.0
Natural family planning		
Withdrawal	4.0	18.0
Postcoital douche		40.0
Periodic abstinence		20.0
Calendar	9.0	
Ovulation method	3.0	
Symptothermal	2.0	
Postovulation	1.0	
Postcoital contraception/emergency (Yuzpe method and progestin-only method, plan B)		25.0
Permanent—sterilization		
Male	0.1	0.15
Female	0.2	0.4

[a]Best performance/compliance; theoretical.
[b]Usual performance/compliance; usual or actual.
IUD, intrauterine device.
Modified with permission from Speroff, L., Darney, P. D.: *A Clinical Guide for Contraception.* 2nd Ed. Baltimore: Williams & Wilkins, 1996:5.

patches (Ortho Evra), and contraceptive rings (NuvaRing).

About one third of all sexually active, fertile women in the United States use oral contraceptives, with over one half of young women 20 to 24 years old using these contraceptives.

But, despite this use, "the pill" is often mistrusted or misunderstood (up to two-thirds of women polled said that they thought the pill was more dangerous than pregnancy, and up to one-third thought that the pill caused cancer). These misunderstandings about such a

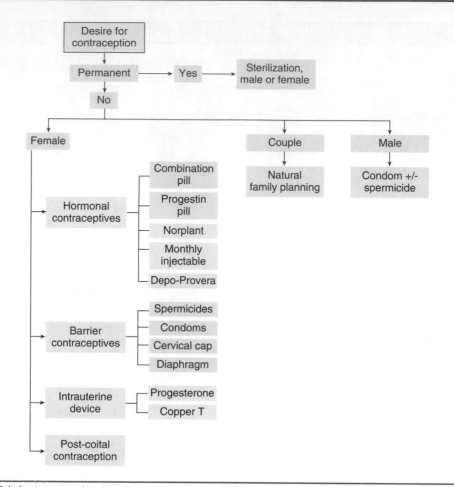

Figure 25.1. Decision tree for choosing a contraceptive method.

commonly used contraceptive method underscore the importance of patient education by those who care for women.

Hormone-based contraceptives provide the most effective reversible pregnancy prevention available. Theoretical failure rates for oral contraceptives are in the range of 1% or less. Longer-acting hormonal methods (injections, patches, and rings) have effectiveness rates that equal or even surpass those of sterilization. Because "oral contraceptive pill (OCP) failures" are usually related to missed pills, injectable long-acting agents, patches, and rings share the additional advantage of lack of a need for daily compliance.

Biochemistry and Methods of Action

Most of the oral contraceptives are *combinations of an estrogen and a progestin*, although there are also progestin-only products (Table 25.2).

Combination oral contraceptive preparations contain *ethinyl estradiol* (estradiol with an ethinyl group at the 17 position, rendering the estradiol active orally) or *mestranol* as the estrogen component, and one of the *19-nortestosterones* as the progestin product. The progestational component provides the major contraceptive effect, acting primarily by suppression of luteinizing hormone secretion and, in turn, ovulation. The estrogenic component acts by suppression of follicle-stimulating hormone secretion (thus preventing selection and emergence of a dominant follicle) as well as by potentiation of the action of the progestational agent, probably by increasing the number of intracellular progesterone receptors. Additional effects of the progestational component include thickening of the cervical mucus and altered fallopian tube peristalsis. Thus, the min-

Table 25.2. Common Oral Contraceptive Preparations

Preparation	Estrogen	μg	Progestin	Days	mg
Combination oral contraceptives					
Alesse	Ethinyl estradiol	20	Levonorgestrel		1
Brevicon	Ethinyl estradiol	35	Norethindrone		0.5
Cyclessa	Ethinyl estradiol	25	Desogestrel	1–7	0.1
				8–14	0.125
				15–21	0.15
Demulen	Ethinyl estradiol	50	Ethynodiol diacetate		1
Demulen 1/35	Ethinyl estradiol	35	Ethynodiol diacetate		1
Desogen	Ethinyl estradiol	30	Desogestrel		0.15
Estrostep	Ethinyl estradiol	20	Norethindrone acetate	1–5	1
		30		6–12	1
		35		13–21	1
Genora 0.5/35	Ethinyl estradiol	35	Norethindrone		0.5
Genora 1/35	Ethinyl estradiol	35	Norethindrone		1.0
Levelen	Ethinyl estradiol	30	Levonorgestrel		0.15
Loestrin 1/20	Ethinyl estradiol	20	Norethindrone acetate		1
Loestrin 1.5/30	Ethinyl estradiol	30	Norethindrone acetate		1.5
Lo/Ovral	Ethinyl estradiol	30	Norgestrel		0.3
Mircette	Ethinyl estradiol	20	Desogestrel		0.15
Modicon	Ethinyl estradiol	35	Norethindrone		0.5
Nordette	Ethinyl estradiol	30	Levonorgestrel		0.15
Norinyl 1/ 35	Ethinyl estradiol	35	Norethindrone		1
Norinyl 1/50	Mestranol	50	Norethindrone		1
Norlestrin 2.5/50	Ethinyl estradiol	50	Norethindrone acetate		2.5
Ortho-Cept	Ethinyl estradiol	30	Desogestrel		0.15
Ortho-Cyclen	Ethinyl estradiol	35	Norgestimate		0.25
Ortho-Novum 1/35	Ethinyl estradiol	35	Norethindrone		1
Ortho-Novum 1/50	Mestranol	50	Norethindrone		1
Ortho-Novum 7/7/7	Ethinyl estradiol	35	Norethindrone	1–7	0.5
		35		8–14	0.75
		35		15–21	1.0
Ortho Tri-Cyclen	Ethinyl estradiol	35	Norgestimate	1–7	0.18
		35		8–14	0.215
		35		15–21	0.25
Ortho Tri-Cyclen Lo	Ethinyl estradiol	25	Norgestimate	1–7	0.180
				8–14	0.215
				15–21	0.25
Ovcon	Ethinyl estradiol	35	Norethindrone		0.4
Ovral	Ethinyl estradiol	50	Norgestrel		0.5
Seasonale	Ethinyl estradiol	30	Levonorgestrel		0.15

(continued)

Table 25.2. continued

Preparation	Estrogen	μg	Progestin	Days	mg
Tri-Levlen	Ethinyl estradiol	30	Levonorgestrel	1–6	0.05
		40		7–11	0.075
		30		12–21	0.125
Tri-Norinyl	Ethinyl estradiol	35	Norethindrone	1–7	0.5
		35		8–16	1.0
		35		17–21	0.5
Triphasil	Ethinyl estradiol	30	Levonorgestrel	1–6	0.05
				7–11	0.075
				12–21	0.125
Yasmin	Ethinyl estradiol	30	Drospirenone		3.0
Progestin-only "minipill"					
Micronor			Norethindrone		0.35
Nor-QD			Norethindrone		0.35
Ovrette			Norgestrel		0.075

imal estrogenic component potentiates the progestational effect and provides an additional modest contraceptive effect leading to the full efficacy of the combination oral contraceptive.

Based on human endometrial response and selected biochemical markers, ethinyl estradiol is thought to be about 1.5 times as potent as the same weight of mestranol. The stomach absorbs ethinyl estradiol; peak serum levels are reached within 1 hour of ingestion, with mestranol peaking somewhat later. Common examples of the progestin compounds used include, in descending order of biologic progestin activity, *norgestrel, ethynodiol diacetate, norethindrone acetate, norethynodrel, and norethindrone.* Oral contraceptives using the less androgenic agents *desogestrel* and *norgestimate* are also available if less androgenic activity is desired.

Many oral contraceptives contain a fixed ratio of estrogen and progestin, although "*phasic*" *formulations* have been introduced that vary this ratio during the course of the month. This leads to a slight decrease in the total dose of hormone used per month, but is also associated with a slightly higher rate of bleeding between periods.

Recently, a monophasic ethinyl estradiol/levonorgestrel preparation has become available (Seasonale). This formulation extends the 4-week usage cycle to 12 weeks (that is, "four periods per year"). Some women may prefer this usage pattern, although they should be aware that there is a higher incidence of breakthrough bleeding in the first 12-week cycle as compared with 4-week cycle preparations.

Progestin-only contraceptives (progestin-only "minipill") act primarily by making the endometrium hostile to implantation and the cervical mucus thick and relatively impermeable. Ovulation continues normally in about 40% of patients using the progestin-only formulation. The minipill has a higher failure rate in younger women compared with women older than 40 years of age. As a result, these oral contraceptives are of special usefulness in two clinical situations: lactating women and women older than 40 years. In the former group, the progestin effect coincides with the prolactin-induced suppression of ovulation; in the latter group, the inherent reduced fecundity adds to the progestin effect. There is no effect on the quality or quantity of breast milk or any evidence of short- or long-term adverse effects on infants, and the progestin-only pill may be started immediately after delivery in the breast-feeding mother. The progestin-only pill is also a good choice for women in whom estrogen-containing formulations are contraindicated. Because of the low dosages of progestin, the minipill must be taken at the same time each day, starting on the first day of menses. If a woman is more than 3 hours late in taking the minipill, a back-up contraceptive method should be used for 48 hours.

Effects of Hormonal Contraceptives

Hormonal contraception affects more than just the reproductive system. Estrogens affect lipid metabolism, potentiate sodium and water retention, increase renin substrate, stimulate the cytochrome P-450 system, increase sex hormone-binding globulin, and can reduce antithrombin III. Progestins increase sebum and facial and body hair, induce smooth muscle relaxation, and increase the risk of cholestatic jaundice. The newer progestational agents, desogestrel and norgestimate, have less metabolic impact.

Oral contraceptives have many beneficial effects. As many as 1 in 750 women, or approximately 50,000 women a year in the United States, avoid hospitalization because of the beneficial effects of oral contraceptives. Oral contraceptive users have a lower incidence of endometrial and ovarian cancer, benign breast and ovarian disease, and pelvic infection. Ectopic pregnancy is prevented, along with the complications of intrauterine pregnancies. Menstrual periods are predictable, shorter, and less painful, and as a result, the risk of iron deficiency anemia is reduced. There even appears to be a protective effect against rheumatoid arthritis.

Breakthrough bleeding occurs in 10% to 30% of women taking low-dose oral contraceptives during the first 3 months of use, and is an especially worrisome symptom, although it is not associated with decreased efficacy as long as the pill-taking regimen is maintained. This breakthrough bleeding occurring in the first 3 months of use is best managed by encouragement and reassurance because it resolves spontaneously. Breakthrough bleeding after approximately 3 months is associated with progestin-induced decidualization, with the shallow and fragile endometrium prone to asynchronous breakdown and bleeding. If the bleeding is too worrisome, a short course of exogenous estrogen, usually 1.25 mg conjugated

estrogen daily for 7 days when the bleeding is present, is given while the patient continues the oral contraceptive, no matter where the patient is in her oral contraceptive cycle.

Taking two or three of the low-dose oral contraceptives is not an effective therapy because the progestin component will predominate, often worsening the problem by further decidualizing already asynchronously shedding endometrium. *Amenorrhea* is another worrisome symptom, primarily because of recurrent concern about pregnancy. It is seen in approximately 1% of users of low-dose oral contraceptives in the first year of use, reaching perhaps 5% of users after several years of use. Contraceptive efficacy is maintained if the pill regimen is followed. Exogenous estrogen (1.25 mg conjugated estrogen throughout the 21 days while taking the oral contraceptive) may be used to facilitate menses, if the patient wishes. A pregnancy test should precede any therapy.

Serious complications such as venous thrombosis, pulmonary embolism, cholestasis and gallbladder disease, stroke, and myocardial infarction were more likely for women using the old-style, high-dose formulations of oral contraceptives than for the lower-dose formulations now in use. Nonetheless, these complications are seen now on occasion in patients taking low-dose formulations. Hepatic tumors have also been associated with the use of oral contraceptives; these are rare and have been most closely associated with high-dose mestranol-containing drugs. Although all of these complications are from 2 to 10 times more likely in pill-users, they are still uncommon. Factors such as age, weight, and especially smoking also represent significant risk factors. For example, the risk of thromboembolic disease is greater during pregnancy than in women taking oral contraceptive pills.

Less serious but more common side effects also depend on the dosage and type of hormones used. Estrogens may cause a feeling of bloating and weight gain, breast tenderness, nausea, fatigue, or headache. Progestins are often blamed for symptoms of acne or depression. Altering the dose or composition of the agent used may treat most of these minor side effects.

The therapeutic principle of contraception is to select the method providing effective con-

Table 25.3. The Management of New Symptoms in Patients Using Oral Contraceptives

Discontinue OCP; start nonhormonal methods, immediate evaluation

Loss of vision, diplopia	(Possible retinal artery thrombosis)
Unilateral numbness, weakness	(Possible stroke)
Severe chest/neck pain	(Possible myocardial infarction)
Slurring of speech	(Possible stroke)
Severe leg pain, tenderness	(Possible thrombophlebitis)
Hemoptysis, acute shortness of breath	(Possible pulmonary embolism)
Hepatic mass, tenderness	(Possible hepatic neoplasm, adenoma)

Continue OCP; immediate evaluation

Amenorrhea	(Possible pregnancy)
Breast mass	(Possible breast cancer)
Right upper quadrant pain	(Possible cholecystitis, cholelithiasis)
Severe headache	(Possible stroke, migraine headache)
Galactorrhea	(Possible pituitary adenoma)

OCP, oral contraceptive pill.

traception with the greatest margin of safety, and then to use it as long as the patient wishes contraception. However, after selection, new clinical situations may arise that require either further evaluation or cessation of the chosen contraceptive method and substitution of another method while evaluation is undertaken (Table 25.3).

Patient Evaluation for Oral Contraceptive Use

Before considering oral contraceptives for a patient, a careful evaluation is required. Not only is the pill relatively or absolutely contraindicated in some patients (Table 25.4), but also factors such as previous menstrual history may have an impact on the choice of these agents.

As an example, approximately 3% of patients may experience problems with resumption of their periods after prolonged oral contraceptive use (*postpill amenorrhea*). Younger women and those with *irregular periods* before the use of oral contraceptives are more likely to experience this problem after discontinuing their use, either because of the pills or a resumption of their previous menstrual pattern. These patients deserve counseling about this potential complication, or a consideration of alternative methods.

Oral contraceptives may interact with other medications that the patient is taking. This interaction may reduce the efficacy of either the oral contraceptive or the other medications. Examples of drugs that decrease the effectiveness of oral contraceptives include penicillin-based antibiotics, tetracycline, barbiturates, benzodiazepines, phenytoin, carbamazepine, rifampin, and the sulfonamides. Drugs that may show retarded biotransformation when oral contraceptives are also used include anticoagulants, methyldopa, phenothiazines, reserpine, and tricyclic antidepressants. *Before prescribing medications to women using oral contraceptives, the clinician should consider possible drug interactions.*

Alternative Hormonal Contraceptives

Ortho Evra was approved for use in 2001 and has become the first transdermal contraceptive patch. Containing ethinyl estradiol and norelgestromin, the "patch" remains effective for an entire week. The patient should start Ortho Evra on the first day of her menstrual period and replace it weekly for 3 weeks. The fourth week is patch-free to allow a withdrawal bleed. Placement on clean, dry skin located on the buttocks, upper outer arm, or lower abdomen is recommended. Because of its ease of application and improved compliance the

Table 25.4. Absolute and Relative Contraindications to the Use of Combination Oral Contraceptives*

Absolute

Thrombophlebitis, thromboembolic disease	Undiagnosed abnormal vaginal bleeding
Cerebral vascular disease	Known or suspected pregnancy
Coronary occlusion	Smokers older than the age of 35 years
Impaired liver function	Congenital hyperlipidemia
Known or suspected breast cancer	Hepatic neoplasm

Relative

Severe vascular headache (classic migraine, cluster)

Severe hypertension (if younger than 35–40 years of age and in good medical control, can elect OCP)

Diabetes mellitus (prevention of pregnancy outweighs the risk of complicating vascular disease in diabetics younger than 35–40 years)

Gallbladder disease (may exacerbate emergence of symptoms when gallstones are present)

Obstructive jaundice in pregnancy (some patients will develop jaundice)

Epilepsy (do not exacerbate epilepsy, but antiepileptic drugs may decrease effectiveness of OCPs)

Morbid obesity (must monitor glucose and lipoprotein profiles regularly)

Conditions no longer considered contraindications

Uterine leiomyoma (low-dose formulations not associated with growth; reduced bleeding may help in management)

Sickle cell disease or sickle C disease

Before elective surgery (theoretical association with thrombosis outweighed in most cases by avoiding pregnancy)

OCP, oral contraceptive pill.
*Risk primarily related to the estrogenic component.

"method failure" and "patient failure" of Ortho Evra are almost identical. Caution should be used when prescribing the patch for women weighing more than 90 kg (198 pounds) because of its decreased efficacy. Side effects and contraindications are similar to the oral contraceptive pill. A complaint specific to the patch, however, includes skin irritation from adhesive residue at the application site.

The first contraceptive vaginal ring, *Nuva-Ring*, releases 120 mcg of etonogestrel and 15 mcg of ethinyl estradiol daily. Comparable with oral contraceptives in efficacy, the ring increases compliance because of its once-a-month usage. Placed into the vagina by the patient at the beginning of her menses, it is left in place for 3 weeks. Removal of the device results in a withdrawal bleed. The NuvaRing can be taken out of the vagina for up to 3 hours, if desired, without altering its efficacy. Colorless and odorless with a 2-inch diameter, most patients and their partners, however, are unaware of the presence of the ring. An advantage of the ring over oral contraceptive pills is a decreased incidence of breakthrough bleeding.

Injectable and Implantable Hormonal Contraceptives

Injectable medroxyprogesterone acetate (Depo-Provera) is an injectable progestin presently available in the United States. It is given in 150-mg intramuscular injections every 3 months, with a contraceptive level of progesterone maintained for at least 14 weeks providing a useful "safety" margin. The injection should be given within the first 5 days of the current menstrual period, and, if not, a back-up method of contraception is necessary for 2 weeks. Depo-Provera is not a sustained-release preparation, relying instead on higher peaks and sustained levels of progestin, as seen in Figure 25.2. In addition to thickening of the cervical mucus and

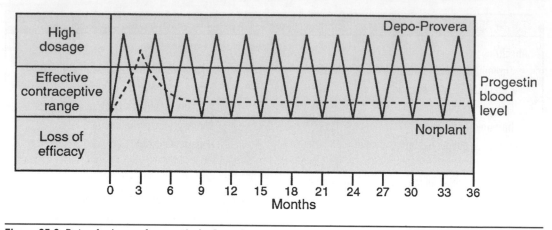

Figure 25.2. Rate of release of progestin for Depo-Provera.

decidualization of the endometrium, Depo-Provera also acts by having a circulating level of progestin high enough to block the luteinizing hormone surge and, hence, ovulation. Follicle-stimulating hormone suppression does not occur as in combination oral contraceptives, with follicular development and maintenance of estrogen production, so that vaginal atrophy, decrease in breast size, and other estrogen-deficiency symptoms do not occur.

Recently, concerns have been raised about adverse effects of Depo-Provera on bone mineral density resulting from alterations in bone metabolism associated with the reduced estrogen levels. Special concern has been raised about this effect during adolescence, a critical period of bone accretion, although the decrease in bone mineral density appears to be substantially reversible after discontinuation of this injectable contraceptive. Nonetheless, the Food and Drug Administration (FDA) has added a warning to this formulation, that use beyond 2 years should be carefully considered and alternate contraceptive methods be evaluated. In addition, women at special risk for osteoporosis should be especially careful when considering the use of Depo-Provera. It is ironic, however, that this concern about the use of Depo-Provera in adolescents is juxtaposed to the advantages of compliance and effective contraception, and the associated reduction in rates of unintended pregnancy and abortion since the formulation's introduction in 1993. In addition, noncontraceptive benefits of depo-medroxyprogesterone include decreased risk of endometrial carcinoma and iron deficiency anemia, and may improve premenstrual dysphoric disorder symptoms, pain associated with endometriosis, endometrial hyperplasia, and dysmenorrhea. This balance of overall risk to benefit for depo-medroxyprogesterone for teens, and for all women, will be the topic of continued research, discussion, and clinical judgment on an individual patient basis.

The efficacy of Depo-Provera is roughly equivalent to that of sterilization (see Table 25.1) and is not affected by weight or altered by patients taking medications that alter hepatic function. Depo-Provera is a popular choice for many and has special advantages for some, with administration contraindicated in only a few situations, as shown in Table 25.5. The most worrisome symptomatic problem with Depo-Provera is irregular vaginal spotting, which decreases with each use so that 80% of women are amenorrheic after 5 years. Because 25% of users discontinue Depo-Provera within the first year of use owing to this problem, treatment with 7 days of conjugated estrogen (1.25 mg/day) may be useful. When Depo-Provera is discontinued, about 50% of patients resume normal menses within 6 months, although perhaps 25% do not resume menses for more than 1 year; these patients should be evaluated because it should not be presumed to be a drug effect.

The *Norplant system,* which is no longer available in the United States, involves the

Table 25.5. Indications and Contraindications for Depo-Provera Contraception

Indications	Discussion
Desire for more than 1 year of contraception has been one of the indications until the recent concerns about effect on bone density. Now, the risk–benefit ratio of use beyond 2 years should be considered carefully.	The delay in pregnancy after the last injection averages about 9 months, with 90% of users achieving pregnancy within 18 months
Women with limited ability to remember contraceptive requirements, those with disorganized lives, and intellectually challenged women	One injection every 3 months, 2-week "safety" interval (i.e., can be delayed up to 2 weeks without loss of efficacy)
Breast feeding	No effect on quality of breast milk or on baby; increases quantity of breast milk; can be administered immediately postpartum
Women for whom estrogen-containing preparations are contraindicated	See Table 25.4, Absolute Contraindications list
Women with seizure disorders	Antiseizure medications unaffected, and sedative effects of progestins may aid in seizure control
Sickle cell anemia	Probable in vivo inhibition of sickling
Anemia secondary to menorrhagia	Decreased menstrual flow

Contraindications

High risk for osteoporosis

Known or suspected pregnancy, or as a diagnostic test for pregnancy

Undiagnosed vaginal bleeding

Known or suspected malignancy of the breast

Active thrombophlebitis, or current or past history of thromboembolic disorders, or cerebral vascular disease

Liver dysfunction or disease

Known sensitivity to Depo-Provera (medroxyprogesterone acetate or any of its other ingredients)

---

subcutaneous implantation of six Silastic rods that permit the continuous release of levonorgestrel, leading to a sustained progestin level and 5 years of contraceptive action (see Figure 25.1). It is used elsewhere in the world to good effect, but was not well accepted in the United States, primarily because of the 5-year interval associated with its use. Another implantable device, _Implanon_, which is currently being investigated for use, releases 40 mcg of etonorgestrel per day in a single rod system. This method maintains its efficacy for 3 years.

Barrier Contraceptives

Among the oldest and most widely used contraceptive methods are those that _provide a_ _barrier between sperm and egg;_ these methods include condoms, diaphragms, and cervical caps. Each of these methods _depends on proper use before or at the time of intercourse and, as such, is subject to a higher failure rate than oral contraceptives. This is the result of inconsistent or incorrect use as well as actual damage to the barrier material itself._ Despite this, _these methods provide relatively good protection from unwanted pregnancy,_ are inexpensive, and most require little or no medical consultation. In addition, condoms and diaphragms provide an estimated 50% reduction in the transmission of sexually transmitted diseases, including gonorrhea, herpes, Chlamydia, HIV virus, and human papillomavirus infection. The use of these methods, however, does not decrease the need for couples to be cautioned about high-risk behaviors.

Condoms

Condoms are sheaths usually worn over the erect penis or inside the vagina to prevent sperm from reaching the cervix and upper genital tract. Although almost one half of all condoms are sold to women, the condom is the only reliable, nonpermanent method of contraception available to men. Condoms are widely available and inexpensive and may be made of latex, nonlatex or, less commonly, animal membrane (usually sheep cecum). They are available with or without lubricants or spermicides, plain or with reservoir tips, in colors, flavors, and with ridges. Although most of these choices are of personal preference only, both lubrication and a reservoir tip reduce the likelihood of breakage.

The condom is well tolerated, with only rare reports of skin irritation or allergic reaction. Some men complain of reduced sensation with the use of condoms, but this may actually be an advantage for those with rapid or premature ejaculation. The slippage and breakage rate in normal use is estimated at 5% to 8%. Couples should be counseled to seek medical care within 72 hours of slippage or breakage so that emergency contraceptive methods may be used.

The introduction of the *female condom* provides another option for some couples. This is a sheath, or vaginal liner, that fits into the vagina before intercourse. Several types are available, including a condom that looks like a G-string panty with a condom rolled within the crotch to be unrolled by the penis, one that is a polyurethane sheath with an open-ringed end to the outside, and a closed internal ring placed over the cervix, much like a diaphragm (Figure 25.3). All have slippage/breakage rates of about 3%, and, like diaphragms and cervical caps, it is recommended that they be left in place 6 to 8 hours after coitus.

Diaphragms and Cervical Caps

The diaphragm is a springy ring with a dome of rubber. Proper use of a diaphragm includes applying a contraceptive jelly or cream containing spermicide to the center and rim of the

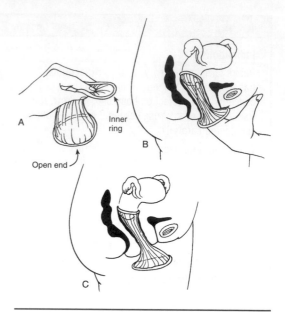

Figure 25.3. The female condom. (**A**) Preparation for insertion. (**B**) Insertion. (**C**) Condom in proper position.

device, which is then inserted into the vagina, over the cervix, and behind the pubic symphysis. In this position, the diaphragm covers the anterior vaginal wall and cervix.

There are three types of diaphragms made in sizes from 50 to 105 mm in 2.5- and 5-mm increments. Most women use 60- to 85-mm diaphragms. The *flat or coil-spring type* is suitable for women with good vaginal tone; it forms a straight line when pinched for insertion. The *arcing spring* diaphragm comes in two types: the *All Flex and the hinged types.* These are easier for most women to insert and are more useful for women with poor vaginal tone, cystoceles, rectoceles, a long cervix, or an anterior cervix with a retroverted uterus. The diaphragm must be inserted up to 1 hour before intercourse and be left in place for 6 to 8 hours afterward. It may then be removed, washed, and stored. If additional intercourse be desired during the 6- to 8-hour waiting time, additional spermicide should be applied without removing the diaphragm, and the waiting time should be restarted.

Diaphragms must be fitted to the individual patient. Fit may change with significant weight change, vaginal birth, or pelvic surgery. The diaphragm should be the largest that can be comfortably inserted, worn, and removed. If the diaphragm is too small, it may slip out during coitus because of vaginal elongation; if it is too large, it may buckle, causing discomfort, irritation, and leakage. The patient must be initially instructed in the proper positioning of the diaphragm, with the correct position subsequently verified by the patient each time it is used. If the cervix can be felt through the dome of the diaphragm, the positioning is correct. If a diaphragm is fitted in the postpartum period, its sizing should be reevaluated in 2 to 3 months because vaginal dimensions and support may change in the interval. The three types of diaphragms and correct positioning of a diaphragm are shown in Figure 25.4.

Women who use diaphragms are approximately twice as likely to have urinary tract infections as women using oral contraceptives. Presumably, this is related to a combination of pressure against the urethra causing a relative urinary stasis and an effect of spermicides on the normal vaginal flora, increasing the risk of *Escherichia coli* bacteriuria and infection.

Fitting a diaphragm involves two steps. The first step is a pelvic examination followed by trial-and-error fitting of various sizes of diaphragms until one meets the criteria noted previously. The second step is to allow the patient to practice insertion, check for proper position, and remove the device, with supervision, until she is comfortable with the process, and both she and the physician know that she is placing the diaphragm properly. Much of

the failure associated with diaphragms may be traced to the patient not using the device because of discomfort with the method and/or improper placement.

The *cervical cap* is a smaller version of the diaphragm that is applied to the cervix itself. This method is associated with a relatively high degree of displacement and, therefore, of failure, as well as association with cervicitis and toxic shock syndrome. It also requires considerable effort to fit.

Spermicides

Although many "spermicidal" chemicals have been tried over the years, today's spermicides rely on one of two agents to immobilize or kill sperm: *nonoxynol-9 and octoxynol-3.* These compounds are inserted into the vagina before intercourse and are delivered in a variety of ways: creams, jellies, foams, films, suppositories, and tablets. They should be applied high into the vagina against the cervix, from 15 to 60 minutes before each act of intercourse, because the duration of maximal spermicidal effectiveness is usually no more than 1 hour. Douching should be avoided for at least 8 hours after use. There is no known association between spermicide use and congenital malformation.

Spermicides are inexpensive, well tolerated, and provide good protection from pregnancy. *For well-motivated couples that wish a greater degree of protection, spermicides are often combined with condoms to achieve failure rates that approach those of hormonal methods.*

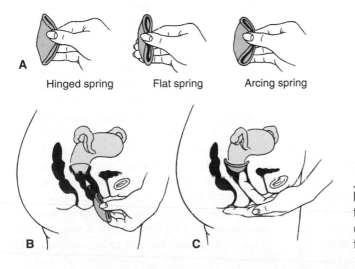

Hinged spring   Flat spring   Arcing spring

Figure 25.4. Diaphragms. **(A)** The three types of diaphragms. **(B)** Insertion of the diaphragm. **(C)** Checking to ensure that the diaphragm covers the cervix.

Intrauterine Devices

Intrauterine contraceptive devices (IUDs) are among the most commonly used and safe methods of interval contraception worldwide, and were used extensively in the United States until the 1980s. At that time a marked increase in pelvic infections in women using a specific IUD, the Dalkon Shield, led to a general rejection of all IUDs by patients and physicians. In fact, the tail of the Dalkon Shield was improperly designed, promoting infection; this is a design not shared by the other IUDs, which were actually safe then and remain safe and effective now. In recent years new, exhaustively tested IUDs have been reintroduced and are again gaining acceptance and use in the United States.

Two "medicated" IUDs are available in the United States (Figure 25.5). The *TCu-380 (ParaGard)* is a T-shaped polyethylene frame holding 380 mm² of exposed copper weighing 176 mg, to which is attached a polyethylene monofilament tied through a 3-mm ball on the stem of the IUD so that two white threads are available for detection and removal. The IUD frame is rendered radiopaque with barium sulfate. The other is the *Mirena*, a T-shaped device whose vertical stem contains the progesterone, levonorgestrel. Two clear monofilament strings are attached at a hole in the base of the stem. The device releases 20 mcg of progesterone per day.

There are many other medicated and unmedicated IUDs used throughout the world.

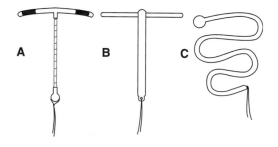

Figure 25.5. Intrauterine devices. The ParaGard (**A**) copper-releasing IUD (approved life span, 10 years) and the Mirena progestin-releasing IUD (**B**) (approved life span, 5 years) are available in the United States. The flexible polyethylene Lippes loop (**C**) is used throughout the world except in the United States.

Perhaps the most common unmedicated variety is the Lippes loop, a barium sulfate impregnated IUD, which was also widely used in the United States until the scare of the 1980s (see Figure 25.5).

Intrauterine contraceptive devices act by rendering the intrauterine environment hostile by means of what has been termed a sterile inflammatory response to the foreign IUD. This environment is spermicidal so few sperm reach the ovum in the fallopian tube, preventing fertilization, and if fertilization does occur, implantation is likewise inhibited when the cleaving ovum reaches the uterine cavity. Thus, IUDs do not act by alteration of ovulation, neither are IUDs abortifacients. In the case of the copper-containing IUD, the copper and copper salts that are released enhance the inflammatory response and, in addition, exert an additional spermicidal effect in the cervical mucus. The progestin-releasing devices add progestin effects, including decidualization of the endometrium and inhibition of implantation, inhibition of sperm capacitation and survival, and thickening of the cervical mucus. An important side effect of the progestin is a decrease in menstrual blood loss (up to 50%) and severity of dysmenorrhea. Serum progesterone levels are not affected. The IUD removal is followed by rapid reversal of the effects and return to a normal intrauterine environment and normal fertility.

The IUDs presently available in the United States are highly effective. The TCu-380A has a recommended life span of 10 years and demonstrates a pregnancy rate of 0.5% to 0.8%. The progesterone-releasing Mirena lasts for up to 5 years and has a pregnancy rate of 0.2%. The overall expulsion rate for IUDs is 1% to 5%, with the greatest likelihood in the first few months of use. Expulsion is often heralded by cramping, vaginal discharge, or bleeding, although it may be asymptomatic with the only evidence being the observed lengthening of the IUD string. Patients should be counseled to see their clinician if expulsion is suspected because the device is not effective in this circumstance, i.e., partially expelled.

Increased *vaginal bleeding and menstrual pain* are experienced by 5% to 10% of women and often result in their request to discontinue IUD use. The progestin IUDs have a lesser incidence of this problem because of the progestin effect on the endometrium. There are two categories of *pelvic infection associated with IUDs*. The first is infection within 6 to 8 weeks of insertion. Such "insertional" infections are presumed to arise from bacteria introduced into the uterus during IUD insertion, and are derived from the endogenous cervicovaginal flora, are polymicrobial, and have a predominance of anaerobes. Doxycycline (200 mg) or azithromycin (500 mg) administered 1 hour prior to insertion can provide significant protection from such infection. Women with rheumatic or valvular heart disease or with prosthetic heart valves may be acceptable candidates for IUD contraception if they are otherwise appropriate candidates. Antibiotic prophylaxis (amoxicillin, 2 g orally) should be given to these women 1 hour before IUD insertion (or removal). Pelvic infection occurring 3 or more months after IUD insertion may be presumed to be an acquired sexually transmitted disease and treated accordingly. Asymptomatic IUD users with positive cervical cultures for gonorrhea or chlamydia, or with bacterial vaginosis, should be treated promptly. The IUD may remain in place unless there is evidence of ascent of the infection to the endometrium or fallopian tubes. In the latter case, the IUD should be removed promptly and the antibiotic regimen used that is appropriate to the patient's clinical diagnosis.

The IUDs do not increase the overall risk of ectopic pregnancy. However, because the IUD offers greater protection against intrauterine than extrauterine pregnancy, the relative ratio of extrauterine pregnancy is greater in a woman who uses an IUD than in a woman not using contraception.

Pregnancy with an IUD in place is a vexing problem. About 40% to 50% of patients will spontaneously abort in the first trimester. Because of this risk, patients should be offered IUD removal if the string is visible, and this is associated with a decreased spontaneous abortion rate of about 30%. If the IUD string is not visible, instrumental removal may be performed, but the risk of pregnancy disruption is increased. If the IUD is left in place, pregnancy may proceed uneventfully and there is no evidence of an increased risk of congenital anomalies, with either medicated or unmedicated devices. There is, however, an approximate twofold to fourfold increase in the incidence of preterm labor and delivery.

Patient selection and skillful insertion are crucial to the successful use of the IUD as a method of contraception. The risk of sexually transmitted diseases is the most important factor in patient selection, not age and parity. Use of IUDs is relatively contraindicated for women with multiple sexual partners, whose partners have multiple partners, who have a history of recurrent or recent episodes of gonorrheal or chlamydial infection, or who are drug or alcohol abusers. Insertion of an IUD is contraindicated when there is a history of current, recent, or recurrent pelvic inflammatory disease. Women with heavy menses, who are anticoagulated, or who have a bleeding disorder may benefit from a progestin IUD but should not use nonmedicated or copper-bearing IUDs. A contraindication specific to the ParaGard is Wilson disease, because of its copper component. Other conditions (i.e., uterine anomalies, leiomyomas, cervical stenosis) can compromise IUD success, and alternate contraceptive methods may be better chosen. Immunosuppressed patients should not use IUDs. Adolescence and nulliparity are not contraindications in properly selected young women in monogamous relationships.

The IUD insertion is best accomplished when the patient is menstruating. The devices may also be inserted in breast-feeding women, who in fact demonstrate a lower incidence of postinsertional discomfort and bleeding. All IUD insertion techniques share the same basic rules: careful bimanual examination before insertion to determine the likely direction of insertion into the endometrial cavity, proper loading of the device into the inserter, careful placement to the fundal margin of the endometrial cavity, and proper inserter removal while leaving the IUD in place. Figure 25.6 demonstrates these techniques. The IUD removal is usually easy; when the patient is on her menses, pull on the IUD string. If the string is not visible, rotating two cotton-tip applicators in the endocervical canal will often retrieve the strings. If this is not possible, a fine probe may

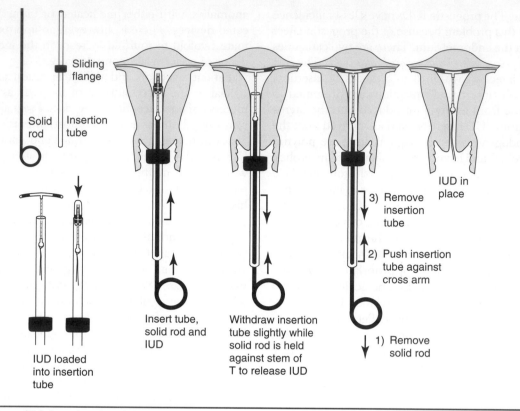

Figure 25.6. Insertion of an IUD.

be inserted, the IUD felt, and then removed with an "IUD hook" or small forceps. Infrequently, IUDs become embedded in the uterine wall and require hysteroscopic removal.

Natural Family Planning

So-called natural family planning (also called "the rhythm method") usually refers to methods that seek to *prevent pregnancy by either avoiding intercourse around the time of ovulation or using knowledge of the time of ovulation to augment other methods,* such as barriers or spermicides. These methods are safe, cost little, and are more acceptable for religious reasons or for those couples who wish a more natural method. For couples who are highly motivated and for women with a regular menstrual cycle, these methods may provide acceptable contraception.

The *estimation of the woman's "fertile" period* is based on calendar calculations, variations in basal body temperature, changes in cervical

mucus, or a combination (sometimes called symptothermic method) of these methods. When the calendar is used, the fertile period would last from days 10 through 17 for a woman with an absolutely regular 28-day cycle. Additional days are added to the fertile period based on the time of shortest and longest menstrual interval. Thus, a woman with periods every 28 ± 3 days would be considered to be fertile from days 7 (10 − 3) to 20 (17 + 3). Basal body temperatures and changes in cervical mucus are used to detect ovulation. A rise in basal body temperature of 0.5°F to 1°F or the presence of thin, "stretchy," clear cervical mucus indicates ovulation.

Couples using these methods avoid intercourse until a suitable period after ovulation, that is, from the start of menses until 2 to 3 days after temperature rise or from the first awareness of the clear, copious mucus associated with ovulation until 4 to 5 days thereafter, indicated by the appearance of the milky or opaque mucus seen in the postovulatory, or "safe," interval. These methods are especially difficult to use in the postpartum time, when menstrual regularity has not yet resumed and cervical secretions are varied in appearance. Resumption of normal pituitary function and ovulation usually occurs some time in the fourth to sixth week postpartum, but can vary with individuals, especially with breast feeding. Ovulation has been reported as early as the fifth week postpartum, however, in a lactating patient.

Postcoital/Emergency Contraception

Postcoital or emergency contraception (ECP) may be used for women who experience an act of unprotected sexual intercourse (e.g., unintended intercourse; IUD expulsion; barrier failure such as condom breakage or diaphragm displacement; or in the case of sexual assault). Making postcoital contraception widely and easily available is one of the most important steps that can be taken to reduce the unacceptable rates of unintended pregnancy and abortion. It is estimated that the regular use of this postcoital regimen would prevent in excess of 1.5 million unintended pregnancies in the United States.

The most frequently used modern method, cited by the Food and Drug Administration as a safe and effective method of postcoital contraception, is the relatively high-dose estrogen-progestin method of Yuzpe, oral contraceptive tablets each containing 0.05 mg ethinyl estradiol and 0.5 mg DL-norgestrel (Ovral). Two tablets are taken within 72 hours of intercourse, followed by two tablets in 12 hours. Alternatively, other regimens cited by the FDA include four tablets within 72 hours of intercourse, followed by four tablets in 12 hours of Lo/Ovral (0.03 mg ethinyl estradiol and 0.30 mg norgestrel), Nordette (0.03 mg ethinyl estradiol and 0.15 mg levonorgestrel), or Triphasil. The regimen is safe, and there are no recognized medical contraindications to its use. Use of an antiemetic (e.g., promethazine hydrochloride [Phenergan], one 25-mg tablet or suppository 1 hour before the first ECP dose and repeated as needed every 8 to 12 hours

thereafter) before beginning this regimen lessens the risk of nausea and emesis, a common side effect. The failure rate for this regimen is estimated at 25%, with up to 98% of the remaining patients menstruating within 3 weeks. Thus, the use of ECP decreases the number of women who become pregnant after a single act of intercourse from 8/100 to 2/100. Multiple unprotected coital events or an interval greater than 72 hours may be associated with an increasing failure rate.

Another approved progestin-only oral emergency contraception method is called "Plan B." It consists of two tablets of levonorgestrel and is associated with a lower incidence of nausea and emesis than the Yuzpe method, and has approximately the same effectiveness. It is believed to act by preventing ovulation and fertilization and, like the Yuzpe method, will not terminate an existing pregnancy.

The total amount of hormone in these regimens is small compared with that when used as interval contraceptive regimens, and is not associated with alterations in clotting factors and similar mechanisms. There are no evidence-based criteria studies suggesting any contraindications to the use of these emergency contraceptive regimens, nor do these studies reveal any teratogenic risk.

The IUD insertion (ParaGard T380 and Mirena within 7 days) is another recommended option for emergency contraception and, in limited studies, has reported a failure rate of approximately 0.1%. An additional advantage of IUD insertion is the contraceptive effect that is provided for up to 10 years.

Ineffective Methods

Just as the clinician must provide and counsel against routine use of less-than-effective, *folklore-based techniques* such as postcoital douching, withdrawal before ejaculation (coitus interruptus), makeshift barriers (such as food wrap), and various contraceptive coital positions, counseling should address effective methods compatible with the patient and her partner.

CHAPTER 26

STERILIZATION

This chapter deals primarily with APGO Educational Topic:

Topic 33: Contraception and Sterilization

Students should be able to list the various types of sterilization by type and describe their mechanisms of action, effectiveness, risks and benefits, indications and contraindications.

Sterilization offers highly effective birth control without continuing expense, effort, or motivation. *It is the most frequently used method of controlling fertility used in the United States.* Approximately one in three married couples has chosen surgical sterilization as their method of contraception. Sterilization is the leading contraceptive method for couples when the wife is older than 30 years and for those who have been married more than 10 years.

All available surgical methods of sterilization prevent the union of sperm and egg, either by preventing the passage of sperm into the ejaculate (vasectomy) or by permanently occluding the fallopian tube (tubal ligation). Although it is possible to reverse some forms of sterilization, the difficulty of doing so, combined with the generally poor rate of success and the financial expense, demands that patients understand the permanent nature of the decision. The physician must be able to accurately counsel couples considering surgical sterilization and assist in determining the best method from those available.

Changes in operative techniques; anesthesia methods; and attitudes of the public, insurance providers, and physicians have contributed to the rapid increase in the number of sterilization procedures performed each year. Modern methods of surgical sterilization are less invasive, less expensive, safer, and as effective–if not more effective–than those used 20 years ago. These factors have combined to decrease concern about the invasive nature of these procedures despite the reality that they are more invasive, per se, than vasectomy. *Counseling of patients must include discussion of the permanent nature of the procedures, the operative risks, and the chance of pregnancy (<1%).*

Despite careful counseling, approximately 1% of patients undergoing sterilization subsequently request reversal of the procedure because of a change in marital status, loss of a child, or desire for more children. If the patient is <30 years of age, she is at greatest risk for regret. *Successful reversal occurs in only 40% to 60% of cases.*

Sterilization of Men

About one-third of all surgical sterilization procedures are performed on men. Because the vas deferens is located outside the abdominal cavity, vasectomy is safer, more easily performed in most cases, and usually less expensive than procedures done on women. Vasectomy is also more easily reversed than most female sterilization procedures (Figure 26.1). Postoperative complications include bleeding, hematomas, and local skin infections, but these occur in <3% of cases. Some authors report a greater incidence of depression and change in body image after vasectomy than after female sterilization. This risk may be minimized with preoperative counseling and education. Concern has been raised about the formation of sperm antibodies in approximately 50% of patients, but no adverse long-term effects of vasectomy have been identified. Likewise, concerns about an increased risk of prostate cancer following vasectomy are not supported in literature; indeed, in countries with the highest rates of vasectomy, there is no increase in the incidence of prostate cancer.

Pregnancy after vasectomy occurs in about 1% of cases. Many of these pregnancies result from intercourse too soon after the procedure, rather than from recanalization. Vasectomy is not immediately effective. Multiple ejaculations are required before the proximal collecting system is emptied of sperm. Couples should use another method of contraception until male sterility is reasonably assured (*6 weeks, or after 15 ejaculations*) and/or postoperative azoospermia is confirmed by semen analysis.

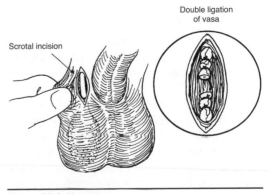

Double ligation of vasa

Scrotal incision

Figure 26.1. Vasectomy.

Sterilization of Women

Surgical sterilization techniques for women may be broadly divided into *postpartum* and *interval* (between pregnancies) procedures, although most techniques may be performed at either time.

Laparoscopy

Performed as an outpatient interval procedure, laparoscopic techniques may be carried out under either local, regional, or general anesthesia. Small incisions, a relatively low rate of complications, and a degree of flexibility in the procedures possible have led to high physician and patient acceptability.

In laparoscopic procedures, a small infraumbilical incision is made in the skin, and a trocar and sheath are placed into the abdominal cavity. Although most operators prefer to create a pneumoperitoneum before trocar placement, safe placement may also be accomplished without this step. The trocar is withdrawn and a laparoscope passed through the sheath into the abdominal cavity. The procedure may be completed using this one port, or two or more smaller trocars may be passed (under direct vision) through the lower abdominal wall. A cannula or uterine manipulator is often used to aid in visualizing pelvic structures and moving them into position for surgery. At the close of the procedure, the pneumoperitoneum is evacuated, and the skin and fascia are closed.

Occlusion of the fallopian tubes may be accomplished through the use of electrocautery (unipolar or bipolar) or the application of a plastic and spring clip (the Hulka clip or Filshie clip) or Silastic band (Yoon or Falope ring) (Figure 26.2). The choice among laparoscopic methods and cautery or occlusive device is often based more on operator experience, training, and personal preference than on outcome data.

Electrocautery-based methods are fast and carry the lowest failure rates, but they carry a risk of inadvertent electrical damage to other structures, poorer reversibility, and greater incidence of ectopic pregnancies when failure does occur. Most operators coagulate at two sites, but whether one or more than one site is coagulated, care should be taken that the coagulation forceps is placed over the entire fallopian tube and onto the mesosalpinx so that the entire tube and its lumen are coagulated over a centimeter in length. Bipolar cautery is preferable over unipolar because it has less risk of spark injury to adjacent tissue because of the current passing directly between the blades of the coagulation forceps.

The Hulka clip is the most readily reversible method because of its minimal tissue damage, but it also carries the greatest failure rate (up to 1%) for the same reason. As in coagulation, care must be taken to place the jaws of the Hulka clip over the entire breadth of the fallopian tube.

The Filshie clip has a lower failure rate than the Hulka clip because of its larger diameter, ease of application, and atraumatic locking device. To maximize effectiveness, this clip should be placed at the isthmic portion of the fallopian tube.

The Falope ring is intermediate for both reversibility and failure rates. Patients may, however, have a higher incidence of postoperative pain, requiring strong analgesics. Care must be taken to draw a sufficient "knuckle" of fallopian tube into the Falope ring applicator so that the band is placed below the outer and inner borders of the fallopian tube, thus occluding the lumen completely.

Laparotomy

The oldest methods of female sterilization have used laparotomy. Whether it is a small infraumbilical incision made in the postpartum period or a small lower abdominal suprapubic incision (minilaparotomy) used as an interval procedure, laparotomy provides ready access to the uterine tubes. Permanent obstruction or interruption of the fallopian tubes may then be accomplished by various means, such as excision of all or part of the fallopian tube or the use of clips, rings, or cautery.

The most common method of tubal interruption done by laparotomy is the Pomeroy tubal ligation (Figure 26.3). In this procedure, a segment of tube from the midportion is elevated, and an absorbable ligature is placed across the base, forming a loop, or knuckle, of tube. This is then excised and sent for histologic confirmation

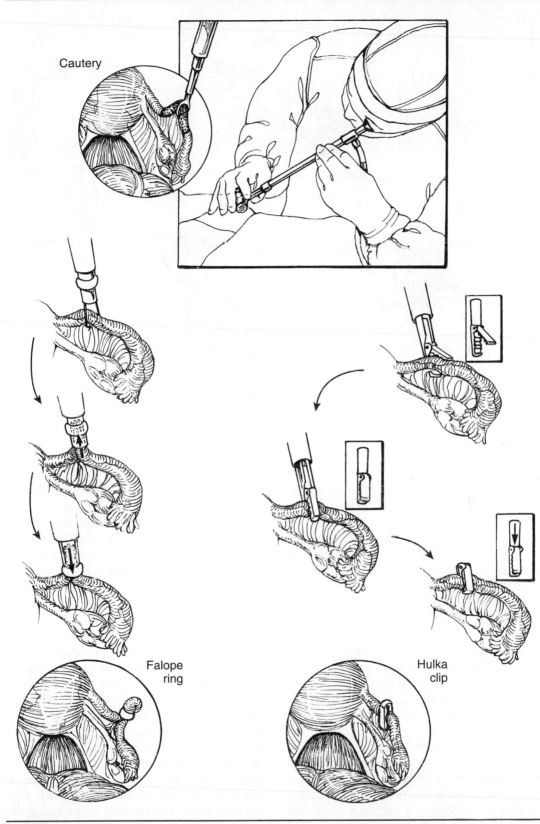

Cautery

Falope ring

Hulka clip

Figure 26.2. Laparoscopic sterilization.

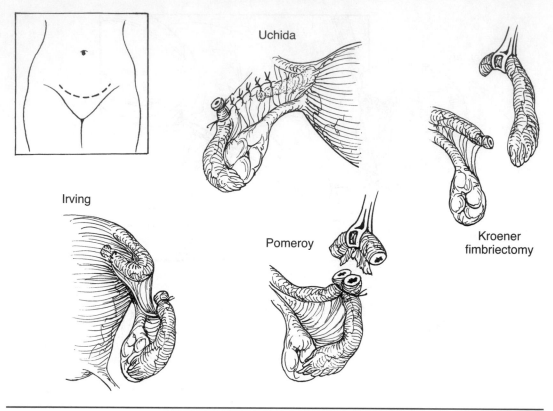

Figure 26.3. Sterilization at laparotomy.

because of the similarity in appearance between the fallopian tube and the round ligament. When healing is complete, the ends of the tube will have sealed closed with a 1- to 2-cm gap between the ends. Failure using this method is *in the range of 1 in 500 procedures.* Many modifications of this technique have been described (Table 26.1). These methods have acceptably low failure rates but are not as popular as the Pomeroy technique. Electrocoagulation or the application of clips or bands may also be accomplished through a laparotomy incision, although these are more widely used with laparoscopy.

Colpotomy
The thin wall of tissue between the vaginal canal and the posterior cul-de-sac also offers a convenient port of entry into the peritoneal cavity for sterilization procedures. Vaginal tubal procedures carry a high rate of vaginal incision site ("cuff") and ovarian infections if

prophylactic antibiotics are not used. Vaginal tubal procedures require restrictions on intercourse and the use of tampons or douches for 2 weeks while healing takes place. Although less popular than in the past, this approach may have some advantage in the retroflexed and retroverted uterus or in the morbidly obese patient.

Hysteroscopy
The possibility of transcervical obstruction of the fallopian tube avoids the inherent risks in penetration of the peritoneal cavity. Methods that have been proposed include the development of formed-in-place silicone plugs, chemical cautery (e.g., phenol), and occlusive agents such as methyl cyanoacrylate. Endometrial ablation by cautery or laser has also been suggested. The only currently available hysteroscopic sterilization method, *Essure,* involves the placement of a titanium-dacron spring device directly into the tubal ostia bilaterally. The

Table 26.1. Techniques of Tubal Ligation at Laparotomy

Technique	Procedure
Madlener	Tube elevated, base crushed in clamp, and crushed area ligated with nonabsorbable suture
Pomeroy	Loop of tube from middle third of tube elevated, ligated with plain gut, and then excised
Irving	Tube divided, proximal stump buried in uterine wall, and distal stump buried in leaves of broad ligament
Cook	Tube divided, proximal stump buried in round ligament, and distal stump buried in leaves of broad ligament
Kroener	Fimbriated end of tube excised
Parkland	Incision of mesosalpinx below the isthmus to create a window, bilateral ligation of segment of tube passing suture through the window, transection of tube
Aldridge	Fimbriated end of tube buried in broad ligament
Uchida	Mesosalpinx injected with saline–epinephrine solution and excised to expose tube, serosa of proximal end stripped off and most of proximal segment removed, stump ligated with nonabsorbable suture and placed in broad ligament, distal end ligated, broad ligament closed with distal stump left outside the broad ligament
Partial salpingectomy	Part of tube removed
Total salpingectomy	All of tube removed
Cornual resection	Tube ligated 1 cm from cornua and excised with cornua, distal end buried in broad ligament, proximal wound covered with round ligament and broad ligament

inserts stimulate a tissue reaction that ultimately leads to tubal occlusion. Patients are instructed to use an additional form of contraception for 3 months after the procedure until the efficacy of the device can be proven with a hysterosalpingogram.

Hysterectomy

Vaginal hysterectomy was once a preferred means of permanent sterilization for the multigravida. Today, the morbidity of this procedure is thought to outweigh the benefits, especially with less aggressive surgical and nonsurgical means of contraception available.

Nonsurgical Methods

A great deal of interest is focused on the development of permanent contraception based on nonsurgical methods. One such approach is the creation of an antipregnancy vaccine. Based on immunization to progesterone, this experimental technique appears promising. As more is learned about the biochemistry of reproduction, other alternatives may become available.

Side Effects and Complications

No surgically based technology is free of the possibility of complications or side effects. Infection, bleeding, injury to surrounding structures, or anesthetic complications may occur with any of the techniques discussed in this chapter. The overall fatality rate attributed to sterilization is about 1.5 per 100,000 procedures, significantly lower than that for childbearing in the United States, estimated at about 10 per 100,000 births. Thus, when the risk of pregnancy from interval contraception is accounted for, sterilization is the safest of all contraceptive methods. Laparoscopic and hysteroscopic techniques carry risks that are unique to their special instrumentation, such as complications of trocar insertion or cervical damage, respectively. *Failure of surgical sterilization occurs in 1%*

or less of all procedures and depends to some extent on the method chosen and operator experience.

Debate continues about the existence of a posttubal ligation syndrome. It has been postulated that disruption of blood flow in the area of the fallopian tubes may influence ovarian function, leading to menstrual dysfunction and dysmenorrhea. Efforts to document or quantify such an effect have not been successful, and the existence of this syndrome remains conjectural.

"Pregnancy after tubal ligation is ectopic until proven otherwise" is still a wise concept for management, but the implication that each pregnancy is usually ectopic is not entirely accurate. Ectopic pregnancy does occur after tubal ligation, more commonly after cautery than mechanical tubal occlusion, probably because of microscopic fistulae in the coagulated segment connecting to the peritoneal cavity. Two or more years after tubal ligation, most pregnancies are ectopic, whereas in the first year only about 10% are ectopic; that is, the overall rate of pregnancy decreases with time after tubal ligation, whereas the ectopic pregnancy rate remains constant. Overall, it appears that approximately one-third of pregnancies after tubal ligation are ectopic, and the rate of ectopic pregnancy is lower in this group than in women who have not had tubal ligation.

Reversal of Tubal Ligation

Reversal of tubal ligation by microsurgical techniques is most successful when minimal damage is done to the smallest length of fallopian tube (e.g., Hulka clip, Filshie clip, or Falope ring), in some series approaching 50% to 75%. In most cases, however, rates of 25% to 50% are more reasonable expectations, so that many specialists in infertility recommend the use of assisted reproductive technology (e.g., in vitro fertilization) rather than attempts at tubal ligation reversal with the attendant low success rates and increased risk of tubal ectopic pregnancy. *Indeed, a patient who has undergone tubal reversal and becomes pregnant is presumed to have an ectopic pregnancy until intrauterine pregnancy is established.*

The Decision for Sterilization

The decision to be permanently sterilized is, obviously, important, emotionally charged, and fraught with risk if it is perceived to have been faulty because of either lack of proper explanation and information or lack of freedom in the decision. The physician has the responsibility to be certain that the following components of this decision-making process occur, and that they are appropriately documented as comprising the "consent."

1. The permanence of the procedure is explained, as well as the failure rates of the procedure and the kinds and rates of complications (e.g., ectopic pregnancy).
2. The risks and benefits and indications and contraindications of the procedure are explained.
3. The risks and benefits and indications and contraindications of alternative interval methods of contraception, including hormonal, barrier, "natural" or timing, and other methods, as well as abstinence, are also explained.
4. The patient (and partner, if appropriate) is given an opportunity to ask questions about this information, and these are fully answered.
5. Finally, given items 1 through 4, the patient freely chooses a given procedure, signing the requisite consent forms.

It is important to remember that it is the patient education and decision-making process described in items 1 through 4, not the documentation described in item 5, that comprise the process of informed patient consent.

CHAPTER 27

VULVITIS AND VAGINITIS

This chapter deals primarily with APGO Educational Topic:

Topic 35: Vulvar and Vaginal Disease

Students should be able to discuss the evaluation and management of vaginitis and dermatoligic disorders of the vulva.

Patients with vulvitis or vaginitis may present with acute, subacute, or indolent symptoms, ranging in intensity from minimal to truly incapacitating. Although generally nonspecific, the patient's history and symptoms may point to chemical, allergic, or other causes rather than infection. Irritation of the well-innervated tissues of the vulva often leads to intense pruritus. Common vaginal infections often present with characteristic patterns (Table 27.1).

Vaginal secretions are always present to some extent and are normal. When abnormal, the amount and character of the secretions also depends on the influence of chemical, mechanical, or pathologic conditions. Understanding the physiologic and pathophysiologic processes responsible for both normal and abnormal discharge makes the diagnosis of vulvitis and vaginitis accurate.

History taking is especially important in patients with vulvar symptoms, including hygiene and sexual practices, use of deodorants and feminine products, changes in detergents, and other contact issues such as new or unusual clothes. Thorough physical examination by inspection and palpation is also important, especially the saline and potassium hydroxide (KOH) wet preparations for evaluations of vaginal secretions and discharges (Figure 27.1). *Inaccurate diagnosis or overtreatment of a physiologic condition is doomed to fail and may even make the patient worse.*

The vulva and vagina are covered by stratified squamous epithelium. The vulva contains hair follicles and sebaceous, sweat, and apoc-

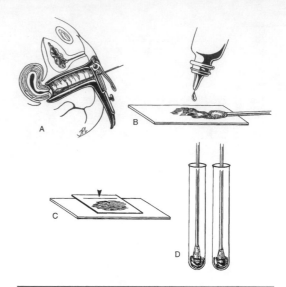

Figure 27.1. Saline and potassium hydroxide (KOH) preparations. A drop of physiologic saline and a drop of 10% to 20% KOH are placed on glass slides. (**A**) Vaginal discharge is collected on a cotton-tipped applicator. (**B**) The discharge is mixed in the droplets. (**C**) The preparations are then covered with a cover slide for microscopic viewing. (**D**) As an alternative, samples of discharge may be collected with two cotton-tipped applicators, which are then placed in small test tubes prepared with a few drops of NaCl and KOH solution. Material from these tubes is examined in a similar manner.

rine glands, whereas the epithelium of the vagina is nonkeratinized and lacks these specialized elements. The skin of the vulva is also vulnerable to secondary irritations from vaginal secretions, and both vulva and vagina are

		Table 27.1. Clinical Aspects of Physiologic Vaginal Secretions and Common Vaginal Infections		
Characteristic	**Physiologic Findings**	**Vaginosis (BV) Bacterial**	**Candidiasis**	**Trichomoniasis**
Vaginal pH	3.8–4.2	> 4.5	≤ 4.5 (usually)	> 4.5
Discharge	White, clear, flocculent	Thin, homogeneous, gray, white, adherent, often increased	White, curdy, "cottage cheese-like," sometimes increased	Green–yellow frothy, adherent, increased
KOH "whiff test" (amine odor)	Absent	Present (fishy)	Absent	Possibly present (fishy)
Patient's main complaints	None	Bad odor, discharge, worse after intercourse, possible itching	Itching/burning, discharge	Frothy discharge, bad odor, dysuria, vulvar pruritus

vulnerable to contact with external irritants (such as soap residue, perfumes, fabric softeners, or infestation by pinworms).

The vulva and vagina are also sites of symptoms and lesions of several sexually transmitted diseases, such as herpes genitalis, human papillomavirus, syphilis, chancroid, granuloma inguinale, lymphogranuloma venereum, and molluscum contagiosum (see Chapter 28).

Vulvitis

Vulvar irritation and itching are the reasons for approximately 10% of all outpatient visits to gynecologists. Erythema, edema, and skin ulcers are all indications of possible *infection.* Ulcerative lesions should suggest the possibility of sexually transmitted disease such as *herpes* or *syphilis.* Other systemic diseases, such as *Crohn's disease,* may also present in this manner. Papillary lesions suggest *condyloma acuminatum* or *condyloma latum.* Screening should be done carefully for these and other sexually transmitted diseases. The vulvar skin is also subject to many common dermatoses, including intertrigo, seborrhea and seborrheic dermatitis, and psoriasis, as well as allergic reactions and infection with parasites such as *Pthirus pubis (the crab louse)* and *Sarcoptes scabiei (the itch mite).* Excoriation caused by the patient's scratching and fissuring of the skin of the vulva are often seen in vulvar irritation secondary to vaginal discharge. Chronic pruritus leads to itching and excoriation, and when chronic this is sometimes called neurodermatitis. In addition to treatment of the underlying cause of the pruritus, these patients may benefit from a time-limited treatment with a topical corticosteroid cream (hydrocortisone 1% twice or three times a day) to relieve the cycle of inflammation and itching, which is neurodermatitis.

Diffuse reddening of the vulvar skin accompanied by itching and/or burning, but without obvious cause, should suggest a *secondary allergic vulvitis.* The list of possible local irritants can be extensive, including feminine hygiene sprays, deodorants, tampons or pads (especially those with deodorants or perfumes), tight-fitting synthetic undergarments, colored or scented toilet paper, and laundry soap or fabric softener residues. Even locally used contraceptives or sexual aids may be the source of irritation. A careful history, combined with the removal of the suspected cause, usually confirms the diagnosis and constitutes the needed therapy. In rare cases, the use of hydrocortisone cream (1% cream applied twice a day to affected areas) may be needed to decrease the local inflammatory response.

Allergic causes of vulvitis are also frequently found in the occasional pediatric patient who presents with vulvovaginal itching. In addition to the causes already noted, pediatric patients often have sources of irritations such as foreign bodies (especially with an accompanying vaginitis or discharge) as well as emotional residual of sexual abuse or infection with pinworms.

Local *Candida* infection is another cause of vulvar pruritus. This etiology must be considered in diabetics and others disposed to such infection and in situations with a suboptimal response to treatment for another problem. The diagnosis and treatment are described later in this chapter.

In older patients, intense itching of the vulva may occur because of *atrophic changes* brought on by reduced estrogen levels. This is typically associated with pale, thin vaginal mucosa, atrophic vaginitis, and the resultant yellowish discharge that has a pH of greater than 5.5. The skin of the vulva and perineum has a symmetrically reddened, smooth, and somewhat shiny look. Biopsy will reflect the hypoplastic nature of this condition and will help to differentiate this from lichen sclerosus, which has a similar appearance. When atrophic change is the cause, estrogen replacement, either locally or systemically, is the treatment of choice (see Chapter 38). In the case of *lichen sclerosus,* local application of clobetasol proprionate 0.05% cream twice a day is generally effective. Alternatives that have been used, although with less effectiveness, include testosterone proprionate 2% in petrolatum base and progesterone cream 3%.

Vulvar itching may be caused by infestation with *P. pubis* or *S. scabiei* (Figure 27.2), especially if itching of the mons is present. This itching is caused by an allergic sensitization from the parasite's bite. The crab louse is a

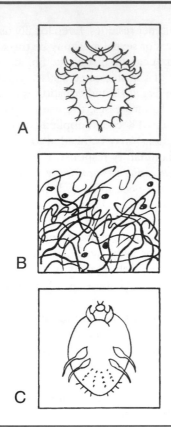

Figure 27.2. (A) *Pthirus pubis* (the crab louse). **(B)** Nits of the crab louse. **(C)** *Sarcoptes scabiei* (the itch mite).

different species from the body or head louse and is acquired by close contact or from bedding or towels. The crab louse is found exclusively in hairy areas, whereas the itch mite, although transmitted similarly, may be found anywhere in the skin surface. The diagnosis is generally made by looking for small black specks (excreta) on the skin, nits and eggs on hair shafts, or the parasites themselves. Local treatment with two applications of a γ-benzene hexachloride lotion (Kwell) is generally successful for infection from either parasite. Clothes, bedding, and those with whom close contact occurs must be disinfected or treated to break the infection cycle. Other specific therapies for both pediculosis pubis and scabies include permethrin and lindane.

The vulva is subject to the same plethora of *dermatologic diseases* as other skin surfaces. *Contact dermatitis* is relatively common, with red, edematous skin surfaces and sometimes with vesicles and secondary infection. Treatment consists of removing the offending substance or material and wet compresses of Burrow's solution, diluted 1 to 20, several times a day followed by drying. Hydrocortisone (0.5% to 1.0%) or fluorinated corticosteroids (Valisone, 0.1%) may be applied several times a day for symptom control. *Psoriasis* affects 1% to 3% of women and seems to have a familial pattern. This generalized pruritic skin disease of unknown cause presents with reddened skin and silvery scales and is often refractory to simple fluorinated corticosteroids, and dermatologic consultation is required. *Hidradenitis suppurativa* is a chronic, unrelenting skin infection causing deep, painful scars and a foul discharge. Its differential diagnosis includes Crohn's disease of the vulva. Treatment with local antibiotics and steroids is sometimes successful, but wide excision of the affected skin areas is often required.

Because of the nonspecific nature of symptoms and physical findings, patients who present with vulvitis and who do not respond to initial therapy should be offered vulvar biopsy to determine histologically the underlying etiology. Particularly in older patients, initial biopsy is often of value, and especially if an initial therapy has failed, a biopsy should usually be performed, as this presentation of one or more failed medical managements without specific diagnosis by biopsy is often noted in unrecognized vulvar malignancy.

Vaginitis

The most common symptom associated with infections of the vagina is discharge. *Discharge from the vagina is normal physiologically; therefore, not all discharges from the vagina indicate infection.* This distinction is important to the diagnostic process but occasionally difficult for the patient to understand or accept.

Vaginal secretions arise from several sources. The majority of the liquid portion consists of mucus from the cervix. A small amount of moisture is contributed by endometrial fluid, exudates from accessory glands such as the Skene's and Bartholin's glands, and from vaginal transudate. Exfoliated squamous cells from the vaginal wall give the secretions a white to off-white color and provide some increase in consistency. The action of the indigenous vaginal flora also can contribute to the secretion. These components together constitute the normal vaginal secretions that provide the physiologic lubrication that prevents drying and irritation. The amount and character of this mixture vary under the influence of many factors, including hormonal and fluid status, pregnancy, immunosuppression, and inflammation. *Asymptomatic women produce, on the average, approximately 1.5 g of vaginal fluid per day. Normal vaginal secretions have no odor.*

After puberty, increased levels of glycogen in the vaginal tissues favor the growth of lactobacilli (Doderlein's bacilli) in the genital tract. These bacteria break down glycogen to lactic acid, lowering the pH from the 6 to 8 range, which is common before puberty (and after menopause), to the *normal vaginal pH range of 3.5 to 4.5* in a reproductive-aged woman. In addition to the lactobacilli, a wide range of other aerobic and anaerobic bacteria may normally be found in the vagina at concentrations of 10^8 to 10^9 colonies per mL of vaginal fluid. Because the vagina is a potential space, not an open tube, a ratio of 5:1 anaerobic: aerobic bacteria is normal.

Increased vaginal discharge is associated with an identifiable microbiologic cause in 80 to 90% of cases. Hormonal or chemical causes account for most of the remaining cases. Most vaginal infections are caused by synergistic bacteria (bacterial vaginosis, nonspecific vaginitis), fungi (candidiasis), and protozoa, such as *Trichomonas vaginalis* (trichomoniasis). Bacterial infections account for approximately 50% of infections, whereas fungi and *Trichomonas* account for roughly 25% each. Through gentle examination and simple microscopic investigation, the etiology of the patient's symptoms generally can be ascertained. *The value of microscopic examination of vaginal smears cannot be overstated. For this reason, any patient who complains of a vaginal discharge or irritation should be evaluated directly before therapy is suggested.* An increase in vaginal discharge is considered physiologic during pregnancy and at the mid-cycle in nonpregnant women. Although the increase in discharge amount is normal at these times, patients who complain of symptoms should be evaluated to rule out a pathologic cause.

Bacterial Vaginosis (BV)

Once thought to be caused by the infection of *Gardnerella vaginalis* (formerly called *Haemophilus* or *Corynebacterium vaginalis*), BV is now understood to be a *symbiotic infection of anaerobic bacteria (Bacteroides, Peptococcus, and Mobiluncus species) and Gardnerella*, both of which contribute to the clinical findings (Table 27.2).

Women with BV generally complain of a *"musty" or "fishy" odor with an increased thin gray–white to yellow discharge.* The discharge may cause some mild vulvar irritation, commonly in approximately one-fifth of the cases. The vaginal discharge is mildly adherent to the vaginal wall and has a pH greater than 4.5. Mixing some of these secretions with KOH (10%) liberates amines that may be detected by their fishy odor (positive "whiff test"). Microscopic examination made under saline wet mount shows a slight increase in white blood cells, clumps of bacteria, and characteristic *"clue cells,"* which are epithelial cells with numerous coccoid bacteria attached to their surface, making them appear to have indistinct borders and a "ground-glass" cytoplasm (Figure 27.3). The diagnosis of BV is defined by any three of the following four criteria: (1) homogeneous discharge, (2) pH greater then 4.5, (3) positive "whiff test," and (4) presence of clue cells.

BV may be treated with oral metronidazole (Flagyl, 500 mg twice a day for 7 days) or by intravaginal creams, using metronidazole (MetroGel) 0.75% vaginal gel twice daily for 5 days or clindamycin (Cleocin) 2% vaginal

Table 27.2. Vaginitis—Altered Ecology		
Finding	Normal	Bacterial Vaginosis
Organisms	10^8	10^{11}
Anaerobes:aerobes	5:1	1000:1
H_2O_2 production	High	Low
Lactobacillus	96%	35%
Gardnerella	5–60%	95%
Mobiluncus	0–5%	50–70%
Mycoplasma hominis	15–30%	60–70%

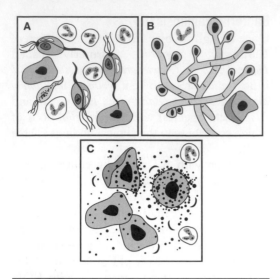

Figure 27.3. (A) Trichomonads; a flagellated protozoan is easy to identify on NaCl wet mount because of its movement. **(B)** Monilial infection; slide shows hyphae and budding yeast. **(C)** Clue cells, which are epithelial cells with clumps of bacteria on their surfaces.

cream once a day for 7 days or a 100-mg suppository at bedtime for 3 consecutive nights. Alternative options include metronidazole 2 g in a single oral dose and clindamycin orally 300 mg twice daily for 7 days. Whether BV is transmitted sexually continues to be debated. Although treatment of sexual partner(s) of patients with frequent recurrences is not recommended by the Centers for Disease Control, it is common practice among physicians to treat the partners.

Trichomonas Vaginitis

Trichomonas vaginalis is a flagellate protozoan that *lives only in the vagina, Skene's ducts, and male or female urethra* and may be freely transmitted by sexual intercourse. More than 60% of partners of women with *Trichomonas* infections will also be infected. Despite the large number of cases of symptomatic vaginitis caused by the organism, up to one-half of women with *Trichomonas* in the vaginal canal are asymptomatic. *Symptoms of Trichomonas infection* vary from mild to severe and may include vulvar itching or burning, copious *discharge* with rancid odor, dysuria, and dyspareunia. Although not present in all women, the discharge associated with

Trichomonas infections is generally "frothy," thin, and yellow–green to gray in color, with a pH above 4.5. *Examination* may reveal edema or erythema of the vulva. "Characteristic" petechiae, or strawberry patches, are described as present in the upper vagina or on the cervix, but are actually found in only about 10% of affected patients.

The *diagnosis* is confirmed by *microscopic examination* of vaginal secretions suspended in normal saline. This wet smear will show large numbers of mature epithelial cells, white blood cells (WBCs), and the *Trichomonas* organism. *Trichomonas* is a fusiform protozoa just slightly larger than a WBC. The organism has three to five flagella extending from the narrow end. These flagella produce active movement that may facilitate identification of the organism (see Figure 27.3).

Treatment of Trichomonas infections is by oral *metronidazole*. Because *Trichomonas* is sensitive to metronidazole, 1-day therapy, with 2 g orally, generally gives a 90% cure rate. Treatment with 500 mg twice a day for 7 days or 250 mg three times a day for 7 days gives comparable results. Many physicians prefer the single-day therapy because of its reduced cost and greater compliance. Vaginal metronidazole gel twice daily for 5 days is also now recommended. Treating sexual partners of women with *Trichomonas* infections is recommended and is often undertaken using the single-day therapy. Abstinence from alcohol use when taking metronidazole is necessary to avoid a possible disulfiram-like reaction. The use of metronidazole during pregnancy is not recommended because of reports of teratogenic effects. Many physicians, however, use the drug in the latter half of pregnancy for highly symptomatic patients.

Even though the pH generally associated with *Trichomonas* infections is different from that found with bacterial vaginosis, estimates show up to a *25% prevalence of bacterial vaginosis in those patients with Trichomonas*. Because of the overlap in metronidazole therapy for these two conditions, this debate is not significant for most patients. It may, however, be worthy of consideration in patients who receive alternative therapies or in those with frequent recurrences of vaginal infections.

Although follow-up examination of patients with *Trichomonas* for test of cure is often advocated, they are usually not cost effective, except in the rare patient with a history of frequent recurrences. In these patients, reinfection or poor compliance must be considered as well as the possibility of infection with more than one agent or other underlying disease.

Candida (Monilial) Vaginitis

Monilial infections of the vagina are caused by ubiquitous *airborne fungi*. Approximately 90% of "yeast" infections are caused by *Candida albicans* with <10% caused by *Candida glabrata, Candida tropicalis,* or *Torulopsis glabrata*. *Candida* infections generally do not coexist with other infections and are not considered to be sexually transmitted, even though 10% of male partners have concomitant penile infections. Candidiasis is more likely to occur in women who are pregnant, diabetic, obese, immunosuppressed, on oral contraceptives or corticosteroids, or have had broad-spectrum antibiotic therapy. Practices that keep the vaginal area warm and moist, such as wearing tight clothing or the habitual use of panty liners, may also increase the risk of *Candida* infections.

The most common presenting complaint for women with candidiasis is *itching*, although up to 20% of women may be asymptomatic. Burning, external dysuria, and dyspareunia are also common. The vulva and vaginal tissues are often bright red in color and excoriation is not uncommon in severe cases. *A thick, adherent "cottage cheese" discharge with a pH of 4 to 5 is* generally found. *This discharge is odorless.*

The *diagnosis* of candidiasis is based on history and physical findings and confirmed by the identification of hyphae and buds in wet mounts of vaginal secretions made with 10% KOH solution, which lyses most epithelial and white cells (see Figure 27.3). No direct correlation is shown between the degree of symptoms and the number of organisms present. Because false-negative wet preps are not uncommon, culture confirmation may be obtained using Nickerson's or Sabouraud's media. Latex agglutination tests may be of particular use for non-*Candida albicans* strains because they do not demonstrate the pseudohyphae on wet prep.

Treatment of Candida infections is primarily with the topical application of one of the synthetic imidazoles (Table 27.3). These agents

Table 27.3. Topical Treatments for *Candida* Vaginitis

Agent	Formulation	Dose
Imidazole		
Miconazole (Monistat)	2% cream	5 g bid for 14 days
	200 mg vaginal suppository	1 g qd for 3 days
Butoconazole (Femstat)	2% cream	5 g qd for 3 days
Clotrimazole		
(Gyne-Lotrimin)	1% cream	5 g qd for 7 days
	100 mg vaginal suppository	1 qd for 7 days
(Mycelex-G)	500 mg vaginal suppository	1 dose
Tioconazole (Vagistat-1)	6.5% cream	5 g in 1 dose
Polyene		
Nystatin	200,000 U vaginal tablet	1 qd for 14 days
Trazole		
Terconazole (Terazol)	0.4% cream	5 g qd for 7 days
	0.8% cream	5 g qd for 3 days
	80 mg vaginal suppository	qd for 3 days

give good cure rates after 3 to 7 days of treatment. Despite greater than 90% relief of symptoms with these therapies, 20% to 30% of patients experience *recurrences* after 1 month. Treatments based on nystatin or povidone-iodine have proved to be less effective than the imidazoles. Resistant strains of *C. tropicalis* or *T. glabrata* may respond to therapy with terconazole or gentian violet. Because noncompliance is the most frequent cause of recurrence and because some women find the topical agents inconvenient or difficult to apply, treatment with the oral agent fluconazole (Diflucan), 150 mg as a single dose, has become widely used. Patients with frequent recurrences should be carefully evaluated for possible risk factors such as diabetes or immune defects. For recurrence or resistance, ketoconazole 100 mg twice daily for 10 days can be effective. Prophylactic local therapy with an antifungal agent should be considered when systemic antibiotics are prescribed.

Chronic Vaginitis

A problem for both physicians and patients is "chronic" or "recurrent" vaginitis. Patients complain, often bitterly, of persistent vaginal discharge, odor, or both, without a readily identifiable cause or satisfactory response to treatment. These patients have frequently "tried everything" and visited several physicians without success. A careful history must be obtained, covering medical conditions and sexual and hygienic habits. A methodical physical examination and microscopic evaluation are also required.

In addition to the three most common causes previously listed, one must evaluate alternative explanations for the patient's complaints. Chlamydial infections may present as vulvovaginitis. Because *Chlamydia trachomatis* is the most common sexually transmitted organism in the United States, its role in recurrent/chronic cases should be evaluated (see Chapter 28). *Cytolytic vaginitis* is a common but underrecognized cause of *cyclic* vulvovaginitis. Although the exact pathophysiology is not known, it is thought to be caused by an overgrowth of the lactobacilli in the vagina, resulting in increased vaginal acidity, with subsequent cytolysis, vaginal discharge, and vulvovaginal irritation. This diagnosis should be considered when more common etiologies have been ruled out. A high index of suspicion should be present if the vaginal pH is between 3.5 and 4.5 and symptoms worsen during the luteal phase. Therapy includes using pads rather than tampons, discontinuing previous antifungal medications, and use of baking soda sitz baths (4 tablespoons in 1–2 inches of warm water) twice daily and douches (30–60 g of sodium bicarbonate in a liter of warm water) every 2–3 weeks.

Desquamative inflammatory vaginitis is characterized by purulent discharge, exfoliation of epithelial cells with vulvovaginal burning and erythema. relatively little lactobacilli and overgrowth of gram-positive cocci, usually streptococci are seen. Vaginal pH is greater than 4.5. Initial therapy is clindamycin cream 2% applied daily for 1 week.

Victims of sexual assault (recent or far in the past) may present in this manner. A frank explanation of the possibility of reinfection must be carried out in individuals with true recurrent infections. The existence of additional sexual contacts for the patient or her partner should be explored in an appropriately nonjudgmental way. Alternate sources of excessive vaginal moisture, such as chronic cervical infections, must be evaluated. When the patient's complaints seem to exceed her physical and microscopic findings, the possibility of inappropriate expectations, inaccurate information, or psychological dysfunction must be entertained.

CHAPTER 28

SEXUALLY TRANSMITTED DISEASES

This chapter deals primarily with APGO Educational Topic:

Topic 36: Sexually Transmitted Diseases

Students should be able to discuss diagnosis, evaluation, and management of the common sexually transmitted diseases and of urinary tract infection. Students should also be able to discuss the evaluation and management of salpingitis and urinary tract infection.

Sexually transmitted diseases run the gamut from vaginitis to life-threatening conditions such as acquired immune deficiency syndrome (AIDS). The increasing prevalence of sexually transmitted disease (STD) has resulted in increased awareness among physicians and patients and, in some cases, changes in attitudes about acceptable behaviors and standards. The impact of STDs for the individual and for society cannot be overlooked or overemphasized. Although some of these diseases can be acquired through nonsexual means, sexual transmission represents the major route by which most are spread.

The sexual habits, modes of expression, and frequency of sexual interactions that individuals choose affect their risk of infection as well as the site and presentation of infections. For this reason, a detailed sexual history is requisite for any in whom an STD is either likely or suspected. Most of these infections require skin-to-skin contact or exchange of body fluids for transmission. Nonsexual activities that meet these criteria may also put the patient at risk. All patients who are (or might be) sexually active should be examined with an awareness of the possibility of an STD. This is not a condemnation of the patient's lifestyle or personal choices, but rather a simple fact of life in today's society. Complicating the issue, most sexually transmitted diseases are asymptomatic in women. This further emphasizes the importance of a detailed sexual history and thorough physical examination. The inguinal region should be inspected for rashes, lesions, and adenopathy. The vulva should be inspected for lesions, ulcerations, or abnormal discharge and palpated for thickening or swelling. The Bartholin's glands, Skene's ducts, and urethra cannot be overlooked because these are frequent sites of infection (e.g., gonorrhea). In patients with urinary symptoms, the urethra should be gently "milked" to express any discharge. The vagina and cervix must be inspected for lesions and abnormal discharge. When suspicion or risk is high, cultures of the urethra and cervix for gonorrhea, chlamydia, or other infections should be obtained. Last, the perineum and perianal areas must also be evaluated for signs of STDs. Cultures of the rectum for gonorrhea should be

obtained in those patients who engage in anal intercourse. For completeness, the oral cavity as well as cervical and other lymph nodes must be evaluated and cultures taken if indicated by the patient's modes of sexual expression. The findings obtained by this process, combined with the patient's history, generally make the establishment of the proper diagnosis much easier. Furthermore, the sexual partner(s) of patients diagnosed with or suspected of having an STD should receive their own evaluation. It is vital to remember that *20% to 50% of patients with an STD have one or more coexisting infections. When one venereal disease is found, others must be suspected.*

Specific Infections

Herpes Genitalis

Office visits for this infection have increased tenfold in the past 10 years. Seroepidemiologic studies estimate that approximately 500,000 new cases are identified per year. Herpes simplex infections are highly contagious. Roughly 75% of sexual partners of infected individuals contract the disease. Approximately 85% of genital herpes lesions are caused by herpes simplex virus type 2 (HSV_2); this type differs slightly from the type 1 virus (HSV_1), which usually causes the cold sore lesions of the mouth but is also responsible for the balance of genital lesions. Both are DNA viruses.

Clinical Course

The development of the classic vesicular lesions is often preceded by a prodromal phase of mild paresthesia and burning beginning approximately 2 to 5 days after infection in symptomatic patients. This progresses to painful vesicular and ulcerated lesions 3 to 7 days after exposure, usually resolving in approximately one week (Figure 28.1). Dysuria caused by vulvar lesions or urethral and bladder involvement may lead to urinary retention. Roughly 10% of patients with initial lesions require hospitalization for pain control or management of urinary complications. Primary infections are also characterized by malaise, low-grade fever, and inguinal adenopathy in 40% of patients. Aseptic meningitis with fever, headache, and

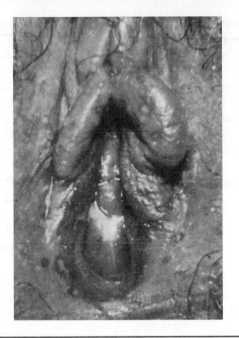

Figure 28.1. Herpes simplex virus infection. Note the small serpiginous, superficial lesions and edema of the vulva and urethral area.

meningismus can be found in some patients 5 to 7 days after the appearance of the genital lesions.

Physical Examination

Findings consist of clear vesicles that lyse and progress to shallow, painful ulcers with a red border. These may coalesce and frequently become secondarily infected and necrotic. These lesions may be found on the vulva, vagina, cervix, or perineal and perianal skin, often extending onto the buttocks. Recurrent lesions are similar in character but milder in severity and shorter in duration, generally lasting 2 to 5 days. However, although often similar in appearance, recurrent lesions can be unilateral rather than bilateral and present as fissures or vulvar irritation as opposed to vesicular in appearance.

Diagnosis

The diagnosis is based on characteristic history and physical findings, although it may be confirmed through the use of viral cultures taken by swab from the lesions. Culturing is

the most sensitive method of diagnosis and allows confirmation in as little as 48 hours. Viral shedding occurs for up to 3 weeks after lesions appear. Scrapings from the base of vesicles may be stained by immunofluorescence techniques for viral particles. This technique provides results faster than cultures and carries approximately 80% agreement with culture results. Smears may also be stained with Wright's stain to visualize the characteristic giant multinucleated cells with eosinophilic intranuclear inclusions. The lesions of herpes simplex infections are distinguishable from the ulcers found in chancroid, syphilis, or granuloma inguinale by their appearance and extreme tenderness.

Treatment

Management of local lesions and symptoms is the focus. The lesions should be kept clean and dry. Sitz baths, followed by drying with a heat lamp or hair dryer, work well for this purpose. The use of a topical anesthetic, such as 2% Xylocaine jelly, may be required. If secondary infections occur, therapy with a topical antibacterial cream such as Neosporin may be of help. Oral medication can reduce the duration of viral shedding and shorten the initial symptomatic disease course. Treatments include acyclovir (Zovirax) 200 mg 5 times/day or 400 mg 3 times/day, famciclovir (Famvir) 250 mg 3 times/day, and valacyclovir (Valtrex) 1 g 2 times/day. These therapies do not decrease the likelihood of recurrence, and the decrease in symptom duration is often minimal.

Recurrences occur in 30% of patients. After the primary infection, the virus migrates via the nerve fibers to remain dormant in the dorsal root ganglia. Recurrences are triggered by unknown stimuli, resulting in the virus traveling down the nerve fiber to the affected area. Episodic recurrences may be treated by oral antiviral therapy, including oral acyclovir (200 mg 5 times a day, or 400 mg 3 times a day, or 800 mg twice daily, all for 5 days); famciclovir 125 mg twice daily for 5 days; or valacyclovir 500 mg twice daily for 5 days. For women with frequent recurrences, suppressive antiviral therapy is useful to decrease the frequency and severity of these flare-ups. Regimens include acyclovir 400 mg twice daily; or valacyclovir

250 mg twice daily, 500 mg once daily, or 1000 mg once a day; or famciclovir 250 mg twice a day. These regimens are not thought to eliminate viral shedding nor the potential for transmission.

Severe episodes may require hospitalization for parenteral analgesia and intravenous antiviral therapy (e.g., intravenous acyclovir [5 mg/kg] infused at a constant rate over 1 hour, administered every 8 hours for 5 days) in adult patients with normal renal function. Such therapy is generally recommended for immunosuppressed or otherwise compromised patients. These patients are best managed in consultation with an infectious disease specialist, and other regimens may be applied to their care, including the use of foscarnet sodium (Foscavir, 40 mg/kg intravenous every 8 hours in patients with normal renal function) or cidofovir (Vistide, 5 mg/kg intravenously every 2 weeks in patients with normal renal function).

In pregnant patients with active herpes infections and intact membranes, cesarean delivery should be considered. Vaginal delivery, when herpetic lesions are present, is associated with a 50% chance that the baby will acquire the infection, which is associated with significant morbidity and an almost 80% mortality rate.

Pelvic Inflammatory Disease

Pathogenesis

Infection of the upper female genital tract is predominantly by direct spread along the mucosal surfaces from initial infection of the cervix. The predominant organisms are *Chlamydia trachomatis* and *Neisseria gonorrhoeae*. A mucopurulent cervicitis is more common in *C. trachomatis* infection, as *N. gonorrhoeae* seems able to reside in the endocervical cells without always promoting a purulent inflammatory response. The endocervical mucus resists upward spread, especially during the progesterone-dominant part of the menstrual cycle. Oral contraceptives mimic this effect, which explains in part their action to limit pelvic inflammatory disease (PID). The cervical mucus may be penetrated by the bacteria, either di-

rectly or as riders on sperm or trichomonads or up the string of an intrauterine device. When the cervicitis traverses the cervical barrier, endometrial infection occurs, followed rapidly in most cases by spread to the fallopian tube mucosa. Occasionally, an indolent endometritis develops with further extension, more commonly with *Chlamydia* infection. Tubal ligation usually provides a barrier to spread, although in some cases small microchannels facilitate continued spread. The salpingitis that results may be localized, or it may spread causing peritonitis, adhesion formation, and abscess formation. The relative mobility of the fallopian tube probably contributes to the rapid and widespread extension of infection. In this anaerobic environment, anaerobes also thrive so that the infection in the upper portions of the genital tract is actually often polymicrobial, with a mixture of aerobic and anaerobic organisms. However, as poor correlation is shown between the diverse organisms cultured and the clinical patterns of disease, the models of *C. trachomatis* and *N. gonorrhoeae* serve well as disease models.

Chlamydia Trachomatis

Chlamydia trachomatis is the most common sexually transmitted disease. Because chlamydiae lack the metabolic and biochemical ability to produce adenosine trophosphate (ATP), they are obligate intracellular parasites that preferentially infect columnar epithelcal cells. Chlamydial infections are manifested by mucopurulent cervicitis, acute urethritis, salpingitis, or PID, and are caused by serotypes different from those strains causing other chlamydial infections such as lymphogranuloma venereum (LGV). LGV has three stages: (1) primary lesions, consisting of papules or ulcers; (2) regional lymphadenopathy, the bubonic stage; and (3) when the buboes suppurate, they develop draining fistulas and lymphatic obstruction. More common than *N. gonorrhoeae* by as much as 10:1 in some studies, infections by *C. trachomatis* can be the source of significant morbidity, including chronic infection, chronic pelvic pain, and infertility. Infection rates are five times higher in women with three or more sexual partners and four times higher in women using no contraception or nonbarrier methods.

In industrialized countries, series report asymptomatic cervical infection in 5 to 20% of women of childbearing age, with perhaps 5 to 10% of these developing ascending infection. Between 20 and 40% of sexually active women have antibodies to *Chlamydia.*

Clinically mild cases of cervicitis or pelvic infection by *Chlamydia* may be virtually asymptomatic yet culminate in infertility or ectopic pregnancy. Infection of the fallopian tubes causes a mild form of salpingitis with insidious symptoms. Once the infection is established, it may remain active for many months, with increasing tubal damage. Perihepatitis (Fitz Hugh-Curtis syndrome), which consists of inflammation leading to localized fibrosis with scarring of the anterior surface of the liver and adjacent peritoneum, may be caused by chlamydial infections more often than by *N. gonorrhoeae* infection, with which it was originally described (Figure 28.2). *Chlamydia* is also frequently found coexisting with or mimicking *N. gonorrhoeae* infection. Chlamydial infections are also responsible for nongonococcal urethritis and inclusion conjunctivitis.

Physical findings in infections caused by *Chlamydia* are often subtle and nonspecific. Eversion of the cervix with mucopurulent

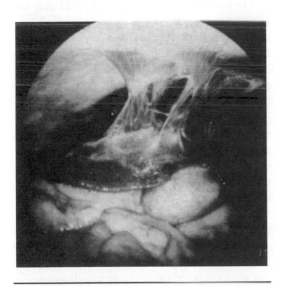

Figure 28.2. Fitz-Hugh-Curtis syndrome. Laparoscopic view of perihepatitis, showing scarring and stringlike perihepatic adhesions associated with both gonococcal and chlamydial salpingitis.

cervicitis may suggest the diagnosis. Any patient with acute PID or who is suspected of having gonorrhea should also be evaluated for *Chlamydia.*

The diagnosis of *Chlamydia* infection is suspected on clinical grounds. Cultures are generally used only to confirm the diagnosis, because it takes 48 to 72 hours to obtain culture results. Two screening tests have recently gained clinical popularity: (1) an enzyme-linked immunosorbent assay (ELISA) performed on cervical secretions and (2) a monoclonal fluorescent antibody test carried out on dried specimens. The immunoassay technique is easy to do and has a 95% specificity. The monoclonal technique is faster, has an 85 to 90% sensitivity and 95% specificity, but requires precision in making the slide and using the fluorescent microscope for interpretation.

Outpatient treatment of suspected or confirmed infections with *Chlamydia* is with azithromycin (Zithromax, 1 g po), doxycycline (Doxycycline or Vibramycin, 100 mg po bid for 7 days), or ofloxacin (Floxin, 300 mg bid for 7 days). Erythromycin base, 500 mg/day for 7 days, or erythromycin ethylsuccinate, 800 mg qid for 7 days, are also alternative treatment options. In pregnant patients, recommended treatment includes either erythromycin base 500 mg/day or amoxicillin 500 tid for 7 days. Alternative treatments in pregnancy include erythromycin base, 250 mg qid or erythromycin ethylsuccinate, 400 mg qid either for 14 days, or a one-time dose of azithromycin 1 g. Follow-up evaluation with culture or other tests as well as screening for other STDs should be performed. Partners should either be treated or referred for immediate treatment.

Neisseria Gonorrhoeae (Gonorrhea)

Infections with *N. gonorrhoeae,* a gram-negative intracellular diplococcus, continue to be common, and the incidence is increasing. The emergence of penicillin-resistant strains, an increased frequency of asymptomatic infections, and changing patterns of sexual behavior have all contributed to the problem. The damage caused by *N. gonorrhoeae* infections and the anaerobic organisms that grow with them in the pelvic environment can lead to recurrent infection, chronic pelvic pain, or infertility

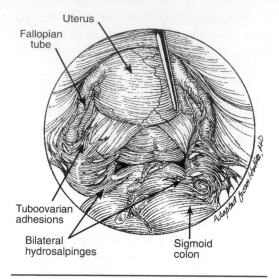

Uterus

Fallopian
tube

Tuboovarian
adhesions

Bilateral
hydrosalpinges

Sigmoid
colon

Figure 28.3. Sequelae of pelvic inflammatory disease. Laparoscopic view of multiple pelvic adhesions, including tuboovarian adhesions and bilateral hydrosalpinges.

caused by adhesion formation, tubal damage, and hydrosalpinx formation (Figure 28.3). Infertility occurs in approximately 15% of patients after a single episode of salpingitis and increases to 75% after three or more episodes. The risk of ectopic pregnancy is increased 7 to 10 times in women with a history of salpingitis. It is estimated that PID results in $2.7 billion in direct medical costs and an additional $4 billion in indirect medical costs per year.

Infections with *N. gonorrhoeae* are easily acquired and can affect almost any part or organ of the body. Infection of the pharynx is found in 10% to 20% of heterosexual women with gonorrhea, and this site should not be overlooked when cultures are taken. For women, a single encounter with an infected partner leads to infection 80% to 90% of the time. Most commonly, the first signs or symptoms of infection occur 3 to 5 days after exposure but are often mild enough to be overlooked. Infection in the lower genital tract is characterized by a malodorous, purulent discharge from the urethra, Skene's duct, cervix, vagina, or anus. Anal intercourse is not always a prerequisite to anal infection. Greenish or yellow discharge from the cervix ("mucopus") should alert the physician to the possibility of either *N. gonorrhoeae*

or *C. trachomatis* infection. Infection of the Bartholin's glands is frequently encountered and can lead to secondary infections, abscesses, or cyst formation. When the gland becomes full and painful, incision and drainage are appropriate (Figure 28.4).

Approximately 15% of women with *N. gonorrhoeae* infections of the cervix will develop acute pelvic infections (PID). *N. gonorrhoeae* infection of the fallopian tubes, adnexa, or pelvic peritoneum generally results in pain and tenderness, fever or chills, and an elevated white blood count (Table 28.1). Peritoneal involvement can also include perihepatitis (Fitz-Hugh-Curtis syndrome). *N. gonorrhoeae* is the causative agent in roughly 50% of patients with salpingitis. Many patients require hospitalization for adequate care (Table 28.2). In severe cases or in patients with one or more prior episodes of PID, tuboovarian abscess (TOA) formation may occur. These patients are acutely ill, with fevers of up to 39.5°C, tachycardia, severe pelvic and abdominal pain, and nausea and vomiting. Findings in PID are often nonspecific (Figure 28.5), and patients presenting with these symptoms must be differentiated from those with septic incomplete abortions, acute appendicitis, diverticular abscesses, and adnexal torsion (Table 28.3).

On examination, patients with PID may exhibit muscular guarding, cervical motion tenderness, and/or rebound tenderness. A purulent cervical discharge is often seen, and the adnexa are usually moderately to exquisitely tender with a mass or fullness potentially palpable.

The laboratory diagnosis of *N. gonorrhoeae* infection is made by culture on Thayer-Martin agar plates kept in a CO_2-rich environment. Cultures should be obtained from the cervix, urethra, anus, and pharynx when appropriate. Cultures provide 80 to 95% diagnostic sensitivity. A solid-phase enzyme immunoassay for the detection of *N. gonorrhoeae* antigen is also available. Gram stain of any cervical discharge for this gram-negative intracellular diplococcus may support the presumptive diagnosis.

Aggressive therapy for patients with either suspected or confirmed *N. gonorrhoeae* infection should be tailored to the site of infection and the individual patient. Initial treatment

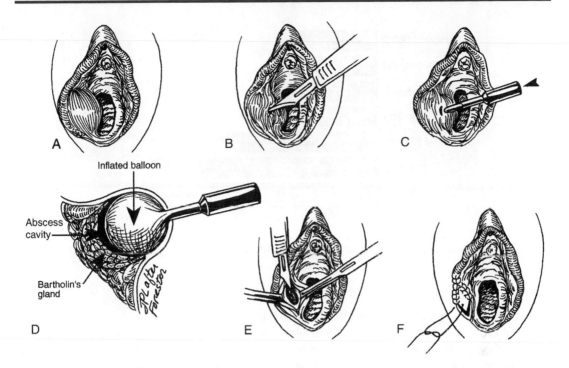

Figure 28.4. Surgical treatment of Bartholin's abscess. (**A**) Unruptured right Bartholin's abscess that is "pointing" (i.e., a prominent area is seen where only a thin layer of tissue covers the abscess). (**B**) A small incision is made with a scalpel on the medial aspect of the abscess. (**C**) The Word catheter, a short catheter with an inflatable balloon tip, is inserted into the incision. (**D**) The balloon is inflated while in the abscess cavity and left in place at least 1–2 weeks to allow epithelialization of the drainage tract. (**E**) An alternative technique of drainage is marsupialization, in which a larger incision is made to allow drainage. (**F**) The marsupialization technique is completed by sewing the incision open to facilitate drainage.

Table 28.1. Clinical Criteria for Diagnosis of Acute Salpingitis
All 3 of the following necessary:
1. Abdominal tenderness with/without rebound
2. Adnexal tenderness
3. Cervical motion tenderness
PLUS
1 or more of the following:
1. Gram stain of endocervix positive for gram-negative, intracellular diplococci
2. Temperature > 38°C
3. WBC > 10,000
4. Pus on culdocentesis or laparoscopy
5. Pelvic abscess on bimanual exam or sonogram
WBC = white blood cell

Table 28.2. Factors Suggesting Hospitalization for Patients with PID
Nulliparity
Peritonitis in upper abdomen
Pregnancy
Intrauterine contraceptive device use
Previous treatment failure
Significant gastrointestinal symptoms
Tuboovarian abscess
Uncertain or complicated differential diagnosis
Unreliable patient
White blood count > 20,000 or < 4000
All adolescents
Concurrent HIV infection
Immunosuppressed patients
HIV = human immunodeficiency virus; PID = pelvic inflammatory disease

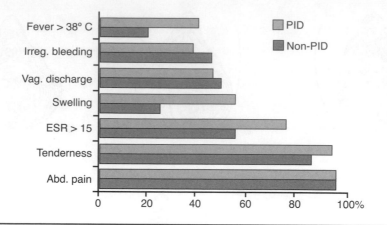

Figure 28.5. Frequency of symptoms in pelvic inflammatory disease (PID).

should not be predicated on the results of cultures but rather on clinical suspicion. General guidelines for treatment are shown in Table 28.4. Hospitalized patients require high-dose intravenous antibiotic therapy with an antimicrobial spectrum that covers aerobic and anaerobic organisms. Surgical drainage of an abscess or even hysterectomy, depending on the reproductive status and desires of the patient, may be warranted in patients who fail an aggressive course of parenteral antibiotics. Rupture of a TOA with septic shock is a life-threatening complication with mortality approaching 10% and should be treated surgically. After successful medical therapy, follow-up cultures and examination of the patient should be performed 3 to 5 days after completion of therapy.

Table 28.3.	Correct Diagnosis in Cases of Misdiagnosis of PID
Acute appendicitis	28% of cases
Endometriosis	17% of cases
Corpus luteum bleeding	12% of cases
Ectopic pregnancy	11% of cases
Adhesions	7% of cases
"Other"	28% of cases
PID = pelvic inflammatory disease	

Tuberculosis

Pelvic tuberculosis (TB) may be associated with either *Mycobacterium tuberculosis* or *Mycobacterium bovis*. It almost always results from miliary hematogenous or lymphatic spread from tuberculosis elsewhere, usually the lungs. Typically, the initial involvement is tubal, with spread to ovaries and endometrium occurring in approximately 30% to 50% of cases. Tuberculosis is a relatively uncommon infection in the United States, although its incidence is increasing in some immigrant and migrant groups, in those who are immunosuppressed, and in those who abuse drugs. The diagnosis is suspected on clinical grounds and confirmed by culture, with the endometrium being the most easily accessible tissue. The TB skin test indicates exposure but not location or current infection. Medical treatment is effective in most cases and consists of the use of one or more of five common agents: isoniazid (INH), rifampin, streptomycin, ethambutol, and pyrazinamide. Surgical treatment is sometimes required for persistent disease, abscess formation, and pelvic pain. The operation of choice in these circumstances is total abdominal hysterectomy with bilateral salpingo-oophorectomy after stringent medical therapy.

Human Papillomavirus

Infection by the human papillomavirus (HPV) is responsible for almost as many cases of STD as *N. gonorrhoeae*. This DNA virus is found in

Table 28.4. Gonorrhea and PID Therapy

Disease	Preferred Treatment	Alternative Treatment
Gonorrhea	Ceftriaxone 125 mg IM (single dose)	Spectinomycin 2 g IM
	Or	*Or*
	Cefixime 400 mg (single dose)	Ceftizoxime 500 mg IM *or* cefotaxime 500 mg IM *or* cefotetan 1 g IM
	Or	*Or*
	Ofloxacin 400 mg (single dose)	Enoxacin 400 mg *or* lomefloxacin 400 mg *or* norfloxacin 800 mg
	Or	
	Ciprofloxacin 500 mg (single dose)	
	Plus	
	Regimen effective against *Chlamydia trachomatis* (e.g., Doxycycline 100 bid for 7 days)	
PID[a]		
Outpatient	Cefoxitin 2 g IM	Ofloxacin 400 mg po bid for 14 days
	Plus	*Plus*
	Probenecid 1 g po	Clindamycin 450 mg po qid
	Or	*Or*
	Ceftriaxone 250 mg IM	Metronidazole 500 mg po bid for 14 days
	Plus	
	Doxycycline 100 mg po bid for 14 days	
Inpatient[b]	Cefoxitin 2 g IV q 6 h	Ofloxacin 400 mg IV q 12 h
	Or	*Plus*
	Cefotetan 2 g IV q 12 h	Metronidazole 500 mg IV q 8 h
	Plus	*Or*
	Doxycycline 100 mg IV or po q 12 h[c]	Ampicillin/sulbactam 3 g IV q 12 h
	Or	*Or*
	Clindamycin 900 mg IV q 8 h	Ciprofloxacin 200 mg IV q 12 h
	Plus	*Plus*
	Gentamicin 2 mg/kg IV *or* IM loading dose followed by maintenance dose of 1.5 mg/kg q 8 h	Doxycycline 100 mg IV q 12 h
		Plus
		Metronidazole 500 mg IV q 8–9 h
		Then
		Doxycycline 100 mg bid for 14 days
		Or
		Clindamycin 450 mg 5 X day for 10–14 days

[a]The indications for outpatient and inpatient treatment based on the need for parenteral administration are less clear nowadays, as parenteral medications can be given on an outpatient basis, either in outpatient care facilities or by home health agencies.
[b]Given for ≥ 48 hours after patient clinically improves.
[c]Doxycycline to be continued for 14 days.
PID = pelvic inflammatory disease

2.5% to 4% of women. Interestingly, HPV is species specific and only infects humans. Over the past 15 years, the number of infected individuals has increased more than fivefold. Unlike other STDs, sequelae of HPV infection may take years to develop. More than 70 subtypes have been identified, with at least 25 identified in genital infections. As with other viral infections, manifestations may be subclinical or clinically obvious. Types 16, 18, 45, and 56 have a relatively higher association with cervical neoplasia.

Infection by HPV after a single contact with an infected partner results in a 65% transmission rate. Following a 6-week to 3-month incubation period, infection by HPV causes soft, fleshy growths on the vulva, vagina, cervix, urethral meatus, perineum, and anus. They may occasionally also be found on the tongue or oral cavity. These growths are termed condyloma acuminata or venereal warts (Figure 28.6). These distinctive lesions may be single or multiple and generally cause few symptoms. They are often accompanied by *Trichomonas* or other STDs. Because HPV is spread by direct skin-to-skin contact, symmetrical lesions across the midline are common (often called "kissing lesions"). Condylomas are commonly associated with HPV types 6 and 11.

The diagnosis of condyloma acuminata is made based on physical examination but may be confirmed through biopsy of the warts. Although cytologic changes typical of HPV can be found on Pap smears, Pap smears of the cervix diagnose only approximately 5% of patients with the virus. Thorough inspection of the external genitalia and anogenital region should be performed during the routine gynecologic exam and especially in patients with known cervical or vaginal lesions. Because the condyloma lata of syphilis may be confused with venereal warts, some care must be taken in making the diagnosis in patients at high risk for both infections. Venereal warts are usually characterized by their narrower base and more "heaped-up" appearance, whereas condyloma lata lesions have a flattened top.

Management options include chemical, cautery, and immunologic treatments. Patient-applied products include Podofilox 0.5% gel or solution and Imiquimod 5% cream. The safety of use during pregnancy for either drug is yet to be established. Treatments that are administered by a health-care provider include application of trichloroacetic acid (TCA), application of podophyllin resin in tincture of benzoin, cryosurgery, surgical excision, laser surgery, or intralesional interferon injections. Lesions exceeding 2 cm respond best to cryotherapy, cautery, or laser treatment.

Lesions are more resistant to therapy during pregnancy, in diabetic patients, in patients who smoke, or in patients who are immunosuppressed. In patients with extensive vaginal or vulvar lesions, delivery via cesarean section may be required to avoid extensive vaginal lacerations and problems suturing tissues with these lesions. Cesarean delivery also decreases the possibility of transmission to the infant, which can cause subsequent development of laryngeal papillomata, although the risk is small and in and of itself not an indication for cesarean section.

Any patient with a history of condyloma should have at least yearly Pap smear evaluations of the cervix. The sexual partners of patients with HPV should also be screened for the development of genital warts.

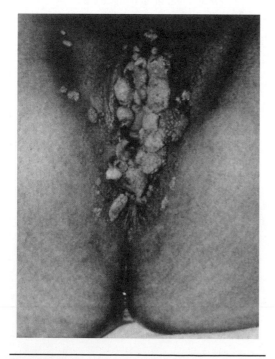

Figure 28.6. Condyloma acuminata.

Syphilis

Since antiquity, syphilis has been the proto-typic venereal disease. The incidence of syphilis has been increasing in the past several years. Early syphilis is a reportable disease. In 2002, there were 6,862 cases reported, approx-imately 2.4 cases per 100,000 population. This represented an increase from the 6,103 cases reported in 2001 as well as increases from the all-time low of 5,979 reported cases in 2000 (2.2 cases per 100,000 population). Contribut-ing perhaps to this incidence rise is today's in-creased use of nonpenicillin antibiotics to treat resistant gonorrhea, whereas in the past, peni-cillin treatment of gonorrhea provided treat-ment for coexisting syphilis.

Treponema pallidum, the causative organism of syphilis, is one of a small group of spirochetes that are virulent for humans. Because this motile anaerobic spirochete can rapidly invade intact moist mucosa, resulting in infection and chancre formation, the most common sites of entry for women are the vulva, vagina, and cervix. Chancres may also be found in or near the anus, rectum, pharynx, tongue, lips, fingers, or other areas. Transplacental spread may oc-

cur at any time during pregnancy and can result in congenital syphilis (see Chapter 16).

Approximately 10 to 60 days after infection with *T. pallidum,* a painless ulcer appears. This is *the chancre of primary syphilis.* The chancre has a firm, punched-out appearance and has rolled edges (Figure 28.7). Even though it is of-ten accompanied by adenopathy, the chancre is commonly asymptomatic and missed. Sero-logic testing at this stage of syphilis generally is negative. Healing of the chancre occurs spon-taneously in 3 to 9 weeks.

At 4 to 8 weeks after the primary chancre ap-pears, manifestations of *secondary syphilis* de-velop. This stage is characterized by low-grade fever, headache, malaise, sore throat, anorexia, generalized lymphadenopathy, and a diffuse, symmetric, asymptomatic maculopapular rash. This rash is often seen over the palms and soles and is sometimes referred to as "money spots." Highly infective secondary eruptions, called *mu-cous patches,* occur in 30% of patients during this stage. In moist areas of the body, flat-topped papules may coalesce, forming condyloma lata (Figure 28.8). These may be distinguished from

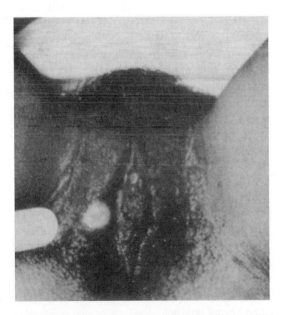

Figure 28.7. Chancre of the vulva. The chancre of syphilis, a rounded or ovoid raised lesion with indurated edges and a depressed center. The surface is reddish or reddish brown.

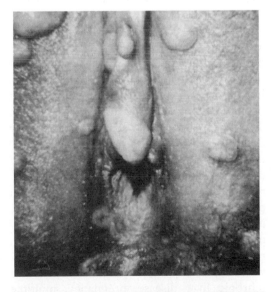

Figure 28.8. Condyloma lata of the vulva. The typical lesion of secondary syphilis, slightly raised, round or oval, plateaulike lesions of various sizes, often occur-ring in clusters. The edges are slightly indurated, and the surface is moist and covered with a grayish necrotic exudate. These lesions are highly infectious.

Table 28.5. Types of Serologic Tests for Syphilis

Nontreponemal

Venereal Disease Research Laboratory (VDRL)

Rapid plasma reagin (RPR) card test

Automated reagin test (ART)

Treponemal

Fluorescent treponemal antibody absorption (FTA–ABS)

Microhemagglutination assay for antibodies to *Treponema pallidum* (MHA–TP)

venereal warts by their broad base and flatter appearance. In untreated individuals, this stage, too, passes spontaneously in 2 to 6 weeks as the disease enters into the latent phase.

In the late stages of the disease, transmission of the infection is unlikely, except via blood transfusion or placental transfer. However, crippling damage to the central nervous system, heart, or great vessels often develops. Destructive, necrotic, granulomatous lesions called *gummas* may develop 1 to 10 years after infection.

The diagnosis of syphilis may be made by identifying motile spirochetes on darkfield microscopic examination of material from primary or secondary lesions or lymph node aspirates. For most patients, the diagnosis is established on the basis of serologic testing (Table 28.5). The Venereal Disease Research Laboratory (VDRL) and rapid plasma reagin (RPR) are nonspecific tests that are rapid, inexpensive, and useful for screening. False-positive tests may result from bacterial causes (pneumococcal pneumonia, scarlet fever, malaria, tuberculosis, mycoplasma pneumonia), viral causes (chickenpox, human immunodeficiency virus [HIV], measles, mononucleosis, mumps, viral hepatitis, various vaccinations), and noninfectious causes (chronic liver disease, pregnancy, multiple myeloma, connective tissue disease, multiple blood transfusions). These tests are used to screen for the disease and also to monitor response to treatment. The biologic false-positive tests are associated with low titers, typically less than 1:8.

The fluorescent treponemal–antibody absorption (FTA–ABS) and microhemagglutination assay for antibodies to *T. pallidum* (MHA–TP) tests are specific treponemal antibody tests that are confirmatory or diagnostic but not used for routine screening. Even these latter tests have sources of false-positive results (e.g., Lyme disease, malaria, leprosy, mononucleosis, systemic lupus erythematosus). A woman with a positive treponemal test will usually have this positive result for life, irrespective of treatment or activity of the disease. When neurosyphilis is suspected, a lumbar puncture, with a VDRL performed on the spinal fluid, is required.

The treatment of choice for syphilis is benzathine penicillin G, as outlined in Table 28.6. The patient should be followed by quantitative VDRL titers and examinations at 3, 6, and 12 months.

AIDS

Acquired immune deficiency syndrome (AIDS) is the advanced manifestation of infection by Human Immunodeficiency Virus (HIV-1), an RNA retrovirus. The virus targets "helper" lymphocytes (those with CD4 marker) and monocytes. Depletion of CD4 (Helper T cells) is an important manifestation of HIV infection. The progression of HIV-1 infection varies from individual to individual. In addition to the quantitative depletion of CD4 (Helper T cells), a qualitative abnormality is seen in CD4 cells. HIV-1 specific T Helper cell function is weak or absent in infected individuals. This renders the host immune system unresponsive to control viral replication during the chronic phase of HIV-1 infection. This lack of HIV-1 specific T Helper cell function is unique to HIV-1 infections. AIDS is now one of the top five causes of death in reproductive-age women. It is estimated that approximately 0.3% of the general population is infected with HIV. The three primary methods of contracting the virus are: (1) use of contaminated needles or blood products, (2) perinatal transmission from mother to child, and (3) intimate sexual contact.

The screening test for AIDS is an ELISA (enzyme-linked immunosorbent assay) that tests for antibodies against HIV. Although rare, false-positive tests are possible and are more

Table 28.6. Treatment of Syphilis

Type	Preferred Treatment	Alternative Treatment
Primary, secondary, early latent	Benzathine penicillin G, 2.4 million units, IM	Doxycycline 100 mg bid for 14 days *Or* Tetracycline 500 mg qid for14 days *Or* Erythromycin 500 mg qid for 14 days
Late latent or syphilis of unknown duration	Benzathine penicillin G, 2.4 million units IM weekly for 3 weeks	Doxycycline 100 mg bid for 14 days *Or* Tetracycline 500 mg qid for 14 days
Neurosyphilis	Aqueous crystalline penicillin G, 3–4 million units IV q 4 h for 10–14 days	Procaine penicillin, 2.4 million units IM daily for 10–14 days *Plus* Probenecid 500 mg qid for 10–14 days

common in multiparous women and women taking oral contraceptives. Confirmation is achieved with the more specific Western blot technique. Because of the accuracy of standard HIV testing, polymerase chain reaction (PCR) and HIV viral load testing are, despite their specificity, rarely needed.

Management of HIV focuses on prevention and chemotherapy. The former emphasizes use of latex condoms and spermicides containing nonoxynol 9. The latter includes various classes of anti-HIV drugs, including the nucleoside reverse transcriptase inhibitors (NRTI) such as zidovudine, nonnucleoside reverse transcriptase inhibitors (NNRTI), and protease inhibitors. Monotherapy is not advocated because of development of drug resistance. Instead, HAART (highly active antiretroviral therapy) combination therapy consisting of at least three agents has shown promise.

Minor Sexually Transmitted Diseases

Chancroid, granuloma inguinale, LGV, molluscum contagiosum, parasite infections (such as pediculosis pubis or scabies), enteric infections, and some types of vaginitis (e.g., trichomoniasis) are infections that are spread through sexual activities. Pertinent information about these infections, some of which are seldom seen, is summarized in Tables 28.7 and 28.8.

Table 28.7. Minor Sexually Transmitted Diseases

Disease	Causative Agent	Main Symptom	Diagnosis	Treatment
Chancroid	*Haemophilus ducreyi*	Painful "soft chancres," adenopathy	Clinical, smears culture	Azithromycin, 1 g single dose Erythromycin base, 500 mg qid for 7 days
				Or Ceftriaxone, 250 mg IM
				Or
				Ciprofloxacin, 500 mg bid for 3 days
Granuloma inguinale	*Calymmato- bacterium granulomatis*	Raised, red lesions	Clinical, smears	Doxycycline, 100 mg bid for a minimum of 3 weeks Trimethoprim/ sulfamethoxazole, 1 double strength tablet bid for 3 weeks
				Or
				Ciprofloxacin, 750 mg bid for 21 days
Lymphogran- uloma venereum (LGV)	*Chlamydia trachomatis*	Vesicle, progressing to bubo	Clinical, complement fixation test	Doxycycline, 100 mg bid for a minimum of 3 weeks Erythromycin base, 500 mg qid for 21 days Permethrin cream/rinse
Molluscum contagiosum	*Poxviridae*	Raised papule with waxy core	Clinical, inclusion bodies	Desiccation, cryotherapy, curettage
Parasites	*Pediculus, Sarcoptes scabiei*	Itching	Inspection	Lindane 1%
Enteric infections	*Neisseria gonorrhoeae, Chlamydia trachomatis, Shigella, Salmonella, protozoa*	Diarrhea	Culture	Based on agent
Vaginitis	*Trichomonas*	Odor, irritation	Microscopic examination of secretions	Metronidazole, 1 g AM and PM for 1 day or 500 mg bid for 7 days

Table 28.8. Genital Lesions in Sexually Transmitted Diseases[a]

Characteristic	Herpes	Genital Warts	Syphilis	Chancroid	LGV	Granuloma Inguinale
Organism	Herpes simplex virus	Human papillomavirus	*Treponema pallidum*	*Haemophilus ducreyi*	*Chlamydia trachomatis*	*Calymmatobacterium granulomatis*
Incubation	3–7 days	1–8 months	10–60 days	2–6 days	1–4 weeks	8–12 weeks
Primary lesion	**Vesicle**	Papule/polypoid	Papule (chancre)	Papule/pustule	Papule/pustule/vesicle	Papule
Number	**Multiple coalesce**	Variable	1	1–3	Single	Single or multiple
Pain	**Yes**	No	**Rare**	**Often**	No	**Rare**
Shape	Regular	Irregular	Regular	Irregular	Regular	Regular
Margins	Flat	Raised	Raised	**Red, undermined**	Flat	**Rolled, elevated**
Depth	Superficial	Raised	Superficial	**Excavated**	Superficial	Elevated
Base	Red, smooth	Normal, pink, white	Red, smooth	**Yellow, gray**	Variable	Red, **rough**
Induration	None	None	**Firm**	Rare, soft	None	**Firm**
Secretions	Serous	None	Serous	**Purulent, hemorrhagic**	Variable	Rare, hemorrhagic
Lymph nodes	Firm, tender	**Normal**	Firm, nontender	Tender, suppurative	Tender, suppurative	Pseudoadenopathy
Duration	5–10 days, **recurrent**	**Months**	Weeks	Weeks	Days	Weeks

[a]Scabies, molluscum contagiosum, *Candida*, and other dermatologic conditions (e.g., hidradenitis suppurativa) may also cause genital lesions. Items in boldface are of particular help in making a differential diagnosis. LGV = lymphogranuloma venereum

CHAPTER 29

PELVIC RELAXATION, URINARY INCONTINENCE, AND URINARY TRACT INFECTION

This chapter deals primarily with APGO Educational Topic:

Topic 37: Pelvic Relaxation and Urinary Incontinence

Students should be able to discuss the types of pelvic relaxation, urinary incontinence, urinary tract infection, and their causes and presentations, evaluation, and managements (behavioral, medical, or surgical).

Pelvic relaxation is a nondescript term that refers to a variety of conditions related to loss of connective tissue support surrounding the reproductive tract organs This includes loss of uterine support, paravaginal tissue support, bladder wall and urethrovesical angle support, and support overlying the distal rectum. Patients with pelvic relaxation present in many different and often subtle ways. To identify patients who would benefit from therapy, the physician should be familiar with the types of pelvic relaxation and the approach to the patient with symptoms suggestive of this problem. The physician must also be aware of other common urinary tract conditions that affect women. Although pelvic relaxation and urinary tract disorders are frequently symptomatic, patients are often reluctant to voice their complaints. The physician must be sensitive to these complaints as well as to the physical findings that suggest a problem.

Pelvic Relaxation

Although not exclusively a condition of advancing age, pelvic relaxation is more common as tissues become less resilient and the accumulated stresses of life have an effect. As a greater proportion of our patients move into their later years, more and more women will be at risk for pelvic relaxation and its attendant problems. Pelvic pressure and pain, dyspareunia, bowel and bladder dysfunction, and urinary incontinence may all result from loss of support for the pelvic organs. Almost half of all women have had the involuntary loss of small amounts of urine at some time in their life; 10 to 15% of women suffer significant, recurrent urinary loss. Loss of pelvic support can have both medical and social implications that necessitate evaluation and intervention.

Causes of Pelvic Relaxation

The pelvic organs are supported by a complex interaction of muscles (e.g., levator muscles), fasciae (e.g., urogenital diaphragm, endopelvic fascia), and ligaments (e.g., the uterosacral and cardinal ligaments). Each of these structures can lose its ability to provide support through birth trauma, chronic elevations of intraabdominal pressure (e.g., obesity, chronic cough,

or repetitive heavy lifting), intrinsic weaknesses, or atrophic changes caused by aging or estrogen loss. Underlying most of these associated factors, the most significant contribution to pelvic relaxation may be intrinsic weaknesses in collagen matrix as a result of genetic factors. Loss of adequate support for the pelvic organs may be manifest by descent or prolapse of the urethra (*urethral detachment* or *urethrocele*), bladder (*cystocele*), or rectum (*rectocele*). A true hernia at the top of the vagina allowing the small bowel to herniate through (*enterocele*) can also occur. These anatomic defects are illustrated in Figure 29.1. A descriptive manner to visualize these defects is as follows. The anterior vaginal wall is a hammock. With good support, the hammock is pulled tight allowing the bladder to rest on the hammock. When support is lost, the hammock sinks, as if someone is now sitting in the hammock. The bladder now forces the anterior vaginal wall down and out, creating the anterior wall defect or cystocele. A similar force occurs in creating the posterior wall defect or rectocele. The posterior vaginal wall loses the lateral support, and thus the pressure from the rectum forces the posterior vaginal wall in an upward direction. Loss of support for the uterus can lead to varying degrees of descent of the uterus (*uterine prolapse*). When the uterus descends beyond the vulva, it is termed *procidentia*. Loss of tissue support can also result in prolapse of the vaginal vault in patients who have had a hysterectomy. Although such loss of support (*pelvic relaxation*) may affect any of the pelvic organs individually, multiple organ involvement is most common.

Evaluation

The evaluation of patients with pelvic relaxation rests primarily on the history and physical examination. Pelvic relaxation is best demonstrated by observing the vaginal area while having the patient strain. This may be done in either or both the supine and standing positions. A urethrocele or cystocele may be demonstrated by separating the labia and asking the patient to "strain down" or cough. When a urethrocele or cystocele is present, a downward movement and rotation of the anterior vaginal wall toward the introitus will be seen. To more fully evaluate a cystocele, recto-

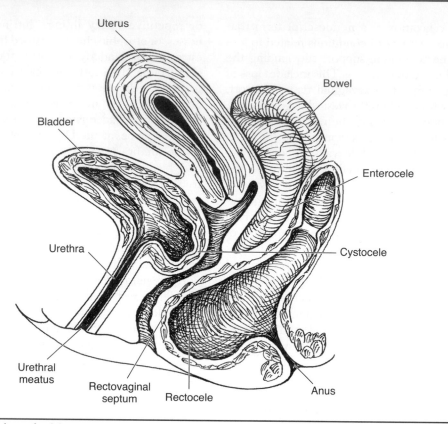

Figure 29.1. Loss of pelvic support.

cele, or enterocele, inspection should be carried out using a Sims or the lower half of a Graves speculum to retract the posterior vaginal wall. The extent of urethral hypermobility may be assessed by the Q-tip test With the patient in the lithotomy position place a cotton-tipped swab with lidocaine jelly into the bladder and pull back until resistance is met. This will be the urethral–vesicular junction (UVJ). Once placed, ask the patient to Valsalva. If urethral hypermobility is present, the UVJ will deflect down, thus causing the swab to rise. The angle is measured from the resting position to the location at maximum Valsalva. An angle greater than 35 degrees is considered a positive test. Urodynamic testing may also be useful. (Urodynamic testing is further discussed later in the chapter.)

The degree of prolapse is classified in degrees or grades (Figure 29.2). A grade 3 prolapse occurs when the leading part of the prolapse reaches the hymenal ring. A grade 4 prolapse is past the hymenal ring. At times

one may see a patient with a grade 3 or 4 prolapse without incontinence. This patient may have experienced leaking in the past, but now the urethra is kinked, and urination is often incomplete. This patient may present with urgency or incomplete bladder emptying. The medical issue of greatest concern for this patient with a significant prolapse is hydronephrosis/hydroureter. The insertion of the ureter into the trigone becomes kinked, and urine begins to back up into the collecting system. A renal ultrasound is helpful to evaluate this scenario.

Differential Diagnosis

The presumptive diagnosis of pelvic relaxation is based on the evaluation of the structural integrity of pelvic support by physical examination. Often the characteristics of the patient's complaint may suggest a diagnosis. Even though the differential diagnosis of pelvic relaxation is generally simple, other processes must be considered. Urinary tract infection

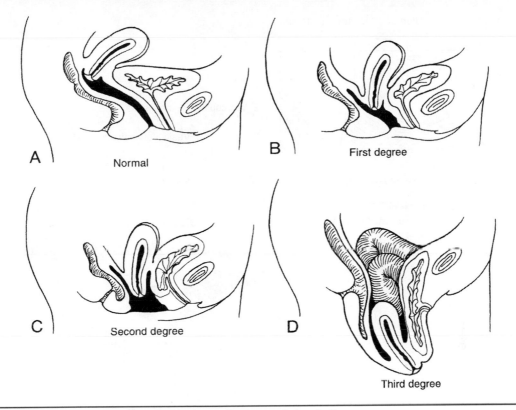

Figure 29.2. Pelvic relaxation classifed by degree (**A–D**) or grade (see text).

may lead to urgency. Urethral diverticulum or Skene's gland abscesses may mimic a cystourethrocele and, in the case of diverticula, may be a source of incontinence. These can be identified through symptoms, careful "milking" of the urethra, or cystoscopy. The complaint of urinary loss may stem from mechanical factors (such as a cystourethrocele), irritation (mechanical, neoplastic, or inflammatory trigonitis), neurologic causes (such as diabetes or detrusor instability), the effects of medications, or mental and psychosocial conditions. In patients who have had a history of recent pelvic surgery or radiation, a vesicovaginal or ureterovaginal fistula must also be considered in the differential diagnosis. It is occasionally difficult to differentiate between a high rectocele and an enterocele. This distinction may be facilitated through rectal examination or the identification of small bowel in the hernia sac. It is common for the diagnosis of an enterocele not to be established until surgical repair is undertaken.

Most pelvic relaxation is the result of structural failure of the tissues involved, but other contributing factors should be considered in the complete care of the patient. Has there been a change in intraabdominal pressure and why? Why does the patient have a chronic cough that has precipitated her symptoms? Is a neurologic process (such as diabetic neuropathy) complicating the patient's presenting complaint? Each of these issues should be considered prior to the selection of a diagnostic or therapeutic plan.

In the evaluation of involuntary loss of urine, the physician must also consider the possibility of fistulae. Fistulae between the vagina and the bladder (vesicovaginal), urethra (urethrovaginal), or ureter (ureterovaginal) are generally the result of surgical trauma, irradiation, or malignancy. A communication between the bladder and the uterus (vesicouterine) may also be found on rare occasions. In addition, fistulae may occur between the rectum and vagina (rectovaginal fistulae),

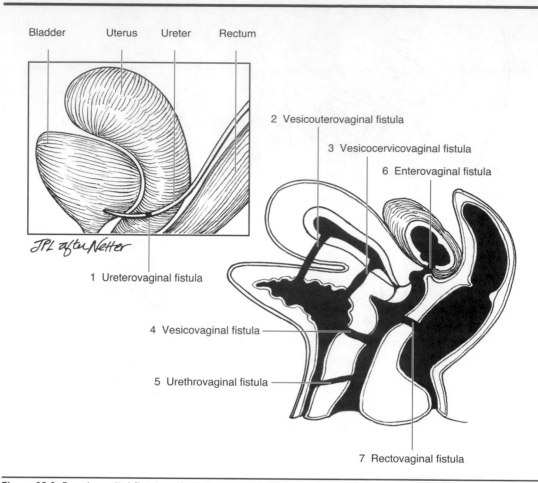

Bladder Uterus Ureter Rectum

JPL after Netter

1 Ureterovaginal fistula

2 Vesicouterovaginal fistula

3 Vesicocervicovaginal fistula

6 Enterovaginal fistula

4 Vesicovaginal fistula

5 Urethrovaginal fistula

7 Rectovaginal fistula

Figure 29.3. Female genital fistulae. (1) Ureterovaginal. (2) Vesicouterovaginal. (3) Vesicocervicovaginal. (4) Vesicovaginal. (5) Urethrovaginal. (6) Enterovaginal. (7) Rectovaginal.

resulting in the passage of flatus or feces from the vagina (Figure 29.3).

Urinary Incontinence

Causes of Urinary Incontinence

The normal voiding "reflex" is initiated when the stretch receptors within the detrusor muscle send a signal to the brain. The brain then decides if it is socially acceptable to void. The detrusor muscle contracts, thus elevating the bladder pressure to exceed the urethral pressure. The external urethral sphincter, under voluntary control, relaxes, and voiding is completed.

A common complaint of patients with a cystocele or urethrocele is urinary incontinence. This does not occur in all patients, and the degree of incontinence is often not commensurate with the degree of pelvic relaxation. Several types of urinary incontinence have been identified; stress, urge, mixed, and overflow are the most common. Stress incontinence is the most common form of urinary incontinence

Types of Urinary Incontinence

Stress Urinary Incontinence

Normal physiology and anatomy allow for increased abdominal pressure to be transmitted along the entire urethra. In addition, the endopelvic fascia that extends beneath the urethra allows for the urethra to be compressed against the endopelvic fascia, thus maintaining a closed system and maintaining the bladder neck in a stable position.

Table 29.1. Characteristics of Urinary Incontinence

Characteristic	Stress Incontinence	Urge Incontinence	Overflow Incontinence
Associated symptoms	None (occasional pelvic pressure)	Urgency, nocturia	Fullness, pressure frequency
Amount of loss	Small, spurt	Large, complete emptying	Small, dribbling
Duration of loss	Brief, corresponds to stress	Moderate, several seconds	Often continuous
Associated event	Cough, laugh, sneeze, physical activity	None, change in position, running water	None
Position	Upright, sitting; rare supine or asleep	Any	Any
Cause	Structural (cystocele, urethrocele)	Loss of bladder inhibition	Obstruction, loss of neurologic control

Pathophysiology With increased intraabdominal pressure the urethral–vesicle angle cannot be maintained because of endopelvic fascia defect. The bladder neck descends, the bladder pressure is elevated above the intraurethral pressure, and urine is lost.

Clinical Presentation Stress incontinence presents with loss of urine with cough, laugh, sneeze, (increased abdominal pressure/Valsalva) that is *viewed as a problem by the patient* (Table 29.1). When stress incontinence is demonstrated with urodynamic testing, the diagnosis is urodynamic stress incontinence.

Nonsurgical Treatment Options An understanding of the anatomic defects that lead to stress incontinence allows the student to clearly understand the nonsurgical and surgical treatment modalities.

Pelvic muscle training (Kegel exercises) is extremely effective. The exercises work to strengthen the pelvic floor and thus decrease the degree of urethral hypermobility. The patient is instructed to contract her pelvic diaphragm. This educational process is imperative, as many women perform these exercises faithfully, but, unfortunately, ineffectively. Biofeedback techniques and even weighted vaginal cones are available to assist patients. When performed correctly the success rate is about 85%. Success is defined as decreased "wet episodes." However, once the patient stops her exercise regimen she will revert to her original status.

Various pessaries and continence tampons can be placed vaginally to aid in urethral compression. In addition, urethra "plugs" and caps can be placed and removed by the patient to inhibit leaking in social situations.

Current research is directed toward medical therapy for the treatment of stress incontinence.

Surgical Therapy The aim of surgical therapy is to restore normal pelvic anatomy. Many different surgical approaches are available to accomplish this goal. These corrections replace or strengthen the support beneath the urethra and bladder neck. These surgical procedures can be completed either vaginally with tension-free vaginal tape, transobturator tape, or bone anchor supports or through an abdominal approach such as the Burch suspension. Retropubic needle procedures place a needle through the space of Retzius, passing just laterally to the urethra on either side, thus creating the support to "hang" the hammock (Table 29.2). Pubovaginal slings have superior durability to needle suspensions. Needle suspensions and Burch are effective; however, these procedures are more invasive than vaginal procedures.

A patient with a coexistent cystocele should have the bladder neck repair along with cystocele correction. The vaginal epithelium should be dissected meticulously to allow the endopelvic fascia to remain along the bladder serosa. The fascia that remains should then be plicated in layers to allow for correction of the fascial defect. The Burch

Table 29.2. Surgical Therapy for Urinary Incontinence

Type	Intent	Approach
Anterior vaginal repair (colporrhaphy, Kelly plication)	Provide support to the bladder and urethra by reinforcing the endopelvic fascia and vaginal epithelium	Vaginal
Retropubic suspension (Marshall-Marchetti-Krantz, Burch, paravaginal repair)	Repair defects in the endopelvic fascia and its attachments	Abdominal
Sling procedure (Pereyra, Stamey)	Supplement or replace the support of the bladder neck and urethra using suture or fascial slings	Combined abdominal and vaginal

suspension allows for cystocele repair and bladder neck support. Through an abdominal incision the space of Retzius is opened, the urethral–vesicular junction (UVJ) is identified, and sutures are placed just lateral to the UVJ to Cooper's ligament.

Success rates vary. Tension-free vaginal tape and the Burch suspension have 85% success rate at five years.

It is imperative that preoperative counseling includes not only the risks of the procedures, but also the goals. The patient must understand that the procedure may not allow her to be always dry, as overcorrection (making the sling too tight) may lead to urinary retention. The surgeon should always err on the side of caution. In addition, studies only show 5-year data; thus, telling the patient that surgery is a permanent solution would be wrong

If lifestyle modification would enhance the success of the procedure, the patient must be counseled to stop smoking and work to achieve weight reduction (Figure 29.4).

Detrusor Overactivity (Urge Incontinence)

Normal physiology allows the detrusor muscle to accommodate filling in a low- resistance setting. The volume increases within the bladder, but the pressure within the bladder should stay low. Patients with an overactive detrusor muscle have uninhibited detrusor contractions. These contractions cause a rise in the bladder pressure that overrides the urethral pressure, and the patient will leak urine without evidence of increased intra-abdominal pressure.

Idiopathic detrusor overactivity has no organic cause. Neurogenic detrusor instability has a relevant neurogenic component.

Clinical Presentation The patient will present with the feeling that she must run to the bathroom frequently. When the "urge" comes she has to run, or she may not make it in time. This may or may not be associated with nocturia.

These symptoms may occur after bladder surgery to correct stress incontinence or after extensive bladder dissection during pelvic surgery. In these cases the symptoms are usually transient.

Evaluation Certainly a medical and pharmacological history may elicit details that would lead to similar symptoms. Is there an excessive caffeine intake? Is the patient using diuretics? Is there excessive oral intake of fluids?

To assess the patient's true oral fluid consumption and to gain a clear picture of her voiding habits, a voiding diary for at least 3 days is tremendously helpful. The patient records when and what she drinks and how often and how much she voids. Once completed, formal or single-channel urodynamic testing is warranted.

Single-channel urodynamic (eyeball testing) The patient voids, and the volume is recorded. A urinary catheter is then placed and the postvoid residual (PVR) urine is recorded. The bladder is filled in a retrograde fashion. The patient is asked to note her first sensation that her bladder is being filled. She then is

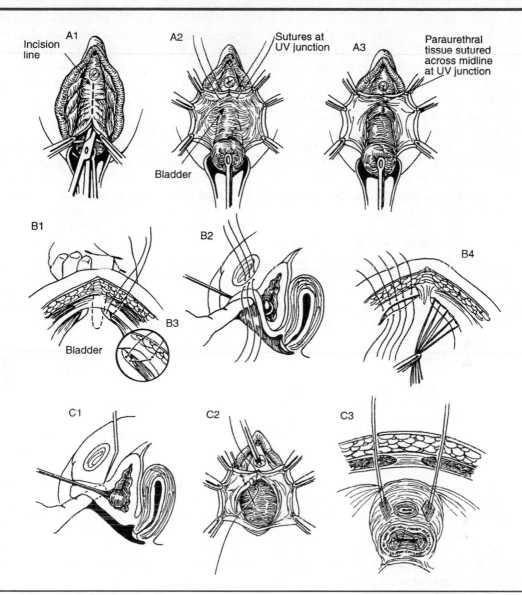

Figure 29.4. Surgical therapy for urinary incontinence. **(A1–A3)** Anterior vaginal wall repair, the Kelly-Kennedy procedure. **(A1)** Anterior vaginal wall is opened and undermined. **(A2)** Paraurethral tissue lateral to the urethrovesical (UV) junction is sutured. **(A3)** This creates a firm bar of tissue that supports the UV junction. **(B1–B4)** Retropubic suspension procedures, the Marshall-Marchetti-Krantz procedure. **(B1)** The suture is placed in the periurethral tissue and then into the pubic periosteum so that **(B2)** the urethra may be advanced upward into an intra-abdominal position. **(B3)** The Burch procedure, by which the tissue adjacent to the UV angle is sutured to the iliopectineal (Coopers) ligament. **(B4)** The Richardson paravaginal repair, by which the sutures are placed between the superior sulcus of the vagina and lateral pelvic side wall at the level of the iliopectineal line. **(C1–C3)** Sling procedures. **(C1)** The Pereyra procedure, by which a needle is guided transabdominally into the paraurethral tissue and back through **(C2)** to be tied suprapubically, thus supporting the UV angle. **(C3)** The Stamey procedure, by which a Dacron support material is used in the paraurethral tissue to buttress the tissue.

asked to note when she has a desire to void, and when she can no longer hold her urine. For the "normal patient," first sensation that the bladder is filling happens when 100–150 cc of fluid have been instilled into the bladder; first strong desire to void at about 250 cc of fluid instilled; and "maximum capacity" ("I can't hold this any longer!") is between 500 and 600 cc of fluid instilled. If at any time during the filling phase the meniscus within the catheter bumps up, this may indicate an uninhibited detrusor contraction.

Multichannel Urodynamic Testing This form of testing provides an assessment of the entire pelvic floor. A transducer is placed in the vagina or rectum to measure intra-abdominal pressure. A transducer is placed in the bladder, and EMG pads are placed along the perineum. An uninhibited bladder contraction can be clearly documented.

Treatment For patients with urgency incontinence, effective therapy may include bladder training, biofeedback, or medical therapy. Bladder training programs are directed toward increasing the patient's bladder control and capacity by gradually increasing the amount of time between voids. Often successful by itself, this may be augmented in difficult cases by biofeedback when available. Treatment with anticholinergic drugs such as Pro-Banthine (propantheline bromide), Ditropan (oxybutynin chloride), Detrol (tolterodine tartrate), and Oxytrol (transdermal oxybutynin chloride); β-sympathomimetic agonists such as Alupent (metaproterenol sulfate); musculotropic drugs such as Urispas (flavoxate hydrochloride) and Valium (diazepam); antidepressants such as Tofranil (imipramine hydrochloride); or dopamine agonists such as Parlodel (bromocriptine mesylate) have had some success based on the character of the patient's problem.

Mixed Incontinence

In many cases, the patient's clinical picture seems to incorporate symptoms from urgency as well as stress. The patient indeed coughs, or laughs, or sneezes, and leaks. However, anatomically, the cough may cause the UVJ to descend while, at the same time, stimulate the detrusor to fire, thus leading to an uninhibited contraction. This may be treated as stress or as detrusor instability. It is not clear which treatment offers the best outcome.

Overflow Incontinence

The detrusor muscle must be viewed as no different than any other muscle. Congestive heart failure will occur when the heart muscle is stretched to the point of no return. The actin and myosin can no longer meet, and the inotropic ability of the heart is lost. The bladder is no different. If an outlet obstruction blocks the urethra, urine will continue to fill the bladder. The bladder will stretch to accommodate the increased volume. The patient may lose the ability to perceive the need to void, either because of anesthesia (spinal or epidural) or a neurologic deficit.

The detrusor will lose the ability to contract. The urine will leak out only after the bladder pressure exceeds the urethral pressure. Usually the patient will only "leak" small amounts of urine. The diagnostic evaluation is relatively straightforward. The patient records the amount that she is able to void. A urinary catheter is placed, and the postvoid residual is measured. Generally the PVR should be less than 75 cc.

The condition is treated by identification of the underlying cause. The treatment is then timed self-catheterization until the detrusor is able to return to spontaneous function.

Other Issues: Relationship to Hysterectomy; Surgical Appropriateness; and Fistulae

Because of the frequent concurrence of defects in pelvic support and uterine descent, vaginal hysterectomy is often performed simultaneously with the reconstruction procedure. This corrects any symptoms referable to the descensus, provides access to the uterine support mechanisms to reinforce other repairs, and prevents the uterus from contributing to the need for subsequent anterior and posterior repairs should further descent occur.

For patients whose medical conditions preclude long surgical procedures and who are not sexually active, partial or complete obliteration of the vaginal canal (LeFort procedure, colpocleisis) may be done to provide support to the pelvic structures.

Therapy for fistulae is primarily surgical. Occasionally fistulae that occur following surgery spontaneously heal when adequate drainage or diversion of the urinary or fecal flow is provided. In all other cases, the only successful therapy consists of meticulous dissection of the fistulous tract and careful reapproximation of tissues. Recurrence is a common problem, especially in patients who have had radiation therapy for malignancies.

Urinary Tract Infections

Women experience urinary tract infections roughly 10 times more often than men. Approximately 15% of women experience at least one urinary tract infection in their lifetime. This necessitates the physician having a familiarity with the diagnosis and treatment of several urologic disorders common to women.

Most urinary tract infections in women ascend from bacterial contamination of the urethra. Except in the case of tuberculosis or immunosuppressed patients, infections are rarely acquired by hematogenous or lymphatic spread. The relatively short female urethra, exposure of the meatus to vestibular and rectal pathogens, and sexual activity that may induce trauma or introduce other organisms all increase the potential for infection. Estrogen deficiency also causes a decrease in urethral resistance to infection, which contributes to ascending contamination. This increased susceptibility explains the almost 10% prevalence of asymptomatic bacteriuria found in postmenopausal women.

Clinical Aspects of Urinary Tract Infections

Approximately 95% of urinary tract infections are symptomatic, uncomplicated, do not ascend to the kidneys, and produce no permanent damage. Of first infections, 90% are caused by *Escherichia coli,* and these respond readily to antibiotic therapy. Anaerobic bacteria and yeasts are rare causes of infections, except in diabetic or immunosuppressed patients or those with chronic indwelling catheters.

Patients with urinary tract infections typically present with symptoms of frequency, urgency, nocturia, or dysuria. The symptoms found vary somewhat with the site of the infection. Symptoms caused by irritation of the bladder or trigone include urgency, frequency, and nocturia. Irritation of the urethra leads to frequency and dysuria. The physical examination generally is nonspecific, although some patients may report suprapubic tenderness.

Evaluation

The evaluation of the patient suspected of having a urinary tract infection should include a urinalysis and a urine culture and sensitivity. These are generally obtained through a "clean-catch midstream" urine sample, which involves cleansing the vulva and catching a portion of urine passed during the middle of uninterrupted voiding. Urine obtained from catheters or suprapubic aspiration may also be used.

Laboratory analysis of the urine may be conducted or the sample examined microscopically by the clinician. This microscopic evaluation is carried out using a drop of urine or the precipitate from a centrifuged specimen. For uncentrifuged samples, more than one white blood cell per high-power field carries 90% accuracy in detecting infection. Centrifuged specimens may be scanned with low power for large numbers of white cells. Pyuria is defined as more than five white cells per high-power field in the centrifuged specimen. Gram stain of urine samples or sediments may also be helpful in establishing the diagnosis of infection. "Dipstick" tests for infection based on leukocyte esterase are also useful.

Cultures of urine samples that show colony counts of more than 100,000 for a single organism generally indicate infection. Colony counts as low as 10,000 for *E. coli* are associated with infection when symptoms are present. When a culture report indicates multiple organisms, contamination of the specimen should be suspected.

Recurrent urinary tract infections should prompt a reevaluation. Possible causes that must be considered include incorrect or incomplete (i.e., noncompliant) therapy, mechanical factors such as obstruction, or compromised host defenses.

Therapy

The selection of therapy for patients with urinary tract infections is simple and generally successful. Hydration, urinary acidification (with ascorbic acid, ammonium chloride, or acidic fruit juices), and urinary analgesics (Pyridium [phenazopyridine hydrochloride]) are helpful in most cases. Once confirmation by urinalysis or culture has been obtained, antibiotic therapy should be instituted. Nitrofurantoin (Macrodantin) produces good urinary antibiosis without undue alteration of other flora, although it is not effective against *Proteus* infections. Antibiotics such as ampicillin, tetracycline, and trimethoprim–sulfamethoxazole (Septra, Bactrim) provide good coverage in the urinary tract but risk more alteration of vaginal or intestinal flora. Vaginal yeast infections may result from these antibiotic treatments. When pyelonephritis is suspected, aggressive antibiotic therapy with cephalosporins such as Keflex (cephalexin) or Duricef (cefadroxil) is indicated.

Patients who have been treated for urinary tract infections should have follow-up urinalysis and culture done 10 to 14 days after the initial diagnosis. This will document cure in most patients and identify those at risk for recurrence because of incomplete or ineffective therapy.

CHAPTER 30

ENDOMETRIOSIS

This chapter deals primarily with APGO Topic:

Topic 38: Endometriosis

Students should be able to describe the theories of pathogenesis of endometriosis and the signs and symptoms, evaluation, and medical and surgical management of endometriosis. Students should be able to explain the relationship between infertility and endometriosis and how to evaluate and manage the combined problem and the relationship to chronic pelvic pain.

Incidence and Prevalence

Endometriosis may be suspected based on history, symptoms, physical examination, and laboratory and imaging information. At laparotomy or laparoscopy engendered by these findings, lesions consistent with endometriosis may be observed. However, only proven tissue biopsy diagnosis is definitive, as lesions may be small or atypical and thus missed or caused by pathology other than endometriosis. Further, many women with endometriosis are asymptomatic with the diagnosis made at surgery for other indication. Thus, the true incidence of endometriosis is difficult to establish.

It is estimated that 1 to 2% of women in the general population have endometriosis, and 30 to 50% of infertile women have it. Endometriosis occurs primarily in women in their 20s and 30s, although this may actually be a function of the frequency of evaluation of women in this age range for infertility and pelvic pain. Endometriosis is less frequently described in postmenopausal women. In adolescents, congenital anomalies that promote retrograde menstruation may be a common associated finding.

It has been thought that certain patient groups are at higher risk for developing endometriosis, such as those who delay childbearing to pursue careers. This stereotypical description has not been proved valid. Evidence shows, however, that women whose first-degree relatives have had endometriosis have a genetic predisposition to also develop it. A first-degree relative of a woman with endometriosis has an approximately 7% chance of being similarly affected.

Pathogenesis

The exact mechanisms by which endometriosis develops are not clearly understood. Three major theories are commonly cited.

1. *Direct implantation of endometrial cells*, typically by means of retrograde menstruation. This appears consistent with the occurrence of pelvic endometriosis and its predilection for the ovaries and pelvic peritoneum, as well as sites such as an abdominal incision or episiotomy scar. Direct implantation is commonly referred to as Sampson's theory because of his experimental work that showed the possibility of such a mechanism.

2. *Vascular and lymphatic dissemination of endometrial cells* (Halban's theory). Distant sites of endometriosis can be explained by this process (i.e., endometriosis in locations such as lymph nodes, the pleural cavity, and kidney).

3. *Coelomic metaplasia of multipotential cells in the peritoneal cavity* (Meyer's theory) states that, under certain conditions, these cells can develop into functional endometrial tissue. This could even occur in response to the irritation caused by retrograde menstruation.

It is probable that more than one theory is necessary to explain the diverse nature and locations of endometriosis. Underlying all these possibilities is the yet undiscovered immunologic factor that would explain why some women develop endometriosis whereas others with similar characteristics do not.

Pathology

Endometriosis is found on the ovaries in 60% of patients and is typically bilateral. Other common pelvic structures involved include the pouch of Douglas (particularly the uterosacral ligaments and rectovaginal septum), the round ligament, the fallopian tubes, and the sigmoid colon (Table 30.1). On rare occasions, distant endometriosis is found in abdominal surgical scars, the umbilicus, and various organs outside the pelvic cavity.

The gross appearance of endometriosis varies considerably. Subtle, minimal findings that have been proven by biopsy to be endometriosis include 1-mm vascular hemorrhagic areas, white-opaque plaques on the peritoneal surfaces, and more classically, spots that have been described as "mulberry" or "raspberry" in appearance. These small areas may also be rust colored, dark brown, or like "powder burns" in appearance. Frequently, reactive fibrosis surrounds these lesions, which gives a puckered appearance. More advanced, disseminated disease causes further fibrosis and results in the typically dense adhesions found in patients whose pelvic anatomy may be obscured by the disease.

Table 30.1. Sites of Endometriosis

Site	Frequency (Percentage of Patients)
Most common	
Ovary (frequently bilateral)	60
Pelvic peritoneum over the uterus	
Anterior and posterior cul-de-sacs	
Uterosacral ligaments	
Fallopian tubes	
Pelvic lymph nodes	30
Infrequent	
Rectosigmoid	10–15
Other gastrointestinal tract sites	5
Vagina	
Rare	
Umbilicus	
Episiotomy or surgical scars	
Kidney	
Lungs	
Arms	
Legs	
Nasal mucosa	

Endometriomas may reach 15 to 20 cm in diameter and are filled with thick, chocolate-appearing fluid, which is primarily old blood. These "chocolate cysts" are associated with endometriosis, although hemorrhagic cysts of the ovary may also have this gross appearance.

The definitive microscopic diagnosis of endometriosis is made when endometrial glands, stroma, and hemosiderin-laden macrophages are present. The glands and stroma do function histologically and physiologically like uterine mucosa, with cyclic changes in response to hormones noted. It is not, however, as well ordered as that which occurs in the endometrial cavity. In as many as one third of cases, the microscopic diagnosis is not conclusive, despite a "classic" clinical appearance.

Clinical Features

Symptoms

Women with endometriosis demonstrate an exceptionally wide variation of symptomatology, the nature and severity of which may be surprisingly independent of both the location and extent of the disease. Women with extensive endometriosis may have few symptoms, whereas, paradoxically, those with minimal gross endometriosis may have severe pain. *The classic symptoms of endometriosis include dysmenorrhea, deep thrust dyspareunia, infertility, abnormal bleeding, and pelvic pain.*

Pelvic pain is a common finding in patients with endometriosis. In some cases, the patient's pain is not solely associated with the menstrual period (dysmenorrhea) or to coital activity (dyspareunia) but, rather, is a chronic, unremitting low pelvic discomfort. Chronic pelvic pain may be related to the adhesions and pelvic scarring found in association with endometriosis, although endometriosis may just as often be asymptomatic.

The *dysmenorrhea* associated with endometriosis is not directly related to the amount of visible disease. Patients who present with dysmenorrhea that does not respond to oral contraceptives or nonsteroidal anti-inflammatory agents should have endometriosis considered as a possible etiology. The *dyspareunia* is often associated with uterosacral or vaginal involvement with endometriosis. In addition, the uterus may be retroverted and fixed in the cul-de-sac because of the extensive adhesions. The dyspareunia is typically reported on deep penetration, although there is no correlation between dyspareunia and the extent of endometriosis.

Infertility is more frequent in women with endometriosis. With extensive disease, pelvic scarring and adhesions may be responsible, but the exact mechanism for the infertility is unclear in patients with minimal endometriosis. Prostaglandins and autoantibodies have been implicated, but these relations remain unproved. *Infertility may, in some cases, be the only complaint.* In these cases, endometriosis is discovered at the time of laparoscopic evaluation as part of the infertility workup.

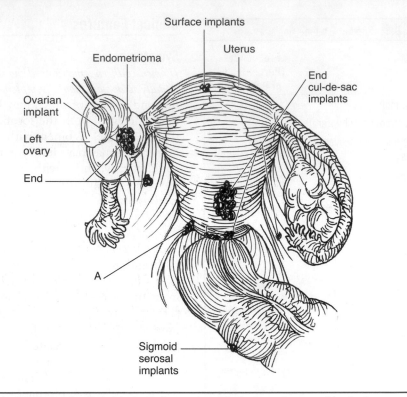

Figure 30.1. Clinical features of endometriosis. End = endometriosis; A = uterosacral implants.

Intermenstrual bleeding occurs in approximately one third of women with endometriosis. In many cases, premenstrual spotting is a symptom, possibly the result of an associated luteal phase inadequacy.

Other, less-common symptoms of endometriosis include gastrointestinal symptoms such as rectal bleeding and dyschezia in patients with endometrial implants on the bowel and urinary symptoms such as hematuria in patients with endometrial implants on the bladder or ureters. Occasionally, patients may present with an acute abdominal emergency, which may be associated with the rupture or torsion of an endometrioma.

Signs

The classic description of uterosacral nodularity on rectovaginal examination is consistent with significant gross disease involving that area, but it is often not present with even substantial gross endometriosis discovered at surgery. The uterus is often relatively fixed and

retroflexed in the pelvis. Ovarian endometriomas may be tender, palpable, and freely mobile in the pelvis or adhered to the posterior leaf of the broad ligament, the lateral pelvic wall, or in the posterior cul-de-sac.

Physical findings in early endometriosis may be subtle or even nonexistent. In cases of unexplained pelvic pain or infertility, the diagnosis of endometriosis should be entertained and diagnostic laparoscopy considered. It is recommended that visual and, ideally, histologic confirmation of endometriosis be obtained before institution of medical therapy for endometriosis. Typical clinical features of endometriosis are shown in Figure 30.1.

Differential Diagnosis

Depending on the symptoms, the differential diagnosis will change. In patients who present with chronic abdominal pain, consideration should be given to diagnoses such as chronic pelvic inflammatory disease, pelvic adhesions, gastrointestinal dysfunction, and other etiologies of chronic pelvic pain. In patients who present primarily with dysmenorrhea, both primary dysmenorrhea and etiologies for secondary dysmenorrhea should be considered. In patients who present with dyspareunia, other considerations should include chronic pelvic inflammatory disease, ovarian cysts, and symptomatic uterine retroversion. If abnormal bleeding is the primary presentation, investigation should rule out conditions such as anovulation, hypothyroidism, and hyperprolactinemia. If premenstrual spotting is the primary symptom, luteal phase defect, polyps, or cervical lesions should be considered. If the patient presents with sudden abdominal pain, considerations other than a ruptured endometrioma include ectopic pregnancy, acute pelvic inflammatory disease, adnexal torsion, and rupture of a corpus luteum cyst or ovarian neoplasm.

Diagnosis

Because of the diverse ways in which patients with endometriosis present, *history taking and physical examination can be considered only preliminary in nature. Establishing a diagnosis requires direct visualization at the time of diagnostic laparoscopy, or on occasion, at laparotomy, and for definitive diagnosis, tissue biopsy demonstrating endometriosis.* The importance of diagnostic laparoscopy is underscored for adolescent patients when it is recognized that endometriosis is discovered in about one half of teenagers undergoing laparoscopy for evaluation of chronic pelvic pain or dysmenorrhea. Should rectal bleeding occur, barium enema and colonoscopy should be undertaken to exclude other primary gastrointestinal disorders and to evaluate for endometriosis involving these structures. Pelvic ultrasound and/or CAT cannot definitively make the diagnosis of endometriosis, nor are any laboratory studies of value except to help rule out other conditions.

Once the diagnosis is made, the extent of the endometriosis should be properly documented. The most widely accepted classification system has been established by the American Fertility Society (Figure 30.2). This system standardizes the extent of the disease and aids in tracking progression or regression of endometriosis after therapy has been instituted.

Prevention

No known method is available to prevent endometriosis. Instead, the prevention of the spread of this disease or continued tissue damage should be the goal once the diagnosis has been established. A high index of suspicion can lead to early diagnosis, resulting in treatment before the endometriosis has progressed extensively. For example, conditions of the lower genital tract that may predispose to retrograde menstruation should be corrected as soon as they are found. Diagnostic procedures that require retrograde insufflation of dye or gas through the fallopian tubes (e.g., hysterosalpingography) should not be done while the patient is menstruating. Because endometriosis appears to be suppressed by the prolonged progestational effect of pregnancy, conception has traditionally been recommended as a way to prevent or minimize the effects of endometriosis. Unfortunately, no scientific data support this latter recommendation.

Treatment

The diagnosis should be as firmly established as possible before instituting either medical or surgical therapy. The choice of therapy depends on the patient's individual circumstances, which include (a) presenting symptoms and their severity, (b) location and severity of endometriosis, and (c) desire for future childbearing. All the medical treatments for endometriosis are temporizing measures to some extent. None can be expected to provide a permanent cure until extirpative surgery is undertaken or the hormonal stimulation is permanently removed.

Observation

Patients can be treated expectantly (i.e., without either medical or surgical therapy) in some selected cases. These include patients with limited disease whose symptoms are minimal or nonexistent and/or those who are trying to get pregnant. In the occasional patient in her mid- to late 40s with mild symptoms, consideration may be given to withholding therapy with the expectation that the decrease in menstrual hormones associated with menopause may not stimulate growth of disease.

THE AMERICAN FERTILITY SOCIETY
REVISED CLASSIFICATION OF ENDOMETRIOSIS

Patient's Name _____ Date_____

Stage I   (Minimal)   · 1-5
Stage II   (Mild)   · 6-15
Stage III (Moderate) · 16-40
Stage IV   (Severe)   · >40
Total_____

Laparoscopy_____ Laparotomy_____ Photography_____
Recommended Treatment_____

Prognosis_____

PERITONEUM	ENDOMETRIOSIS	<1cm	1-3cm	>3cm
	Superficial	1	2	4
	Deep	2	4	6
OVARY	R Superficial	1	2	4
	Deep	4	16	20
	L Superficial	1	2	4
	Deep	4	16	20

	POSTERIOR CULDESAC OBLITERATION	Partial	Complete
		4	40

	ADHESIONS	<1/3 Enclosure	1/3-2/3 Enclosure	>2/3 Enclosure
OVARY	R Filmy	1	2	4
	Dense	4	8	16
	L Filmy	1	2	4
	Dense	4	8	16
TUBE	R Filmy	1	2	4
	Dense	4*	8*	16
	L Filmy	1	2	4
	Dense	4*	8*	16

*If the fimbriated end of the fallopian tube is completely enclosed, change the point assignment to 16.

Additional Endometriosis: _____

Associated Pathology: _____

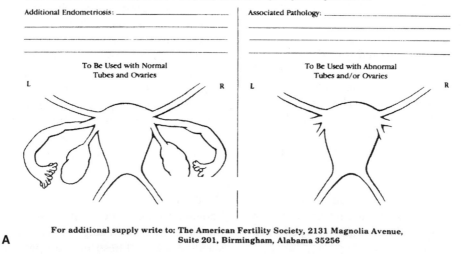

To Be Used with Normal
Tubes and Ovaries

To Be Used with Abnormal
Tubes and/or Ovaries

For additional supply write to: The American Fertility Society, 2131 Magnolia Avenue,
Suite 201, Birmingham, Alabama 35256

A

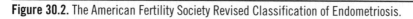

Figure 30.2. The American Fertility Society Revised Classification of Endometriosis.

EXAMPLES & GUIDELINES

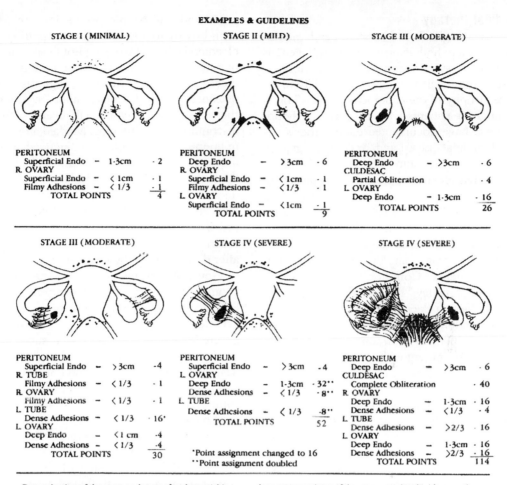

| STAGE I (MINIMAL) | STAGE II (MILD) | STAGE III (MODERATE) |

PERITONEUM
Superficial Endo – 1-3cm - 2
R. OVARY
Superficial Endo – < 1cm - 1
Filmy Adhesions – < 1/3 - 1
    TOTAL POINTS   4

PERITONEUM
Deep Endo – >3cm - 6
R. OVARY
Superficial Endo – < 1cm - 1
Filmy Adhesions – < 1/3 - 1
L. OVARY
Superficial Endo – < 1cm - 1
    TOTAL POINTS   9

PERITONEUM
Deep Endo – >3cm - 6
CULDESAC
Partial Obliteration - 4
L. OVARY
Deep Endo – 1-3cm - 16
    TOTAL POINTS   26

| STAGE III (MODERATE) | STAGE IV (SEVERE) | STAGE IV (SEVERE) |

PERITONEUM
Superficial Endo – >3cm -4
R. TUBE
Filmy Adhesions – < 1/3 - 1
R. OVARY
Filmy Adhesions – < 1/3 - 1
L. TUBE
Dense Adhesions – < 1/3 - 16*
L. OVARY
Deep Endo – < 1 cm -4
Dense Adhesions – < 1/3 -4
    TOTAL POINTS   30

PERITONEUM
Superficial Endo – >3cm - 4
L. OVARY
Deep Endo – 1-3cm - 32**
Dense Adhesions – < 1/3 - 8**
L. TUBE
Dense Adhesions – < 1/3 -8**
    TOTAL POINTS   52

*Point assignment changed to 16
**Point assignment doubled

PERITONEUM
Deep Endo – >3cm - 6
CULDESAC
Complete Obliteration - 40
R. OVARY
Deep Endo – 1-3cm - 16
Dense Adhesions – < 1/3 - 4
L. TUBE
Dense Adhesions – >2/3 - 16
L. OVARY
Deep Endo – 1-3cm - 16
Dense Adhesions – >2/3 - 16
    TOTAL POINTS   114

Determination of the stage or degree of endometrial involvement is based on a weighted point system. Distribution of points has been arbitrarily determined and may require further revision or refinement as knowledge of the disease increases.

To ensure complete evaluation, inspection of the pelvis in a clockwise or counterclockwise fashion is encouraged. Number, size and location of endometrial implants, plaques, endometriomas and/or adhesions are noted. For example, five separate 0.5cm superficial implants on the peritoneum (2.5 cm total) would be assigned 2 points. (The surface of the uterus should be considered peritoneum.) The severity of the endometriosis or adhesions should be assigned the highest score only for peritoneum, ovary, tube or culdesac. For example, a 4cm superficial and a 2cm deep implant of the peritoneum should be given a score of 6 (not 8). A 4cm deep endometrioma of the ovary associated with more than 3cm of superficial disease should be scored 20 (not 24).

In those patients with only one adnexa, points applied to disease of the remaining tube and ovary should be multiplied by two. **Points assigned may be circled and totaled. Aggregation of points indicates stage of disease (minimal, mild, moderate, or severe).

The presence of endometriosis of the bowel, urinary tract, fallopian tube, vagina, cervix, skin etc., should be documented under "additional endometriosis." Other pathology such as tubal occlusion, leiomyomata, uterine anomaly, etc., should be documented under "associated pathology." All pathology should be depicted as specifically as possible on the sketch of pelvic organs, and means of observation (laparoscopy or laparotomy) should be noted.

B

Figure 30.2. continued

Medical Therapy

Because the glands and stroma of endometriosis respond to both exogenous and endogenous hormones, suppression of endometriosis is based on a medication's potential ability to induce atrophy of the endometrial tissue. This is optimal for patients who are currently symptomatic, have documented endometriosis beyond minimal disease, and/or desire pregnancy sometime in the future. The patient should be aware that recurrence after the completion of medical therapy is common and that medical therapy does not have an effect on adhesions and fibrosis caused by the endometriosis.

Beneficial effects have been obtained using combined estrogen and progestin oral contraceptive agents. Commonly referred to as "pseudopregnancy," the use of oral contraceptives induces a decidual reaction in the functioning endometriotic tissue. Patients can also be maintained on oral contraceptive agents without intermittent withdrawal bleeding, thus avoiding secondary dysmenorrhea.

Progestins alone have also been administered by both the oral and parenteral routes (e.g., Provera [medroxyprogesterone acetate] 20 to 40 mg/day; Depo-Provera [depomedroxyprogesterone acetate] 100 mg IM every 2 weeks, then 200 mg monthly after 8 weeks). Progestins suppress gonadotropin release and, in turn, ovarian steroidogenesis; they also directly affect the uterine endometrium and endometrial implants. Recently low-dose subcutaneous medroxyprogesterone has been approved for amelioration of pain associated with proven endometriosis.

A state of "pseudomenopause" can also be induced with danazol, a 17 α-ethinyl testosterone derivative. Danazol suppresses both luteinizing hormone (LH) and follicle-stimulating hormone (FSH) midcycle surges so the ovary no longer produces estrogen, which stimulates endometriosis. At a dosage of up to 800 mg/day, amenorrhea occurs within 4 to 8 weeks after the onset of therapy. The desired endometrial atrophy results, but side effects are also significant. Despite the term *pseudomenopause,* FSH and LH levels are suppressed rather than elevated as they would be in the physiologic menopausal state. Side effects of danazol are related to its hypoestrogenic and androgenic properties, including acne in 15% to 20% of patients; spotting and bleeding in 10% of patients; hot flushes in 15% of patients; oily skin, growth of facial hair, decreased libido, and atrophic vaginitis in approximately 5% of patients; and deepening of the voice, not all of which will reverse with the discontinuation of therapy. Marked alterations of lipoprotein metabolism are induced, including a 60% decrease in serum high-density lipoprotein (HDL) cholesterol level and a 40% decrease in low-density lipoprotein (LDL). Danazol provides relief from symptoms in approximately 80% of patients, with symptoms recurring in 5 to 20% of patients within 1 year after discontinuing the medication.

Gonadotropin-releasing hormone (GnRH) agonists such as monthly or quarterly leuprolide acetate (Lupron) injections, nafarelin acetate nasal spray, and monthly injected goserelin acetate have also been successfully used to down-regulate the pituitary gland. Marked suppression of LH and FSH are noted, and the side effects are somewhat less troublesome than those of danazol because patients may have hypoestrogenic symptoms without androgenic side effects. However, the therapy is expensive, and parenteral administration is required. Efficacy for each of these agents appears comparable with that of danazol.

Surgical Therapy

The surgical management of endometriosis can be classified as either conservative or extirpative. *Conservative surgery* includes excision, cauterization, or ablation (by laser or electrocoagulation) of visible endometriotic lesions and preservation of the uterus and other reproductive organs to allow for a possible future pregnancy. Conservative surgery is often undertaken at the time of the initial diagnosis. Whether the initial laparoscopy is performed for pain or infertility, attempts to remove the existent endometriosis are undertaken by the surgeon. If extensive disease is found, conservative surgery involves lysis of adhesions, removal of active endometriotic lesions, and possibly reconstruction of reproductive organs. Success rates of conservative surgery appear to correlate with the severity of the disease at the time of surgery. Medical therapy is often added either before surgery, to reduce the amount of endometriosis with which the surgeon has to contend, or after surgery, to attempt to facilitate healing and avoid recurrence of the endometriosis. Pregnancy is also possible after conservative surgical therapy, with pregnancy rates of 60, 50, and 40% reported after conservative surgery for mild, moderate, and severe disease, respectively.

Extirpative surgery for endometriosis is reserved only for cases in which the disease is so extensive that conservative medical or surgical therapy is not feasible or when the patient has completed her family and wishes definitive therapy. Definitive surgery includes total abdominal hysterectomy, bilateral salpingo-oophorectomy, lysis of adhesions, and removal of endometriotic implants. The ramifications of not being able to conceive in the future must be thoroughly explored with the patient. Assuming that all the ovarian tissue is removed at the time of surgery, it is unlikely that any residual endometriosis will be stimulated by further endogenous hormonal production. Occasionally, in younger patients, ovarian tissue may be left to avoid the need for long-term estrogen-replacement therapy. This should be done only with the understanding that further surgery may be necessary to remove the remaining ovary should endometriosis recur. Estrogen replacement therapy after definitive extirpative surgery for endometriosis should not be avoided for fear of stimulating recurrent disease. Only rarely is reactivation of endometriosis noted, a far smaller risk than that associated with prolonged estrogen deficiency (i.e., osteoporosis and cardiovascular disease).

CHAPTER 31

DYSMENORRHEA AND CHRONIC PELVIC PAIN

This chapter deals primarily with APGO Educational Topics:

Topic 46: Dysmenorrhea

Students should be able to define primary and secondary dysmenorrhea and assess the evaluation and management of each.

Topic 39: Chronic Pelvic Pain (CPP)

Students should be able to define chronic pelvic pain and list the possible causes. Students should be able to describe an approach to the diagnosis and management of CPP, including the psychosocial issues associated with CPP.

Millions of hours each year are lost from school, work, and productive daily life because of pelvic pain, symptoms of dysmenorrhea, and chronic pelvic pain. Painful menstruation (*dysmenorrhea*) may be caused by clinically identifiable causes (*secondary dysmenorrhea*) or by an excess of prostaglandins, leading to painful uterine muscle activity (*primary dysmenorrhea*). The term *chronic pelvic pain* is generally applied to pelvic discomfort (not solely associated with menstruation*) of more than 6 months'* duration.

For most patients, diagnosis can be accomplished by a careful evaluation through history and physical examination. In some instances, evaluation using other modalities, including laparoscopy, may be needed. Once the diagnosis is established, specific and usually successful therapy may be instituted.

Dysmenorrhea

Primary and secondary dysmenorrhea represent a source of recurrent disability for approximately 10 to 15% of women in their early reproductive years. It is uncommon for primary dysmenorrhea to occur during the first three to six menstrual cycles, when rhythmic ovulation is not yet well established. *The incidence of primary dysmenorrhea is greatest in women in their late teens to early twenties and declines with age. Secondary dysmenorrhea becomes more common as a woman ages,* because it accompanies the rising prevalence of causal factors. Childbearing does not affect the occurrence of either primary or secondary dysmenorrhea.

Secondary Dysmenorrhea

The *causes of secondary dysmenorrhea* may be conveniently categorized into those processes that are outside the uterus, those that are within the wall of the uterus, and those that are internal or within the uterine cavity (Table 31.1). The mechanism by which these processes bring about menstrual pain is generally apparent when one considers that pain anywhere in the body occurs when there is inflammation, ischemia, stretch or distention, hemorrhage, or perforation. Pain results when these processes alter pressure in or around the pelvic structures, change or restrict blood flow, or cause irritation of the pelvic peritoneum. This may occur in

Table 31.1. Secondary Dysmenorrhea
Extrauterine causes
Endometriosis
Tumors (benign, malignant)
Inflammation
Adhesions
Psychogenic (rare)
Nongynecologic causes
Intramural causes
Adenomyosis
Leiomyomata
Intrauterine causes
Leiomyomata
Polyps
Intrauterine contraceptive devices
Infection
Cervical stenosis and cervical lesions

combination with the normal physiology of menstruation, creating discomfort, or it may arise independently, with symptoms becoming more noticeable during menstruation. *When symptoms continue between menstrual periods, these processes may be the source of chronic pelvic pain.*

Primary Dysmenorrhea

In patients with *primary dysmenorrhea,* no clinically identifiable cause of pain exists. Instead, there is *an excess of prostaglandin $F_2\alpha$ produced in the endometrium.* This potent smooth muscle stimulant causes intense uterine contractions, resulting in intrauterine pressures that can exceed 400 mm Hg and baseline intrauterine pressures in excess of 80 mm Hg. Prostaglandin $F_2\alpha$ also causes contractions in smooth muscle elsewhere in the body, resulting in the nausea, vomiting, and diarrhea reported by many women (Table 31.2). Prostaglandin production in the uterus normally increases under the influence of progesterone, reaching a peak at, or soon after, the start of menstruation. With the onset of menstruation, formed prostaglandins are released from the shedding endometrium. In addition, the necrosis of endometrial cells provides increased substrate arachidonic acid

Table 31.2. Pain and Associated Systemic Symptoms in Primary Dysmenorrhea

Symptom	Estimated Incidence (%)
Pain: spasmodic, colicky, laborlike; sometimes described as an aching or heaviness in lower middle abdomen; may radiate to the back and down the thighs; starts at onset of menstruation; lasts hours to days	100
Associated symptoms	
Nausea and emesis	90
Tiredness	85
Nervousness	70
Dizziness	60
Diarrhea	60
Headache	45

from cell walls for prostaglandin synthesis. In addition to prostaglandin F$_2\alpha$, prostaglandin E$_2$ is produced in the uterus. Prostaglandin E$_2$, a potent vasodilator and inhibitor of platelet aggregation, has been implicated as a cause of primary menorrhagia.

Clinical Evaluation

Patients with *primary dysmenorrhea* present with recurrent, month-after-month, spasmodic lower abdominal pain, which occurs on the first 1 to 3 days of menstruation. The pain is often diffusely located in the lower abdomen and suprapubic area, with radiation around or through to the back. The pain is described as "coming and going" or laborlike. The patient often illustrates her description with a fist opening and closing. This pain is frequently accompanied by moderate to severe nausea, vomiting, and/or diarrhea. Fatigue, low backache, and headache are also common. Patients often assume a fetal position in an effort to gain relief, and many report having used a heating pad or hot water bottle in an effort to decrease their discomfort. Dyspareunia is generally not found in patients with primary dysmenorrhea and, if present, should suggest a secondary cause.

In patients with *secondary dysmenorrhea*, symptoms may be slightly milder and are often more general in nature. The specific complaint that an individual patient has is determined by the underlying abnormality. Frequently, a careful history suggests the possibility of an ongoing problem and helps direct further evaluations. Complaints of heavy menstrual flow, combined with pain, suggest uterine changes such as adenomyosis, myomas, or polyps.

Adenomyosis is islands of endometrial tissue within the myometrium, resulting in a usually tender, symmetrically enlarged, "boggy" uterus. Menses are especially uncomfortable. The diagnosis is supported by exclusion of other causes of secondary dysmenorrhea, but definitive diagnosis can be made only by histologic examination of a hysterectomy specimen. Pelvic heaviness or a change in abdominal contour should raise the possibility of large *leiomyomata* or *intra-abdominal neoplasia*. Fever, chills, and malaise should suggest an *inflammatory process*. A coexisting complaint of infertility may suggest *endometriosis or chronic pelvic inflammatory disease.*

Assessment

For patients with dysmenorrhea, the physical examination is directed toward uncovering possible causes of secondary dysmenorrhea. Asymmetry or irregular enlargement of the uterus should suggest myomas or other tumors. Symmetrical enlargement of the uterus is often found in patients with adenomyosis. Painful nodules in the posterior cul-de-sac and restricted motion of the uterus should suggest endometriosis. Restricted motion of the uterus is also found in cases of pelvic scarring from adhesions or inflammation. Thickening and tenderness of the adnexal structures caused by inflammation may suggest this diagnosis as the cause of secondary dysmenorrhea. Cultures of the cervix for *Neisseria gonorrhoeae* or *Chlamydia trachomatis* should be obtained if infection is suspected.

In evaluating the patient thought to have primary dysmenorrhea, the most important differential diagnosis is that of secondary dysmenorrhea. Although the patient's history is often characteristic, a diagnosis of primary dysmenorrhea should not be made without a thorough evaluation to eliminate other possible causes. *Physical examination of patients with primary dysmenorrhea should be normal.* There should be no palpable abnormalities of the uterus or adnexa, and no abnormalities should be found on speculum or abdominal examinations. Patients examined while experiencing symptoms often appear pale and "shocky," but the abdomen is soft and nontender, with a normal uterus.

In patients with chronic pain, the clinician must always consider nongynecologic causes as a possibility. In some patients, a final diagnosis may not be established without invasive procedures, such as laparoscopy.

Therapy

In patients with dysmenorrhea in whom no other clinically identifiable cause is apparent, it is appropriate to presume a diagnosis of primary dysmenorrhea. Therapy with nonsteroidal anti-inflammatory agents is generally so successful that, if some response is not evident, the diagnosis of primary dysmenorrhea should be reevaluated. Other useful components of therapy for primary dysmenorrhea include the application of heat; exercise, psychotherapy, and reassurance; and on occasion, endocrine therapy (i.e., oral contraceptives to induce anovulation).

Patients with primary dysmenorrhea generally experience exceptional pain relief through the use of nonsteroidal anti-inflammatory drugs (NSAIDs), which are prostaglandin-synthetase inhibitors. Treatments include 500 mg of mefenamic acid (Ponstel) followed by 250 mg every 4 to 6 hours, 1200 to 1600 mg of ibuprofen (Motrin) followed by 600 to 800 mg three times a day, or 150 mg of diclofenac (Voltaren) followed by 75 mg three times a day (Table 31.3). For a time, the cyclo-oxygenase inhibitors (COX-2 inhibitors) were becoming the NSAID of choice because of their targeted action. However, recently these drugs have virtually left the methodology of treatments because of associations of the drugs with life-threatening cardiovascular and gastrointestinal effects. Further, similar albeit less-stringent concerns over all NSAIDs make it likely that all these effective medications will soon cease to be used in the treatment of pelvic pain (or pain in general). Recent studies suggest that continuous low-level topical heat therapy (such as ThermaCare) can provide pain relief comparable to that offered by NSAID therapy without the concerns of systemic side effects that may occur with NSAIDs.

In the rare patient who does not respond to medical and other therapy and whose pain is so severe as to be incapacitating, *presacral neurectomy* may be a consideration. The procedure involves surgical disruption of the "presacral nerves," the superior hypogastric plexus, which is found in the retroperitoneal tissue from the fourth lumbar vertebra to the hollow over the sacrum. It is associated with considerable morbidity if the adjacent venous structures are disrupted.

As in other areas of medicine, the best therapy is one directed toward the cause of the patient's problems. Hence, for secondary dysmenorrhea when a specific diagnosis is possible, therapy tailored to that process is the most likely to succeed. Specific treatments for many of these processes are discussed in their respective chapters. When definitive therapy cannot be used (e.g., in the case of a patient with adenomyosis in whom fertility is to be preserved, thereby making hysterectomy inappropriate), symptomatic therapy in the form of analgesics and/or modification of the menstrual cycle may be effective. The dysmenorrhea may be improved with the use of low-dose oral contraceptives in those patients who desire contraception and have no contraindications to their use.

Chronic Pelvic Pain

The *prevalence* of chronic pelvic pain is less than that of dysmenorrhea but still represents a source of significant disability. It often demands a great deal of time and resources, from both physician and patient, to make a diagnosis and

Table 31.3. Nonsteroidal Anti-inflammatory Drugs That Have Been Used for the Treatment of Dysmenorrhea

Drug	Initial Dose	Subsequent Dose
Diclofenac (potassium)	50–100 mg	50 mg t.i.d.
Diclofenac (sodium)	75–150 mg	75 mg t.i.d.
Diflunisal	1000 mg	500 mg q 12 h
Etodolac	400 mg	400 mg q 4–6 h
Fenoprofen calcium	200 mg	200 mg q 4–6 h
Flurbiprofen	50 mg	50 mg t.i.d.
Ibuprofen	1200–1600 mg	600–800 mg q 4 h
Indomethacin	25 mg	25 mg t.i.d.
Ketoprofen	75 mg	75 mg t.i.d.
Ketorolac	10 mg	10 mg q 4–6 h
Meclofenamate	100 mg	50–100 mg q 4–6 h
Mefenamic acid	500 mg	250 mg q 4–6 h
Naproxen	500 mg	250 mg q 4–6 h
Naproxen sodium	550 mg	275 mg q 6–8 h
Sulindac	200 mg	200 mg b.i.d.
Suprofen	200 mg	200 mg q 4 h
Tolmetin	400 mg	40 mg t.i.d.

(From Smith RP: *Gynecology in Primary Care.* Baltimore: Williams & Wilkins, 1996, p. 398.)

establish treatment. In these patients, the pathophysiology involved can be variable (Table 31.4). In many patients, the pain itself becomes the disease. Indeed, in approximately one third of patients with chronic pelvic pain who undergo laparoscopic evaluation, no identifiable cause is found. However, two thirds of these patients have potential causes identified where none was apparent before laparoscopy. A wide-ranging, often multidisciplinary approach to these patients yields the best results.

The *history* reported in chronic pelvic pain can be varied. In general, it relates to the underlying etiology. As with the evaluation of any pain, attention must be paid to the description and timing of the symptoms involved. Gastrointestinal symptoms, urinary difficulties, or back problems should suggest the possibility of nongynecologic causes. The history must include a thorough medical, surgical, menstrual, and sexual history. Inquiries should be made into the patient's home and work status, social history, and family history (past and present). The patient should be questioned about sleep disturbances and other signs of depression.

Assessment

As in patients with dysmenorrhea, the *physical examination* of patients with chronic pain is directed toward uncovering possible causative pathologies. The patient should be asked to indicate the location of the pain. This acts as a guide to further evaluation and provides some indication of the character of the pain by the way in which the patient points. For example, if the location of the pain is indicated with a single finger, you are probably dealing with a different process than when the patient uses a sweeping motion of the whole hand. Maneuvers that duplicate the patient's complaint should be noted, but undue discomfort should be avoided to minimize guarding, which would limit a thorough examination. Many of the same conditions that cause secondary dysmenorrhea may cause

Table 31.4. Causes of Chronic Pelvic Pain

Gynecologic Causes
  Adnexal
    Adhesive disease (adhesions from any cause)
    Chronic infection
    Chronic ectopic pregnancy
    Torsion of pelvic mass or organ (generally a cause of acute pain)
    Ovarian cyst (generally not painful without bleeding or growth)
  Uterine
    Fibroid tumors (uncommon cause of pain)
    Infection
    Retrodisplacement (rate)
  Urologic causes
    Infection
    Calculi
    Tumors
  Gastrointestinal causes
    Inflammatory
      Chronic appendicitis
      Gastroenteritis
      Ulcerative colitis
      Ulcer disease
      Irritable bowel syndrome
      Diverticulitis
      Mesenteric adenitis
      Biliary disease
    Mechanical
      Constipation
      Herniation
      Obstruction
      Torsion
      Intussusception
    Other
      Neoplasia
      Parasites

Other causes
  Aneurysm
  Musculoskeletal
    Chronic back pain
    Radiculopathy
    Spondylolisthesis
    Ankylosing spondylitis
    Strains
    Rectus hematoma
  Biochemical
    Sickle cell disease/crisis
    Acute intermittent porphyria
    Heavy metal poisoning
    Black widow spider bites
  Neurologic
    Tabes
    Herpes zoster (shingles)
  Psychosocial
    Somatization
    Sleep disorders
    Substance abuse
    Physical or sexual abuse
    Family or economic stress

chronic pain states. As in the evaluation of patients with dysmenorrhea, cervical cultures should be obtained if infection is suspected.

For most patients, a reasonably accurate differential diagnosis can be established through the history and physical examination. *The wide range of differential diagnoses possible in chronic pelvic pain lends itself to a multidisciplinary approach,* which might include psychiatric evaluation and/or testing. Consultation with social workers, physical therapists, gastroenterologists, anesthesiologists, orthopaedists, and others should be considered. The use of imaging technologies or laparoscopy may also be required to determine a diagnosis.

The evaluation should begin with the presumption that there is an organic cause for the pain. Even in patients with obvious psychosocial stress, organic pathology can and does occur. Only when other reasonable causes have been ruled out should psychiatric diagnoses such as somatization, depression, or sleep and personality disorders be entertained.

Irritable Bowel Syndrome

Irritable bowel syndrome (IBS) is three times more common in women than in men, and symptoms of the syndrome are found in about 15% of adults. Because it is so common and more common in women, the evaluation and management of pelvic pain includes diagnosing this syndrome and treating it or ruling it out prior to gynecologic therapy such as surgery.

The diagnosis of IBS is defined by the Rome criteria: abdominopelvic pain that cannot be explained by known disease for 12 weeks (not necessarily consecutive) in the preceding 12 months, having at least two of three features. These features are pain (1) relieved with defecation, (2) associated with a change in the frequency of bowel movements (diarrhea or constipation), or (3) onset associated with a change in the form of stool (loose, watery, with mucus, or pelletlike). IBS is often usefully subcategorized for purposes of treatment depending on the predominant complaint: pain, diarrhea, constipation, or alternating constipation and diarrhea. The pathophysiology of the syndrome is not clearly identified, but factors proposed to be involved include altered bowel motility, visceral hypersensitivity, psychosocial factors (especially stress), an imbalance of neurotransmitters (especially serotonin), and infection (often indolent or subclinical). A history of childhood sexual or physical abuse is highly correlated with the severity of symptoms experienced by those with IBS.

The diagnosis is made by history and flexible sigmoidoscopy in women less than about 50 years old or history and colonoscopy or flexible sigmoidoscopy plus barium enema in women over about 50 years of age. When the predominant symptom is diarrhea, a biopsy of the mucosae of the descending colon should be considered to rule out microscopic colitis.

Use of a food diary to identify and eliminate foods that are associated with symptoms combined with the nurturing physician–patient relationship, to avoid "doctor shopping" and episodic care, are the mainstays of treatment. The limiting of caffeine, alcohol, fatty foods, and gas-producing vegetables is often helpful. If constipation is a major symptom, the addition of 20–30 g of fiber or the use of osmotic laxatives such as lactulose (10 mg/15 mL of syrup, 15–30 mL per day) is often useful. When diarrhea is a major symptom, antidiarrheals such as Loperamide (4 mg/day initially, then 4–8 mg/day in single or divided doses) have been useful.

Therapy

Patients with chronic pelvic pain offer a therapeutic challenge. In these patients, care must be taken that the therapy offered does not potentiate the underlying problem. Analgesics may be used, but sparingly, and every effort must be made to reduce the risk of both emotional and physical dependence. When used, analgesics should be given on a fixed time schedule that is independent of symptoms. Frequent follow-up is required and should be scheduled separate of fluctuations in pain. Suppression of ovulation may be useful as either a therapeutic modality or as a diagnostic tool to assist in ruling out ovarian or cyclic processes. Surgical therapies are appropriate only when specific surgically treatable pathologies are present and thought to be the specific cause of the patient's complaints. Alternate treatment modalities such as transcutaneous electrical nerve stimulation (TENS), biofeedback, nerve blocks, laser ablation of the uterosacral ligaments, and pre-sacral neurectomy may be used in selected patients. *In some cases, the goal in treatment may not be a cure (i.e., elimination of chronic pain), but rather successful management of the symptoms to allow maximal function and quality of life.*

Follow-up

Patients begun on therapy for pelvic pain (dysmenorrhea or chronic pain states) should be carefully monitored for success and the possibility of complications from the therapy itself. Patients on oral contraceptives for the first time should be asked to return for follow-up after 2 months and again after 6 months. Once successful therapy is established, routine periodic health maintenance visits should continue. *Patients with chronic pain should be encouraged to return for follow-up on a periodic basis, rather than only when pain is present, thus avoiding reinforcing pain behavior as a means to an end.*

CHAPTER 32

DISORDERS OF THE BREAST

This chapter addresses APGO Educational Topic:

Topic 40: Disorders of the Breast.

> Students should understand the evaluation of common symptoms associated with the breast.

In our society, the female breast is associated with a series of highly charged and somewhat contradictory symbolic meanings. On the one hand, the female breast is positively associated with adult female sexuality and maternal nurturance. On the other hand, it is perceived as a potential source of life-threatening carcinoma. It is against this complex cultural background that women present for routine breast examinations as well as with various symptoms referable to the breast, including pain (*mastalgia*), nipple discharge, and palpable masses. The maintenance of breast health and the management of breast disease are therefore uniquely challenging for women and their health-care providers.

The adult female breast is actually a modified sebaceous gland, located within the superficial fascia of the chest wall (see Figure 1.3). Histologically, the breast is composed primarily of lobules or glands, milk ducts, connective tissue, and fat. The relative amounts of these tissue types vary considerably with age. In younger women, the breast consists predominantly of glandular tissue. With age, the glands involute and are replaced by fat, a process accelerated by menopause. Differences in palpable consistency and in radiographic density between the glands and fat are key components of breast cancer detection programs.

Architecturally, the breast is organized into 12 to 20 lobes, with a disproportionate amount of the glandular or lobular tissue present in the upper outer quadrants of each breast. The lobules consist of clusters of secretory cells arranged in an alveolar pattern and surrounded by myoepithelial cells. These glands drain into a series of collecting milk ducts that course through the breast, ultimately coalescing into approximately five to ten collecting ducts that lead to and drain at the nipple. Congenital anomalies of the breast can include absence of the breast as well as accessory breast tissue located anywhere along the "milk lines," which extend from the axilla to the groin in the fetus. Extra nipples (*polythelia*) are more common than true accessory breasts (*polymastia*).

The breast has a rich blood supply and lymphatic system, which support milk production and overall breast health. The blood supply comes from perforating branches of the internal mammary artery, the lateral thoracic artery, the thoracodorsal artery, the thoracoacromial artery, and various intercostal perforating arteries. The lymphatic vessels lead to several superficial and deep nodal chains throughout the trunk and neck, including those located in the axilla, deep to the pectoralis muscles, and caudal to the diaphragm. (Figure 32.1). These pathways facilitate the metastasis of breast malignancies.

Breast tissue is very sensitive to hormonal changes, especially the glandular cells. In fact, the transition from the immature, pediatric breast to the mature, adult breast is orchestrated by the changes in circulating levels of estrogen and progesterone that accompany puberty (Figure 1.4) Tissue responsiveness to circulating hormones is also responsible for the changes that occur during the normal menstrual cycle and for the symptoms often reported by patients receiving hormones in pharmacologic doses.

Each of the tissues in the breast may undergo pathologic transformation. The connective tissue of the breast may give rise to fibrocystic changes and fibroadenomas. Fatty tissues may undergo necrosis in response to trauma or may harbor lipomas. The duct system of the breast may become dilated (duct ectasia or galactocele), contain papillary neoplasms, or undergo malignant transformation. Although more common in nursing mothers, infection of the breast (mastitis) may also occur.

Ranking only behind skin cancer, *breast cancer is the second-most-common malignancy of women,* accounting for roughly one third of all malignancies in women. It is the second leading cause of death from cancer for American women, after lung cancer. *Currently a woman living in the United States has a 12.5%, or 1 in 8, lifetime risk of developing breast cancer.* It is estimated that there are over 210,000 new cases of invasive breast cancer and 40,000 breast cancer deaths annually. An additional 56,000 new cases of in situ breast cancer are also expected.

Benign Breast Disease

Fibrocystic Change

The term *fibrocystic change* encompasses more than 35 different processes, including the misnomer "fibrocystic disease." Fibrocystic changes

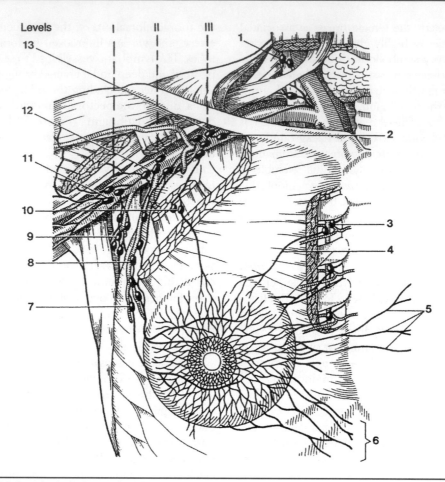

Figure 32.1. Lymphatic drainage of the breast. (*I*), Low axillary nodes; (*II*), central axillary nodes; (*III*), subclavian nodes; (*1*), deep cervical nodes; (*2*), infraclavicular nodes; (*3*), sternal nodes; (*4*), pathway to the mediastinal nodes; (*5*), pathway to the contralateral breast; (*6*), pathway to the subdiaphragmatic nodes and liver; (*7*), anterior pectoral lymph nodes; (*8*), central axillary nodes; (*9*), subpectoral axillary nodes; (*10*), interpectoral nodes (Rotter's); (*11*), brachial vein nodes; (*12*), axillary vein nodes; (*13*), subclavian vein nodes.

are the *most common of all benign breast conditions.* They may be present in one third to one half of premenopausal women and are a source of symptoms for roughly half of these women. The alterations associated with fibrocystic change may arise from an exaggerated response to hormones. Consequently, fibrocystic changes are most common during the reproductive years or occasionally during hormone replacement after menopause. Disturbed ratios of estrogen and progesterone and an increased rate of prolactin secretion have both been suggested as causes for these changes. Neither of these theories has been conclusively proven, nor is there any evidence that fibrocystic changes are caused by oral contraceptives.

Histologically, fibrocystic changes occur in three stages. Initially, there is a *proliferation of stroma,* especially in the upper outer quadrants of the breast, leading to the induration and pain experienced by the patient. In the second stage, *adenosis* occurs, leading to cyst formation. During this phase, cysts range from microscopic to 1 cm in diameter. Marked proliferation of the ducts and alveolar cells occurs during this stage. In the late stages of fibrocystic change, *larger cysts* are present and *less pain* occurs, unless there is rapid change in a particular cyst.

Proliferative changes may be marked in any of the involved tissues. When atypia is found in hyperplastic ducts or apocrine cells, most experts agree that risk of developing carcinoma in the future is severalfold higher.

Fibrocystic changes most commonly present as cyclic, bilateral pain (mastalgia) and engorgement. The pain associated with fibrocystic changes is diffuse, often with radiation to the shoulders or upper arms. Occasionally, well-localized pain occurs when a cyst expands rapidly. On examination, diffuse bilateral nodularity is typical, with larger cysts taking on the characteristics of a fluid-filled balloon. These symptoms are most prominent just before menstruation.

Studies are conflicting regarding the efficacy of dietary modifications in the management of cyclic mastalgia. Interventions have included the restriction of caffeine and foods containing methylxanthines, reversion to a low-salt diet, and use of vitamin E. Some women respond well to intermittent dosing of mild diuretics such as hydrochlorothiazide (25 to 50 mg per day for 7 to 10 days before menses). Danazol is effective in severe cases, but symptoms often resume after discontinuation of the medication. In unusual cases, surgery may be required to relieve intractable, incapacitating pain.

The office management of fibrocystic changes may include fine-needle aspiration of palpable or ultrasound-identifiable cysts. Aspiration can be diagnostic as well as therapeutic. If the fluid retrieved is bloody, cytologic evaluation of the aspirate and possible follow-up biopsies are warranted. Core and/or excisional biopsies are also considered when mammographic findings suggest neoplasia, when a residual mass remains even after aspiration, or when the cyst recurs.

Fibroadenoma

Fibroadenomas are the second-most-common form of benign breast disease, occurring in 10% to 20% of women. Occurring most often in young women, these firm, painless, freely movable breast masses average 1 to 3 cm wide and consist of a mixture of proliferating epithelial and supporting fibrous tissues. Although usually solitary, multiple fibroadenomas develop in 15% to 20% of patients. These tumors do not change during the menstrual cycle and are usually slow growing. They are often found during physical examination or during breast self-examination. Histologically, they are characterized by monolayers of benign ductal cells associated with dense stroma.

The management of these lesions begins with the physical examination complemented by diagnostic imaging. Histologic evaluation of tissue obtained via office biopsy or excision typically follows to rule out malignancy. The combination of ultrasound and fine-needle biopsy usually distinguishes fibroadenomas from cysts. Fibroadenomas can be conservatively managed by periodic clinical examinations and imaging, without excision. Surgical excision is considered if the mass causes pain or grows rapidly, if the fine-needle aspirate is inconclusive or suspicious for malignancy, or if the patient needs more reassurance than biopsy can provide.

Lipomas and Fat Necrosis

The fatty tissue of the breast may be the source of benign tumors that are difficult to distinguish from malignancy. Both lipomas and fat necrosis may present as ill-defined tumors of the breast. Lipomas are usually nontender, but their diffuse character may raise suspicions of malignancy. Secondary signs suggestive of cancer (e.g., skin and nipple changes) usually are absent. Biopsy or excision is often required. *Fat necrosis* is uncommon and most often the result of trauma, although the causative event frequently cannot be identified. The patient usually presents with a solitary, tender, ill-defined mass. Skin retraction is present in some patients. Direct evidence of trauma is most often lacking. Even with a history of trauma, the similarity of physical examination and mammographic findings between fat necrosis and cancer often mandates biopsy or excision to establish the diagnosis.

Intraductal Papilloma

Intraductal papillomas are polypoid epithelial tumors arising in the ducts of the breast. These fibrovascular tumors are covered by benign ductal epithelium. Although these tumors may range from 2 to 5 mm in diameter, they are typically not palpable. The patient presents with a *spontaneous bloody, serous, or cloudy nipple discharge*. Although these polyps are most often benign, excisional biopsy is typically required to differentiate the lesions from malignancies.

Mammary Duct Ectasia and Galactocele

Mammary duct ectasia may arise from chronic intraductal and periductal inflammation, which causes *dilation of the ducts and inspissation of breast secretions*. Most common in the fifth decade of life, this condition presents with a thick gray to black nipple discharge, pain, and nipple tenderness. Palpation around the nipple elicits discharge and may reveal thickening that may be difficult to distinguish from cancer. Nipple retraction is common. Biopsy confirms the diagnosis, and, once established, no further therapy is needed unless warranted by the patient's symptoms.

Ductal obstruction and inflammation during or soon after lactation may lead to the development of a *galactocele*. Galactoceles are cystic dilations of a duct or ducts. These ducts contain inspissated, milky secretions that may become infected and lead to acute mastitis or abscess formation. When uncomplicated by infection, needle aspiration and decompression of the ducts is curative, and excision is rarely required.

Breast Cancer

Demographics

A woman who lives to the age of 90 in the United States has a cumulative overall risk of 1 in 8 of developing breast cancer. After her gender, increasing age is a woman's greatest risk factor for developing breast cancer. Approximately 1 in 2,000 women in their 20s develop breast cancer, as compared with 1 in 25 women at or above the age of 70 (Table 32.1). Roughly 25% of women diagnosed with breast cancer ultimately succumb to their disease.

Factors other than age that are associated with developing breast cancer are summarized in Table 32.2. A *relative risk* compares the risk of disease among people with a specific exposure to those without that same exposure. Relative risks above 1.0 equate with a higher risk. Approximately 70% of women who develop breast cancer, however, do not have currently identifiable risk factors. Many of the risk fac-

Table 32.1. Probability of Developing Breast Cancer by Age for Women

Age	Probability, 1 in
20–29	2,187
30–39	258
40–49	67
50–59	38
60–69	29
70 or more	25

tors listed share endogenous estrogen exposure as a common denominator. These include earlier menarche, later menopause, fewer pregnancies, and no history of breast feeding.

Currently, risk factor identification is often used to plan and execute targeted breast cancer detection and management strategies. A classic example involves carriers of mutations in the breast cancer susceptibility genes BRCA1 and BRCA2. These mutations appear in less than 1% of the general population, but are associated with as many as 3% to 10% of breast cancers. Women with these mutations may benefit from initiating screening mammography at a younger age than is recommended for the general population. Other interventions for these women, such as prophylactic therapy with selective estrogen receptor modulators or surgery, are highly individualized and should be undertaken only after careful evaluation and counseling by clinicians with expertise in this field.

General Clinical Approach

The contemporary management of breast cancer as a public health issue includes reduction of modifiable risk factors, early identification of lesions through a combination of breast examination and mass screening, and treatment of identified malignancies. Superimposed on this approach to the general population are efforts to identify patients at especially high risk who might benefit from more intensive screening and prophylactic therapy. The controversies surrounding each of these elements taken alone as well as in combination are the subject of ongoing research and debate.

Table 32.2. Relative Risk Factors for Developing Breast Cancer in Women

Relative Risk	Factor
0–1.0	Menarche >17 years old
	Menopause before age 45
	Oophorectomy before age 35
	Term pregnancy before age 35
1.1–2.0	Menarche <12 years old
	Menopause after age 55
	First full-term pregnancy after age 35
	No full-term pregnancies (for cancer diagnosed after age 40)
	Personal history of cancer of the endometrium, ovary, or colon
	Never breast-fed a child
	Recent oral contraceptive use*
	Recent hormone replacement therapy*
2.1–4.0	One first-degree relative with breast cancer (pre- or postmenopausal, unilateral disease)
	Atypical hyperplasia on breast biopsy
	Personal history of cancer of major salivary glands
	Ovaries not surgically removed at less than 35 years of age
	Nodular densities occupy more than three fourths of mammogram
>4	Personal history of breast cancer
	Two or more first-degree relatives with breast cancer
	Age greater than 65
	Inherited genetic mutations for breast cancer
>8	Premenopausal first-degree relative with bilateral breast cancer

*See text for discussion.

Symptoms

Approximately 80% of breast cancers present as a mass. In the early stages of cancer growth, the tumor is usually painless and may feel mobile. As the tumor grows, the borders become less distinct, and fixation to the supporting ligaments or underlying fascia occurs. Nipple discharge and skin changes (*peau d'orange,* or "orange peel skin") are late occurrences and are associated with a poor prognosis.

The Medical Interview and Physical Examination

A complete reproductive, medical, and family history should be obtained and reviewed during all routine gynecologic visits. Significant breast cancer risk factors can thereby be identified and addressed. Modifiable risk factors

such as obesity and a sedentary lifestyle can be discussed and behavior modification plans implemented. The identification of certain nonmodifiable risk factors can lead to appropriate referral for more intensive management.

During the medical interview, patients should be asked whether they practice breast self-examination. Because *90% of breast cancers are found by the patient,* discussion of the risks, benefits, and techniques of breast self-examination should be routine.

The Gail Model Risk Assessment Tool helps clinicians estimate an individual's short- and long-term risks of developing breast cancer by collecting specific information about her personal and family medical history. For women age 40 and over who undergo routine mammography, relevant personal history data includes her race, age at first menses, age at first live birth, number of previous breast biopsies, and a history of atypical hyperplasia on those biopsies. Relevant family history information includes the number of first-degree relatives who have breast cancer. Entry of this data into existing calculators provides the patient with her 5-year and lifetime risks of developing breast cancer. Women at high risk, defined as a 5-year risk of 1.7% or more, can be referred for possible prophylactic therapy with selective estrogen receptor modulators, such as tamoxifen.

For a patient presenting with a specific breast problem, information about pain, tenderness, fever, mass, or discharge should be sought. Other important aspects include the duration of and any temporal changes in symptoms, changes related to the menstrual cycle or use of exogenous steroid hormones, and results of recent imaging studies or biopsies.

With as many as one fourth of all breast cancers found during routine examination, the role of the physical examination cannot be overemphasized, particularly in older and high-risk women. *A careful breast examination is a part of every routine gynecologic examination, particularly as women age.*

Screening and Evaluation

The *evaluation of any breast complaint* is based on the history and physical examination, augmented by imaging and microscopic evaluation of biopsy material and aspirates.

Imaging

Breast imaging modalities typically include mammography and ultrasound. Additional techniques such as digital mammography, magnetic resonance imaging (MRI), and positron emission tomography (PET) scans are currently being investigated as screening and diagnostic tools.

Mammography is able to detect lesions roughly 2 years before they become clinically palpable (Figure 32.2). Mammography currently provides the best available mode of screening for early lesions and has been

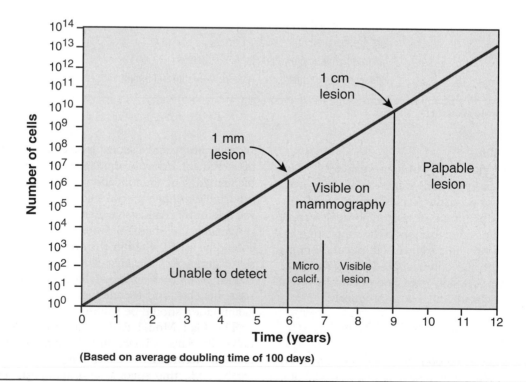

Figure 32.2. Mammographic and clinical detection of breast mass. With a presumed doubling time of 100 days, breast cancer may be detected by mammography significantly earlier than it can be identified clinically. Micro calcif. = microcalcification.

credited with reducing the mortality rate from breast cancer by up to 30%.

Mammography uses ionizing radiation exposure of approximately 0.5 rads to image the breasts. Screening mammography involves compression of the breast tissue against an imaging plate in two projections per breast. Two craniocaudal and two mediolateral images therefore comprise the standard four-image screening mammogram. Compression of the breast tissue is necessary to encompass the tissue and provide clear visualization of the tissue. The axillary tail is sometimes not fully visualized, and this must be kept in mind in the interpretation of screening mammograms. The resultant images are reviewed for changes suspicious for malignancy, including discrete nonpalpable lesions, microcalcifications, and distortions of the normal breast architecture (Figures 32.3 and 32.4).

The guidelines for screening mammography remain controversial with differing recommendations as to the age at which screening should start and the frequency with which mammograms should be obtained. Current recommendations in the United States typically call for screening mammograms every 1 to 2 years between the ages of 40 and 50, with annual screening mammography thereafter.

One limitation of any screening test is the false-positive rate, or the rate at which a test

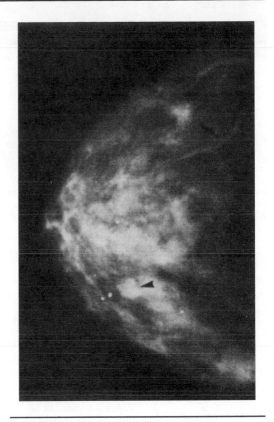

Figure 32.4. Cephalocaudal film-screen mammogram. Small scirrhous carcinoma (*arrow*) is contrasted with well-marginated fibroadenoma (*arrowhead*).

result erroneously indicates that a disease-free individual has the condition in question. In addition to causing undue psychological distress, these false results typically lead to follow-up testing, which incurs additional morbidity and cost. To reduce the rate of false-positive readings on mammograms, the American College of Radiology developed the Breast Imaging Reporting and Data System, or BI-RADS nomenclature (Table 32.3). The six overarching report categories include one for normal results, two for findings that are probably benign, two for findings concerning malignancy, and a final category that simply calls for additional imaging. Familiarity with these categories helps clinicians plan and implement appropriate follow-up.

Although screening mammograms are not routinely recommended for women who are pregnant or breast feeding, mammography may be an appropriate modality for evaluating

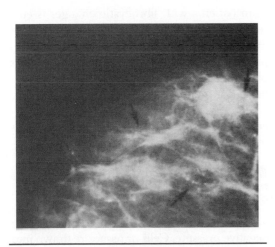

Figure 32.3. Multifocal duct carcinoma. Close-up shows multiple clusters of calcifications (*arrows*) and two masses. Only the larger mass was palpable.

Table 32.3. BI-RADS Classification of Screening Mammograms*

BI-RADS Classification	Summary Recommendation	Explanation
Category 0	Additional imaging evaluation	A finding is noted that warrants further imaging (spot compression films, magnification, special views, etc.)
Category 1	Negative	No abnormalities noted: breasts are symmetrical and no masses, architectural disturbances, or suspicious calcifications are present
Category 2	Benign finding	A negative mammogram, but the mammographer wishes to describe a finding such as a calcified fibroadenoma, multiple secretory calcifications, impants, and so forth, while still concluding that there is no mammographic evidence of malignancy
Category 3	Probably benign finding—short interval follow-up suggested	The finding has a high probability of being benign, but the mammographer would prefer to establish its mammographic stability over a short interval, usually 3 to 6 months; the interval is determined on a case-by-case basis
Category 4	Suspicious abnormality—biopsy is recommended	Lesions are noted that do not have the characteristic morphologies of breast cancer but have a definite probability of being malignant; biopsy is recommended
Category 5	Highly suggestive of malignancy—appropriate action should be taken	Lesions have morphologies characteristic of malignancy and the probability of malignancy is high; appropriate action means referral to a gynecologic oncologist or breast surgeon

*BI-RADS: Breast Imaging Reporting and Data System, American College of Radiology, 1995.

symptomatic lesions during both of these physiologic states.

Ultrasonography has come to play an important part in the evaluation of breast lesions. It is commonly used to distinguish fluid-filled (cystic) from solid masses and help guide cyst aspiration and fine-needle biopsy. The combination of fine-needle aspiration and ultrasound guidance is especially useful in distinguishing fibroadenomas from cysts, and in the histologic evaluation of the former to exclude carcinoma.

Needle Aspiration

A simple diagnostic tool, *needle aspiration* (Figure 32.5) is appropriate when a patient has a discrete breast mass that feels cystic. Aspiration with a 22- to 25-gauge needle may be both diagnostic and therapeutic. Fluid aspirated

from patients with fibrocystic changes is customarily straw colored. Fluid that is dark brown or green occurs in cysts that have been present for a prolonged period of time. Unless blood is present in the aspirate, cytologic evaluation of the fluid obtained is usually of little value. This technique is also useful for differentiating discrete cystic from solid lesions, as no fluid will be obtained from the latter.

Fine-Needle Aspiration

Fine-needle aspiration of cells from a breast mass involves inserting into the lesion a 16- to 22-gauge needle attached to a syringe and applying negative pressure. Cells or tissue are drawn into the syringe by making multiple passes through the mass (Figure 32.6). The material thus collected is examined histologically or cytologi-

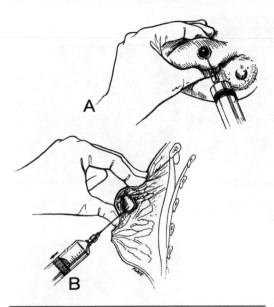

Figure 32.5. Needle aspiration of cystic breast mass. The needle is passed into the cyst, which is stabilized as shown. The cyst's contents are removed by gentle suction.

cally for signs of malignancy. This technique is 70% to 90% accurate, with a 20% false-negative rate. Therefore, if the aspiration is negative, open biopsy should still be performed. This technique depends heavily on the availability of expert cytopathology services.

Advanced Biopsy Techniques

Advanced breast biopsy techniques are typically carried out by qualified radiologists and general surgeons. One such technique is the *stereotatic core needle biopsy.* Information from multiple mammographic images is analyzed by a computer program that guides an automated biopsy tool, allowing multiple cuts of core tissue from a suspicious area, often one that is not associated with physical findings.

The ultimate method of evaluation of any breast mass is open biopsy. For lesions difficult to localize clinically, surgeons and radiologists work in teams to perform needle-localized biopsies. Radiographic imaging allows the team to place a radiopaque guide wire within the lesion preoperatively. The tissue adjacent to the needle is then excised. Images taken of the resultant specimen postoperatively confirm that the targeted tissue was adequately excised (Figure 32.7).

Histologic Types of Breast Cancer

Malignant tumors of the breast may arise from any of the major components of the breast. The American Joint Committee on Cancer classifies most breast malignancies into one of three histologic categories according to their corresponding cells of origin: ductal, lobular, and nipple. Ductal carcinoma in situ (DCIS) and lobular carcinoma in situ (LCIS) consist of malignant cells confined to the mammary ducts and lobules, respectively. Seventy to eighty percent of breast cancers are invasive ductal carcinomas. These are most common among women in their 50s and have a tendency to spread to regional lymph nodes. Invasive lobular carcinomas comprise 5% to 50% of breast cancers. This type is often multifocal and bilateral. A final, notable type of breast cancer is Paget's disease of the nipple. Paget's disease presents as a superficial skin lesion similar to eczema.

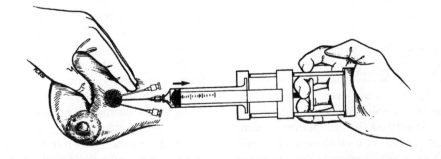

Figure 32.6. Fine-needle aspiration of solid breast mass. The needle is passed into the solid mass and withdrawn at several different angles and in several different places while suction is maintained.

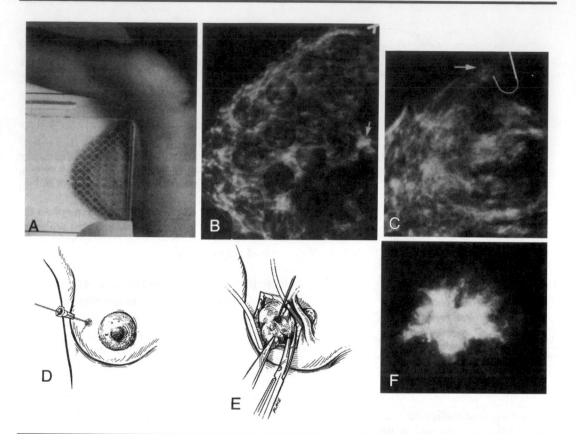

Figure 32.7. Prebiopsy mammographic needle localization of nonpalpable lesion. (***A***) A hole plate is applied to the breast surface closest to the lesion. (***B***) A mammogram identifies the hole over the nonpalpable stellate lesion suggestive of malignancy. (***C, D***) A guide wire is inserted under mammographic direction. (***E***) Excision of the specimen along the needle. (***F***) Demonstration by mammogram of the specimen that the stellate lesion has been removed for evaluation.

Breast Cancer Staging

The American Joint Committee on Cancer stages breast malignancies according to characteristics of the primary tumor, involvement of regional lymph nodes, and distant metastasis. Such systems are commonly referred to as TNM systems.

Breast Cancer Management and the Obstetrician/Gynecologist

Breast malignancies are managed principally by surgeons, radiologists, oncologists, and their associated health-care delivery teams. Various modalities are used alone or in combination to treat patients with breast cancer. These include surgical excision, radiation therapy, chemotherapy, and systemic therapy with selective estrogen receptor modulators and/or aromatase inhibitors. Factors governing therapeutic decisions include the overall health of the patient, her menopausal status, the size of her tumor, whether or not nodal spread was detected, and the histologic presence of estrogen and progesterone receptors in the primary tumor. For some patients, breast reconstruction is undertaken.

Many chemotherapeutic agents have a deleterious effect on the ovaries and can induce premature menopause. Acceptable strategies for managing menopausal vasomotor symptoms depend largely on the tumor type and, for patients with hormonally responsive tumors, typically include nonhormonal therapies such as clonidine, Bellergal-S, or SSRI antidepressants. Among women whose ovaries still function, pregnancy remains possible. Patients not interested in future childbearing need to select their contraceptive methods carefully, avoiding systemic hormonal methods when indicated. Most women interested in additional childbearing can be reassured that a pregnancy will not adversely affect their overall survival. The management of women diagnosed with breast cancer during an ongoing pregnancy is understandably complex. Women receiving chemotherapy in the postpartum period are often counseled against breast feeding.

Many patients with estrogen receptor positive tumors are placed on selective estrogen receptor modulators (SERMs) for several years after their breast cancers are initially diagnosed and treated. The goal of such therapy is to reduce recurrence and improve overall mortality. The role of such therapy in other groups of patients remains under investigation. At least one of these agents, tamoxifen, has been associated with proliferative changes in the endometrium. Patients on tamoxifen may present with vaginal bleeding. If this occurs, endometrial sampling is important to rule out endometrial hyperplasia and carcinoma.

Differential Diagnosis by Complaint

The most common presenting complaints referable to the breast are pain and the presence of a mass. Both of these complaints represent sources of great distress and perceived emergency to the patient. They therefore deserve prompt and considerate attention.

Diffuse, bilateral breast pain occurring before menstruation is most often caused by fibrocystic changes. Dorsal radiculitis or inflammatory changes in the costochondral junction (Tietze's syndrome) may also present this way. Well-localized breast pain may result

from rapid expansion of a cyst, obstruction of a duct, or inflammation (such as mastitis). Breast pain is a presenting complaint in less than 10% of patients with breast cancer.

Masses in the breast, with the attendant fear of cancer, represent one of the most emotionally charged and difficult differential diagnoses the clinician must make. Masses that are firm, round, and well demarcated are most likely to be fibroadenomas. Areas with a flattened, rubbery consistency are suspect for malignancy, although other conditions such as fat necrosis may cause similar changes. In either case, further evaluation (such as tissue confirmation by open or needle biopsy) is mandatory.

Although bloody discharge from the nipple is the hallmark of intraductal papillomas, any unilateral, spontaneous nipple discharge requires a thorough evaluation. The color or clarity of the fluid does not rule out carcinoma. Cytologic evaluation of the nipple discharge is associated with a false-negative rate of almost 20%, significantly reducing its value. Mammography and biopsy are required to establish the diagnosis.

Nipple discharge associated with burning, itching, or nipple discomfort in older patients is suggestive of ductal ectasia. In these patients, the discharge is thick or sticky and gray to black in color. As with other sources of nipple discharge, excisional biopsy is often required.

Patients with diffuse tenderness and no dominant mass may be safely rechecked at a different time in the menstrual cycle. Patients who have undergone aspiration of a cyst (with clear fluid and disappearance of the palpable mass) should be rechecked in 2 weeks. Any recurrence of the cyst should prompt biopsy or additional evaluation. Some authors advocate a follow-up mammogram after cyst aspiration to delve for other lesions, although this is best individualized based on the needs and history of each patient.

CHAPTER 33

GYNECOLOGIC PROCEDURES

This chapter deals primarily with APGO Educational Topic:

Topic 41: Gynecologic Procedures

Students should be familiar with the risks and benefits of the various procedures needed to diagnose and treat gynecologic disorders.

Imaging

The ability to image various parts and organs of the body has dramatically enhanced our diagnostic capabilities. These methods do not replace a careful and thoughtful history and physical evaluation but can add more detail, which assists in both medical and surgical management. The effective use of these modalities requires that the physician be familiar with the benefits and limitations of each.

Ultrasonography

Ultrasonography is based on the use of high-frequency sound reflections to identify different body tissues and structures. The term *sonography* literally means "sound writing" and is often described as using sound waves to make a picture. Short bursts of low-energy sound waves are sent into the body. When these waves encounter the interface between two tissues that transmit sound differently, some of the sound energy is reflected back toward the sound source (Figure 33.1). The returning sound waves are detected, and the distance from the sensor is deduced using the elapsed time from transmission to reception.

This information is displayed graphically as a cross-sectional view of the structure encountered by the beam.

Because ultrasonography uses low-energy sound waves, it is safe in all patients, both pregnant and nonpregnant. In obstetrics, measurement of fetal anatomy to allow estimation of fetal age and weight is routinely performed with ultrasonography. Detailed evaluations of fetal structures such as heart, brain, spinal column, and kidneys can be performed. Fetal gender is frequently determined as well.

In gynecology, ultrasonography is used to distinguish the character of pelvic masses (solid versus cystic) to provide accurate measurement of tumors such as fibroids or to assess blood flow to structures. Ultrasonography should be used to evaluate pelvic masses when an adequate examination is not possible (e.g., extreme obesity), if findings are in doubt, or when the information gathered will alter patient management. Routine ultrasonography to confirm pelvic examination findings is not appropriate.

Improved resolution for imaging intrauterine and adnexal structures may be obtained by placing the ultrasound transducer inside the

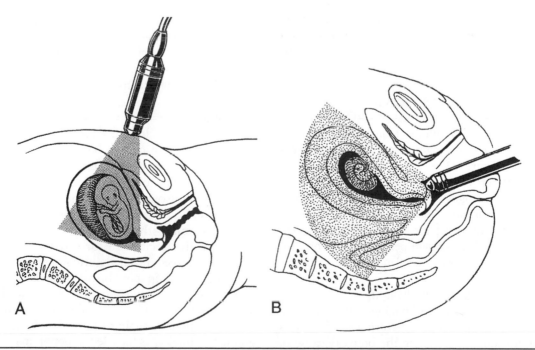

Figure 33.1. Transabdominal (**A**) and transvaginal (**B**) ultrasonography.

vagina, much closer to the structures to be examined than is possible with transabdominal positioning of the ultrasound transducer. The higher frequencies of sound used for transvaginal imaging allow enhanced details to be seen but limit the depth of penetration of the sound. Therefore, transvaginal ultrasound is especially useful for conditions located near the apex of the vagina (e.g., early gestations, possible ectopic pregnancies) and for ovarian follicle monitoring during assisted reproduction. Measurements of the thickness of the endometrium may be of help in the assessment of the patient with bleeding but do not replace traditional histological methods of evaluation. The sonographic assessment of intrauterine pathology may be enhanced by the infusion of a small amount of sterile saline into the uterine cavity (hysterosonography or sonohysterography). Saline infusion sonohysterography is particularly useful in defining intracavitary lesions such as endometrial polyps and submucous fibroids.

Doppler ultrasound is a form of ultrasonography that uses changes in the frequency of the reflected sound to infer motion of the reflecting surface. This can be useful in detecting cardiac motion or assessing blood flow. A growing application of Doppler ultrasound has been the evaluation of blood flow patterns in the umbilical vessels and cerebral blood vessels, because changes in these patterns may be an indication of fetal stress.

Computed Axial Tomography

Computed axial tomography (CT or CAT) scanning uses computer algorithms to construct cross-sectional images based on x-ray information (Figure 33.2). This technique involves slightly greater radiation exposure than a conventional single-exposure radiograph but provides significantly more information. With the use of contrast agents, this modality can help the physician evaluate pelvic masses, look for signs of adenopathy, or plan radiation therapy.

Magnetic Resonance Imaging

Magnetic resonance imaging (MRI) is based on the magnetic characteristics of various atoms and molecules in the body. Because of the variations in chemical composition of body

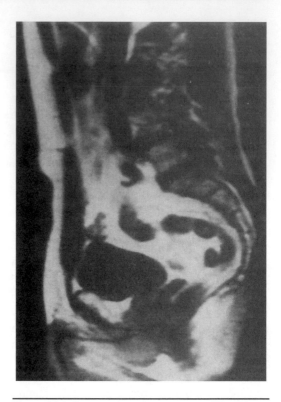

Figure 33.2. Computed axial tomography (CT) of the pelvis.

tissues (especially the content of hydrogen, sodium, fluoride, or phosphorus), MRI offers exceptional images of many soft tissues. Emerging areas of clinical applicability are in the assessment of lesions in the breast and in the staging of cervical malignancy.

Mammography

The need to develop an effective screening method for breast cancer has prompted the evaluation of many imaging technologies such as thermography (based on skin temperature patterns), ultrasonography, transillumination by light, and radiograph. It has been the latter (mammography) that has proved to be the most effective technique for screening and evaluation of recognized abnormalities (Figure 33.3). In mammography, breast tissue is compressed against an imaging plate, and a small amount of radiation is used to form the image. Improved films, imaging screens, and xerographic technologies have led to better images with lower radiation exposures, usually less

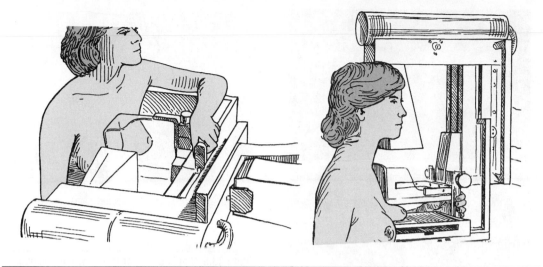

Figure 33.3. Technique of screening mammography.

than 0.5 rad per image set. Breast ultrasonography is a valuable adjunctive examination, especially to differentiate cystic from solid masses or lucent images on mammography.

Hysterosalpingography

For hysterosalpingography, contrast material is introduced through the cervix into the uterine cavity, and radiographs are taken at specific intervals to reveal the progression of the dye through the uterus, fallopian tubes, and into the abdominopelvic cavity (Figure 33.4). This technique is useful for assessment of the size, shape, and configuration of the uterine cavity as part of the evaluation for infertility or genital anomalies. The contrast material flows through the fallopian tubes and spills into the peritoneal cavity, which can be a good indicator of tubal patency and allow examination of tubal anatomy.

Hysterosalpingography is associated with the risk of infection of the uterus or pelvis as well as bleeding or pain. As a result, other techniques are also being used for evaluation of the uterine cavity, including hysteroscopy as well as hysterosonography

Genital Tract Biopsy

Tissue from genital tract lesions for histological study may be safely obtained from the vulva, vagina, cervix, and endometrial cavity.

Usually performed in the office, most of these procedures require little or no anesthetics and are associated with minimal risk.

Vulvar biopsies are generally accomplished with the use of a local anesthetic. Tissue may be removed by circumscribing the biopsy specimen with a Keyes biopsy instrument (a sharp, hollow punch), elevating the tissue, and cutting across the base or by simple excision with a scalpel (Figure 33.5). This allows for full-thickness histopathologic assessment and may also serve to fully excise small lesions. Local pressure or the use of styptics such as Monsel's solution (ferric subsulfate) is usually adequate for hemostasis; sutures are seldom required.

Biopsy of *vaginal* lesions is generally carried out using biopsy forceps and is most often done at the vaginal apex in cases of cellular atypia found on Pap smears in patients who have had prior hysterectomy. The biopsy forceps is also used for cervical biopsy. Local anesthesia is usually not required for vaginal or cervical biopsies.

An *endometrial* biopsy may be obtained in several ways. A small, hollow tube may be passed through the cervix and tissue fragments aspirated using the suction pressure generated by removal of the stylet (Figure 33.6). Larger, more rigid cannula may be used to aspirate or even curette the endometrium.

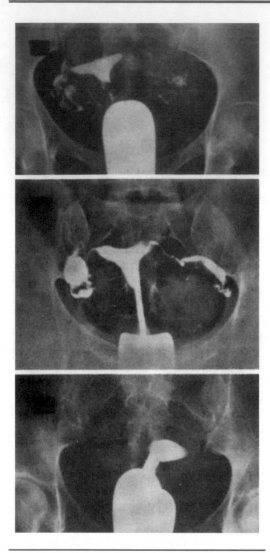

Figure 33.4. Hysterosalpingography.

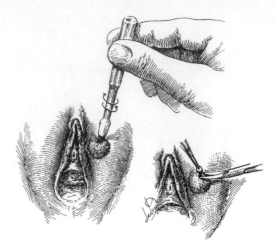

Figure 33.5. Biopsy of vulvar lesion with Keyes punch. Instrument is rotated in place to incise tissue.

Cryotherapy

Cryotherapy is the term used to describe tissue destruction by freezing. Liquid carbon dioxide or nitrogen is run through a metal probe that is placed on the tissue to be treated, allowing freezing of the tissue. Cryotherapy is most frequently used to treat dysplastic changes and benign lesions such as condyloma (Figure 33.7). The formation of ice crystals within the cells of the treated tissue leads

Colposcopy

A colposcope is a fixed stereomicroscope with an internal light source used to facilitate detailed evaluation of the surface of the cervix, vagina, and vulva when malignancy is suspected based on history, physical examination, or cytologic report. It is used to facilitate directed biopsies of suspicious areas and is an improvement over random biopsies in the face of abnormal cytology. Colposcopy may be performed in the office—almost always without the need for analgesia or anesthesia—and has minimal morbidity.

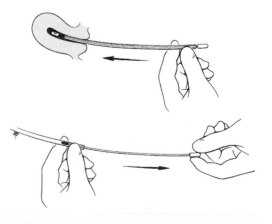

Figure 33.6. Endometrial biopsy using Pipelle. Hollow tube held in uterine cavity as stylet is withdrawn generating aspiration.

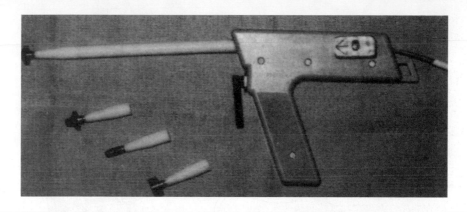

Figure 33.7. Cryosurgical equipment.

to tissue destruction and subsequent sloughing. As a result, patients who have had cryotherapy of the cervix can be expected to have a watery discharge for several weeks as the tissue sloughs and healing occurs. Cryotherapy is inexpensive and generally effective, but it is less precise than other tissue destruction procedures such as laser ablation or electrosurgical techniques.

Laser Vaporization

Highly energetic coherent light beams (light amplification by stimulated emission of radiation [LASER]) may be directed onto tissues, facilitating tissue destruction or incision, depending on the specific wavelength of light used and the power density, or intensity, of the light beam. Great precision is possible with these systems, allowing specific tissue destruction (margins and depth of destruction) or incision selection. Infrared (CO_2) lasers are commonly used in gynecology, used alone, coupled to colposcopes, or transmitted through laparoscopes and hysteroscopes for intra-abdominal and intrauterine procedures, respectively.

Dilation and Curettage

The *dilation* of dilation and curettage (D&C) refers to opening the cervix to allow access to the endometrial cavity. This is usually done by gently using a series of graduated dilators to stretch the cervical opening. Because stretching of the cervix is painful, D&C is usually performed under a local (paracervical), regional, or general anesthetic in an operating room. *Curettage* is a scraping of the uterine lining.

For the purpose of obtaining a representative sample of the uterine cavity (i.e., endometrial biopsy), D&C has been supplanted by more easily accomplished office endometrial biopsy techniques, such as the Novak or Pipelle endometrial biopsy technique, or by biopsy under direct hysteroscopic visualization. Removal of polyps and other tumors may be accomplished by blind D&C, although removal under direct hysteroscopic visualization is more commonly chosen. D&C is also used to evacuate the uterus in cases of incomplete spontaneous abortion.

Hysteroscopy

Improved optics have led to the availability of small endoscopes that allow a direct view of the endocervix and endometrial cavity (Figure 33.8). These endoscopes may be used for diagnosis (e.g., the evaluation of bleeding or congenital malformations, the location of missing intrauterine devices) or for therapy (e.g., polypectomy, myomectomy, endometrial ablation, removal of a uterine septum). Usually done as an outpatient procedure under local, regional, or general anesthesia, hysteroscopy shares most of the same problems and complications found in D&C. Fluid may be used to

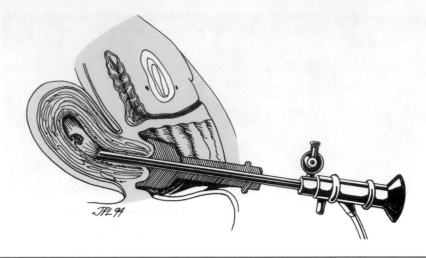

Figure 33.8. Hysteroscopy.

distend the uterine cavity to improve visualization or the endometrium may be directly visualized (contact hysteroscopy).

Endometrial Ablation

Several techniques have been developed to resect or ablate the endometrial lining to reduce or eliminate menstrual bleeding. This is generally accomplished under hysteroscopic visualization using heat, cold, electrosurgical, or laser energy to destroy the endometrial tissue. The ability to accomplish these procedures in an ambulatory setting is attractive, but complete control of menstrual bleeding is not always accomplished, and although fertility is impaired, the technique should not be seen as a reliable form of sterilization.

Pregnancy Termination

Pregnancy termination refers to the planned interruption of a pregnancy before viability and is often referred to as induced abortion. It is generally accomplished surgically through dilation of the cervix and evacuation of the uterine contents accomplished under local anesthetics.

Removal of the products of conception in the first and early second trimester uses either a suction or a sharp curette. Suction curettes are often preferred because they are less likely to cause uterine damage such as endometrial scarring or perforation. In the second trimester, destructive grasping forceps may be used to remove the pregnancy through a dilated cervix (*dilation and evacuation [D&E]*). Alternatively, termination of pregnancy using medical rather than surgical techniques can be performed in the first and second trimester.

Cervical Conization

Conization is a surgical procedure performed for either diagnostic or therapeutic purposes in which a cone-shaped sample of tissue, encompassing the entire cervical transformation zone and extending up the endocervical canal, is removed from the cervix (Figure 33.9). Conization is required for the definitive evaluation of patients with abnormal Pap smears for whom adequate colposcopic examinations are impossible or are inconsistent with Pap smear data.

Conization may be performed using various techniques, including sharp dissection (cold knife cone), laser excision, and electrosurgery (large loop excision of the transformation zone [LLETZ] or loop electrosurgical excision procedure [LEEP]). An early complication of conization is excessive bleeding, which can occur 5 to 10 days after surgery. Cervical stenosis or incompetence is an infrequent complication.

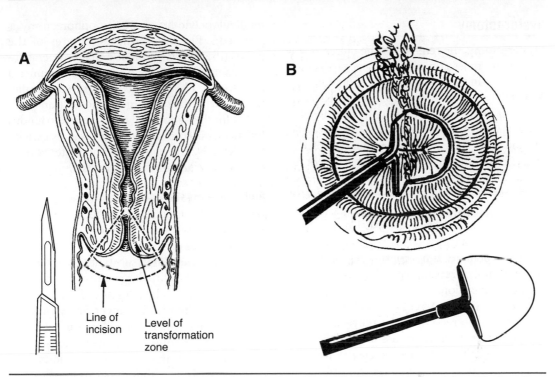

Figure 33.9. Conization of the cervix. (**A**) Cold knife technique. (**B**) LLETZ/LEEP (large loop excision of the transformation zone/loop electrosurgical excision procedure) technique.

Laparoscopy

Laparoscopy (or pelviscopy) involves inspection and manipulation of tissue within the abdominal cavity using endoscopic instruments. The laparoscope is inserted into the abdominal cavity, usually through a periumbilical incision. To facilitate viewing and to decrease the chance of bowel injury, the abdominal cavity may be distended with either carbon dioxide or nitrous oxide gas. Additional incisions in the lower abdomen may be made to allow supplementary instruments to be placed into the abdominal cavity for surgical or other manipulations (Figure 33.10). A probe or other device is often inserted into the uterine cavity to facilitate uterine manipulations.

Laparoscopy is used for diagnostic or therapeutic purposes. Laparoscopic inspection of the pelvis can be invaluable in the diagnosis of pelvic pain, infertility, congenital abnormalities, or small pelvic masses. Operative laparoscopy may be used to perform lysis of adhesions, treat endometriosis, or carry out surgical sterilizations and other gynecologic procedures.

Serious complications from injury to the bowel or great vessels can occur. Intraperitoneal bleeding or injuries such as damage to bowel during fulguration or laser also pose a risk. Anesthetic complications are possible, as are infections and bleeding at the incision site.

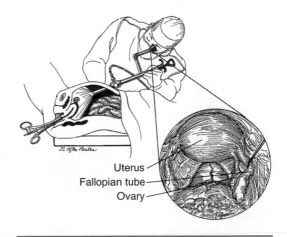

Uterus
Fallopian tube
Ovary

Figure 33.10. Laparoscopy.

Hysterectomy

Hysterectomy, the removal of the uterus, is still one of the most common surgical procedures performed. In the United States, approximately 500,000 hysterectomies are performed each year. Removing the uterus may be indicated for patients with benign or malignant changes in the uterine wall or cavity, abnormalities of the cervix, or menstrual disturbances that do not respond to more conservative therapy. Hysterectomy essentially eliminates the possibility of pregnancy, causes cessation of menses, and removes the risk of cervical disease. Despite these apparent advantages, hysterectomy is sufficiently expensive, time consuming, and risky that it cannot be recommended for the sole purpose of sterilization.

In discussing hysterectomy with patients, it is important to recognize the correct use and common misuse of terms associated with the procedure. When physicians use the term *total* hysterectomy, they are referring to the removal of the entire uterus, including cervix and uterine corpus. The term does not indicate removal of the ovaries (oophorectomy) or fallopian tubes (salpingectomy). These distinctions are important and should be emphasized when taking the patient's history and providing preoperative counseling. A *subtotal,* or *supracervical,* hysterectomy is one in which the body of the uterus is removed near the level of the internal cervical os, leaving the cervix in place. A *radical* hysterectomy is a cancer-related surgery procedure in which the uterus is removed with wide margins of surrounding tissues.

Removal of the uterus may be accomplished by entering the abdominal cavity from above (abdominal hysterectomy) or by extracting the uterus through the vagina (vaginal hysterectomy). Each has advantages and disadvantages that must be evaluated for each patient. With either approach, certain steps must be accomplished to allow the safe removal of the uterus. The blood supply to the uterus is interrupted by ligation of the uterine arteries and the anastomotic connections to the vaginal and ovarian blood supplies. The latter is ligated at the level of the uteroovarian ligament (if the ovaries are to be preserved) or at the level of the in-

fundibulopelvic ligament (if oophorectomy is planned). The supporting structures of the uterus (the round, cardinal, and uterosacral ligaments and the leaves of the broad ligament) are severed. The sequence of these steps is dictated by the route of surgery chosen (fundus to cervix for the abdominal route; cervix to fundus for the vaginal route) and the local exigencies mandated by the pathology encountered (e.g., distortion of anatomy by fibroids).

Abdominal Hysterectomy

Removal of the uterus through an abdominal incision allows the surgeon maximal exposure and latitude in performing the procedure. This approach is used when substantial pathology is anticipated (as with large fibroids or pelvic scarring), when wide margins or further exploration is required (as in cancer surgery), when additional abdominal procedures are contemplated (such as some forms of bladder suspension), or when surgery is done at the time of cesarean delivery. Abdominal hysterectomies generally involve longer operating times because of the time spent making and repairing the abdominal wall incision. This route also is associated with a greater rate of morbidity and a longer hospital stay.

Vaginal Hysterectomy

Vaginal hysterectomy is generally associated with a faster recovery period and less patient discomfort than an abdominal hysterectomy. Offsetting this is the higher incidence of fever and infection, although the use of prophylactic antibiotics has reduced this to a minimum. Vaginal hysterectomy is often chosen when the uterus is not enlarged and other adnexal or pelvic pathology is not anticipated. This procedure is especially appropriate for patients who require repair of a cystocele, rectocele, or enterocele. Vaginal hysterectomy is typically avoided when the uterus is larger than 10 to 12 weeks' size, scarring or endometriosis restricts movement of the pelvic organs, or further abdominal exploration is required.

Laparoscopically Assisted Vaginal Hysterectomy

The role of laparoscopic-assisted vaginal hysterectomy (LAVH)–in which some of the initial stages of hysterectomy are done with laparo-scopic instrumentation, but the uterus is ulti-mately removed transvaginally–remains to be fully established. Advocates of the procedure point to the advantages of avoiding an abdominal incision by facilitating vaginal delivery of the uterus or adnexal mass in situa-tions where such was impossible or inadvisable: pelvic adhesions, uterus size >10 to 12 weeks, an adnexal mass, and poor uterine descent as may be found in women of low gravidity. Con-cerns that have been raised about the procedure include its technical difficulty, increased opera-tive time, and increased anesthesia exposure.

UNIT IV

REPRODUCTIVE ENDOCRINOLOGY AND INFERTILITY

CHAPTER 34

REPRODUCTIVE CYCLE

This chapter deals primarily with APGO Educational Topic:

Topic 45: Normal and Abnormal Uterine Bleeding

The student should understand the normal menstrual cycle in order to diagnose and treat common abnormalties.

In the female reproductive cycle, ovulation is followed by menstrual bleeding in a recurring, predictable sequence. This recurring sequence is established at puberty (around age 12.5) and continues until the time of menopause at around age 51. A regular, predictable ovulation cycle is usually established by age 15 and continues (except during pregnancy) until age 45. Thus a woman has approximately 30 years of optimal reproductive function. In healthy women, reproductive cycles occur at approximately 28-day intervals with a range of 24 to 35 days from the beginning of menses to the begining of the next menses. This cycle may be interrupted by endogenous conditions such as pregnancy, lactation, illness, gynecologic abnormalities or endocrine disorders, or exogenous factors (e.g., hormone-based contraceptive use or other medications).

The reproductive cycle depends on the complex cyclic interaction between hypothalamic gonadotropin-releasing hormone (GnRH), the pituitary gonadotropins follicle-stimulating hormone (FSH) and luteinizing hormone (LH), and the ovarian sex steroid hormones estradiol and progesterone. Through positive and negative feedback loops, these hormones stimulate ovulation, facilitate implantation of the fertilized ovum, or bring about menstruation. Feedback loops between the hypothalamus, pituitary gland, and ovaries are depicted in Figure 34.1. If the levels or a relationship of any one (or more) of the above hormones become altered, the reproductive cycle becomes disrupted, and ovulation and/or menstruation cease.

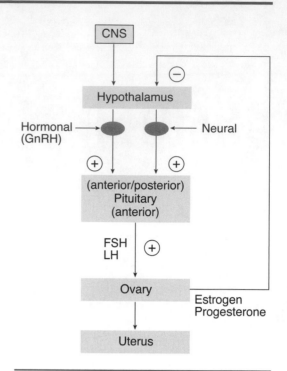

Figure 34.1. Traditional block diagram of feedback and control of menstruation. Traditionally, control of menstruation is based on a simple feedback loop involving the "hypothalamic–pituitary–ovarian axis." This view is giving way to evidence that the follicle itself controls the cyclic process. CNS = central nervous system; FSH = follicle-stimulating hormone; GnRH = gonadotropin-releasing hormone; LH = luteinizing hormone. (From Smith RP: *Gynecology in Primary Care.* Baltimore: Williams & Wilkins, 1996, p. 26.)

Hypothalamic GnRH Secretion

GnRH (a decapeptide) is secreted in a pulsatile manner from the arcuate nucleus of the hypothalamus. The hypothalamus serves as the pulse generator of the reproductive clock. Ovarian function requires the pulsatile secretion of GnRH at 70- to 90-minute intervals. The mechanism for stimulation of GnRH secretion is unknown; however, GnRH secretion is influenced by estradiol and catecholamine neurotransmitters. The latter influence may help explain psychogenic influences on the reproductive cycle. GnRH reaches the anterior pituitary gland through the hypothalamic-

pituitary portal plexus. Pulsatile secretion of GnRH stimulates and modulates pituitary gonadotropin secretion.

Pituitary Gonadotropin Secretion

The pituitary gonadotropins FSH and LH are glycoprotein hormones secreted by the anterior pituitary gland. FSH and LH are also secreted in pulsatile fashion in response to the pulsatile release of GnRH; the magnitude of secretion and the rates of secretion of FSH and/or LH are determined largely by the levels of ovarian steroid hormones and other ovarian factors. When a woman is in a state of relative estrogen deficiency, as in the early follicular phase, the principal gonadotropin secreted is FSH. The ovary responds to FSH secretion with estradiol production, with subsequent negative feedback on the pituitary inhibiting FSH secretion and positive feedback facilitating LH secretion.

Ovarian Sex Steroid Hormone Secretion

Ovarian follicles respond to pituitary gonadotropin secretion by synthesizing the principal ovarian hormones *estradiol* and *progesterone*. Increasing levels of estradiol influence the pituitary gland via a negative feedback mechanism, resulting in decreased secretion of FSH, but also via a positive feedback mechanism leading to increased secretion of LH. At midcycle there is a marked increase in LH secretion (the LH surge), which triggers ovulation. With ovulation, the ovarian follicle is converted into a corpus luteum and begins secreting progesterone.

At birth, the human ovary is filled with approximately one million *primordial follicles.* Each follicle contains an oocyte that is arrested in prophase of the first meiotic division. The oocyte is surrounded by a single layer of pregranulosa cells, which become the granulosa cells. The pregranulosa cells are surrounded by a matrix of cells that become the theca cells. Some primordial follicles partially respond to pituitary FSH during childhood, and the others undergo atresia resulting in 300,000 to 400,000 oocytes by menarche. The process of ovulation does not occur until the onset of positive feedback mechanism during puberty.

During a full reproductive cycle, one oocyte is brought to maturity before ovulation, though a number of oocytes are stimulated to partial maturation but subsequently undergo atresia before reaching ovulation.

During the process of follicular maturation, pregranulosa cells are stimulated by FSH to become *granulosa cells,* which begin secreting *estradiol.* Binding of FSH to receptors in the granulosa cells causes granulosa cell proliferation, increased binding of FSH, and increased production of estradiol. The follicle with the greatest number of granulosa cells, FSH receptors, and the highest estradiol production becomes the dominant follicle from which ovulation occurs.

As a primordial follicle is stimulated, the pretheca cells surrounding the granulosa cells

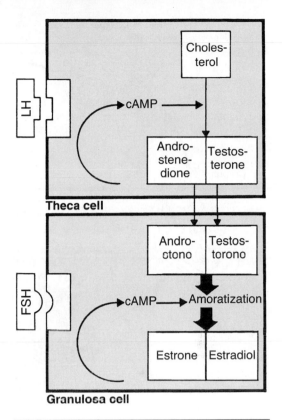

Figure 34.2. Two-cell theory of estradiol production.

become *theca cells.* The theca cells secrete *androgens,* which serve as the precursors for estradiol production by the granulosa cells (Figure 34.2). These androgens enter the granulosa cells by diffusion, where they are aromatized to estradiol.

After ovulation, the dominant follicle becomes the *corpus luteum,* which secretes *progesterone* to complete preparation of the endometrium for implantation of a fertilized oocyte. If pregnancy does not occur, the corpus luteum undergoes involution, menstruation begins, and the cycle repeats. The changes in the follicle during the follicular phase of the cycle are presented in Figure 34.3.

Reproductive Cycle

For purposes of discussion, *the reproductive cycle is divided into three phases: menstruation and the follicular phase, ovulation, and the luteal phase.* These three phases refer to the status of the ovary during the reproductive cycle.

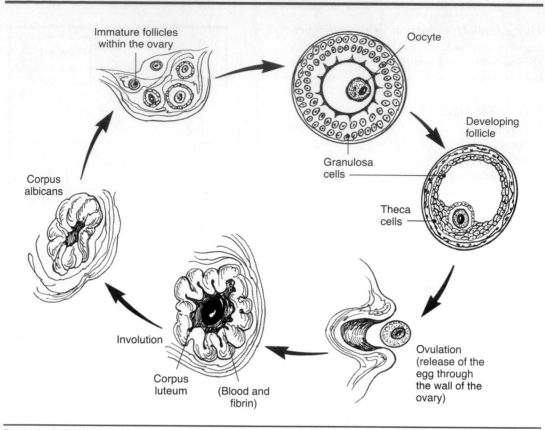

Figure 34.3. Cyclic changes in ovarian follicle development. (From Smith RP: *Gynecology in Primary Care.* Baltimore: Williams & Wilkins, 1996, p. 29.)

Phase I: Menstruation and the Follicular Phase

The first day of menstrual bleeding is considered day 1 of the menstrual cycle. During menstruation, the endometrium is sloughed in response to progesterone withdrawal. This is accompanied by the development of a new follicle during the follicular phase, with renewal of the endometrial lining of the uterus in preparation for implantation of an embryo. Women usually menstruate for 3 to 5 days. A woman sheds approximately 30 to 50 mL of dark, nonclotting menstrual blood during menstruation. Occasionally, tissue elements of endometrium can be identified in the menstrual effluent.

There may be uterine cramps during the first day or two of menstrual bleeding. These cramps are a result of the action of prostaglandins liberated from the endometrium during menstruation (Figure 34.4). At the time of menstruation, prostaglandins are formed and released, and they produce contractions of the uterine musculature and vasculature, causing contractile and ischemic pain (Figure 34.5). These prostaglandin-associated uterine contractions also aid the normal expulsion of the menstrual effluent.

Menstruation marks the beginning of the follicular phase of the cycle. With the beginning of menstruation, plasma concentrations of estradiol, progesterone, and LH reach their lowest point. In response to this reduction in negative feedback at the pituitary gland, FSH is increased at the beginning of menstruation. The increase in FSH begins approximately 2 days before the onset of menstruation and is involved in the maturation of another group of ovarian follicles with selection of a dominant follicle for ovulation in the next cycle. FSH binds to receptors located in the granulosa cells of the primary oocyte stimulating their differentiation from a stratified squamous-type cell into a cuboidal cell. Moreover, FSH stimulates mitosis of the granulosa cells, thereby

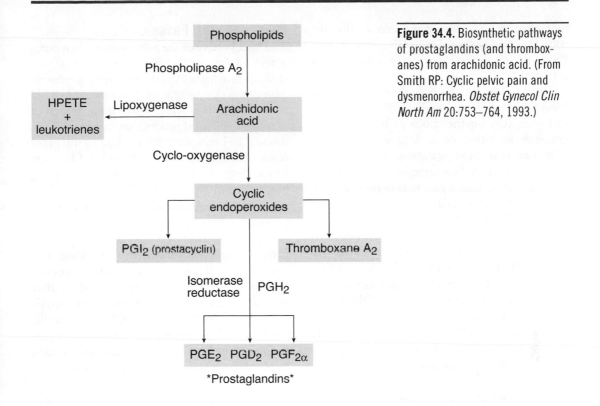

Figure 34.4. Biosynthetic pathways of prostaglandins (and thromboxanes) from arachidonic acid. (From Smith RP: Cyclic pelvic pain and dysmenorrhea. *Obstet Gynecol Clin North Am* 20:753–764, 1993.)

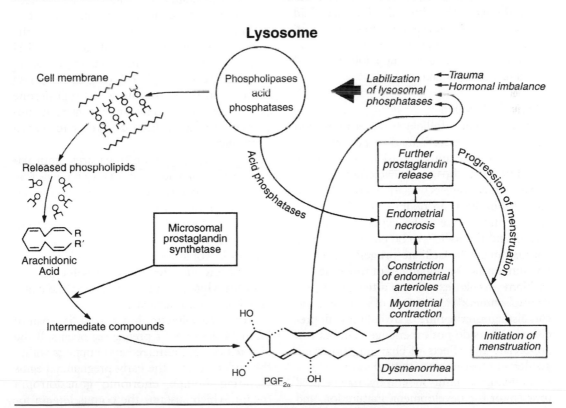

Figure 34.5. Menstrual-associated prostaglandin release and uterine contractions.

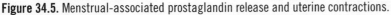

increasing the number of granulosa cells surrounding the oocyte. Under the influence of FSH, the granulosa cells begin to secrete estradiol.

Estradiol begins to rise in plasma by the fourth day of the cycle. Estradiol stimulates LH receptors on the theca cells, further increasing secretion of androgen precursors, which are converted by aromatase to estradiol in granulosa cells. This upregulation of LH receptors and hormone production prepares the granulosa and theca cells for progesterone synthesis after ovulation.

With rising estradiol, there is negative feedback on the pituitary gland to decrease the release of FSH and positive feedback on the pituitary gland to increase the release of LH. During the early follicular phase of the cycle, the FSH:LH ratio is >1; as the cycle progresses, the FSH:LH ratio becomes <1, demonstrating both positive and negative feedback effects of estradiol on the pituitary gland.

As follicles enlarge, they secrete both androgens and estrogens; however, if the estradiol:androgen ratio within the follicular fluid becomes <1, that follicle becomes atretic and never becomes a dominant follicle. The dominant follicle is the one that has a follicular fluid estradiol:androgen ratio of >1.

Phase II: Ovulation

As the dominant follicle secretes more and more estradiol, there is marked positive feedback to the pituitary gland to secrete LH. By days 11 to 13 of the normal cycle, an LH surge occurs, which triggers ovulation. Ovulation occurs within 30 to 36 hours of the LH surge, causing the oocyte to be expelled from the follicle and the follicle to be converted into a corpus luteum to facilitate progesterone production during the remainder of the cycle.

Many women experience a twinge of pain ("mittelschmerz") at the time of ovulation and can distinguish the time of ovulation with precision. Others do not experience pain but can appreciate the effects of changing hormone production that occur with ovulation.

Transvaginal ultrasonography may be used to monitor the development, maturation, and collapse of the dominant follicle.

Phase III: Luteal Phase

The luteal phase of the menstrual cycle is characterized by a change in secretion of sex steroid hormones from estradiol predominance to progesterone predominance. As FSH rises early in the cycle, stimulating mitosis of granulosa cells and production of estradiol, additional LH receptors are created in the granulosa cells and theca cells. With the LH surge at the time of ovulation, these LH receptors bind LH and convert the enzymatic machinery of the granulosa and theca cells to facilitate production of progesterone.

The production of progesterone begins approximately 24 hours before ovulation and rises rapidly thereafter. A maximal production of progesterone occurs 3 to 4 days after ovulation and is maintained for approximately 11 days following ovulation. If fertilization and implantation do not occur, progesterone production diminishes rapidly, initiating events leading to the beginning of a new cycle.

Adequate progesterone production is necessary to facilitate implantation of the fertilized oocyte into the endometrium and to sustain pregnancy into the early first trimester. If the initial rise in FSH is inadequate and if the LH surge does not achieve maximal amplitude, an "inadequate luteal phase" (i.e., luteal phase defect) can occur, resulting in progesterone production that is inadequate to facilitate implantation of a fertilized oocyte or to sustain pregnancy.

The corpus luteum measures approximately 2.5 cm wide and has a characteristic deep yellow color. It can be seen on gross inspection of the ovary if laparoscopy or laparotomy is performed during the luteal phase of the cycle. As the corpus luteum fails, it decreases in volume and loses its yellow color. After a few months, the corpus luteum becomes a white fibrous streak within the ovary called the corpus albicans.

The corpus luteum has a fixed life span of 13 to 14 days unless pregnancy occurs. If the oocyte becomes fertilized and implants within the endometrium, the early pregnancy begins secreting human chorionic gonadotropin (hCG), which sustains the corpus luteum for another 6 to 7 weeks.

Progesterone has negative feedback on pituitary secretion of both FSH and LH. During the luteal phase of the cycle, both FSH and LH are suppressed to low levels. As the corpus luteum fails and progesterone secretion diminishes, FSH begins to rise to prepare a woman for the next reproductive cycle.

The cyclic changes in FSH, LH, estradiol, and progesterone along with the changes in the follicle, endometrium, vagina, and cervix are summarized in Figure 34.6.

Perimenopause

As a woman ages, the ovarian follicles diminish in number and become less sensitive to FSH. The process of ovulation becomes increasingly inefficient, less regular, and less predictable than in earlier years. A woman may begin to notice changes in her reproductive cycle in her late 30s or early 40s. Initially, she may notice a shortening of the cycle length. With increasing inefficiency of the reproductive cycle, the follicular phase shortens, but the luteal phase is maintained at normal length. With the passing of time, some cycles become anovulatory.

As menopause approaches, the remaining follicles become almost totally resistant to FSH. The process of ovulation ceases entirely, and cyclic hormone production ends with menopause.

With diminishing ovarian function one will see serum FSH levels start to rise. With advancing age elevated FSH levels are first detected in the follicular phase. This early follicular phase rise in FSH has developed into an endocrine test of ovarian functional reserve in which one draws an FSH level on cycle day 3. With a further decrease in ovarian function, the FSH level will be elevated throughout the menstrual cycle.

Clinical Manifestations of Hormonal Changes

The endometrium and endocervix, the breasts, the vagina, and the hypothalamic thermoregulating center all undergo cyclic changes in response to hormonal control. The changes in the endocervix and breasts can be directly observed, and the changes in the hypothalamic thermoregulatory center can be measured by recording the basal body temperature. The changes in the vagina can be identified by cytological examination of the vaginal epithelium, and the changes in the endometrium can be evaluated by endometrial biopsy followed by histological examination of the biopsy sample. Other changes can be ascertained through a careful history. Some of these changes include abdominal bloating, fluid retention, mood changes, and uterine cramps at the onset of menstruation.

Endometrium

The endometrial lining of the uterus undergoes dramatic histological changes during the reproductive cycle. During menstruation, the endometrium is sloughed to a basal level, consisting of compact stroma cells and short, narrow endometrial glands. Estrogen is a mitogenic hormone, which stimulates cell growth. With rising estradiol production during the follicular phase of the cycle, the endometrial stroma thickens and the endometrial glands become elongated; this is a proliferative endometrium. The endometrium reaches a maximal thickness at the time of ovulation. If ovulation does not occur and a woman remains in an estrogenic state, the endometrium continues to slowly thicken and the endometrial glands continue to elongate until the endometrium outgrows its blood supply and sloughs. This abnormal condition is the basis for dysfunctional uterine bleeding (see Chapter 36).

When ovulation occurs, the hormonal balance changes from an estrogenic state to a progestational state. Progesterone is not a mitogen, but causes differentiation of the tissues that contain progesterone receptors. Progesterone converts the proliferative endometrium into a secretory endometrium. The endometrial stroma becomes loose and edematous, and blood vessels entering the endometrium become thickened and twisted. The endometrial glands, which were straight and tubular in the proliferative phase of the endometrium, become tortuous and contain secretory material within the lumina. Following ovulation, distinct, recognizable changes occur within the endometrium at almost daily intervals. Therefore, the quality of the corpus luteum and stage of the

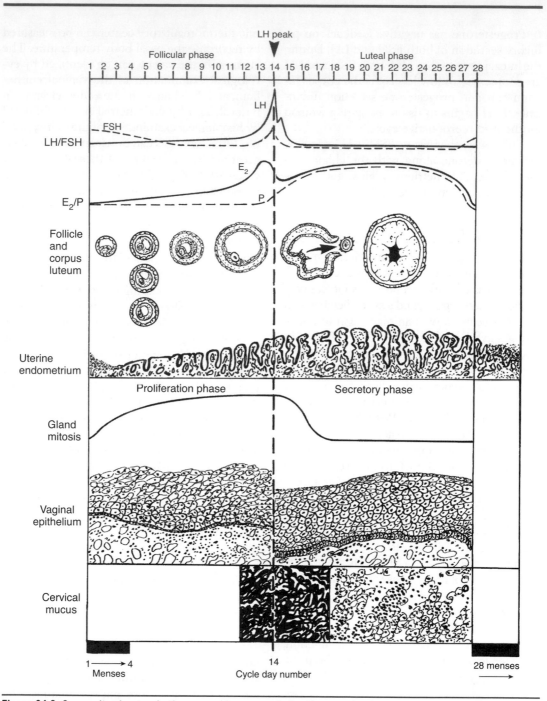

Figure 34.6. Composite changes in tissues and hormones during the reproductive cycle.

reproductive cycle can be evaluated by histological examination of a sample of endometrium. With the withdrawal of progesterone at the end of the luteal phase, the endometrium undergoes breakdown and is sloughed during menses.

Endocervix

The endocervix contains glands that secrete endocervical mucus in response to hormonal changes. Under the influence of estradiol, the endocervical glands secrete large quantities of thin, clear, watery, mucus. This mucus facilitates sperm capture, sperm storage, and sperm transport. Sperm can be stored in the crypts of the endocervical glands for up to 7 days (average 2 days) and then released into the upper genital tract for fertilization of an oocyte. Endocervical mucous production is maximal at the time of ovulation. With ovulation and the shift in hormone production from estradiol to progesterone, the endocervical mucus becomes thick, opaque, and tenacious. This type of mucus is an impediment to sperm capture, storage, and transport. Some women monitor their mucus to assist in trying to conceive or avoid conception; however, the timing of these changes is nonspecific, and it tends to be unreliable for contraception.

Breasts

The ductal elements of the breasts, nipples, and areolae respond to progesterone secretion. After ovulation, progesterone stimulates the acinar (milk-producing) glands. Because the acinar glands are located in the tails of the breasts, this gives the breasts a more rounded configuration. Moreover, progesterone makes the venous pattern on the surface of the breasts appear more prominent and accentuates the small Montgomery glands contained within the areolae. Some patients will complain of more breast tenderness in the luteal phase due to these progestin-mediated changes.

Vagina

Estradiol stimulates vaginal thickening and maturation of the surface epithelial cells of the vaginal mucosa. Estradiol also facilitates vaginal transudation during sexual excitement, creating a moist, lubricated vagina for sexual intercourse. During the luteal phase of the cycle, the vaginal epithelium retains its thickness, but the secretory changes are markedly diminished.

Hypothalamic Thermoregulating Center

Progesterone shifts the basal body temperature upward by 0.6°F to 1.0°F. This shift occurs abruptly with the beginning of the progesterone secretion and wanes abruptly with loss of progesterone secretion. The changes in the basal body temperature reflect the changing plasma progesterone concentration. To be useful for the evaluation of ovulatory function, the patient must have a normal night's sleep (without interruption), and the temperature must be taken when the patient first awakens and before any activity (see Figure 39.3).

CHAPTER 35

PUBERTY

This chapter deals primarily with APGO Educational Topic:

Topic 42: Puberty

Students should be able to discuss normal puberty, including the physiological events involving the neuroendocrine axis and end organs and how they are expressed in the stages of puberty and the psychosocial issues of puberty and adolescence. Students should also be able to discuss the abnormalities of pubertal development and their evaluation and management.

Puberty is the physical, emotional, and sexual transition from childhood to adulthood, occurring gradually in a series of well-defined events and milestones. Few individuals have problems with this endocrine process. However, when puberty is delayed or advanced, an understanding of the hormonal events of puberty and the sequence of physical changes is essential. Moreover, an understanding of puberty is essential for an understanding of the process of reproduction.

Normal Pubertal Development

The endocrine events that initiate the onset of secondary sexual maturation are only partially understood. The hypothalamic–pituitary–gonadal axis functions during fetal life and during the first few weeks following birth, after which the axis becomes quiescent. This suppression of hypothalamic–pituitary–gonadal axis is because of enhanced negative feedback at the pituitary and the presence of a central inhibitor factor. At approximately the age of 8 in boys and 6 to 8 in girls, the adrenal glands begin to secrete increasing quantities of dehydroepiandrosterone; approximately 2 years later, the gonads begin secreting sex steroid hormones. The process of secondary sexual maturation requires approximately 4 years from its beginning until full sexual maturation has been achieved; this process takes place in an orderly, predictable sequence (Figure 35.1). The events, age, and hormone(s) responsible for the sequence of *sexual maturation* in girls are presented in Table 35.1. The initial event is acceleration in growth; however, this may be subtle, and breast budding is easier to detect as the first event. The sequence of breast development (*thelarche*) and the pubic hair growth (*adrenarche*) is presented in Figure 1.4 and is often referred to as the *sexual maturation index*. About 10% of girls (more commonly in African Americans) will have adrenarche prior to thelarche.

Three known critical elements play a role in the timing of *secondary sexual maturation*. These are adequate body fat, adequate sleep, and vision (optic exposure to sunlight). Girls must

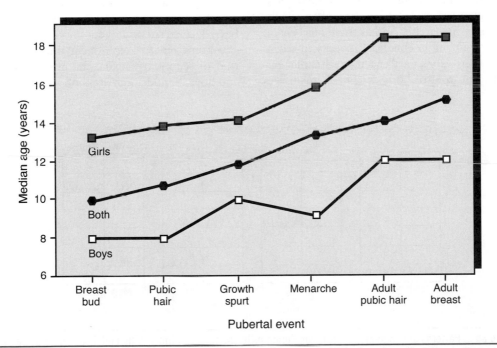

Figure 35.1. Expected sequence of events in puberty. The median age at which six major milestones in the process of puberty occur is shown. Each event may occur over a wide range of "normal" ages, making prediction difficult. When events fall outside these age ranges, however, further evaluation is indicated. (From Smith RP. *Gynecology in Primary Care.* Baltimore: Williams & Wilkins, 1996, p. 169.)

Table 35.1. Sequence of Sexual Maturation in Girls

Event	Age (Years)	Hormone(s)
Breast budding	10–11	Estradiol
Sexual hair growth	10.5–11.5	Androgens
Growth spurt	11–12	Growth hormone
Menarche	11.5–13	Estradiol
Adult breast development	12.5–15	Progesterone
Adult sexual hair	13.5–16	Androgens

attain a *critical body weight*–irrespective of height–before breast development begins. Moreover, a body weight of *85 to 106 pounds* must be achieved before menses begins, and a proportion of *body fat of 16% to 24%* is required to sustain ovulatory cycles. Girls who engage in strenuous exercise programs before puberty often have delayed sexual development, and those who are obese as children often experience early menarche. And as there has been at least a doubling in childhood obesity in recent times, there is also a trend toward earlier puberty. The role of body weight in male secondary sexual maturation and reproductive function is not well defined.

Sleep has varying effects on the gonadotropin secretory pattern in prepubertal children, intrapubertal children, and sexually mature adolescents (Figure 35.2). In prepubertal children, there is no correlation between sleep cycle and gonadotropin secretion. In intrapubertal adolescents–girls who have breast development and sexual hair growth but who have not menstruated and boys who have penile and testicular enlargement but who have not ejaculated–there is a sleep-entrained gonadotropin secretory cycle. That is, during sleep, there is a marked increase in the secretion of follicle-stimulating hormone (FSH) and luteinizing hormone (LH), though the amounts vary depending on gender. In sexually mature adolescents, the release of gonadotropins bears no relationship to the sleep cycle. Instead, gonadotropins are released at 6- to 8-hour intervals, a pattern that is maintained for the remainder of a person's reproductive life unless reproductive dysfunction occurs.

Optic exposure to sunlight is essential for timely secondary sexual development. Blind girls have delayed menarche, and blind boys have delayed spermatogenesis and ejaculation.

Abrupt *mood changes* occur during the period of secondary sexual maturation in girls and boys. Periods of depression, euphoria, and

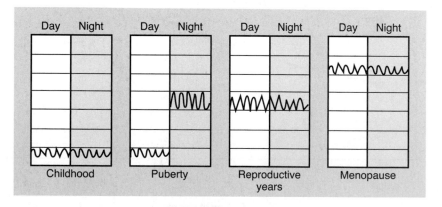

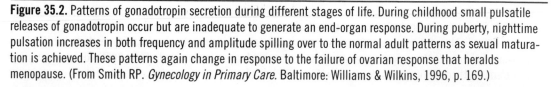

Figure 35.2. Patterns of gonadotropin secretion during different stages of life. During childhood small pulsatile releases of gonadotropin occur but are inadequate to generate an end-organ response. During puberty, nighttime pulsation increases in both frequency and amplitude spilling over to the normal adult patterns as sexual maturation is achieved. These patterns again change in response to the failure of ovarian response that heralds menopause. (From Smith RP. *Gynecology in Primary Care.* Baltimore: Williams & Wilkins, 1996, p. 169.)

even violent behavior occur to some extent in many intrapubertal adolescents. Once full sexual maturation—with release of gametes—is completed, these mood changes disappear, so the physician can reassure the young person and concerned parents that the mood changes will abate with time.

Abnormalities of Pubertal Development

The abnormalities of puberty include delayed sexual maturation, incomplete sexual maturation, primary amenorrhea, and precocious puberty. The presence of any of these disorders requires investigation of *both* the hypothalamic–pituitary–gonadal axis *and* the reproductive outflow tract. The initial investigation must begin with measurement of pituitary gonadotropins (FSH and LH). These hormones distinguish a hypothalamic-pituitary etiology from a gonadal etiology.

Delayed Sexual Maturation

The first noticeable step in sexual maturation is breast budding in 90% of girls, which usually begins at a mean age of 10.5 years. The earliest normal breast development occurs at 6 or 7 years, and this falls within the range of normal. However, if breast budding does not begin by 13 years, puberty may be delayed or may not begin spontaneously. *Failure to establish a breast bud by age 13* should cause the physician to initiate an endocrine evaluation to elucidate the cause of pubertal delay. In about 10% of girls, sexual hair growth may precede breast budding. However, *if sexual hair growth precedes breast budding by more than 6 to 9 months,* the physician should likewise initiate an endocrine evaluation. The most *common causes of delayed puberty* are presented in Table 35.2.

Premature Ovarian Failure

Ovarian failure can occur anytime before the expected time of menopause. *Ovarian failure is characterized by diminished or absent estrogen production in association with elevated gonadotropins.* The most common etiology of premature ovarian failure seen in prepubertal and pubertal girls is *Turner syndrome.* The features of Turner syndrome are failure to establish secondary sexual development along with so-

Table 35.2. Causes of Delayed Puberty or Menstruation

Premature ovarian failure
- Turner syndrome
- Long-arm X chromosomal deletion
- Alkylating chemotherapy

Inadequate gonadotropin-releasing hormone secretion
- Olfactory tract hypoplasia (Kallmann syndrome)
- Constitutional delayed puberty
- Craniopharyngioma
- Hypothalamic hamartoma
- Marijuana use

Inadequate gonadotropin secretion
- Isolated gonadotropin deficiency
- Prolactin-secreting pituitary adenoma
- Other space-occupying lesions of the sella turcica

Inadequate body fat
- Anorexia nervosa
- Exercise-induced hypothalamic dysfunction

Genital tract abnormalities
- Imperforate hymen
- Cervical agenasis
- Transverse vagianl septum
- Vaginal and uterine agenesis (Rokitansky-Küster-Hauser syndrome)

Other
- Pelvic radiation
- Galactosemia
- Idiopathic

matic changes such as short stature, a webbed neck (pterygium colli), a shield chest with widely spaced nipples, and an increased carrying angle of the elbows (cubitus valgus) among others. There is a window of gonadotropin suppression between about 2 years of age through the initiation of puberty. So even Turner's patient will have low FSH and LH values during this prepubertal window and then the FSH will rise at puberty.

The fundamental genetic defect in girls with Turner syndrome is the absence of an X chro-

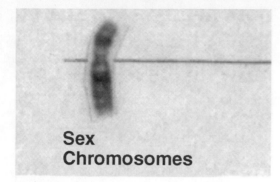

Sex Chromosomes

Figure 35.3. Karyotype of Turner syndrome: 45,X, one of the X chromosomes is missing. Approximately 50% of people with Turner syndrome have this 45,X karyotype; 15% have 46,X,i [XqO]; 25% have 45,X/46,XX;46,XY;47,XXX; and 2% to 3% each have 46,X,Xp- and 46,X,r[X].

mosome (45,X, Figure 35.3). On buccal smear there are no Barr bodies seen. Genetic information that regulates the rate of ovarian follicular atresia is carried on the long arm of the X chromosome, whereas somatic information is carried on the short arm of the X chromosome. The absence of the entire X chromosome leads to loss of ovarian function and to the somatic features described earlier.

Partial deletions of the long arm of the X chromosome cause premature ovarian failure to occur at varying chronological ages. For example, complete loss of the long arm of the X chromosome results in premature ovarian failure before puberty, whereas a small fragmentary loss of the X chromosome may not result in ovarian failure until many years after a normal puberty. Other karyotypical abnormalities, though rare, may also lead to premature ovarian failure.

When breast development fails to occur at the expected age or when breast development begins and then fails to be completed, the clinician should consider premature ovarian failure. This diagnosis is established easily by the finding of elevated gonadotropins in association with decreased levels of ovarian sex hormones. Any time elevated gonadotropins are noted in women under 40, a Karyotype should be performed. Estrogen administration should be initiated at the normal time of initiation of puberty, and growth hormone should be initiated very

early (often prior to estrogen therapy) and aggressively to normalize adult height. Estrogen is necessary to stimulate breast development, genital tract maturation, and the beginning of menstruation. Administration of a low dose of estrogen is used to initiate secondary sexual maturation. Estradiol-17β (Estrace), 0.5 mg/day, or conjugated equine estrogens (Premarin), 0.3 mg/day, is an appropriate starting dose. Once breast budding begins, the dosage may be doubled. The usual dose of estrogen to initiate menarche is estradiol-17β, 2 mg/day or conjugated equine estrogens, 1.25 mg/day. Once menarche occurs, medroxyprogesterone (Provera), 5 to 10 mg for 10 to 14 days every month will complete breast development and produce cyclic uterine bleeding. If an excessive amount of estrogen is administered initially, epiphyseal closure may begin, and long bone growth will be truncated and adult height compromised. A delay in estrogen administration can lead to the development of osteoporosis beginning during the teenage years. Progestins should not be started until the patient has reached Tanner Stage IV because premature progestin therapy may blunt the full development of the breast and may result in an abnormal contour (a more tubular breast).

Hypothalamic Dysfunction

The arcuate nucleus of the hypothalamus secretes gonadotropin-releasing hormone (GnRH) in cyclic bursts (or a pulsatile fashion), which stimulates release of gonadotropins from the anterior pituitary gland. Dysfunction of the arcuate nucleus disrupts the short hormonal loop between the hypothalamus and pituitary, resulting in absent FSH or LH secretion. Consequently, the ovaries are not stimulated to secrete estradiol, and secondary sexual maturation is delayed.

An unusual cause of hypothalamic dysfunction is *Kallmann syndrome*. In this disorder, the olfactory tracts are hypoplastic, and the arcuate nucleus does not secrete GnRH. Young women with Kallmann syndrome have little or no sense of smell and fail to have breast development. The diagnosis of this condition can be made on initial physical examination by challenging olfactory function with known odors such as coffee or rubbing alcohol. Once recognized, the prognosis for successful secondary sexual maturation and reproduction is excellent in Kallmann syndrome: Secondary sexual maturation can be stimulated by the administration of exogenous hormones or by the administration of pulsatile GnRH. Ovulation can be induced by exogenous gonadotropin administration or by administration of pulsatile GnRH. Once pregnancy is established, the lack of pituitary secretions has no adverse effects. After ovulation, the luteal phase needs to be supported by progesterone to enable a pregnancy to implant. After the pregnancy is well established and no longer relies on progesterone (8 to 10 weeks) this may be discontinued.

Other causes of hypothalamic amenorrhea include simple weight loss, strenuous exercise (such as ballet dancer or long-distance runner), anorexia nervosa, or bulimia. These conditions all result in suppressed gonadotropin levels with low estrogen levels. The correction of the underlying abnormality (such as weight gain in the simple weight-loss patient) results in restoration of normal gonadotropin levels, stimulating ovarian steroidogenesis, and resumption of pubertal development.

Less-common causes of hypothalamic dysfunction are *neoplasms and inflammatory disorders of the hypothalamic–pituitary axis.* Examples are craniopharyngioma, hamartoma of the pituitary stalk, and sarcoidosis of the hypothalamus. More than 70% of sarcoid cases are associated with calcifications in the suprasellar region on plain skull radiograph. In a child with delayed puberty and evidence of hypogonadotropic hypogonadism, it is important to evaluate the pituitary for its remaining functions. A magnetic resonance image of the hypothalamic–pituitary area is indicated to rule out a sellar or suprasellar neoplasm.

Use of marijuana by prepubertal and intrapubertal boys and girls delays the onset of puberty. Marijuana blocks the release of GnRH from the hypothalamus; thus marijuana truncates gonadotropin secretion by the pituitary gland, which in turn delays gonadal function. With the increasing incidence of drug abuse by adolescents, this must be considered in the differential diagnosis of hypogonadotropic-hypogonadism.

Genital Tract Anomalies

During fetal life, müllerian ducts develop and fuse in the female fetus to form the upper reproductive tract (i.e., the fallopian tubes, uterus, and upper vagina). The lower and midportion of the vagina develop from the canalization of the genital plate. Approximately 1 in 10,000 females has a birth defect of the reproductive tract that presents as primary amenorrhea and normal secondary sexual characteristics. The simplest genital tract anomaly is *imperforate hymen.* In this condition, the genital plate canalization is incomplete, and the hymen is, therefore, closed. Menarche occurs at the appropriate time, but because there is obstruction to the passage of menstrual blood, it is not apparent. This condition presents with pain in the area of the uterus and a bulging bluish-appearing vaginal introitus. Hymenotomy is the definitive therapy.

This may be confused with a transverse vaginal septum. Transverse vaginal septa can occur along the vagina at any level and result in obstruction to outflow of menses. A vaginal septum can be resected and primarily repaired with a Z-vaginoplasty. Prolonged obstructions to menstruation are associated with a high rate of endometriosis.

In *müllerian agenesis (Rokitansky–Küster–Hauser syndrome),* the uterus is absent along with the cervix and vagina. All the secondary sexual characteristics of puberty occur at the proper time, as ovarian development is unaffected. The young woman establishes normal breast development, sexual hair growth, and ovulation. Yet, there is no menstruation. Physical examination leads to the diagnosis of müllerian agenesis. Renal anomalies (e.g., reduplication of the ureters, horseshoe kidney, or unilateral renal agenesis) occur in 25% to 35% of cases. Skeletal anomalies such as scoliosis occur in 15% to 25% of these women. Rokitansky–Küster–Hauser syndrome is generally sporadic in expression, although families displaying autosomal recessive inheritance have been documented. If there is an affected child, the estimated risk of recurrence in future female siblings is approximately 4%; there is no way to determine whether the inheritance is familial or sporadic.

There are several therapeutic approaches to this condition. Nonsurgical approaches should be tried first using dilators and pressure on the dimple between the urethra and the rectum, twice a day. This tissue is quite pliable and with increasing dilator size, a normal-length vagina can be achieved. Ingram developed a bicycle seat for such use by the patient at home. An artificial vagina may be created by repetitive pressure by vaginal dilators to the perineum or by surgical construction followed by a split-thickness skin graft. After creation of a vagina, these women are able to have sexual intercourse. With the advances in assisted reproductive technologies, including in vitro fertilization (IVF) and use of a surrogate mother (gestational carrier), it is possible for women with this condition to have a genetic child by using her oocytes.

Precocious Puberty

If physical signs of *secondary sexual development appear before the age of 6 to 8 years,* the physician should consider the diagnosis of precocious puberty. Precocious puberty occurs in girls more frequently than in boys. Most precocious puberty is isosexual (i.e., the sequence of pubertal events is appropriate for sexual development and leads to full sexual maturation). Precocious puberty is secondary to either GnRH dependent or GnRH independent sex hormone production. In girls, the most common etiology is idiopathic, and CNS tumors are much lower in incidence. In boys, it is much more likely that a CNS tumor is present. Hamartomas secreting FSH and LH are fairly common. Surgical therapy is indicated. Some data suggests that hamartomas may be observed without surgery. *Idiopathic isosexual precocious puberty* has no serious pathology and is GnRH dependent with premature activation of the arcuate nucleus in the hypothalamus. It causes an advance in sexual maturation with early reproductive capability and carries the risk of short stature because of premature closure of the epiphyseal plates. These individuals are also at high risk for sexual abuse and have psychosocial issues related to their early development.

Occasionally, GnRH dependent, isosexual precocious puberty results from *neoplasms of the hypothalamic–pituitary stalk or transient inflammatory conditions of the hypothalamus.* In these situations, although sexual development be-

gins early, the rate of sexual development is slower than the usual rate. In the case of inflammatory conditions, sexual development may begin and end abruptly. Laboratory studies show either an appropriate rise in gonadotropins or a steady gonadotropin level in the prepubertal range.

GnRH independent precocious puberty may be the result of *inappropriate secretion of androgens or estrogens.* The most common cause of inappropriate androgen secretion is *congenital adrenal hyperplasia of the 21-hydroxylase type.* In this disorder, the adrenal glands are unable to produce adequate amounts of cortisol as a result of a partial block in the conversion of 17-hydroxyprogesterone to desoxycorticosterone. The degree of the block in 21-hydroxylase determines the phenotypic characteristics of salt wasting or simple virilizing types. Deficiency of this enzyme leads to an accumulation and release of precursor adrenal androgens, which results in precocious adrenarche. In girls, there is premature development of pubic hair followed by axillary hair called premature adrenarche. Breast development either does not occur or is incomplete for the stage of sexual development. Measurement of elevated adrenal androgens–such as dehydroepiandrosterone (DHEA), dehydroepiandrosterone sulfate (DHEA-S), and androstenedione–are supportive of the diagnosis. A pathognomonic finding for 21-hydroxylase deficiency is an elevated 17-hydroxyprogesterone level. Medical therapy consists of steroid replacement, a standard regimen being hydrocortisone (10–15 mg/M2/day) in divided doses (or its equivalent), with fludrocortisone 0.1 mg/day (higher dose in the neonatal period) for those afflicted with salt wasting. Therapy should be instituted as early as possible to achieve maximum benefit and to avoid reduced adult height (Figure 35.4). Surgical therapy is often also required in the classical form of this disease, which presents at birth with ambiguous genitalia, depending on the degree and nature of the effect, including removal of redundant erectile tissue with preservation of the sensitive glans clitoris and vulvoplasty to allow for menstruation and sexual intercourse. In the nonclassical form of congenital adrenal hyperplasia (CAH), patients present with premature adrenarche present at

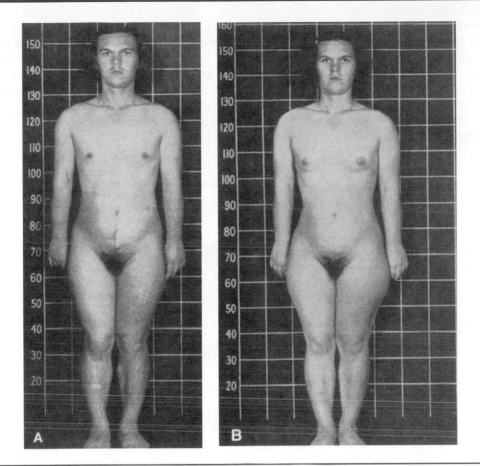

Figure 35.4. Medical treatment of congenital adrenal hyperplasia. (**A**) Untreated 16-year-old with characteristic short stature, short arms and legs, absence of breast development, and growth of hair on body and face. (**B**) Same patient after 3 months of cortisone therapy. Note alteration of body habitus to a more feminine configuration and reduction of hirsutism.

puberty with anovulation and hyperandrogenism, appearing somewhat like polycystic ovarian syndrome (PCO) patients.

In boys with this condition, there is premature enlargement of the phallus and the appearance of axillary and pubic hair. However, the testicles remain small because the source of androgens is of adrenal rather than of testicular origin. Again, adrenal hormones are elevated.

Another rare cause of GnRH independent precocity is *inappropriate secretion of estrogens* in girls. This can result from ovarian neoplasms or from McCune–Albright syndrome. McCune–Albright syndrome is characterized by café-au-lait spots, polyostotic fibrous dysplasia of the bones, and precocious puberty. The

molecular basis of McCune–Albright syndrome is a somatic, activating mutation in the G protein, resulting in constitutive activation of the G-protein-coupled-receptors of affected cells. If these mutations occur in the ovary, they produce autonomously functioning follicular cysts with hormone production. In these conditions, there is rapid breast development without sexual hair growth. Menarche may be established within a few months of thelarche. In males chorionic gonadotropin production by hepatic, gonadal, or pineal neoplasms can result in precocious puberty. In this scenario the hCG stimulates the testicular Leydig cells and results in testosterone production. In males an activating mutation in the LH receptor also can result in precocious puberty.

Isosexual precocious puberty can be treated by the tonic administration of an exogenous GnRH agonist. These agents block the periodic secretion of GnRH and suppress pituitary gonadotropin secretion. If precocious puberty is within a few months of the expected time of normal puberty, it is probably wise to allow puberty to progress. However, if puberty or the bone age is advanced by several years, the process should be arrested. If the events of puberty do not progress in the expected way, an evaluation for hormonal abnormalities and/or hypothalamic–pituitary tumors is advised. If an abnormality is found, it should be treated specifically.

CHAPTER 36

AMENORRHEA AND DYSFUNCTIONAL UTERINE BLEEDING

This chapter deals primarily with APGO Educational Topics:

Topic 43: Amenorrhea

Students should be able to discuss the endocrine and anatomic causes of the absence of menstruation (amenorrhea) and irregular menstruation (oligomenorrhea) and their evaluation and management.

Topic 45: Normal and abnormal uterine bleeding

Students should be able to discuss the normal menstrual cycle and the evaluation and management of the causes of menses at times other than expected (abnormal uterine bleeding).

Amenorrhea and dysfunctional uterine bleeding are the most common gynecologic disorders of reproductive-age women. *Absence of menstruation is amenorrhea; irregular menstruation without anatomic lesions of the uterus is dysfunctional uterine bleeding.* Amenorrhea and dysfunctional uterine bleeding are discussed as separate topics in this chapter. However, the pathophysiology underlying amenorrhea and dysfunctional uterine bleeding are often the same.

Amenorrhea

If a young woman has never menstruated by age 14 without secondary sexual development or by 16 with secondary sexual development, this is classified as having *primary amenorrhea.* If a menstrual-aged woman has previously menstruated but has failed to menstruate for 6 months, she is classified as having *secondary amenorrhea.* The designation of primary or secondary amenorrhea has no bearing on the severity of the underlying disorder or on the prognosis for restoring cyclic ovulation. Terms often confused with these include *oligomenorrhea,* defined as a reduction of the frequency of menses, with the interval being >40 days but <6 months, and *hypomenorrhea,* defined as a reduction in the number of days or the amount of menstrual flow. Amenorrhea not caused by pregnancy occurs in 5% or less of all women during their menstrual lives.

Causes of Amenorrhea

When there is disruption of hypothalamic–pituitary–ovarian endocrine function or alteration of the genital outflow tract (obstruction of the uterus, cervix, or vagina or scarring of the endometrium), menstruation ceases. Causes of amenorrhea are divided into those arising from (1) pregnancy, (2) hypothalamic–pituitary dysfunction, (3) ovarian dysfunction, and (4) alteration of the genital outflow tract.

Pregnancy

Because the most common cause of amenorrhea is pregnancy, it is essential to exclude pregnancy in the evaluation of amenorrhea. A history of breast fullness, weight gain, nausea, and a "feeling of being pregnant" suggest the diagnosis of pregnancy, whereas the diagnosis is confirmed by a positive human chorionic gonadotropin assay. It is important to rule out pregnancy to allay the patient's anxiety and to avoid unnecessary testing. Also, some of the treatments for other causes of amenorrhea can be harmful to an ongoing pregnancy.

Hypothalamic–Pituitary Dysfunction

Release of hypothalamic gonadotropin-releasing hormone (GnRH) occurs in a pulsatile fashion, modulated by catecholamine secretion from the central nervous system and by feedback of sex steroids from the ovaries. When this pulsatile secretion of GnRH is disrupted or altered, the anterior pituitary gland is not stimulated to secrete follicle-stimulating hormone (FSH) and luteinizing hormone (LH). The result is an absence of folliculogenesis despite estrogen production, no ovulation, and lack of corpus luteum, with its usual production of estrogen and progesterone. Because of the lack of sex hormone production with no stimulation of the endometrium, there is no menstruation.

Alterations in catecholamine secretion and metabolism in sex steroid hormone feedback or an alteration of blood flow through the hypothalamic–pituitary portal plexus can disrupt the signaling process that leads to ovulation. This latter disruption can be caused by tumors or infiltrative processes that impinge on the pituitary stalk and alter blood flow.

The most common causes of hypothalamic–pituitary dysfunction are presented in Table 36.1. Most hypothalamic–pituitary amenorrhea is of functional origin and can be corrected by modifying causal behavior, by stimulating gonadotropin secretion, or by giving exogenous human menopausal gonadotropins.

The physician cannot differentiate hypothalamic–pituitary causes of amenorrhea from ovarian or genital outflow causes by medical history or even physical examination alone. However, there are some clues in the medical history and physical examination that would suggest a hypothalamic–pituitary etiology for amenorrhea. A history of any condition listed in Table 36.1 should cause the physician to consider hypothalamic–pituitary dysfunction.

Table 36.1. Causes of Hypothalamic–Pituitary Amenorrhea
Functional causes
Weight loss
Excessive exercise
Obesity
Drug-induced causes
Marijuana
Tranquilizers
Neoplastic causes
Prolactin-secreting pituitary adenomas
Craniopharyngioma
Hypothalamic hamartoma
Psychogenic causes
Chronic anxiety
Pseudocyesis
Anorexia nervosa
Other causes
Head injury
Chronic medical illness

The way to definitively identify hypothalamic–pituitary dysfunction is to measure FSH, LH, and prolactin in blood. In these conditions, FSH and LH are in the low range. Prolactin is normal in most conditions but is elevated in prolactin-secreting pituitary adenomas.

Ovarian Dysfunction

In ovarian failure, the ovarian follicles are either exhausted or are resistant to stimulation by pituitary FSH and LH. As the ovaries fail, *blood concentrations of FSH and LH increase.* Women with ovarian failure experience the symptoms and signs of estrogen deficiency.

A summary of causes is presented in Table 36.2. A detailed description of these causes is presented in Chapter 38.

Obstruction of the Genital Outflow Tract

Obstruction of the genital outflow tract prevents overt menstrual bleeding even if ovulation occurs. Most cases of outflow obstruction result from congenital *abnormalities in the development and canalization of the müllerian ducts.*

Imperforate hymen and no uterus and/or vagina are the most common anomalies that result in primary amenorrhea. Surgical correction of an imperforate hymen allows for menstruation and fertility. Less-commonly encountered anomalies such as a transverse vaginal septum are more difficult to correct, and even with attempted surgical correction, menstruation and fertility are often not restored.

Scarring of the uterine cavity (Asherman's syndrome) is the most frequent anatomic cause of secondary amenorrhea. Women who undergo dilation and curettage (D&C) for retained products of pregnancy are at risk for developing scarring of the endometrium. Cases of mild scarring can be corrected by surgical lysis of the adhesions performed by hysteroscopy and D&C. However, severe cases are often refractory to therapy. Estrogen therapy should be added to the surgical treatment postoperatively to stimulate endometrial regeneration of the denuded areas. In some cases, a balloon or IUCD may be placed in the uterine cavity to help keep the uterine walls apart during healing.

Treatment of Amenorrhea

It is essential to first establish a cause for the amenorrhea. The progesterone "challenge test" is commonly used to determine whether or not the patient has adequate estrogen, a competent endometrium, and a patent outflow

Table 36.2. Causes of Ovarian Failure
Chromosomal causes
Turner's syndrome (45,X gonadal dysgenesis)
X chromosome long-arm deletion (46,XX q5)
Unknown causes
Gonadotropin-resistant ovary syndrome (Savage's syndrome)
Premature natural menopause
Immunologic cause
Autoimmune ovarian failure (Blizzard's syndrome)
Iatrogenic causes
Ovarian failure because of effects of alkylating chemotherapy
Menopause ("normal, or physiologic")

tract. An injection of 100 mg of progesterone in oil or a 5- to 14-day course of oral medroxyprogesterone acetate or micronized progesterone is expected to induce progesterone withdrawal bleeding within a few days of completing the oral course. If this does occur, the patient is likely to be anovulatory or oligoovulatory. If withdrawal bleeding does not occur, the patient is felt to be hypoestrogenic or have an anatomic condition such as Asherman's syndrome or outflow tract obstruction.

The *hyperprolactinemia associated with some pituitary adenomas* results in amenorrhea and galactorrhea. Approximately 80% of all pituitary tumors secrete prolactin, causing galactorrhea, and these are treated with either cabergoline (Dostinex) or the dopamine agonist *bromocriptine (Parlodel)*. In approximately 5% of patients with hyperprolactinemia and galactorrhea, the underlying etiology is hypothyroidism. A low serum thyroxine (T_4) level results in a lack of negative feedback to the hypothalamic–pituitary axis with increased TRH (thyrotropin-releasing hormone). In addition, there is a lack of positive feedback on dopamine. Elevated TRH stimulates release of prolactin from the pituitary gland. The reduced dopamine secretion results in elevated levels of TSH (thyroid-stimulating hormone) and prolactin.

In patients who desire pregnancy, ovulation can be induced through use of clomiphene citrate, human menopausal gonadotropins, pulsatile GnRH, or aromatase inhibitors. In patients who are oligo-ovulatory or anovulatory (polycystic ovary syndrome), ovulation can usually be induced with clomiphene citrate. In patients with hypogonadotropic hypogonadism ovulation can be induced with pulsatile GnRH or human menopausal gonadotropins. (see Chapter 39). Women with genital tract obstruction require surgery to create a vagina or to restore genital tract integrity. Menstruation will never be established if the uterus is absent. Women with premature ovarian failure require exogenous estrogen replacement. Hormone replacement regimens are discussed in Chapter 38.

Dysfunctional Uterine Bleeding

Failure to ovulate results in either amenorrhea or irregular uterine bleeding. *Irregular bleeding,*

unrelated to anatomic lesions of the uterus, is referred to as dysfunctional uterine bleeding. Dysfunctional uterine bleeding is most likely to occur in association with anovulation as found in polycystic ovarian disease, exogenous obesity, or adrenal hyperplasia.

Women with hypothalamic amenorrhea (hypothalamic–pituitary dysfunction) and no genital tract obstruction are in a state of estrogen deficiency. Estrogen is inadequate to stimulate growth and development of the endometrium. Therefore, there is inadequate endometrium for uterine bleeding to occur. In contrast, *women with oligo-ovulation and anovulation with dysfunctional uterine bleeding* have constant, noncyclic blood estrogen concentrations that stimulate growth and development of the endometrium. Without the predictable effect of ovulation, there are no progesterone-induced changes. Initially these patients have amenorrhea because of the chronic, constant estrogen levels, but eventually, the endometrium outgrows its blood supply and sloughs from the uterus at irregular times and in unpredictable amounts.

When there is chronic stimulation of the endometrium from low plasma concentrations of estrogens, the episodes of dysfunctional uterine bleeding are infrequent and light. Alternatively, with chronic stimulation of the endometrium from increased plasma concentrations of estrogens, the episodes of dysfunctional uterine bleeding can be frequent and heavy. Because amenorrhea and dysfunctional uterine bleeding both result from anovulation, it is not surprising that they can occur at different times in the same patient.

Dysfunctional uterine bleeding can occasionally occur in association with ovulation. Although this may seem a contradiction, subtle alterations in the mechanisms of ovulation can produce abnormal cycles, even when ovulation occurs (e.g., the luteal phase defect). In the *luteal phase defect,* ovulation does occur; however, the corpus luteum of the ovary is not fully developed to secrete adequate quantities of progesterone to support the endometrium for the usual 13 to 14 days and is not adequate to support a pregnancy if conception does occur. The menstrual cycle is shortened, and menstruation occurs earlier than expected. Although this is not classical dysfunctional uterine bleeding, it is considered to be in the same category. Another example is mid-cycle spotting in which patients report bleeding at the time of ovulation. Without demonstrable pathology, this self-limited bleeding can be attributed to the sudden drop in estrogen level at this time of the cycle.

Diagnosis of Dysfunctional Uterine Bleeding

Dysfunctional uterine bleeding should be suspected when vaginal bleeding is not regular, not predictable, and not associated with the premenstrual molimina that usually accompanies ovulatory cycles. Moliminal symptoms include breast fullness, abdominal bloating, mood changes, edema, weight gain, and menstrual cramps.

Before a diagnosis of dysfunctional uterine bleeding is made, anatomic causes of abnormal uterine bleeding must be excluded. In a reproductive-aged female, one wants to exclude complications of pregnancy as a cause of irregular vaginal bleeding. Other anatomic causes of irregular vaginal bleeding include uterine leiomyomata, inflammation/infection of the genital tract, carcinoma of the cervix or endometrium, cervical erosions, cervical polyps, and lesions of the vagina (Table 36.3). Pelvic ultrasonography or sonohysterography may assist in diagnosing these lesions. Women with organic causes for bleeding typically have regular ovulatory cycles with superimposed irregular bleeding.

If the diagnosis is uncertain from history and physical examination alone, a woman may keep a basal body temperature chart for 6 to 8 weeks to look for the shift in the basal temperature that occurs with ovulation or an ovulation kit may be used. A luteal phase progestin may also be measured. In the cases of anovulation and irregular bleeding, an endometrial biopsy may reveal endometrial hyperplasia. Because dysfunctional uterine bleeding results from chronic, unopposed estrogenic stimulation of the endometrium, the endometrium appears proliferative or, with prolonged estrogenic stimulation, hyperplastic. Without treatment, these women are at increased risk for developing endometrial cancer.

Table 36.3. Anatomic Causes of Irregular Bleeding

Uterine lesions
  Myomas
  Polyps
  Endometrial carcinoma
Cervical lesions
  Neoplasia
  Polyps
  Cervical eversion
  Cervicitis
  Cervical condyloma
Vaginal lesions
  Carcinoma, sarcoma, or adenosis
  Laceration or trauma
  Infections
  Foreign bodies (diaphragm, tampons)
  Pessaries
Bleeding from other sites
  Urethral caruncle
  Infected urethral diverticulum
  Gastrointestinal bleeding
  Labial lesion (neoplasm, trauma, infection)

Treatment of Dysfunctional Uterine Bleeding

The risks to a woman with dysfunctional uterine bleeding include anemia, incapacitating blood loss, endometrial hyperplasia, and/or carcinoma. Uterine bleeding can be severe enough to require hospitalization. Both hemorrhage and endometrial hyperplasia can be prevented by appropriate management.

The primary goal of treatment of dysfunctional uterine bleeding is to convert the proliferative endometrium into secretory endometrium, which results in predictable uterine withdrawal bleeding. This goal can be achieved by administration of a progestational agent for a minimum of 10 days, the most commonly used being medroxyprogesterone acetate. When the progestational agent is discontinued, uterine withdrawal bleeding ensues, thereby mimicking physiologic withdrawal of progesterone.

As an alternative, administration of oral contraceptives suppresses the endometrium and establishes regular, predictable withdrawal cycles. No particular oral contraceptive preparation is better than any of the others for this purpose. Women who take oral contraceptives as treatment of dysfunctional uterine bleeding often resume dysfunctional uterine bleeding after therapy is discontinued.

If a patient is being treated for a particularly heavy bleeding episode, once organic pathology has been ruled out, treatment should focus on two issues: (1) control of the acute episode and (2) prevention of future recurrences. Both high-dose estrogen and progestin therapy as well as combination treatment (oral contraceptive pills, four per day) have been advocated for management of heavy dysfunctional bleeding in the acute phase. Long-term preventive management may include either intermittent progestin treatment or oral contraceptives.

In the patient with irregular vaginal bleeding, especially long-term bleeding, an endometrial biopsy can be helpful in ruling out endometrial hyperplasia or endometrial carcinoma. Dysfunctional uterine bleeding that does not respond to medical therapy often is managed surgically with hysterectomy or endometrial ablation. Before proceeding with endometrial ablation, one must rule out endometrial carcinoma.

CHAPTER 37

HIRSUTISM AND VIRILIZATION

This chapter deals primarily with APGO Educational Topic:

Topic 44: Hirsutism and Virilization

Students should be able to describe normal and abnormal variations in secondary sexual characteristics and hirsutism and virilization. Students should be able to discuss the evaluation and management of each of these issues.

Hirsutism and virilization may be clinical clues to an underlying *androgen excess disorder.* When evaluating and treating hirsutism and virilization, one should consider the sites of androgen production and the mechanisms of androgen action. Idiopathic (constitutional or familial) hirsutism (a diagnosis of exclusion) is the most common nonpathologic etiology, representing about one-half of all cases. *The most common pathologic cause of hirsutism is polycystic ovarian syndrome; the second-most-common, congenital adrenal hyperplasia.* These conditions must be diagnosed by laboratory evaluations. *Treatment of androgen excess should be directed at suppressing the source of androgen excess or blocking androgen action at the receptor site.*

Hirsutism is defined as excess terminal hair in a male pattern of distribution. It is manifested initially by the appearance of midline *terminal hair.* Terminal hair is darker, coarser, somewhat kinkier than vellus hair, which is soft, downy, and fine. Care must be taken to evaluate the possibility that excess terminal hair is familial, not pathological, in origin. When a woman is exposed to excess androgens, terminal hair first appears on the lower abdomen and around the nipples, next around the chin and upper lip, and finally between the breasts and on the lower back. Usually a woman with hirsutism also has *acne.* For women in Western cultures, terminal hair on the abdomen, breasts, and face is considered unsightly and presents a cosmetic problem. As a result, at the first sign of hirsutism, women often consult their physician to seek a cause for the excess hair growth and seek treatment to eliminate it.

Virilization is defined as masculinization of a woman and is associated with a marked increase in circulating *testosterone.* As a woman becomes virilized, she first notices enlargement of the clitoris followed by temporal balding, deepening of the voice, involution of the breasts, and a remodeling of the limb–shoulder girdle as well as hirsutism. Over time, she takes on a more masculine appearance.

Androgen Production and Androgen Action

In women, *androgens are produced in the adrenal glands, the ovaries, and adipose tissue,* where there is extraglandular production of testosterone from androstenedione. The following three androgens may be measured when evaluating a woman with hirsutism and virilization.

1. *Dehydroepiandrosterone* (DHEA): a weak androgen secreted principally by the *adrenal glands.* (This is generally measured as the sulfate (DHEA-S) because of its longer half-life, making it a more reliable measure.)
2. *Androstenedione:* a weak androgen secreted in equal amounts by the *adrenal glands and ovaries.*
3. *Testosterone:* a potent androgen secreted by the *adrenal glands and ovaries* and produced in *adipose tissue* from the conversion of androstenedione.

The sites of androgen production and proportions produced are presented in Table 37.1. In addition, testosterone is also converted within hair follicles and within genital skin to *dihydrotestosterone* (DHT), which is an androgen even more potent than testosterone. This metabolic conversion is the result of the local action of 5α-reductase on testosterone at these sites. This is the basis for *constitutional hirsutism,* which is discussed later.

Adrenal androgen production is under classic feedback regulation through pituitary secretion of adrenocorticotropic hormone (ACTH). ACTH stimulates the adrenal cortical production of cortisol. In the metabolic sequence of

Table 37.1. Sites of Androgen Production

Site	DHEA-S (%)	Androstenedione (%)	Testosterone (%)
Adrenal glands	90	50	25
Ovaries	10	50	25
Extraglandular	0	0	50

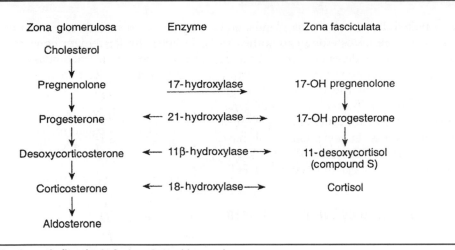

Figure 37.1. A schematic flowchart of adrenal steroidogenesis.

cortisol production, DHEA is one precursor hormone. In enzymatic deficiencies of adrenal steroidogenesis (21-hydroxylase deficiency and 11β hydroxylase deficiency), DHEA accumulates and is further metabolized to androstenedione and testosterone. The flow of adrenal hormone production is shown in Figure 37.1.

Ovarian androgen production is largely under the control of luteinizing hormone (LH) secretion from the pituitary gland. LH stimulates theca-lutein cells surrounding the ovarian follicles to secrete androstenedione and, to a lesser extent, testosterone. These androgens are precursors for estrogen production by granulosa cells of the ovarian follicles. In conditions of sustained or increased LH secretion, androstenedione and testosterone increase. The metabolic relationship between androgens and estrogens is shown in Figure 37.2.

Extraglandular testosterone production occurs in adipocytes (fat cells) and depends on the magnitude of adrenal and ovarian androstenedione production. When androstenedione production increases, there is a dependent increase in extraglandular testosterone production. When a woman becomes obese, the conversion of androstenedione to testosterone in adipocytes increases.

Testosterone is the primary androgen that causes increased hair growth, acne, and the physical changes associated with virilization. After testosterone is secreted, it is bound to a carrier protein—*sex hormone–binding globulin* (SHBG)—and primarily circulates in plasma as a bound steroid

hormone. Bound testosterone is unable to attach to testosterone receptors and is, therefore, metabolically inactive. Only a small fraction (1% to 3%) of testosterone is unbound (free). This small fraction of free hormone exerts the effects. The liver produces SHBG. Estrogens stimulate hepatic production of SHBG. Greater estrogen production is associated with less free testosterone, whereas decreased estrogen production is associated with increased free testosterone. Therefore, measurement of total testosterone alone may not reflect the amount of biologically active testosterone.

Testosterone receptors are scattered throughout the body. For the purpose of this discussion, testosterone receptors are considered

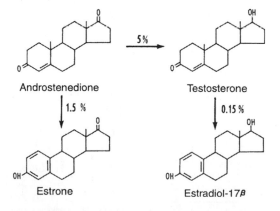

Figure 37.2. The metabolic interrelationships between androgens and estrogens. The percentages indicate the extent of metabolism in adipocytes.

only in hair follicles, sebaceous glands, and genital skin. Free testosterone enters the cytosol of testosterone-dependent cells. There it is bound to a testosterone receptor and carried into the nucleus of the cell to initiate its metabolic action. *When testosterone is excessive,* increased hair growth, acne, and rugation of the genital skin is seen. Some individuals have increased 5α-reductase within hair follicles, resulting in excessive local production of DHT.

Conditions Caused by Ovarian Androgen Excess

Polycystic Ovarian Syndrome

Polycystic ovarian syndrome (PCOS) is the *most common cause of androgen excess and hirsutism.* The etiology of this disorder is unknown. Some cases appear to result from a genetic predisposition, whereas others seem to result from obesity or other causes of LH excess. One proposed mechanism for PCOS is shown in Figure 37.3.

PCOS is a syndrome primarily defined by excess androgen. The definition of PCOS has varied in the past resulting in the NIH conven-ing consensus conferences in 1990 and 2000. In 2003 the Rotterdam consensus workshop developed a more encompassing definition of PCOS that included two of the three following criteria:

- Oligo-ovulation or anovulation usually marked by irregular menstrual cycles
- Biochemical or clinical evidence of hyper-androgenism
- Polycystic appearing ovaries on ultrasound.

It is also important to rule out other endocrine disorders that can mimic PCOS, such as congenital adrenal hyperplasia, Cushing's syndrome, and hyperprolactinemia.

In many women with PCOS, obesity seems to be the common factor, and the acquisition of body fat coincides with the onset of PCOS. In fact, Stein and Leventhal first described PCOS as women with hirsutism, irregular cycles, and obesity. PCOS is related to obesity by the following mechanism: LH stimulates the theca-lutein cells to increase androstenedione production. Androstene-dione undergoes aromatization to estrone within adipocytes. Although estrone is a

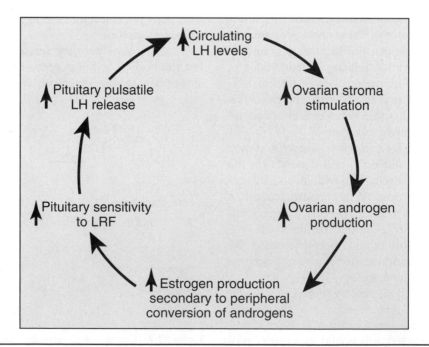

Figure 37.3. A mechanism for polycystic ovarian syndrome proposed by Yen. LH = luteinizing hormone; LRF = luteinizing-releasing factor.

weak estrogen, it has a positive-feedback action or stimulating effect on the pituitary secretion of LH. LH secretion is, therefore, stimulated by increased estrogen. With increasing obesity comes increased conversion of androstenedione to estrone. With the increased rise in androstenedione, there is coincident increased testosterone production, which causes acne and hirsutism. Hormonal studies in women with PCOS show the following: (1) increased LH:FSH (follicle-stimulating hormone) ratio, (2) estrone in greater concentration than estradiol, (3) androstenedione at the upper limits of normal or increased, and (4) testosterone at the upper limits of normal or slightly increased. One approach to the evaluation of these women is shown in Figure 37.4.

The symptoms of PCOS include *oligomenorrhea or amenorrhea, acne, hirsutism, and infertility.* The disorder is characterized by chronic anovulation or extended periods of infrequent ovulation (oligo-ovulation).

Unopposed long-term elevated estrogen

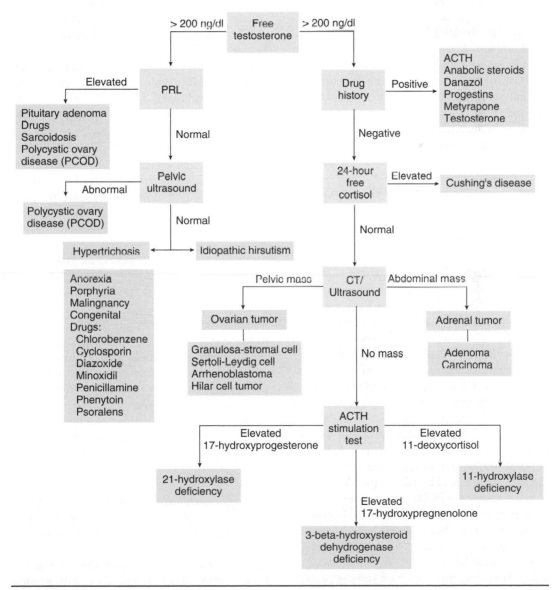

Figure 37.4. Scheme for the evaluation of hirsutism.

levels characterize PCOS. This unopposed estrogen increases the risk of abnormal uterine bleeding, endometrial hyperplasia, and in some cases the development of endometrial carcinoma.

The typical woman with PCOS has many of the manifestations of the Dysmetabolic syndrome (Syndrome X). Approximately 30% of patients with PCOS have impaired glucose tolerance, and 8% have overt type 2 diabetes mellitus. Screening for diabetes with a fasting glucose level or glucose tolerance test in these patients is a cost-effective test. Classic lipid abnormalities include elevated triglyceride levels, low high-density lipoproteins (HDL levels), and elevated low-density lipoproteins (LDL) levels. Hypertension is also common in individuals with this condition. The combination of the preceding abnormalities potentially increases the risk of cardiovascular disease.

Acanthosis nigricans has also been found in a significant percentage of these patients. The HAIR-AN syndrome (hyperandrogenism, insulin resistance, acanthosis nigricans) constitutes a defined subgroup of patients with PCOS. Administration of the insulin-sensitizing agent metformin also reduces androgen and insulin levels.

PCOS is a functional disorder whose treatment should be targeted to interrupt the disorder's positive-feedback cycle. The most common therapy for PCOS is the *administration of oral contraceptives,* which suppresses pituitary LH production. Suppressing LH causes decreased production of androstenedione and testosterone. The ovarian contribution to the total androgen pool is thereby decreased. Acne clears, new hair growth is prevented, and there is decreased androgenic stimulation of existing hair follicles. By preventing estrogen excess, oral contraceptives also prevent endometrial hyperplasia, and women have cyclic, predictable, withdrawal bleeding episodes.

If a woman with PCOS wishes to conceive, oral contraceptive therapy is not a suitable choice. If the patient is obese, a *weight-reduction* diet designed to restore the patient to a normal weight should be instituted. With body weight reduction alone, many women resume regular ovulatory cycles and conceive spontaneously.

In some women, ovulation induction with clomiphene citrate is needed and is facilitated by weight reduction. Insulin sensitizers (metformin) alone or with clomiphene citrate may be used to reduce insulin resistance, control weight, and induce ovulation.

Hyperthecosis

Hyperthecosis is a *more severe form of polycystic ovarian syndrome(PCOS).* In cases of hyperthecosis, *androstenedione* production may be so great that testosterone reaches concentrations such that *virilization* appears. Women with this condition may exhibit temporal balding, clitoral enlargement, deepening of the voice, and remodeling at the limb–shoulder girdle. Hyperthecosis is often refractory to oral contraceptive suppression. It is also more difficult to successfully induce ovulation in women with this condition.

Sertoli–Leydig Cell Tumors

Sertoli–Leydig cell tumors (also called androblastoma and arrhenoblastoma) are ovarian neoplasms that secrete testosterone. These tumors constitute < 0.4% of ovarian tumors and usually occur in women between the ages of 20 and 40. The tumor is most often unilateral and may reach a size of 7 to 10 cm wide.

The history and physical examination give critical clues in diagnosing subjects who present with hirsutism and testosterone-secreting ovarian tumors. Testosterone-secreting tumors usually have a more rapid onset and more severe hirsutism with virilizing signs. Women with a Sertoli–Leydig cell tumor have a rapid onset of *acne, hirsutism* (three-fourths of patients), *amenorrhea* (one-third of patients), and *virilization.* A characteristic clinical course of two overlapping stages is described: first, the stage of *defeminization,* characterized by amenorrhea, breast atrophy, and loss of the subcutaneous fatty deposits responsible for the rounding of the feminine figure; and second, the stage of *masculinization,* characterized by clitoral hypertrophy, hirsutism, and deepening of the voice. These changes may occur over 6 months or less.

Laboratory studies of this disorder show suppression of FSH and LH, low-plasma androstenedione, and marked elevation of testosterone. An ovarian mass may be palpable on pelvic examination. Once the diagnosis is suspected, there should be no delay in *surgical removal* of the involved ovary. The contralateral ovary should be inspected, and if it is found to be enlarged, it should be bisected for gross inspection.

Following surgical removal of a Sertoli–Leydig cell tumor, ovulatory cycles return spontaneously, and further progression of hirsutism is arrested. If the clitoris has become enlarged, it does not revert to its pretreatment size. However, temporal hair is restored, and the body habitus becomes feminine once again. However, terminal hair in a sexual distribution will not revert to vellus hair, but the growth and pigmentation will slow. Most patients will require mechanical removal of excess hair following removal of the ovarian tumor. The 10-year survival rates for this low-grade malignant ovarian tumor approximate 90% to 95%.

Uncommon Virilizing Ovarian Tumors

Gynandroblastoma is a rare ovarian tumor, having both granulosa cell and arrhenoblastoma components. The predominant clinical feature is masculinization, although estrogen production may simultaneously produce endometrial hyperplasia and irregular uterine bleeding.

Lipid (lipoid) cell tumors are usually small ovarian tumors containing sheets of round, clear pale-staining cells with a differential histologic diagnosis of hilus cell tumors, stromal luteoma of pregnancy, and Sertoli–Leydig cell tumors. The clinical presentation is *masculinization* or *defeminization* associated with elevated 17-ketosteroids in many cases.

Hilus cell tumors arise from an overgrowth of mature hilar cells or from ovarian mesenchyme and are typically found in postmenopausal women. They are characterized clinically by masculinization that supports the idea that hilar cells are the homologs of the interstitial or Leydig cells of the testis. Histologically, the tumors contain pathognomonic Reinke albuminoid crystals in most cases, and grossly, they are always small, unilateral, and benign. Treatment is surgical removal for these three rare tumors.

Adrenal Androgen Excess Disorders

Congenital Adrenal Hyperplasia

DHEA is a precursor for androstenedione and testosterone. The most common cause of increased adrenal androgen production is adrenal hyperplasia as a result of *21-hydroxylase deficiency;* 21-hydroxylase catalyzes the conversion of progesterone and 17α-hydroxyprogesteroneto desoxycorticosterone and compound S. When 21-hydroxylase is deficient, there is an accumulation of progesterone and 17α-hydroxyprogesterone, which are metabolized subsequently to DHEA. This disorder affects approximately 2% of the population and is caused by an alteration in the genes for 21-hydroxylase, which are carried on chromosome 6. The genetic defect is autosomal recessive and has variable penetrance.

In the most severe, classic form of 21-hydroxylase deficiency, the newly born female infant is simply virilized (ambiguous genitalia) or is virilized and suffers from life-threatening salt wasting. However, milder forms are more common and can appear at puberty or even later in adult life. A mild deficiency of 21-hydroxylase is frequently associated with terminal body hair, acne, subtle alterations in menstrual cycles, and infertility. These patients can also have sonographic evidence of polycystic appearing ovaries. *When 21-hydroxylase deficiency is manifested at puberty,* adrenarche may precede thelarche. The history of pubic hair growth occurring before the onset of breast development may be a clinical clue to this disorder. The *diagnosis of 21-hydroxylase deficiency* is made by measuring *increased 17-OH progesterone* in plasma during the follicular phase. Patients with classic 21-hydroxylase deficiency will have significantly elevated plasma 17-OH progesterone levels, usually over 2000 ng/dL. Those with nonclassic 21-hydroxylase deficiency may have mildly elevated basal levels, ≥200 ng/dL, and an increase to usually >1000 ng/dL in response to ACTH stimulation. Dehydroepiandrosterone sulfate (DHEA-S) and androstenedione will also be elevated and contribute to the hirsutism and virilizing signs.

A less-common cause of adrenal hyperplasia is *11β-hydroxylase deficiency.* 11β-hydroxylase catalyzes the conversion of desoxycorticosterone to cortisol. A deficiency in this enzyme also results in increased androgen production. The clinical features of 11β-hydroxylase deficiency are mild hypertension and mild hirsutism. The *diagnosis* of 11β-hydroxylase deficiency is made by demonstrating increased plasma desoxycorticosterone.

Treatment of Congenital Adrenal Hyperplasia

In congenital adrenal hyperplasia, the adrenal glands have a reduction in cortisol production secondary to the enzymatic block. This decreased cortisol production results in a compensatory increase in ACTH secretion that stimulates cortisol production. This increased ACTH production results in the oversecretion of precursor molecules proximal to the enzymatic block, which results in oversecretion of androgens. In patients with a high-grade enzymatic block, inadequate amounts of glucocorticoids and mineralocorticoids are made, resulting in salt loss, which can be life threatening. Nonclassic congenital adrenal hyperplasia can be managed easily by *supplementing glucocorticoids*. Usually, prednisone, 2.5 mg daily (or its equivalent), suppresses adrenal androgen production to within the normal range. When this therapy is instituted, facial acne usually clears promptly, ovulation is restored, and there is no new terminal hair growth.

Medical therapy for adrenal and ovarian disorders cannot resolve hirsutism; it can only suppress new hair growth. Hair that is present must be controlled by shaving, bleaching, the use of depilatory agents, by electrolysis or laser hair ablation.

Cushing Syndrome

Cushing syndrome is a major adrenal disease resulting in adrenal excess. As a result of an adrenal neoplasm or ACTH-producing tumor, the patient demonstrates signs of corticosteroid excess (i.e., truncal obesity, moonlike facies, glucose intolerance, skin thinning with striae, osteoporosis, and proximal muscle weakness in addition to evidence of hyperandrogenism and menstrual irregularities).

Adrenal Neoplasms

In androgen-secreting adrenal adenomas, there is a rapid increase in hair growth associated with severe acne, amenorrhea, and sometimes virilization. In androgen-secreting adenomas, DHEA-S is usually elevated above 6 mg/mL. The diagnosis of this rare tumor is established by computed axial tomography or magnetic resonance imaging of the adrenal glands. Adrenal adenomas must be removed surgically.

Constitutional Hirsutism

Occasionally after a diagnostic evaluation for hirsutism, there is no explanation for the cause of the disorder. By exclusion, this condition is often called *constitutional hirsutism*. Data support the hypothesis that women with constitutional hirsutism have *greater activity of 5α-reductase* than do unaffected women.

Treatment of constitutional hirsutism is primarily androgen blockade and mechanical removal of the excess hair. Spironolactone 100 mg/day is the most commonly used androgen blocker. Spironolactone also inhibits testosterone production by the ovary and reduces 5α-reductase activity. Other androgen blockers include flutamide and cyproterone acetate. The activity of 5α-reductase can also be inhibited directly through the use of drugs such as finasteride (5 mg po daily). Eflornithine hydrochloride 13.9% is an irreversible inhibitor of L-ornithine decarboxylase, which slows and shrinks hair. This cream has been approved for facial use with satisfactory local effects. Patients taking an androgen receptor or 5α-reductase blocker should be placed on concomitant oral contraceptives because of the teratogenic and demasculinizing effects on a fetus should pregnancy occur. Oral contraceptives may also improve the efficacy of these treatments through the decreased androgen and increased sex hormone–binding globulin production effects associated with their use.

Iatrogenic Androgen Excess

Danazol

Danazol is an *attenuated androgen used for the suppression of pelvic endometriosis*. It has androgenic properties, and some women develop hirsutism, acne, and deepening of the voice while taking the drug. If these symptoms develop, the value of the danazol should be weighed against the side effects before continuing therapy. Preg-nancy should be ruled out before initiating a course of danazol therapy because it can produce virilization of the female fetus.

Oral Contraceptives

The progestins in oral contraceptives are impeded androgens. Rarely, a woman taking oral contraceptives develops acne and even hirsutism. If this occurs, another product with a less-androgenic progestin should be selected or the pill should be discontinued. Moreover, evaluation for the coincidental development of late-onset adrenal hyperplasia should be done.

CHAPTER 38

MENOPAUSE

This chapter deals primarily with APGO Educational Topic:

Topic 47: Climacteric

Students should be able to define perimenopause and menopause and describe the neuroendocrine changes associated with each and the results of these changes, and evaluation and management of each of these life stages, including counseling and hormonal and nonhormonal management regimens.

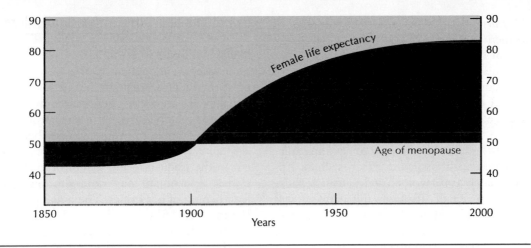

Figure 38.1. Age of menopause and female life expectancy.

The cessation of menses is *menopause*. The *climacteric* and *perimenopause* are the periods of waning ovarian function before menopause (i.e., the transition from the reproductive to the nonreproductive years). An increasing proportion of American women are included in these groups because the female life expectancy has lengthened and the number of women in this age group is expanding (Figure 38.1). If a woman reaches the menopausal age of approximately 50 years, she can expect to live another 30 to 35 years and thus spend approximately one-third of her life after menopause

Menstruation and Menopause

Unlike the male who is able to renew gametes on a daily basis, the female has a fixed number of gametes for her reproductive life. At the time of birth, the female infant has approximately 1 to 2 million oocytes; by puberty, she has approximately 400,000 oocytes remaining. By age 30 to 35, the number of oocytes has decreased to approximately 100,000. For the remaining reproductive years, the process of oocyte maturation and ovulation becomes increasingly inefficient.

A woman ovulates approximately 400 oocytes during her reproductive years. The process of *oocyte selection* is poorly understood. During the reproductive cycle, a cohort of oocytes is stimulated to begin maturation, but

only 1 or 2 dominant follicles complete the process and are eventually ovulated.

Follicular maturation is induced and stimulated by the pituitary release of follicle-stimulating hormone (FSH) and luteinizing hormone (LH). FSH binds to its receptors in the follicular membrane of the oocyte and stimulates follicular maturation, providing estradiol (E_2), which is the major estrogen of the reproductive years. LH stimulates the theca luteal cells surrounding the oocyte to produce androgens as well as estrogens and serves as the triggering mechanism to induce ovulation. With advancing reproductive age, the remaining oocytes become increasingly resistant to FSH. Thus plasma concentrations of FSH begin to increase several years in advance of actual menopause, when the FSH is generally found to be >30 mIU/mL (Table 38.1).

Menopause marks the end of a woman's natural reproductive life. *The average age for menopause in the United States is between 50 and*

Table 38.1. Relative Changes in FSH as a Function of Life Stages

Life Stages	FSH (mIU/mL)
Childhood	<4
Prime reproductive years	6–10
Perimenopause	14–24
Menopause	>30

52 *years of age (median 51.5),* with 95% of women experiencing this event between the ages of 44 and 55. The age of menopause is not influenced by the age of menarche, number of ovulations or pregnancies, lactation, or the use of oral contraceptives. Race, socioeconomic status, education, and height also have no effect on the age of menopause. Undernourished women and smokers do tend to have an earlier menopause, although the effect is slight. Approximately 1% of women undergo menopause before the age of 40. When this happens, it is generally referred to as "premature ovarian failure" rather than "menopause" because of the social implications inherent in the latter.

Menopause is a physiologic process. However, the consequences of ovarian failure can diminish a woman's quality of life and can predispose her to osteoporosis and an increased risk of bone fracture among other things, including an increased risk of cardiovascular disease.

The postmenopausal ovary is not quiescent. Under the stimulation of LH, theca cell islands in the ovarian stroma produce hormones, primarily the androgens testosterone and androstenedione. Testosterone appears to be the major product of the postmenopausal ovary. Testosterone concentrations decline after menopause but remain two times higher in menopausal women with intact ovaries than in those whose ovaries have been removed or are premenopausal. Estrone is the predominant endogenous estrogen in postmenopausal women and is termed extragonadal estrogen because the concentration is directly related to body weight and androstenedione is converted to estrone in fatty tissue (Table 38.2).

Symptoms and Signs of Ovarian Failure

Menstrual Cycle Alterations

Soon after an adolescent woman has her first menstrual cycle, regular, predictable menstrual cycles are established that continue until approximately 40 years of age. Around 40 years, the number of ovarian follicles becomes substantially depleted, and subtle changes occur in the frequency and length of menstrual cycles. A woman may note shortening or lengthening of her cycles. The luteal phase of the cycle remains constant at 13 to 14 days, whereas the variation of cycle length is related to a change in the follicular phase. Women in their 20s and 30s ovulate 13 to 14 times per year. Several years in advance of menopause, the frequency of ovulation decreases to 11 to 12 times per year and, with advancing reproductive age, may decrease to 3 to 4 times per year.

With the change in reproductive cycle length and frequency, there are concomitant changes in the plasma concentration of FSH and LH. More FSH is required to stimulate follicular maturation. Beginning in the late 30s and early 40s, the concentration of FSH begins to increase. This is the first chemical evidence of ovarian failure. The 5- to 10-year period before menopause is termed *perimenopause.* During the perimenopausal years, women begin to experience symptoms and signs of estrogen deficiency as reproductive function becomes increasingly inefficient (Table 38.3). Relative changes in FSH as a function of stage of life are presented in Table 38.1.

Table 38.2.	Steroid Hormone Serum Concentrations in Premenopausal Women, Postmenopausal Women, and Women After Oophorectomy		
Hormone	**Premenopausal (Normal Ranges in Parentheses)**	**Postmenopausal**	**Postoophorectomy**
Testosterone (ng/dL)	325 (200–600)	230	110
Androstenedione (ng/dL)	1500 (500–3000)	800–900	800–900
Estrone (pg/mL)	30–200	25–30	30
Estradiol (pg/mL)	35–500	10–15	15–20

Table 38.3. Signs and Symptoms Associated with Menopause in Women Not on Estrogen Therapy

Vulva and vagina	Skeleton
Dyspareunia (atrophic vaginitis)	Fracture of hip or wrist
Blood: stained discharge (atrophic vaginitis)	Backache
Pruritus vulvae	Breasts
Bladder and urethra	Reduced size
Frequency, urgency	Softer consistency
Stress incontinence	Reduced support
Uterus and pelvic floor	Emotional symptoms
Uterovaginal prolapse	Fatigue or diminished drive
Skin and mucous membranes	Irritability
Dryness or pruritus	Apprehension
Easily traumatized	Altered libido
Loss of resilience and pliability	Insomnia
Dry hair or loss of hair	Feelings of inadequacy or nonfulfillment
Minor hirsutism of face	Headache, tension
Dry mouth	Metabolic
Voice changes: reduction in upper register	Vasomotor symptoms: hot flushes
Cardiovascular system	Diaphoresis
Angina and coronary heart disease	

Hot Flushes and Vasomotor Instability

Coincident with the change in reproductive cycle length and frequency, *the hot flush is the first physical manifestation of ovarian failure.* Occasional hot flushes begin several years before actual menopause. *The hot flush is the most common symptom of impending ovarian failure.* More than 95% of perimenopausal and menopausal women experience hot flushes.

Hot flushes have rapid onset and resolution. When a hot flush occurs, a woman experiences a sudden sensation of warmth. The skin of the face and the anterior chest wall become flushed for approximately 90 seconds. With resolution of the hot flush, a woman feels cold and breaks out into a "cold sweat." The entire phenomenon lasts less than 3 minutes. The hot flush is the result of declining estradiol-17β secretion by the ovarian follicles. As a woman approaches menopause, the frequency and intensity of hot flushes increase. Hot flushes may be disabling, producing *diaphoresis,* especially at night. When perimenopausal and postmenopausal women receive estrogen replace-

ment, hot flushes usually resolve in 3 to 6 weeks. If a menopausal woman does not receive estrogen-replacement therapy, hot flushes usually resolve spontaneously within 2 to 3 years.

Sleep Disturbances

Ovarian failure with consequent declining estradiol induces a change in a woman's sleep cycle so that restful sleep becomes difficult and for some, impossible. The latent phase of sleep (i.e., the time required to fall asleep) is lengthened; the actual period of sleep is shortened. Therefore, perimenopausal and postmenopausal women complain of having difficulty falling asleep and of waking up soon after going to sleep. This is one of the most disabling and least appreciated adverse effects of menopause. Women with marked sleep aberration are often tense and irritable and have difficulty with concentration and interpersonal relationships. During estrogen therapy, the sleep cycle is restored to the premenopausal state.

Vaginal Dryness and Genital Tract Atrophy

The vaginal mucosa, cervix, endocervix, endometrium, myometrium, and uroepithelium are estrogen-dependent tissues. With decreasing estrogen production, these tissues become atrophic, resulting in various symptoms. The vaginal epithelium becomes thin and cervical secretions diminish. Women experience vaginal dryness while attempting or having sexual intercourse, leading to diminished sexual enjoyment and dyspareunia. *Atrophic vaginitis* also may present with itching and burning. The thinned epithelium is also more susceptible to becoming infected by local flora.

The endometrium also becomes atrophic, sometimes resulting in postmenopausal spotting. The paravaginal tissues that support the bladder and rectum become atrophic, resulting in loss of support for the bladder (cystocele) and rectum (rectocele). In addition, uterine prolapse is more common in the hypoestrogenic patient. Because of atrophy of the lining of the urinary tract, there may be symptoms of dysuria and urinary frequency. *Senile urethritis* often improves dramatically with estrogen-replacement therapy, leading to loss of the symptoms of urgency, frequency, and dysuria. Loss of support to the urethrovesical junction may result in stress urinary incontinence.

Therapy with replacement estrogens restores the integrity of the vaginal epithelium, relieving symptoms of vaginal dryness and dyspareunia. Sexual pleasure is often restored. Estrogen therapy partially restores the integrity and support of the tissues surrounding the vagina. If a menopausal woman has symptomatic pelvic relaxation, estrogen therapy is often administered for several months before surgical correction is considered. In some cases, estrogen therapy plus pelvic muscle (Kegel) exercises reverse the changes sufficiently to reestablish continence without surgery.

Mood Changes

Perimenopausal and postmenopausal women often complain of volatility of affect. Some women experience depression, apathy, and "crying spells." These may be caused directly by estrogen deficiency, by associated sleep disturbance, or by both. Not only are these emotional symptoms disturbing to a woman but also her inability to control these feelings is equally of concern. The physician should provide counseling and emotional support as well as medical therapy. The role of estrogens in central nervous system function is unknown. However, it is well established that sex steroid hormone receptors are present in the central nervous system. Estrogen therapy in perimenopausal and postmenopausal women often diminishes these mood swings.

Skin, Hair, and Nail Changes

Estrogen influences *skin* thickness. With declining estrogen production, skin tends to become thin, less elastic, and eventually more susceptible to abrasion and trauma. Estrogen therapy helps restore the thickness and elasticity of skin and may slow the formation of wrinkles.

Some women notice *changes in their hair and nails* with the hormonal changes of menopause. Estrogen stimulates the production of sex hormone–binding globulin, which binds androgens and estrogens. With declining estrogen production, there is less available sex hormone–binding globulin, which results in more free testosterone. This may result in *increased facial hair*. Moreover, changes in estrogen production affect the rate of hair shedding. Hair from the scalp is normally lost and replaced in an asynchronous way. With changes in estrogen production, hair is shed and replaced in a synchronous way, resulting in the appearance of increased scalp hair loss. This is a self-limiting condition and requires no therapy, but patients do require reassurance. *Nails become thin and brittle* with estrogen deprivation, but are restored to normal with estrogen therapy.

Osteoporosis

Bone demineralization is a natural consequence of aging. Diminishing bone density occurs in both men and women. However, the onset of bone demineralization occurs 15 to 20 years earlier in women than in men by virtue of acceleration after ovarian function ceases. Bone demineralization not only occurs with natural menopause but also has been reported in association with decreased estrogen production in certain groups of young women. Other factors contribute to the risk of osteoporosis (Table 38.4).

Table 38.4. Risk Factors for Osteoporosis
Reduced weight for height
Family history of osteoporosis
Early menopause or oophorectomy
Low calcium intake
Cigarette smoking
Nulliparity
High alcohol intake
High caffeine intake

Estrogen receptors have been demonstrated in osteoblasts. This finding suggests a permissive and perhaps even essential role for estrogen in bone formation. Bone density diminishes at the rate of approximately 1% to 2% per year in postmenopausal women compared with approximately 0.5% per year in perimenopausal women. Estrogen therapy is effective, especially when combined with appropriate calcium supplementation and judicious exercise, in the management of menopausal osteoporosis. Indeed, weight-bearing activity, such as walking, for as little as 30 minutes a day increases the mineral content of older women.

Progressive, linear decrease in bone mineral mass is noted in women who do not receive estrogen therapy in the first 5 years following menopause. When estrogen therapy is initiated before or at the time of menopause, bone density loss is greatly reduced. Estrogen therapy begun in a woman 5 or more years after menopause may still have a positive effect on bone density loss.

Calcium supplementation is beneficial to prevent bone loss, and 1000 to 1500 mg of daily calcium intake for menopausal women is recommended. Calcium therapy combined with estrogen therapy is more effective in most instances.

The recent approval of several bisphosphonates such as alendronate (Fosamax) for the management of menopause-associated osteoporosis and bone loss has provided effective nonhormonal managements. These agents reduce bone resorption through the inhibition of osteoclastic activity and provide good bone response. In addition, a new class of drugs, the selective receptive modulators (SERMs) provides another nonhormonal management option. Most estrogenic responses are mediated in the body by one of two receptors, either ER (alpha) or ER (beta). SERMs are ER ligands, which act like estrogens in some tissues but block estrogen action in others. Examples include tamoxifen and raloxifene, which exhibit ER antagonist activity in the breast but agonist activity in the bone. But, as with the bisphosphonates, they also lack the capabilities of mitigating many of the other estrogen deprivation symptoms such as hot flushes and sleeplessness (Table 38.5).

Cardiovascular Lipid Changes

With approaching ovarian failure, changes occur in the cardiovascular lipid profile. Total cholesterol increases, high-density lipoprotein (HDL) cholesterol decreases, and low-density

Table 38.5. Nonhormal Regimens for Osteoporosis		
Drug	**Mechanism of action**	**Dosage**
Alendronate	Inhibits osteoclast bone resorption	10 mg q day
Calcium carbonate	Inhibits osteoclast bone resorption (bisphosphonate)	1–1.5 gm q day in 3 or 4 divided doses
Raloxifene	Estrogen receptor modulator (SERM); selectively binds to estrogen receptors, inhibiting bone resorption and turnover	60 mg q day with Vitamin D 400 IU q day and calcium supplementation
Risedronate	Inhibits osteoclast bone resorption	5 mg q day

lipoprotein (LDL) cholesterol increases. Estrogen therapy may promote changes in the lipid profile that are favorable to the cardiovascular system. Retrospective case control studies suggest a cardioprotective effect. However, recent data suggest that no such protection exists in placebo control clinical trials. At this time, hormone replacement should not be offered to patients with the primary goal of protection against heart disease.

Premature Ovarian Failure

The diagnosis of premature ovarian failure applies to the approximately 1% of women who experience menopause before the age of 40 years. The diagnosis should be suspected in a young woman with hot flushes and other symptoms of hypoestrogenism and secondary amenorrhea. The diagnosis is confirmed by the laboratory findings of menopausal FSH levels. Interestingly, hot flushes are not as common as might be expected in this group of patients. The diagnosis has profound emotional implications for most patients, especially if their desires for childbearing have not been fulfilled, as well as metabolic and constitutional implications. For some, premature ovarian failure may be the cause of infertility, and for others, the cause for the menopausal symptoms.

There are many causes of premature loss of oocytes and premature menopause (Table 38.6), some of the more common of which are discussed following.

Genetic Factors
Several factors influence a woman's reproductive life span. Genetic information that determines the length of a woman's reproductive life is carried on the distal long arm of the X chromosome. Partial deletion of the long arm of one X chromosome results in premature ovarian failure. Total loss of the long arm of the X chromosome, as seen in Turner's syndrome, results in ovarian failure at birth or in early childhood. When suspected, these diagnoses can be established by careful mapping of the X chromosome.

Gonadotropin-Resistant Ovary Syndrome (Savage's Syndrome)
Some women with premature ovarian failure have an adequate number of ovarian follicles, yet these follicles are resistant to FSH and LH. A number of pregnancies have been reported in women with the gonadotropin-resistant ovary syndrome during the administration of exogenous estrogen. This fact suggests a role for estrogens in stimulating FSH receptors in the ovarian follicles.

Table 38.6. Causes of Premature Loss of Oocytes

Decreased number of germ cells	Congenital thymic aplasia
Failure of germ cell migration	Gonadotropin receptor and/or postreceptor defects (resistant ovary or Savage's syndrome)
Inherited reduction in germ cell number	
Accelerated atresia	Postnatal destruction of germ cells
Inherited tendencies	Physical causes
Chromosomal abnormalities	Chemotherapeutic agents
Gonadal dysgenesis	Viral agents
With stigmata of Turner's syndrome	Surgical extirpation
Pure (46,XX or 46,XY)	Autoimmune disorders
Mixed disorder	With associated endocrine disorders
Trisomy X with or without chromosomal mosaicism	Isolated
Defects in gonadotropin secretion	
Secretion of biologically inactive forms	
Subunit a or b defects	

Autoimmune Disorders

Some women develop autoantibodies against thyroid, adrenal, and ovarian endocrine tissues. These autoantibodies may cause ovarian failure. Some women respond to estrogen-replacement therapy with subsequent resumption of ovulation.

Smoking

Women who smoke tobacco can undergo ovarian failure some 3 to 5 years earlier than the expected time of menopause. It is established that women who smoke metabolize estradiol primarily to 2-hydroxyestradiol. The 2-hydroxylated estrogens are termed *catecholestrogens* because of their structural similarity to catecholamines. The catecholestrogens act as antiestrogens and block estrogen action. The mechanism for premature ovarian failure in women smokers is unknown. However, the effects of smoking should be considered in smokers who are experiencing symptoms of estrogen deficiency.

Alkylating Cancer Chemotherapy

Alkylating cancer chemotherapeutic agents affect the membrane of ovarian follicles and hasten follicular atresia. One of the consequences of cancer chemotherapy in reproductive age women is loss of ovarian function. Young women being treated for malignant neoplasms should be counseled of this possibility and advised that they may be candidates for follicular retrieval and cryopreservation as a means for attempting future pregnancy.

Hysterectomy

Surgical removal of the uterus (hysterectomy) in reproductive-age women is associated with ovarian failure some 3 to 5 years earlier than the expected age. The mechanism for this occurrence is unknown. It is likely to be associated with alteration of ovarian blood flow resulting from the surgery.

Low Body Weight

Because adipocytes play a role in estrogen production and estrogen storage, slender women experience menopausal symptoms earlier than do women of normal body habitus and obese women. Moreover, slender women tend to be more difficult to normalize with exogenous estrogen replacement during the menopausal years. Women who are less than their ideal body weight at the time of menopause should be counseled regarding the clinical implications of their weight.

Management of Menopause

All the signs and symptoms, and adverse effects, of menopause result from declining estradiol-17β production by the ovarian follicles. *Exogenous estrogen administration* to the perimenopausal and postmenopausal woman obviates most of these changes.

Estradiol-17β and its metabolic by-products, estrone and estriol, are used in estrogen therapy, the objective *of which is* to diminish the signs and symptoms of menopause. Several different estrogen preparations are available through various routes of administration (Table 38.7). Conjugated estrogens have been used as oral medication and are unconjugated in the gastrointestinal tract and delivered to the target tissues as estrone. Conjugated estrogens are effective in diminishing the symptoms of estrogen deficiency, maintaining bone mass, and restoring plasma lipids to more nearly normal levels.

Estradiol-17β can be administered orally; however, it then is oxidized in the enterohepatic circulation to estrone. Estradiol-17β remains unaltered if it is administered transdermally, transbucally, transvaginally, intravenously, or intramuscularly. Unfortunately, intramuscular estradiol administration results in unpredictable fluctuations in plasma concentration. When estradiol is administered across the vaginal epithelium, absorption is poorly controlled, and pharmacologic plasma concentrations of estradiol can result. The *transdermal administration* of estradiol results in steady, sustained estrogen blood levels and may be a preferable alternative to oral dosing for many patients.

The administration of continuous *unopposed estrogens* can result in endometrial hyperplasia and an increased risk of endometrial adenocarcinoma. Therefore, it is essential to administer a progestin in conjunction with estrogens in women who have not undergone hysterectomy. Progestins may include any variety of synthetics such as medroxyprogesterone,

Table 38.7. Common Estrogen Preparations and Dose Equivalence of Estrogenic Components

Estrogen	Preparation	Dose Equivalency
Conjugated equine estrogen	Oral: 0.3, 0.625, 0.9, 1.25, and 2.5 mg	0.625 mg
Premarin	Vaginal: 0.625 mg/g of cream	
Conjugated plant based estrogen	Oral: 0.3, 0.625, 0.9, 1.25, and 2.5 mg	0.625 mg
Cenestin	Vaginal: 0.625 mg/g of cream	
Esterified estrogen	Oral: 0.3, 0.625, 1.25, and 2.5 mg	0.625 mg
Estratab	Oral: 0.625 and 1.25 mg methyltestosterone	
Estratest h. s.	1.25 and 2.5 mg methyltestosterone	
Estratest		
Estradiol-17β	0.05, 0.10 mg	0.05 mg
Climara, Vivelle		
(transdermal patch)		
Micronized estradiol	Oral: 0.5, 1.0, and 2.0 mg	1.0 mg
Estrace	Vaginal: 0.1 mg/g	

acetate and norethindrone or micronized progesterone (Table 38.8). To achieve this protective effect, the progestin chosen may be given continuously in low dose or sequentially in higher dose. Sequential dosing is usually for 10 or 12 days each calendar month. If estrogen is administered alone because of unacceptable side effects of progestins, then it is imperative to counsel the patient as to the need for yearly endometrial biopsy.

There are two principal *regimens for estrogen therapy*. Continuous estrogen replacement with cyclic progestin administration results in excellent resolution of symptoms and cyclic withdrawal bleeding from the endometrium. One of the difficulties of this method of therapy is that many postmenopausal women do not want to continue having menstrual cycles. As a result, many physicians and patients choose to avoid the problem of cyclic withdrawal bleeding by the daily administration of both an estrogen and a low-dose progestin.

There is a wide *variety of estrogen preparations available*. The following are comparable dosages: conjugated equine estrogens, 0.625 mg; estrone sulfate, 0.625 mg; estradiol-17β, 1 mg; and transdermal estradiol-17β, 50 mg. Most perimenopausal and menopausal

Table 38.8. Common Progestin Preparations and Dose Equivalence of Progestin Components

Progestin	Preparation	Dose Equivalency
Medroxyprogesterone		10.0 mg
Provera, Cycrin, Amen	Tablets in 2.5, 5.0, and 10.0 mg	
Depo-Provera	Injectable, 100 and 400 mg/mL	
Norethindrone acetate		5.0 mg
Aygestin	Tablet, 5 mg	
Norlutate	Tablet, 5 mg	
Micronized progesterone	Capsules, 100 and 200 mg	400 mg
Prometrium		

women respond to one of these preparations, all of which ameliorate acute menopause symptoms and relieve vaginal atrophy. The administration of progestins given for 10 to 12 days each month converts the proliferative endometrium into a secretory endometrium, brings about endometrial sloughing, and prevents endometrial hyperplasia or cellular atypia. If continuous progestin therapy is used to produce endometrial atrophy, 2.5 mg of medroxyprogesterone acetate or 100 mg micronized progesterone per day is used.

Numerous preparations combining estrogen and progestins are available in both oral and transdermal formulation. The most widely used contain a combination of conjugated equine estrogens and medroxyprogesterone acetate in one tablet. Newer preparations include a combination of micronized estradiol and norethindral acetate or ethinyl estradiol and norethindrone acetate. Transdermal preparations include a combination of micronized estradiol and norethindrone acetate. It is important to remember that current transdermal formulations only contain estradiol, as conjugated estrogen preparations are not absorbed readily through the skin.

Cautions in Hormone Therapy

The results of the Women's Health Initiative (WHI) revealed epidemiologic findings that have modified the contemporary use of hormone therapy. This large multicenter randomized clinical trial (approximately 160,000 women) studied the effects of hormone therapy, dietary modification, and calcium and vitamin D supplementation as related to heart disease, fractures, breast cancer, and colorectal cancer. Although there are features of this study that are not applicable to many younger menopause patients, the overall results suggested that when compared to placebo, a combination of conjugated equine estrogens and low-dose medroxyprogesterone acetate resulted in an increased risk of heart attack, stroke, thromboembolic disease,

and breast cancer with a reduced risk of colorectal cancer and hip fractures. Some of the data contradicted prior large-scale observational studies, and thus many physicians have changed their practice regarding hormone therapy to center more on the relief of short-term symptoms of estrogen deprivation including hot flushes, sleeplessness, and vaginal atrophy.

Hormone therapy in women with prior history of breast and endometrial cancer is controversial. Currently, prospective studies using low-dose estrogen replacement in women with a prior history of limited-lesion, successfully treated breast cancer are underway. Similar studies in women with prior treated limited-lesion endometrial cancer have been completed and show no increased risk of recurrence for estrogen users.

Alternatives to Hormone Replacement Therapy

Because of controversy surrounding hormone therapy, many women are seeking alternative therapies. As women age, their risk for heart disease begins to rise, and thus it is important to advocate heart-healthy lifestyle changes. Likewise, preventive counseling about osteoporosis as previously discussed should also be included.

Alternative therapies do exist for the treatment of common symptoms of menopause. For hot flushes, these include botanical products that contain or act like estrogens such as soy or herbs (e.g., black cohosh). Unfortunately, most well-controlled studies of the common soy-based over-the-counter remedies have not shown dramatic improvements. Some SSRI antidepressants (e.g., paroxetine) and antiseizure medications (e.g., Gabapentin) are also used to provide moderate relief. Lifestyle changes can also offer some relief from hot flushes, including stress reduction, avoidance of triggers such as spicy foods, alcohol, and caffeine; and increased aerobic physical activity.

CHAPTER 39

INFERTILITY

This chapter deals primarily with APGO Educational Topic:

Topic 48: Infertility

Students should be able to define infertility and be able to discuss the causes, evaluation, and management of the male and female infertility as well as the psychosocial issues associated with infertility.

Infertility affects at least 15% of reproductive-age couples in the United States. Infertility is defined as a couple's failure to conceive following 1 year of unprotected sexual intercourse. This definition is emphasized in the cumulative monthly conception rates for fertile couples engaging in unprotected coitus (Figure 39.1).

Reproductive age is synonymous with a woman's reproductive years (generally defined as ages 15 to 44 years, although menarche and pregnancy before age 15 are not uncommon and pregnancy after 44 is no longer rare). When evaluating the infertile woman, one must look not only for disease, such as endometriosis, which causes infertility, but also causes resulting from environmental and lifestyle issues (such as maintaining a low body weight associated with dieting and/or exercise, smoking, the use of drugs such as marijuana, and increased sexual contacts associated with increased incidence of pelvic inflammatory disease). Deferred childbearing is a factor of increasing importance in a society where both husband and wife may have careers outside the home, because female fecundity decreases with increasing age. Indeed, fertility is approximately halved between about the 37th and 45th year of a woman's life.

Today, 85% of couples who are infertile by definition can expect to have a child, with appropriate diagnosis and treatment. However, the price is often high not only in dollars and medical risk, but also emotionally. Indeed, *the inability to conceive a child or carry a pregnancy places a great emotional burden on infertile couples.* The quest to have a child becomes the driving force in the infertile couple's life. Friends, family, and often occupation can be subordinated to this medical problem. Unlike dysfunction of other organ systems, dysfunction of the reproductive system does not directly produce physical or mental abnormalities. Yet, the mental anguish of infertility is nearly as incapacitating as the pain or life restrictions of other diseases. *The emotional needs of infertile couples must be recognized and fully addressed.*

Causes of Infertility

Infertility can be reduced to *three generic causes* that account for 90% of reproductive dysfunction. These causes are:

1. *anovulation (30%)*
2. *anatomic defects of the female genital tract (30%)*
3. *abnormal spermatogenesis (40%)*

Each of these categories can be investigated by a *simple diagnostic procedure* that gives a high probability of establishing a cause.

1. *anovulation–basal body temperature*
2. *anatomic defects–hysterosalpingogram*
3. *abnormal spermatogenesis–semen analysis*

In the initial investigation, it is important to establish the major cause(s) of the infertility, using the least invasive tests possible. For this reason, the sequence generally chosen is based on the most commonly observed causes of infertility: male factors and ovulation disorders (Figure 39.2).

Basal body temperature measurement is an excellent screening test for ovulation and is also often useful for documenting and optimizing the timing of coitus. The characteristic biphasic temperature shift occurs in more than 90% of ovulating women: The temperature drops at the time of menses, then rises 2 days after the peak of the luteinizing hormone (LH) surge, coinciding with a rise in peripheral levels of progesterone to greater than 4 ng/mL. Ovum release probably occurs 1 day before the first temperature elevation, and the

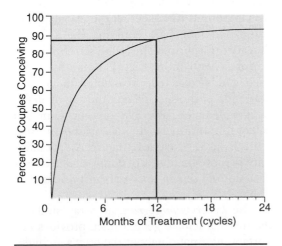

Figure 39.1. Conception rates for fertile couples.

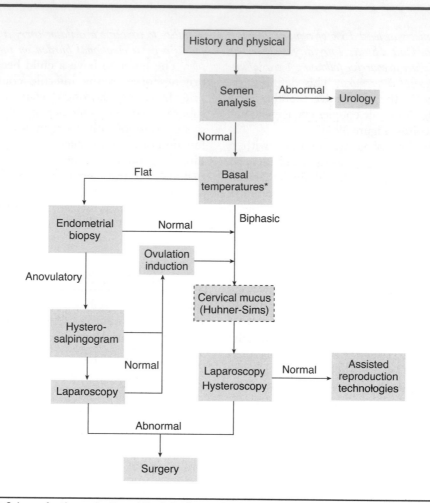

Figure 39.2. Scheme for the evaluation of the infertile couple. (Modified from Smith RP: *Gynecology in Primary Care.* Baltimore: Williams & Wilkins, 1996, p. 344.)
*A luteal phase progestin may also be used.

temperature remains elevated for 13 to 14 days, then drops, with menses beginning 14 to 36 hours thereafter. A temperature elevation of more than 16 days' duration is suggestive of pregnancy (Figure 39.3). *Serum progesterone levels* drawn in midluteal phase are sometimes useful. A value above 15 ng/mL is 80% accurate in distinguishing a normal from an abnormal cycle, whereas values <10 ng/mL are rarely associated with normal cycles.

Analysis of a semen specimen obtained by masturbation provides immediate information about the quantity and quality of seminal fluid, the density of the sperm, the morphology of sperm, and the motility of sperm. The man is instructed to abstain from ejaculation for 2 to 3 days before the test, because ejaculation during this time interval may lower the sperm count. It is important to collect all the ejaculate, because the first part contains the greatest density of sperm. The analysis should be performed no more than 2 hours after the specimen is collected, preferably sooner; thus collection of the specimen at the site of analysis is preferable. Table 39.1 presents common values for a normal semen analysis. A normal semen analysis excludes a male cause for infertility in more than 90% of couples. The causes of abnormal semen analyses are presented in Table 39.2.

The *hysterosalpingogram,* an x-ray study of the internal female genital tract, provides important information about the tract's architecture and integrity. A radiopaque dye is injected

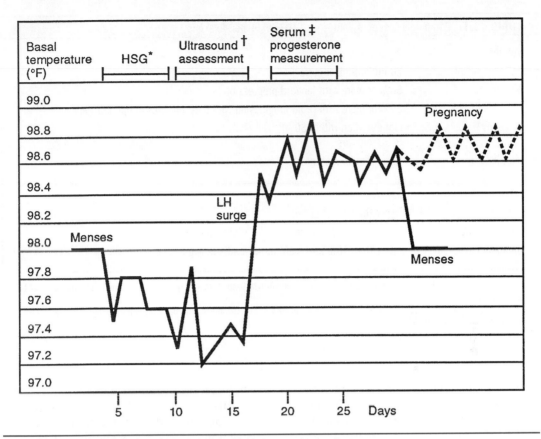

Figure 39.3. Ovulation associated biphasic basal body temperature pattern.
*Preferred time for hysterosalpingogram (HSG) testing.
†Preferred timing for sonographic assessment for ovulation.
‡Optimal interval for serum progesterone measurement for ovulation.

through the cervix into the uterine cavity and fallopian tubes and then into the peritoneal cavity, assuming that the tubes are patent. The internal architecture of all these structures is then outlined on x-ray. The hysterosalpingogram has a diagnostic accuracy of approximately 70% for detecting anatomic abnormalities of the genital tract. Diagnostic hysteroscopy or laparoscopy are additional methods of evaluating the genital tract but are complementary to the hysterosalpingogram (Table 39.3). The internal architecture of the uterus and the general health of the uterine cavity are evaluated by *hysteroscopy*. The pelvic cavity, including visualization of the "external surfaces" of the uterus, ovaries, fallopian tubes, and support structures, is evaluated by *laparoscopy*.

Anovulation

The *secretion of progesterone dominates the luteal phase of the menstrual cycle.* Progesterone acts on the endocervix to convert the thin, clear endocervical mucus into a sticky mucoid material. Progesterone shifts the thermoregulatory center set point of the basal body temperature, resulting in a temperature rise of approximately 0.6°F, remaining elevated until menstruation begins. With involution of the corpus luteum, progesterone production abruptly decreases, and the basal body temperature shifts downward; menstruation ensues soon after.

A history of regular menstrual periods strongly suggests regular ovulation. Characteristically, following ovulation and preceding menstruation, an ovulating woman experiences some fullness and heaviness of the breasts,

Table 39.1. Commonly Accepted Values for a Normal Semen Analysis	
Volume	2.0 mL or more
Sperm concentration	20 million/mL or more
Motility	50% or more with forward progression
	25% or more with rapid progression within 60 minutes of ejaculation
Viscosity	Liquefaction within 30 to 60 minutes
Morphology	30% or more normal forms
pH	7.2–7.8
White blood cells	Fewer than 1 million/mL
Immunobead test*	Fewer than 20% spermatozoa with adherent particles
SpermMar Test†	Fewer than 10% spermatozoa with adherent particles

*Sperm incubated with beads labeled with anti-IgG, anti-IgA, or anti-IgM; beads with anti-IgG adhere to sperm heads, with anti-IgA to sperm tails.
†Mixed agglutination test; uses antiserum to IgG to bridge antibody-coated sperm and latex particles that have been conjugated with human IgG, end point clumping.

decreased vaginal secretions, abdominal bloating, mild peripheral edema with slight increase in body weight, and occasional episodes of depression. These changes do not occur in anovulatory women. Therefore, *a history of these cyclic changes may be interpreted as presumptive evidence of ovulation.*

Diagnostic studies to confirm ovulation, in addition to recording the basal body temperature, include the endometrial biopsy, measurement of luteal phase serum progesterone, and the urinary ovulation-detection kit. The *endometrium* undergoes specific histological changes on an almost daily basis following ovulation. These changes can be detected from an endometrial biopsy. This is a useful procedure for evaluating certain causes of infertility, but it is expensive, is invasive, and provides only static information. *Progesterone* increases in plasma following ovulation and can be measured to confirm that ovulation has occurred. However, a single measurement provides little information that cannot be obtained by a well-kept basal body temperature chart. Ovulation-detection kits are available that measure changes in urinary LH. As the LH surge begins, more LH is excreted in the urine,

which can be measured by qualitative detection kits. This is useful in helping to predict ovulation, but it does not confirm ovulation. Ovulation-detection kits should not be used routinely, but can be useful when ovulation prediction is needed, such as in the timing of artificial insemination.

Symptoms such as irregular, unpredictable menstrual cycles and episodes of *amenorrhea* as well as signs of hirsutism, acne, galactorrhea, and decreased vaginal secretions *suggest anovulation.* A woman with irregular menstrual cycles can be presumed to be oligo-ovulatory or anovulatory. In this case, maintaining a basal body temperature record is not necessary.

Given a history of irregular menstrual cycles, the physician should look for signs of abnormal androgen, prolactin, or gonadotropin secretion. A woman who is anovulatory should have some or all of the following tests drawn, depending on individualized evaluation of the case: follicle-stimulating hormone (FSH), LH, prolactin, androstenedione, total testosterone, and dehydroepiandrosterone sulfate (DHEAS). If thyroid dysfunction is suspected, thyroxin (T_4) and thyroid-stimulating hormone (TSH) should be measured as well. Once the etiology

Table 39.2. Causes of Abnormal Semen Analysis	
Abnormal sperm count	
No sperm (azoospermia)	Klinefelter's syndrome or other genetic disorders
	Sertoli cell only syndrome
	Seminiferous tubule or Leydig cell failure
	Hypogonadotropic-hypogonadism
	Ductal obstruction (e.g., vasectomy)
	Varicocele
Few sperm (oligospermia)	Genetic disorder
	Endocrinopathies, including androgen receptor defects
	Varicocele and other anatomic disorders
	Maturation arrest
	Hypospermatogenesis
	Exogenous factors (e.g., heat)
Abnormal sperm morphology	Varicocele
	Stress
	Infection (mumps)
Abnormal motility	Immunologic factors, male–female incompatibility
	Infection
	Defect in sperm structure or metabolism
	Poor liquefaction of semen
	Varicocele
Abnormal volume	
No ejaculate	Ductal obstruction
	Retrograde ejaculation
	Ejaculatory failure
	Hypogonadism
Low volume	Obstruction of ejaculatory ducts
	No seminal vesicles and vas deferens
	Partial retrograde ejaculation
	Infection

of anovulation is established, a treatment regimen designed to induce ovulation can be developed for the patient.

Anatomic Disorders of the Female Genital Tract

The internal anatomic genital tract serves as more than a simple conduit for sperm and ova. Indeed, these dynamic structures are essential for normal transportation, fertilization, and implantation. The female genital tract *facilitates* the migration of sperm from the posterior vaginal fornix toward the unfertilized egg. *Cervical mucus* secreted by the endocervix traps the coagulated ejaculate, where the sperm are stored and capacitated for immediate or later migration into the endometrial cavity and fallopian tubes.

Table 39.3. Tests in the Infertility Work-up

Possible Cause	Test	Comments
Anovulation	Basal body temperature	Patient must do each morning
	Endometrial biopsy	Office procedure in late luteal phase
	Serum progesterone	Blood test (done in luteal phase)
	Urinary ovulation-detection kit	Home use at midcycle
Anatomic disorder	Hysterosalpingogram	X-ray in proliferative phase
	Diagnostic laparoscopy	View external surfaces of pelvic organs
	Hysteroscopy	Visualize endometrial cavity
Abnormal spermatogenesis	Semen analysis	Normal value >20 million/mL, 2 mL volume, 60% motility
	Postcoital test	Midcycle timing
Immunologic disorder	Antisperm antibodies	Male and female tested

At the time of ovulation, the oocyte is either picked up directly or retrieved from the pelvic cul-de-sac by the fimbriated end of the fallopian tube. The oocyte is then transported to the proximal portion of the fallopian tube, where fertilization occurs. The fertilized oocyte cleaves and forms a zygote and then an embryo. At 3 to 5 days following fertilization, the embryo enters the *endometrial cavity,* where it implants into the secretory endometrium for subsequent growth and development.

Acquired and Congenital Disorders

The most *common disorders* of the female genital tract are acquired during the early reproductive years. The most common cause of fallopian tube disease is *acute salpingitis.* Organisms that infect the fallopian tubes include *Neisseria gonorrhoeae* and *Chlamydia trachomatis.* These organisms alter the functional integrity of the fallopian tubes and can lead rapidly to fallopian tube obstruction. An example of an acquired uterine disorder would be intrauterine scarring (Asherman's syndrome, intrauterine synechiae) associated with excessive denuding of the endometrial lining at the time of curettage or endometritis following such a procedure. This scarring may lead to irregular or absent bleeding and impaired implantation.

Endometriosis, scarring and adhesions from pelvic inflammation or surgery, tumors of the uterus (e.g., leiomyoma) and ovary, and (rarely) sequelae of trauma may also distort the reproductive tract anatomy. Less-common congenital anatomic abnormalities of the female genital tract can range from a simple septum of the upper uterine cavity to a complete reduplication of the genital tract with a double vagina, double cervix, and double uterus. Such abnormalities are more often associated with recurrent pregnancy loss than infertility.

Hysterosalpingography

The hysterosalpingogram is a useful diagnostic tool for evaluation of the internal genital structures. The hysterosalpingogram should be performed between the 7th and 11th day of the menstrual cycle. If it were performed during menses, the risk of iatrogenic retrograde menstruation would be increased. If performed later, it could interfere with the possible ovum transport, fertilization, or implantation.

There are several important characteristics of the normal hysterosalpingogram (Figure 39.4). The endometrial cavity should be smooth and symmetrical. Indentations and irregularities of the endometrial cavity suggest uterine leiomyomata or chronic scarring of the endometrium from previous surgery. The

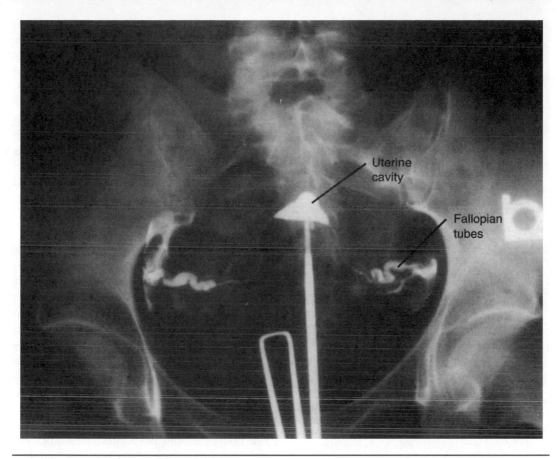

Figure 39.4. A hysterosalpingogram showing normal genital tract anatomy and architecture.

proximal two-thirds of the fallopian tubes should be slender, approximating the diameter of a pencil lead. The distal one-third of the fallopian tubes is the ampulla and should appear dilated compared with the proximal two-thirds. The fimbrial folds should appear as linear radiolucencies along the longitudinal axis of the tube. Examples of hysterosalpingograms, demonstrating two common abnormalities, are shown in Figure 39.5.

During the radiographic study, contrast material should *spill* promptly from the fallopian tubes into the peritoneal cavity. In a pelvis free of adhesions, contrast material intersperses between loops of bowel, producing characteristic crescents throughout the pelvis. Moreover, contrast material should spill freely into the cul-de-sac and dispense throughout the pelvis. Failure to observe these late changes in the hysterosalpingogram suggests the possibility

of adhesions or endometriosis, which restrict normal fallopian tube mobility.

A hysterosalpingogram that shows an abnormality of the fallopian tubes should be followed with a *diagnostic laparoscopy. The hysterosalpingogram provides information about the inner surfaces of the genital tract organs, whereas diagnostic laparoscopy provides information about the external surfaces of these organs.* Hysteroscopy can provide direct visualization of the endometrial cavity as well as access to possible correction of lesions found.

Abnormalities of Spermatogenesis

More than *40% of cases of infertility* are caused by problems of spermatogenesis. Unlike oocytes, which are ovulated periodically, sperm are being constantly produced by the germinal epithelium of the testicles. As sperm develop within the germinal epithelium, they

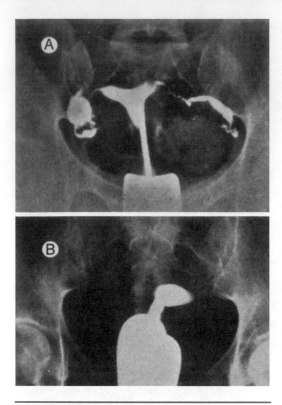

Figure 39.5. Abnormal hysterosalpingograms. (**A**) Bilateral hydrosalpinx obstructing the fallopian tubes at the fimbriated ends; arcuate uterus. (**B**) Bilateral tubal occlusion at the cornu; uterus overdistended with radiopaque medium.

are released into the epididymis, where maturation occurs before ejaculation.

Normal *sperm generation time* is approximately 73 days. Thus an abnormal sperm count is a reflection of events that occurred 73 days before the collection of a semen specimen. Alternatively, a minimum of 73 days is required to observe the change in sperm production following therapy for oligospermia.

Sperm production is thermoregulated. Intratesticular temperature is regulated by contraction and relaxation of the scrotum. Sperm production occurs at a temperature of approximately 1°F less than body temperature. External thermal shock to the testicles can result in reduced sperm production. Examples include spending time in a hot tub, sitting on the testicles for long periods of time with poor heat dispersion, and wearing tight clothing that pulls the testicles against the body for ex-

tended periods of time. In many cases, one of these causes can be discovered from a carefully obtained history. As the follicle of the ovary responds to FSH and LH, the Leydig cells and germinal epithelium of the testicles also respond to gonadotropin stimulation. In some men, the germinal epithelium becomes fibrotic, and sperm production is diminished. In others, testosterone production by Leydig cells is decreased. Men with oligospermia should have gonadotropin hormones measured to exclude testicular failure. Suspected testicular failure should be confirmed by testicular biopsy.

Some men with marginal testicular failure or poor gonadotropin production respond to the administration of clomiphene citrate. This is appropriate therapy for a limited time.

Besides semen analysis, another method to evaluate sperm density and sperm motility has historically been the *postcoital test (Huhner--Sims test)*. The test should be timed to take place during the late follicular phase of the menstrual cycle just before ovulation. At this time of the cycle, cervical mucus is abundant and facilitates sperm survival and transport. The couple should have intercourse approximately 8 hours before the test is scheduled. With a tuberculin syringe, a small sample of endocervical mucus is aspirated from the endocervical canal. This is placed on a glass slide and examined under a microscope. Normally, 8 to 10 motile sperm per high-powered field are seen in the cervical mucus. This simple test provides important information about coitus, ejaculation, sperm pickup, sperm motility, and sperm storage within the endocervical canal. Because scientific support for the usefulness of the postcoital test is lacking, it is no longer as widely used as it once was.

Both men and women can produce *antisperm antibodies*. If the woman produces antisperm antibodies, sperm are immobilized in the cervical mucus. If the man produces antisperm antibodies (3% to 20% of "infertile" men), sperm agglutinate and are unable to penetrate the cervical mucus. The diagnosis of antisperm antibodies is made by performing immunologic studies on both partners. If antisperm antibodies exist in the woman, timed intrauterine insemination using washed sperm may produce a pregnancy. There is no known effective treatment for men with antisperm antibodies, although attempts at therapy include washing and concentration of sperm with either intracervical or intrauterine insemination and high-dose steroid therapy for the man.

For some couples, there may be no biologic explanation for their infertility. These "normal" infertile couples may comprise up to 10% of those seeking treatment of infertility.

Treatment of the Infertile Couple

Anovulation

If *anovulation* is the cause of infertility, therapy should be directed to *restore ovulation by correcting the underlying problem or the administration of ovulation-inducing agents.* The most frequently used therapy is *clomiphene citrate. Clomiphene citrate* is an antiestrogen that combines with and blocks estrogen receptors at the hypothalamic and pituitary level, thus inducing, by negative-feedback inhibition, an increase in FSH release from the pituitary. FSH in turn is one of the major signals stimulating the development of follicles. Progesterone (50 to 100 mg) is given intramuscularly, and clomiphene is begun on the 5th day of menses. Depending on the hormonal milieu of the patient, 50 to 100 mg are given from day 5 to day 9. If the patient ovulates, it occurs approximately 14 days after the first day of clomiphene administration. Ovulation may be monitored through the use of basal body temperatures or sequential assessments of follicular development by ultrasonography. Without ovulation, the schedule of medication may be altered by increasing the daily dosage of clomiphene, increasing the duration of administration, or administering human chorionic gonadotropin (hCG) timed to substitute for the absent LH surge. This is commonly given as 5000 IU of hCG at the time of optimum cervical mucus. The maximum dosage of clomiphene is usually 150 mg/day.

If a woman fails to respond to clomiphene citrate, FSH can be administered directly to stimulate follicular growth. A purified preparation of gonadotropins from the urine of postmenopausal women (*Pergonal [menotropins]*) is usually used. Pergonal contains approximately 75 or 150 IU of both FSH and LH per dose and must be given parenterally because it is inactivated if given orally. If exogenous FSH is administered, monitoring requires frequent measurement of estradiol-17β and frequent imaging of the ovarian follicles by ultrasonography. The therapy is expensive and includes significant risk of three complications: hyperstimulation of the ovaries, multiple gestation, and fetal wastage.

Anatomic Abnormalities

In the event an anatomic abnormality of the genital tract is discovered, a *surgical treatment* is usually recommended. Lysis of pelvic adhesions results in freeing of entrapped internal genital structures. In case of fallopian tube obstruction, the obstruction can be corrected surgically. However, for these operations to be successful, the endosalpinx must be healthy. If the endosalpinx has been damaged such that ovum pickup and transport cannot occur, one of the assisted reproductive technologies—primarily in vitro fertilization—must be considered as an option. Correction of abnormalities of the endometrial cavity can also be accomplished, often at the time of hysteroscopic diagnosis.

Inadequate Spermatogenesis

Problems of spermatogenesis should be addressed by trying to eliminate alterations of thermoregulation. Attempts at induction of spermatogenesis can be made by the administration of clomiphene citrate. However, the response to this therapy is usually < 20%.

If spermatogenesis cannot be improved, couples may choose to use *artificial insemination using donor sperm* (AID); several techniques are in common use (Figure 39.6). Couples may also choose one of the assisted reproductive technologies such as gamete intrafallopian tube transfer (GIFT) or in vitro fertilization (IVF) to facilitate fertilization using the partner's sperm.

Assisted Reproductive Technologies

An explosion of assisted reproductive technologies has occurred in the last decade

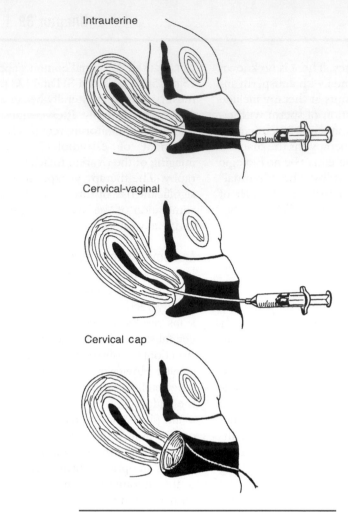

Intrauterine

Cervical-vaginal

Cervical cap

Figure 39.6. Techniques of artificial insemination.

Table 39.4. Commonly Encountered Abbreviations Associated with Assisted Reproduction

Abbreviation	Technique
AID	Artificial insemination, donor (using donor sperm, occasionally referred to as therapeutic donor insemination [TDI])
AIH	Artificial insemination, homologous (using the partner's sperm)
BBT	Basal body temperature
GIFT	Gamete intrafallopian transfer (gametes are placed in the fallopian tube for fertilization
HSG	Hysterosalpingogram, or uterine cavity radiograph
ICSI	Intracytoplasmic sperm injection
IUI	Intrauterine insemination, placement of either donor's or husband's sperm directly into the uterine cavity
IVF/ET	In vitro fertilization with embryo transfer
PCT	Postcoital test or Huhner–Sims test
SPA	Sperm penetration assay (also known as a hamster egg test, or zona-free egg penetration test)
ZIFT	Zygote intrafallopian transfer (fertilization takes place in vitro and the zygote is transferred to the fallopian tube to be transported into the uterine cavity)

From Smith RP: *Gynecology in Primary Care.* Baltimore: Williams & Wilkins, 1996, p. 352.

(Table 39.4). These include IVF, GIFT, and zygote intrafallopian tube transfer (ZIFT). These technologies provide infertility specialists with tools to bypass the normal mechanisms of gamete transportation and fertilization. However, IVF, GIFT, and ZIFT are expensive and place infertile couples on an emotional roller coaster. The expected successful outcome from IVF in properly selected couples is approximately 18% to 22% per cycle. The expected successful outcome for properly selected couples for GIFT and ZIFT is approximately 22% to 28% per cycle. Strict indications for the use of these procedures must be maintained to prevent misuse and exploitation of couples. The probability of pregnancy in a healthy couple is approximately 18% to 20% per cycle. Assisted reproductive technologies do not enhance the possibility of pregnancy in couples who do not have appropriate indications for their use, and they should be used only in carefully selected cases.

CHAPTER 40

PREMENSTRUAL SYNDROME/PREMENSTRUAL DYSPHORIC DISORDER

This chapter deals primarily with APGO Educational Topic:

Topic 49: Premenstrual Syndrome (PMS) and Premenstrual Dysphoric Disorder (PMDD).

The student should have an understanding of the diagnostic measures used to interpret the various manifestations of this condition to plan effective management.

Premenstrual syndrome (PMS) is a group of physical, mood, and behavioral changes that occur in a regular, cyclic relationship to the luteal phase of the menstrual cycle. These symptoms occur in most cycles, resolving near the end of menses with a symptom-free interval of at least 1 week. In patients with PMS, this cyclic symptom complex may be minimally to totally disruptive of the patient's normal daily activities. Literature describing mood and behavioral changes timed just prior to the menses dates back to ancient times. More recently, the *Diagnostic and Statistical Manual of Mental Disorders,* fourth edition (DSM-IV) lists the *premenstrual dysphoric disorder (PMDD)* as a type of depression in which symptoms such as depressed mood, marked anxiety, affective lability, and decreased interest in activities (anhedonia) regularly occur during the luteal phase of menstrual cycle. Whether PMDD is merely the description of a subset of the most severe variations of mood-related PMS is unclear.

Incidence

Because of the wide variability in the signs and symptoms that are considered part of a diagnosis of PMS, the reported incidence of the syndrome ranges from 10% to 90%. Severe, debilitating PMS is reported in approximately 5% of women. PMS appears to be most prevalent in women in their 30s and 40s, with a greater incidence in women with a past history of postpartum depression or other affective disorders. An accurate diagnosis is often difficult for the clinician who must determine if a woman has PMS, PMDD (as opposed to PMS), a psychiatric disorder, or a premenstrual exacerbation of a psychiatric disorder.

Symptoms

Over 200 symptoms have been attributed to PMS. Each patient presents with her own constellation of symptoms, thus making *specific symptomatology less important than the cyclic occurrence of the symptoms.* Somatic symptoms that are most common include breast swelling and pain (mastodynia), bloating, headache, constipation and/or diarrhea, and fatigue. The most common *emotional symptoms* include irritability, depression, anxiety, hostility, and changes in libido. Common *behavioral symptoms* include food cravings, poor concentration, sensitivity to noise, and loss of motor skills. Table 40.1 presents the diagnostic criteria for PMDD. Table 40.2 contrasts diagnostic aspects of PMS and PMDD.

Etiology

Many theories have been proposed to explain PMS, but none provides a single, unified expla-

---

Table 40.1. Diagnostic Criteria for Premenstrual Dysphoric Disorder

All of the following:

1. NOT an exacerbation of another underlying psychiatric disorder
2. MUST be documented with prospective charting for at least 2 months: luteal-phase symptoms that remit a few days after onset of menses
3. MUST interfere with work, school, usual activities, relationships

Plus, five or more of the following (at least one of which is a "core" symptom):

A. "Core" symptoms
   1. Marked affective lability
   2. Marked anxiety or tension
   3. Significantly depressed mood, feelings of hopelessness, or self-deprecating thoughts
   4. Persistent and marked anger or irritability

B. Other symptoms
   5. Decreased interest in usual activities
   6. Difficulty with concentration
   7. Marked lack of energy
   8. Marked change in appetitie, overeating, or food cravings
   9. Sleep disturbances (hypersomnia or insomnia)
   10. Feeling overwhelmed
   11. Other physical symptoms (breast tenderness, bloating, headache, joint pain, etc.)

Table 40.2. Contrasting PMS and PMDD

	PMS	PMDD
Diagnostic Criteria	ICD-10*	DSM-IV**
Providers using criteria	Ob/gyn, primary care	Mental health
Number of symptoms required	1	5 of 11
Functional impairment	Not required	Required
Prospective symptom charting	Not required	Required

*International Classification of Diseases, 10th Revision
**Diagnostic and Statistical Manual of Mental Disorders, 4th Edition

nation that accounts for all the variations that are seen. Currently the data support serotonin regulation as the basis for PMS/PMDD. It appears that normal, cyclic hormonal fluctuations trigger an abnormal serotonin response. Given the high incidence of anxiety, depression, and other mood symptoms, an underlying psychiatric diagnosis must still be ruled out. Historically, it was proposed that a low luteal-phase progesterone level is the cause of what is now recognized as PMS or PMDD, but measurement of serum progesterone values and clinical results of progesterone supplementation have not supported this theory.

The beneficial results of other treatments such as those listed following suggest that other etiologies may also be at play.

Differential Diagnosis

Virtually any condition that results in mood or physical changes in any cyclic fashion may be included in the differential diagnosis of PMS (Table 40.3). As a result, the physician must remain open-minded at the outset so as not to prematurely exclude the primary problem. In general, the physician should consider three major categories: medical problems, psychiatric disorders, and premenstrual exacerbations of medical and/or psychiatric conditions.

Diet Basis

Some patients with PMS seem to have a high intake of salt and refined carbohydrates, resulting in premenstrual hypoglycemic episodes, sometimes associated with outbursts of crying and violent behavior. Diet and evaluation for glucose intolerance are advocated in this subset of patients, though results are unproven.

Endorphin Basis

There is a relative decrease in the luteal-phase endorphin levels in some patients who suffer from PMS. Because these endogenous opiates are associated with a sense of well-being, a decline in their production is seen as a cause for some of the findings in these patients. In addition, PMS symptoms are mimicked by some symptoms of opiate withdrawal. A strong argument in favor of the endorphin basis of PMS comes from patients who describe alleviation of symptomatology when moderate exercise is undertaken, presumably because of an exercise-associated increase in endorphin production.

Serotonin Basis

Premenstrual serotonin levels in PMS patients have been reported to be lower than in control patients. Because lower serotonin levels have been associated with clinical depression, affective changes in PMS may be explained on this basis. In addition, anxiety has been described as a possible state of serotonin excess.

Prostaglandin Basis

Because prostaglandins are produced in the breast, brain, gastrointestinal tract, kidney, and reproductive tract and because these are areas that often present with physical symptoms in patients with PMS, a prostaglandin-associated basis for PMS remains attractive. Nonsteroidal anti-inflammatory agents have provided relief for some symptoms in some studies.

Fluid Retention Basis

Many women both with and without PMS report some premenstrual bloating and edema. Although studies do not demonstrate an increased body weight in these patients, alterations of the renin-angiotensin-aldosterone

Table 40.3. Differential Diagnosis of Premenstrual Syndrome

Allergy	Gynecologic disorders
Breast disorders (fibrocystic change)	Dysmenorrhea
Chronic fatigue states	Endometriosis
Anemia	Pelvic inflammatory disease
Chronic cytomegalovirus infection	Perimenopause
Lyme disease	Uterine leiomyomata
Connective tissue disease (lupus erythematosus)	Idiopathic edema
Drug and substance abuse	Neurologic disorders
Endocrinologic disorders	Migraine
Adrenal disorders (Cushing's syndrome, hypoadrenalism)	Seizure disorders
Adrenocorticotropic hormone-mediated disorders	Psychiatric and psychological disorders
Hyperandrogenism	Anxiety neurosis
Hyperprolactinemia	Bulimia
Panhypopituitarism	Personality disorders
Pheochromocytoma	Psychosis
Thyroid disorders (hypothyroidism, hyperthyroidism)	Somatoform disorders
Family, marital, and social stress (physical or sexual abuse)	Unipolar and bipolar affective disorders
Gastrointestinal conditions	
Inflammatory bowel disease (Crohn's disease, ulcerative colitis)	
Irritable bowel syndrome	

From Smith RP: *Gynecology in Primary Care*. Baltimore: Williams & Wilkins, 1996, p. 434.

axis as well as antidiuretic hormone have been suggested as a basis for PMS.

Vitamin Basis

Particular focus has also been placed on deficiency of vitamins A, B, and E as possible causes of PMS. Of note, vitamin B$_6$ (pyridoxine) is a cofactor in the production of serotonin as well as prostaglandin.

Diagnosis

Because the etiology of PMS is unknown, no definitive historical, physical examination, or laboratory markers are available to aid in diagnosis. At present, the diagnosis of PMS is based on documentation of the relationship of the patient's symptoms to the luteal phase. This is best done by prospective documentation of symptoms using a *menstrual diary in two consecutive menstrual cycles.* Because the patient's memory of daily symptoms cannot be depended on for accuracy given the wide variety and sometimes subtle nature of the symptoms, she is asked to monitor and record key symptoms and their severity on a daily basis. *To confirm the diagnosis of PMS, the patient must demonstrate a symptom-free follicular phase.*

A thorough physical examination to rule out specific organic pathology is essential, although it is also important to understand that no specific physical findings are diagnostic of PMS.

Treatment

Because of the diverse symptoms of patients with PMS, a multidisciplinary team of providers, including a gynecologist, psychiatrist or psychologist, endocrinologist, nutritionist, social worker, and others, is often advocated.

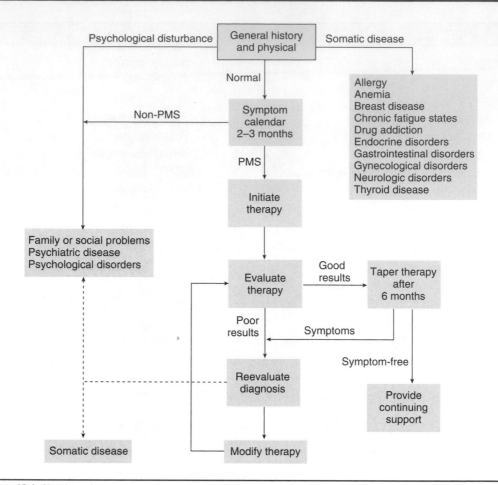

Figure 40.1. Algorithm for the management of premenstrual syndrome (PMS). The diagnosis of PMS is predicated on the elimination of other mimicking physical and psychological conditions, and the use of a 2- to 3-month, prospective calendar of symptoms. Once the diagnosis of PMS is established, pharmacologic and supportive (nonpharmacologic) therapy is begun. If successful, the pharmacologic therapy is withdrawn after 6 months and careful, supportive follow-up continued. Failure of any therapy suggests the need for a critical reevaluation of the diagnosis. If this reassessment continues to support the diagnosis of PMS, the therapy is modified, and the process of monitoring begins anew. (From Smith RP: *Gynecology in Primary Care.* Baltimore: Williams & Wilkins, 1996, p. 433.)

Figure 40.1 provides an approach that allows incorporation of the various potential treatments. Any successful management scheme will include *education of the patient as well as her family* to clarify what is known about PMS as well as what to expect from possible therapies. Education can, in and of itself, be therapeutic for a patient who either lacks insight into the possible causes of her symptoms or has never had her symptoms validated.

The prospective charting of symptoms not only documents the cyclic or noncyclic nature of the patient's symptoms but also allows her to become a part of the diagnostic and management team rather than a victim of her condition. For some, providing a diagnostic label helps relieve the fear that she is "going crazy." Often a patient's symptoms become less unbearable as she gains insight. The symptom calendar is usually continued during the treatment phase to monitor the effectiveness of treatment and to suggest the need for further focused therapy.

In addition to patient education, the following interventions have been shown to be helpful in selected groups of patients. Patients should be advised that no one therapy works for all patients and that a logical sequence of therapeutic manipulations may have to be done to achieve resolution of symptoms. There are two levels of intervention, the first being lifestyle/behavior modification issues (i.e., nonpharmacologic) and the second being pharmacologic.

Nonpharmacologic Treatment

Diet recommendations emphasize fresh rather than processed foods. The patient is encouraged to eat more fresh fruits and vegetables and minimize refined sugars and fats. Eating frequent small meals rather than having three large meals reduces the possibility of hypoglycemia symptoms. Minimizing salt intake may help with bloating, and eliminating caffeine from the diet can reduce nervousness and anxiety.

Exercise has been found to be helpful in some patients, possibly by increasing endogenous production of endorphins. Relaxation techniques such as *reflexology* benefit some patients. *Vitamin therapy,* including administration of pyridoxine (vitamin B$_6$), a cofactor in the synthesis of serotonin, has been shown to be helpful in some patients. Reported side effects include reversible peripheral neuropathy when large doses of pyridoxine are taken. Evening primrose oil, rich in vitamin E, has also been helpful in relieving both breast tenderness and depressive symptoms associated with PMS. *Dietary supplements* such as *calcium carbonate,* often taken in the form of antacid tablets, can help both mood and physical symptoms. Magnesium supplementation and vitex agnus castus have also been helpful in some studies.

Pharmacologic Treatment

In addition to lifestyle/behavior and dietary supplementation, some pharmacologic agents have been shown to provide symptomatic relief. *Nonsteroidal anti-inflammatory agents* have been found in controlled trials to be useful in PMS patients for more symptoms than just dysmenorrhea. This is possibly related to prostaglandin production in various sites in the body. *Diuretics* have been found to help control symptoms of weight gain as well as some psychological symptoms. Bloating is also minimized in patients taking diuretics. Even though the diuretic is only used when the patient is symptomatic, the potential for hypokalemia with certain agents must be monitored.

Because the underlying mechanism appears to be normal hormone fluctuations triggering an abnormal serotonin response, it should be no surprise that reports show *medications to induce anovulation* are sometimes of benefit in PMS/PMDD. Because symptoms are associated with ovulatory cycles, suppressing ovulation is beneficial for some patients. This can be accomplished by using oral contraceptives, danazol, or gonadotropin-releasing hormone (GnRH) agonists. Oral contraceptives are a logical first choice for patients who also require contraception. Some patients, however, find a worsening of their symptoms when taking oral contraceptives. The use of *danazol* and *GnRH* agonists has been demonstrated to be beneficial in short-term studies, but long-term effects of such drugs for PMS have not been fully evaluated. The use of either constitutes a "medical oophorectomy" and may be used as a trial before surgical oophorectomy is considered.

Anxiolytic and *antidepressant medications* have been widely studied and found to be useful in some patients. Patient response is seen in those treated with serotonergic agents, most notably the selective serotonin reuptake inhibitors (SSRIs). Commonly used examples of SSRIs include fluoxetine (Prozac), sertraline (Zoloft), paroxetine (Paxil), and escitalopram (Lexapro). Venlafaxine (Effexor), which inhibits the reuptake of both serotonin and norepinephrine, has also been used. Antidepressants that do not have a serotonergic effect have not been found to be efficacious in PMS/PMDD, adding to the evidence that it is a serotonin-based condition. *Buspirone* (BuSpar) is a nonsedating, nonaddictive anxiolytic found effective in some cases. *Alprazolam* (Xanax) is also an efficacious anxiolytic for selected patients with PMS/PMDD.

UNIT V

NEOPLASIA

CHAPTER 41

CELL BIOLOGY AND PRINCIPLES OF CANCER THERAPY

No specific APGO Educational Topic is given for this chapter, although many chapters, especially those in Unit V, Neoplasia, rely on an understanding of this content.

Treatment of cancers involving the breast and genital organs may involve surgery, chemotherapy, radiation therapy, and hormone therapy, used alone or in combination. The specific treatment plan depends on the type of cancer, the stage of the cancer, and the characteristics of the individual patient. Individualizing treatment is an important characteristic of cancer therapy.

Cell Cycle and Cancer Therapy

Knowledge of the cell cycle is important in understanding cancer therapies. Many treatments are based on the fact that cancer cells are constantly dividing, making them more vulnerable to agents that interfere with the cell division process.

The cell cycle consists of four phases (Figure 41.1). During the G_1 phase, there is synthesis of RNA and protein that prepares the cell for DNA synthesis, which occurs in the S phase. The G_2 phase is a period of additional RNA, protein, and specialized DNA synthesis. This leads to mitosis (M phase), during which cell division occurs. After mitosis, cells can again enter the G_1 phase or can "drop out" of the cell cycle and enter a resting phase (G_0). Cells in G_0 do not engage in the synthetic activities characteristic of the cell cycle and, therefore, are not vulnerable to therapies aimed at actively growing and dividing cells. The *growth fraction* is the number of cells in a tumor that are actively involved in cell division (i.e., not in the G_0 phase). The growth fraction of tumors decreases as they enlarge, because vascular supply and oxygen levels are decreased. *Surgical removal of tumor tissue* (cytoreductive debulking surgery) can result in G_0 cells reentering the cell cycle, thus making them more

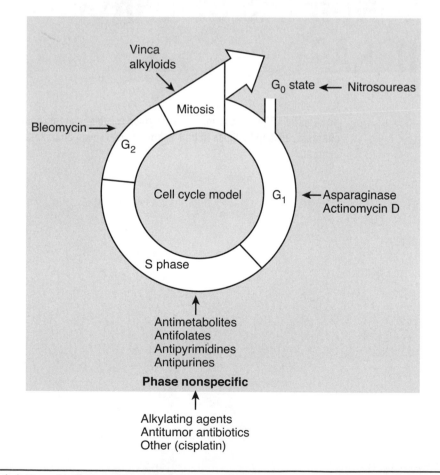

Figure 41.1. Actions of antineoplastic agents within the cell cycle.

vulnerable to chemotherapy and radiation therapy.

The generation time is the length of the cell cycle, from M phase to M phase. For a given cell type, the lengths of the S and M phases are relatively constant, whereas G_2 and, especially, G_1 vary. The variable length of G_1 can be explained by cells entering the resting phase (G_0) for a period and then reentering the cycle.

Chemotherapeutic agents and radiation kill cancer cells by first-order kinetics. This means that each dose kills a constant fraction of tumor cells, instead of a constant number. The implication of this is that several intermittent doses are more likely to be curative than a single large dose.

Chemotherapy

Chemotherapeutic agents can be (a) cell-cycle (phase) nonspecific, which means that they can kill in all phases of the cell cycle and are useful in tumors with a low growth index, or *(b) cell-cycle (phase) specific,* which means that they kill in a specific phase of the cell cycle and are

most useful in tumors that have a large proportion of cells actively dividing. Figure 41.1 illustrates common drugs and their sites of action within the cycle.

Several *classes of antineoplastic drugs* (Table 41.1) are available. *Alkylating agents* possess positively charged alkyl groups that are able to bind to negatively charged sites on DNA. They form DNA adducts, leading to single- and double-strand breaks or cross links. This interferes with DNA, RNA, and protein synthesis. Dividing cells, especially those in the late G_1 and S phases, are most sensitive to the effects of these drugs. The major side effects of the alkylating agents are myelosuppression and immunosuppression. They also may result in amenorrhea.

The *antitumor antibiotics* intercalate between DNA base pairs to inhibit DNA-directed RNA synthesis and also are involved in the formation of free radicals, causing strand breakage. They are phase nonspecific (i.e., they are effective in all phases of the cell cycle). Their general side effects are similar to those of the alkylating agents. Other side effects are drug specific.

Table 41.1. Examples of Antineoplastic Drugs

Alkylating agents	Hydroxyurea (Hydrea)
Carboplatin	Gemcitabine
Cyclophosphamide	Plant alkaloids
Chlorambucil (Leukeran)	Vinblastine (Velban)
Busulfan (Myleran)	Vincristine (Oncovin)
Melphalan (Alkeran, L-PAM)	Paclitaxel (Taxol)
Ifosfamide (Ifex)	Docetaxel
Antitumor antibiotics	Platinum-based drugs
Doxorubicin (Adriamycin)	Cis-diaminedichloroplatinum (cisplatin)
Bleomycin (Blenoxane)	Carboplatin
Actinomycin D (Dactinomycin, Cosmegen)	Topoisomerase-I Inhibitors
Mitomycin C (Mutamycin)	Camptothecin
Mitoxantrone	Topotecan
Antimetabolites	Endocrine therapy
Methotrexate (MTX, Amethopterin)	Tamoxifen
6-Mercaptopurine (6-MP, Purinethol)	Anastrozole
5-Fluorouracil (Fluorouracil, 5-FU)	

The *antimetabolites* are structural analogs of normal molecules necessary for cell function. They competitively interfere with the normal synthesis of nucleic acids and, therefore, are most active during the S phase of cell division. They may cause bone marrow suppression or gastrointestinal mucositis when given in a bolus.

Plant (vinca) alkaloids primarily prevent the assembly of microtubules, thus interfering with the M phase of cell division. They may cause bone marrow suppression or an anaphylactoid reaction.

Platinum-based drugs bind to DNA to cause interstrand and intrastrand cross-links. A major side effect is the impairment of renal tubular function.

Topoisomerase I inhibitors produce single-strand breaks during replication by inhibition of the TOPO-I enzyme. This enzyme normally produces single-strand breaks in DNA molecules during replication to relieve torsional strain. TOPO-I inhibitors complex with the DNA and replication enzymes resulting in double-strand breaks and cellular death.

Endocrine therapy with *selective estrogen receptor modulators* (SERMs) acts in estrogen-sensitive breast tumors to block the interaction of estrogen with estrogen receptors. The therapeutic importance of cellular estrogen receptors (ER) has been well established in breast cancers. There is a good relationship between ER and the response of patients to endocrine therapy. Normally, estrogen enters cells and binds to ER in the cytoplasm. The complex is translocated to the nucleus, where it binds to acceptor sites on chromosomes, resulting in activation of RNA and protein synthesis. SERMs act as competitive inhibitors of estrogen binding. The two available SERMs are tamoxifen and raloxifene-related drugs. The SERM–ER complex also binds to chromosomes but does not activate cell metabolism. This decreases cellular activity and cell division, thus reducing tumor growth. Although relatively nontoxic, the most commonly used drug in this category, tamoxifen, is related to some increased risk for endometrial cancer and an increase in benign endometrial pathology; however, the benefits of decreased risk for recurrence of breast cancer and development of contralateral breast cancer outweigh the risk

of developing endometrial cancer. Aromatase inhibitors (AIs), which suppress intratumor and plasma estrogen levels, are being used in postmenopausal patients for treatment of advanced breast cancer that has progressed beyond tamoxifen therapy.

Progestational agents have been found to be useful in treatment of early stage endometrial cancer when surgery is either not feasible, unsafe, or not desired. Furthermore, progestational therapy is useful for some patients with recurrent disease. The most common progestational agents used are medroxyprogesterone and megestrol acetate. Other hormonal agents that have demonstrated efficacy in cases of recurrent disease include tamoxifen, goserelin acetate, anastrazole (SERM), and arzoxifene (SERM).

Antineoplastic drugs are toxic because they act on normal as well as cancer cells. Table 41.2 describes the major side effects of antineoplastic agents. Rapidly dividing cell types are most sensitive, e.g., the cells of the erythroid, myeloid, and megakaryocytic series are dam-

Table 41.2. Major Side Effects of Antineoplastic Drugs	
Hematologic	Cardiac
Granulocytopenia	Cardiomyopathy
Thrombocytopenia	Urinary
Anemia	Chronic azotemia
Gastrointestinal	Acute renal failure
Mucositis	Neurologic
Necrotizing enterocolitis	Peripheral neuropathies
Immunosuppression	Ototoxicity
Dermatologic	Paresthesias
Alopecia	Reproductive
Local necrosis	Amenorrhea
Allergic/ hypersensitivity reactions	Metabolic abnormalities
Hepatic	Tumor lysis syndrome
Pulmonary	
Interstitial pneumonitis	

aged by common neoplastic drugs. Anemia, granulocytopenia (neutropenia) and thrombocytopenia are predictable side effects. Patients with anemia will often suffer from incapacitating lethargy. Patients with neutropenia are at high risk for fatal sepsis, and those with sustained thrombocytopenia are at risk for spontaneous gastrointestinal or acute intracranial hemorrhage. Prophylactic antibiotics are administered to patients with febrile neutropenia or in neutropenic patients to prevent serious infection. Platelet transfusions can be used to decrease the risk of hemorrhage.

There are limitations in the use of single agents. These include the development of drug resistance and toxicity. As a consequence, combination chemotherapy has come into use.

Several strategies can be used to select drugs for combination chemotherapy. In sequential blockade, the drugs block sequential enzymes in a single biochemical pathway. In concurrent blockade, the drugs attack parallel biochemical pathways leading to the same end product. Complementary inhibition interferes with different steps in the synthesis of DNA, RNA, or protein.

The interactions between drugs used in combination are defined as synergistic (result in improved antitumor activity or decreased toxicity rather than with each agent alone), additive (result in enhanced antitumor activity equal to the sum of each individual agent), or antagonistic (result in less antitumor activity rather than with each individual agent). Drugs used in combinations should (a) be effective when used singly, (b) have different mechanisms of action, and (c) be additive or, preferably, synergistic in action.

Chemotherapy is administered in various regimens. Adjuvant chemotherapy is usually a set course of combination chemotherapy that is given in a high dose to patients with no evidence of residual cancer after radiotherapy or surgery. The purpose is to eliminate any residual cancer cells typically for curative intent. Neoadjuvant chemotherapy aims to eradicate micrometastases or reduce nonoperable disease so as to allow for or prepare patients for surgery and/or radiotherapy. Induction chemotherapy is usually a combination chemotherapy given in a high dose to cause a remission. Maintenance chemotherapy (consolidation chemotherapy) is a long-term and low-dose regimen that is given to a patient in remission to maintain the remission by inhibiting the growth of remaining cancer cells.

Radiation Therapy

Ionizing radiation causes the production of free hydrogen ions and hydroxyl (OH^-) radicals. With sufficient oxygen, H_2O_2 is formed, which affects DNA and, eventually, the cell's ability to divide. As with chemotherapy, killing is by first-order kinetics. Because dividing cells are more sensitive to radiation damage and because not all cells in a given tumor are dividing at any one time, *fractionated doses of radiation are more likely to be effective than a single dose.* Providing multiple lower doses of radiation also reduces the deleterious effects on normal tissues.

The basis of fractionated dosage comes from the *"four Rs" of radiobiology.*

1. *Repair of sublethal injury.* When a dose is divided, the number of normal cells that survive is greater than if the dose were given at one time (higher total amounts of radiation can be tolerated in fractionated as opposed to single doses).
2. *Repopulation.* Reactivation of stem cells occurs when radiation is stopped; thus regenerative capacity depends on the number of available stem cells.
3. *Reoxygenation.* Cells are more vulnerable to radiation damage with oxygen present; as tumor cells are killed, surviving tumor cells are brought into contact with capillaries, making them radiosensitive.
4. *Redistribution in the cell cycle.* Because tumor cells are in various phases of the cell cycle, fractionated doses make it more likely that a given cell is irradiated when it is most vulnerable.

The *rad* has been used as a measure of the amount of energy absorbed per unit mass of tissue. A standard measure of absorbed dose is the *Gray,* which is defined as 1 joule per kilogram; *1 Gray is equal to 100 rad.* Radiation is delivered in two general ways: external irradiation (teletherapy) and local irradiation (brachytherapy). *Teletherapy* depends on the use of high-energy (>1 million eV) beams because this spares the skin and delivers less toxic radiation to the bone. Tolerance for external radiation depends on the vulnerability of surrounding normal tissues. Teletherapy usually is used to shrink tumors before localized radiation. *Brachytherapy* depends on the inverse square law: the dose of radiation at a given point is inversely proportional to the square of the distance from the radiation source. To put the radioactive material at the closest possible distance, brachytherapy uses encapsulated sources of ionizing radiation implanted directly into tissues (interstitial) or placed in natural body cavities (intracavity). *Intracavity devices* can be placed within the uterus, cervix, or vagina and then afterloaded with radioactive sources as either low-dose radiotherapy (cesium-137), high-dose radiotherapy (iridium-192, cobalt-60), or as interstitial implants. This method protects health personnel from radiation exposure. A new method of treating early breast cancer involves high-dose–rate brachytherapy inserted by balloon catheter into the cavity created by lumpectomy. *Interstitial implants* use isotopes (iridium-192, iodine-125) formulated as wires or seeds. These implants are usually temporary, but permanent seed implants are being investigated.

New strategies are being developed for radiation therapy. For example, intraoperative therapy is being used for previously irradiated patients with recurrent disease who would require unacceptable high dosages of external radiation.

Complications associated with radiation therapy can be acute or late (chronic). *Acute reactions* affect rapidly dividing tissues, such as epithelia (skin, gastrointestinal mucosa, bone marrow, and reproductive cells). Manifestations are cessation of mitotic activity, cellular swelling, tissue edema, and tissue necrosis. Early problems associated with irradiation of gynecologic cancers include enteritis, acute cystitis, vulvitis, proctosigmoiditis, topical skin desquamation, and occasionally, bone marrow depression. *Chronic complications* occur months to years after completion of radiation therapy. These include obliteration of small blood vessels or thickening of the vessel wall, fibrosis, and reductions in epithelial and parenchymal cell populations. This results in chronic proctitis, hemorrhagic cystitis, formation of uterovaginal or vesicovaginal fistula, rectal or sigmoid stenosis, and bowel obstructions, as well as gastrointestinal fistulae.

Gene Therapy

In the next decade, it is anticipated that there will be significant progress in so-called gene therapy, therapies designed to modulate gene function and thus many biological processes, including the abnormal cellular proliferation we term cancer. The potential benefits of this therapeutic concept are manifold, whether considered as primary or adjunctive therapy. Work in this area remains in the experimental stage. Clinical trials for ovarian cancer have studied the feasibility of delivering specific agents and identified problems with the delivery of therapy.

CHAPTER 42

GESTATIONAL TROPHOBLASTIC NEOPLASIA

This chapter addresses APGO Educational Topic:

Topic 50: Gestational Trophoblastic Neoplasia.

The student should be familiar with the morbidity and mortality associated with this unique neoplasm.

Gestational trophoblastic neoplasia (GTN) is a *rare variation of pregnancy* of unknown etiology and usually presents as a benign disease called *molar pregnancy*. This disorder includes neoplasms that are derived almost entirely from abnormal placental (trophoblastic) proliferation. Molar pregnancy may, in turn, be divided into *complete mole* (no fetus) and *incomplete mole* (fetus plus molar degeneration). *Persistent* or *malignant disease* will develop in approximately 20% of patients with molar pregnancy. Fortunately, persistent or malignant GTN is responsive to effective chemotherapy.

Key clinical features of GTN include (1) predictable clinical presentation as a pregnancy, (2) reliable means of diagnosis with pathognomonic ultrasound findings, (3) specific tumor marker (quantitative serum human chorionic gonadotropin [hCG]), (4) effective surgical treatment, (5) sensitivity to chemotherapy when GTN is persistent or malignant, and (6) reliable long-term follow-up through assessment of quantitative hCG levels.

The incidence varies among different national and ethnic groups, with the highest occurring among Asian women living in Asia (up to 1 in 200 pregnancies) and the lowest incidence occurring in white women of Western European and U.S. origins (approximately 1 in 2,000 pregnancies). The recurrence rate is approximately 2%. It is more common in very young and older women and is also associated with dietary deficiencies, such as folic acid deficiency. The classification of gestational trophoblastic neoplasia is described in Table 42.1. Because persistent GTN may follow simple molar pregnancy, an appreciation of the latter's clinical presentation, histology, clinical risk factors, and long-term follow-up is necessary to thoroughly treat the patient with this unusual tumor.

Hydatidiform Mole (Molar Pregnancy)

A *hydatidiform mole* includes abnormal proliferation of the syncytiotrophoblast and replacement of normal placental trophoblastic tissue by *hydropic placental villi*. *Complete* moles do not include the formation of a fetus. *Partial moles* are characterized by focal trophoblastic proliferation and degeneration of the placenta and are associated with a chromosomally abnormal fetus. In this form of molar pregnancy, trophoblastic proliferation is largely from the cytotrophoblast (Figure 42.1).

Table 42.1. Classification of Gestational Trophoblastic Neoplasia

   I. Primary nonmetastatic disease; no evidence of disease outside uterus (includes complete and partial mole)

  II. Persistent nonmetastatic gestational trophoblastic neoplasia

 III. Metastatic disease: any disease outside uterus

    A. Good prognosis metastatic disease

       1. Short duration (last pregnancy <4 months)

       2. Low pretreatment hCG titer (<100,000 IU/24 hr or <40,000 mIU/mL)

       3. No metastasis to brain or liver

       4. No significant prior chemotherapy

    B. Poor prognosis metastatic disease

       1. Long duration (last pregnancy >4 months)

       2. High pretreatment hCG titer (>100,000 IU/24 hr or >40,000 mIU/mL)

       3. Brain or liver metastasis

       4. Significant prior chemotherapy

       5. Term pregnancy

    C. Placental site tumors

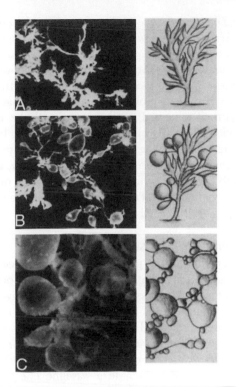

Figure 42.1. Villi gross morphology. **(A)** Normal chorionic villi. **(B)** Partial mole with normal villi admixed with swollen ones (case of triploidy, 69,XXY). **(C)** Complete mole with swollen, vesicular villi.

The *genetic constitutions* of the two types of molar pregnancy are different (Table 42.2). Complete moles are entirely of paternal origin as a result of the fertilization of a blighted ovum by a haploid sperm, which then reduplicates. Accordingly, the karyotype of a com-

plete mole is 46,XX. The fetus of a partial mole is usually a triploidy, the most common being 69,XXY. The triploidy comprises one haploid set of maternal chromosomes and two haploid sets of paternal chromosomes, which arise from dispermic fertilization. The complete mole is more common (approximately 90% of molar pregnancies) and more likely to undergo malignant transformation.

Clinical Presentation

Patients with molar pregnancy of either variety may present with findings consistent with pregnancy but also with uterine size/dates discrepancy, exaggerated subjective symptoms of pregnancy, and bleeding suggestive of spontaneous abortion. Of these symptoms, painless *bleeding* is the most characteristic and occurs in most patients early in the second trimester of pregnancy. The patient also may experience the passage of tissue, as fragments of the edematous trophoblast are passed through the dilated cervical os. Most patients have already been *diagnosed as pregnant*, having had a positive pregnancy test. There is a *uterine dates/size discrepancy* in two-thirds of patients. The uterus may be either too large or too small for gestational age, usually larger than expected. This discrepancy, coupled with late first or early second trimester bleeding, usually leads the clinician to perform ultrasound imaging of the uterus, which confirms the diagnosis of molar pregnancy by its characteristic "snowstorm" appearance (Figure 42.2).

Table 42.2. Complete and Incomplete Hydatidiform Moles		
Characteristic	**Complete**	**Incomplete**
Synonyms	True; classic	Partial
Uterus large for dates	About 50%	Not usually
Villi	All edematous	Some normal
Capillaries	Few, no fetal RBCs	Some; fetal RBCs
Embryo	None	Abnormal fetus
hCG titer	High	Moderately elevated to high
Karyotype	Mostly 46,XX	Triploid (69,XXY)
Malignant potential	15–30%	Slight (<5%)

hCG = human chorionic gonadotropin; RBCs = red blood cells.

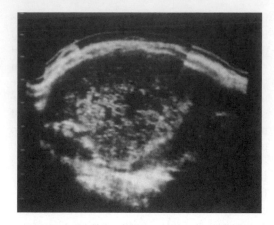

Figure 42.2. "Snowstorm" appearance of complete mole on ultrasound examination.

Molar pregnancies may present with *other signs and symptoms,* including visual disturbances, severe nausea and vomiting, marked pregnancy-induced hypertension (pre-eclampsia), proteinuria, and rarely, clinical hyperthyroidism. Some patients experience tachycardia and shortness of breath, arising from intense hemodynamic changes associated with acute hypertensive changes. In these patients, hyperreflexia may also be found. Physical examination reveals not only the dates/size discrepancy of the uterine fundus and absent fetal heart tones, but also changes associated with developing preeclampsia. Occasionally, bimanual pelvic examination may reveal large *adnexal masses* (theca lutein cysts), which represent marked enlargement of the ovaries as a result of high levels of hCG stimulation.

Histologically identical to complete mole, *invasive mole (chorioadenoma destruens)* is a complete mole invading the myometrium without any intervening endometrial stroma on histologic sample. It is often diagnosed months after evacuation of a complete mole when hCG levels do not fall appropriately. Occasionally, it may be diagnosed on curettage at the time of initial molar evacuation. Untreated, its natural course includes local invasion and, on occasion, vascular invasion and metastasis. It is reported to follow 5% to 15% of complete hydatidiform moles.

The clinical presentation of partial molar pregnancy is similar to that for complete mole, although typically the patient presents at a more advanced gestational age (after the 20th week of pregnancy). Vaginal bleeding is less common than with complete moles. Uterine growth that is less than expected for the gestational age, especially if coupled with rapidly developing hypertension, may be the first clinical indication. Because of the growth/dates discrepancy, ultrasonography is obtained, which reveals molar degeneration of the placenta and frequently a grossly abnormal fetus.

Laboratory Assessment

After the molar pregnancy has been confirmed by imaging studies, laboratory documentation is necessary to ascertain the *level of hCG.* These levels are extremely high in molar pregnancy and not only *help classify risk category but also serve as a sensitive tumor marker in the follow-up* of these patients. Other valuable studies include a baseline chest radiograph to check for metastatic disease, assessment of hemoglobin and hematocrit, and selected other tests depending on clinical evidence of other conditions such as preeclampsia and/or hyperthyroidism. Before treatment, blood should be obtained for blood type and Rh and screened for antibodies in case blood replacement is necessary. Similar laboratory studies should be obtained whether the patient has partial or complete mole.

Treatment

In most cases of *molar pregnancy,* the definitive treatment is prompt *removal of the intrauterine contents.* Uterine evacuation is done most expeditiously by dilation of the cervix followed by *suction curettage.* After suction curettage with an atraumatic plastic cannula, *gentle sharp curettage* may be performed to provide small amounts of myometrial tissue for separate pathologic assessment. This is used to ascertain whether there has been myometrial invasion. The evacuation of larger moles is sometimes associated with uterine atony and excessive blood loss, so that appropriate preparations should be made for oxytocin administration and blood transfusion if they are needed.

In cases of *partial mole,* a similar procedure may be carried out, with the additional need for larger grasping instruments to remove the abnormal fetus. With cases involving enlargement of the uterus beyond 24 weeks' gestational size, an alternative to suction evacuation is induction of labor with prostaglandin vaginal suppositories. In general, *the larger the uterus, the greater the risk of pulmonary complications* associated with trophoblastic emboli, fluid overload, and anemia. This is particularly true in patients with extreme degrees of associated pregnancy-induced hypertension (preeclampsia), because patients may experience concomitant hemoconcentration and alteration in vascular hemodynamics. In these patients, uterine evacuation by prostaglandin stimulation may be safer.

Some patients in the older reproductive age group may be best served by hysterectomy, which ensures removal of the entire primary neoplasm. This is especially true in patients with "high-risk" disease, as described in Table 42.3. This treatment should be reserved for patients who have no interest in further childbearing and/or have other indications for hysterectomy.

The *bilaterally enlarged multicystic ovaries (theca lutein cysts),* resulting from follicular stimulation by high levels of circulating hCG, do not represent malignant changes. This enlargement invariably regresses within a few months after evacuation of the molar pregnancy and therefore does not require surgical removal.

Postevacuation Management

Because of the predisposition for recurrence, patients should be followed closely for at least 1 year. The *removed molar tissue* should be examined carefully to identify hyperplastic and/or anaplastic proliferation. The small tissue sample provided by the sharp curettage specimen is pivotal in determining myometrial invasion. RhoGAM should be given in cases of incomplete mole.

Follow-up consists primarily of *periodic physical examination,* including pelvic examination and the *assessment of quantitative hCG levels,* according to the schedule outlined in Table 42.4. Quantitative serum β-hCG values fall after evacuation in a characteristic manner (Figure 42.3), with plateauing being an indication of persistent disease and the need for further treatment. Following this guideline assures the physician that recurrent disease is not developing; that an intercurrent pregnancy (within 1 year) is not causing an increase in hCG levels; and that for future pregnancy another molar pregnancy is ruled out early, because the *recurrence rate* for these patients is approximately five times the initial rate (1 in 400 in the United States).

Little or no increased risk of congenital anomalies is seen in subsequent pregnancies, but the risk of major obstetric complications is higher in this group, approaching 5% to 9%.

Table 42.3. Conditions That Define High-Risk Gestational Trophoblastic Disease
Uterus >16–week size
Theca lutein cysts
Marked trophoblastic proliferation and/or anaplasia
Hyperthyroidism

Table 42.4. Posttreatment Follow-up for Molar Pregnancy
General physical and pelvic examination and baseline chest radiograph at 2 weeks
Serum quantitative hCG level every 2 weeks until normal (0–5 mIU)
Serum quantitative hCG monthly for 1 year after obtaining first normal level
Assurance of effective contraception for 1 year (oral contraceptives preferred unless contraindicated)
Early ultrasound examination and quantitative hCG level for future pregnancy
hCG = human chorionic gonadotropin.

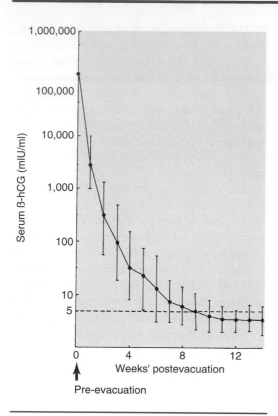

Figure 42.3. Normal regression curve and smoothed 95% confidence limits of serum b-hCG after evaluation of a hydatidiform mole. Time 0 is time of evacuation.

The incidence of placental accreta in particular appears to be increased.

Metastatic/Malignant Gestational Trophoblastic Neoplasia

Recurrent benign GTN occurs in < 10% of patients with antecedent molar pregnancy. Malignant transformation of hydatidiform mole, *choriocarcinoma,* is characterized by rapid myometrial and uterine vessel invasion and systemic metastasis resulting from hematogenous embolization. Lung, vagina, central nervous system, kidney, and liver are common metastatic locations for this tumor. Instead of chorionic villi, the tumor has a red, granular appearance on cut section and consists of intermingled syncytiotrophoblastic and cytotrophoblastic elements with many abnormal cellular forms. Choriocarcinoma may also follow a normal antecedent term pregnancy, an

abortion, or an ectopic pregnancy. In the United States, *choriocarcinoma is associated with approximately 1 in 150,000 pregnancies, 1 in 15,000 abortions, 1 in 5,000 ectopic pregnancies, and 1 in 40 moles.* Early identification and treatment of recurrence are critically important. Failure of quantitative hCG levels to regress after initial therapy suggests that further treatment is needed. Common sites of persistent or metastatic disease include the uterus, adjacent pelvic structures, the lungs, and the brain. Treatment of persistent gestational trophoblastic disease may involve the use of several potentially effective chemotherapeutic agents. What should be remembered is that GTN, even in its malignant form, is highly sensitive to chemotherapy and is considered a "prototype" for tumors that are sensitive to these agents. The indications for chemotherapy for persistent or malignant trophoblastic disease are presented in Table 42.5.

In general, nonmetastatic persistent GTN is completely treated by single-agent chemotherapy. The prognosis for malignant GTN is more complex, divided into good and poor prognostic categories (Table 42.6). The World Health Organization (WHO) has developed a prognostic scoring system for GTN that takes into account a number of epidemiologic and laboratory findings (Table 42.7). Chemotherapeutic regimens include single-agent treatment with either methotrexate or actinomycin D, as well as combination chemotherapy (EMACO: etoposide, methotrexate, actinomycin D, cyclophosphamide, and Oncovin).

Table 42.5. Indications for Chemotherapy for Trophoblastic Disease
Histologic diagnosis of choriocarcinoma
Evidence of metastatic disease
Indications based on quantitative serum β-human chorionic gonadotropin levels
Plateaued or rising titer after evacuation
Titer that has not returned to normal after 12 weeks' postevacuation
Re-elevated level after a normal level has been obtained, exclusive of a new pregnancy

Table 42.6. Clinical Classification of Malignant Gestational Trophoblastic Neoplasia (GTN)

1. Nonmetastatic GTN (not defined in terms of good versus poor prognosis)
2. Metastatic GTN
   a. *Good prognosis:* No high-risk factors

   Pretreatment hCG level < 40,000 mIU/mL serum β-hCG

   <4 months' duration of disease

   No evidence of brain or liver metastasis

   No significant prior chemotherapy

   No antecedent term pregnancy

   b. *Poor prognosis:* any single high-risk factor

   Pretreatment hCG level >40,000 mIU/mL serum β-hCG

   >4 months' duration of disease

   Brain and/or liver metastases

   Failed prior chemotherapy

   Antecedent term pregnancy

Where chemotherapy is indicated, the treatment protocol depends on whether patients fall into the "good" or "poor" prognosis metastatic group. Adjunctive radiation therapy is usually recommended for patients with brain or liver metastases, although the data in support of this therapy are scant.

Placental Site Tumors

Placental site tumor is a rare form of trophoblastic disease. The tumor is composed of monomorphic populations of intermediate cytotrophoblastic cells that are locally invasive at the site of placental implantation. It is different in that it secretes placental lactogen but only small amounts of hCG, is rarely metastatic, and unfortunately is much more resistant to standard chemotherapy. Hysterectomy is the appropriate initial therapy in most cases, although curettage has been effective in some situations.

Table 42.7. WHO Prognostic Scoring System for Gestational Trophoblastic Disease*

Prognostic Factor	0	1	2	3
Age	<39	>39		
Antecedent pregnancy	HM†	Abortion; ectopic	Term	
Interval (months)‡	<4	4–6	7–12	>12
hCG level (IU/L)	$<10^3$	10^3–10^4	10^4–10^5	$>10^5$
ABO blood groups (female H male)		O × A	B	
		A × O	AB	
Largest tumor (cm)	<3	3–5	>5	
Site of metastasis		Spleen, kidney	GI† tract, liver	Brain
Number of metastases		1–3	4–8	>8

*Low risk, 4; intermediate risk, ≤5–7; high risk, ≥8.
†GI = gastrointestinal; hCG = human chorionic gonadotropin; HM = hydatidiform mole.
‡Time between antecedent pregnancy and start of chemotherapy.

CHAPTER 43

VULVAR AND VAGINAL DISEASE AND NEOPLASIA

This chapter deals primarily with APGO Educational Topic:

Topic 51: Vulvar Neoplasms.

Students should be able to describe the risk factors associated with vulvar neoplasms and common vulvar diseases, and their appropriate evaluation and management. Students should also be able to explain the indications for vulvar biopsy and describe the standard techniques.

Appreciation of vulvar symptoms and examination for vulvar disease and neoplasia constitute a significant part of primary health care for women. The vulvar region is particularly sensitive to irritants, more so than other regions of the body. It has been suggested that the layer overlying the vulva, the stratum corneum, may be less of a barrier to irrants, thereby making the vulva more susceptible to irritations and contributing to the "itch-scratch" cycle. Noninflammatory vulvar pathology is found in women of all ages, but is particularly significant in perimenopausal and postmenopausal women because of concern regarding the possibility of vulvar neoplasia. *The major symptoms of vulvar disease are pruritus, burning, nonspecific irritation, and/or appreciation of a mass.* Diagnostic aids for the assessment of noninflammatory conditions are likewise relatively limited in number and include, in addition to careful history, inspection and biopsy. *Because vulvar lesions are often difficult to diagnose, liberal use of vulvar biopsy is central to good care. Cytologic evaluation of the vulva is of limited value as the vular skin is keratinzed, and epithelium shedding does not occur as readily as that of the cervix. Colposcopy is useful for evaluating known vulvar atypia and intraepithelial neoplasia. Punch biopsies of vulvar abnormalities are most helpful to determine if a malignancy is present or to histologically determine the correct etiology of a perceived abnormality of the vulva.*

This chapter provides discussions of a range of vulvar pathologic conditions, including nonneoplastic dermatoses, white lesions (atrophic and hyperkeratotic lesions), benign vulvar mass lesions, vulvar intraepithelial neoplasia, and vulvar cancer. Inflammatory conditions of the vulva are discussed in Chapter 27. Table 43.1 outlines common vulvar diseases.

Common Vulvar Dermatoses

Lichen Simplex Chronicus

In contrast to many dermatologic conditions that may be described as "rashes that itch," lichen simplex chronicus (LSC) can be described as "*an itch that rashes.*" It is thought that most patients develop this disorder secondary to *an irritant dermatitis, which progresses to LSC*

Table 43.1. Common Vulvar Diseases

Common vulvar dermatoses
  Lichen simplex chronicus (LSC)
  Lichen planus
  Psoriasis
  Seborrheic dermatitis
  Vestibulitis
White lesions
  Hyperplastic vulvar dystrophy
Lichen sclerosis (atrophic vulvar dystrophy)
Vulvar intraepithelial neoplasia (VIN)
  Without atypia
With atypia, including carcinoma in situ
Vulvar carcinoma
  Paget's disease
  Squamous cell carcinoma

---

as a result of the effects of chronic mechanical irritation from scratching and rubbing an already irritated area. The mechanical irritation contributes to epidermal hyperplasia and inflammatory cell infiltrate, which, in turn, leads to heightened sensitivity that triggers more mechanical irritation.

Accordingly, the history of these patients is one of *progressive vulvar pruritus and/or burning,* which is temporarily relieved by scratching or rubbing with a washcloth or some similar material. *Etiologic factors* for the original pruritic symptoms often are unknown but may include sources of skin irritation such as laundry detergents, fabric softeners, scented hygienic preparations, and the use of colored or scented tissue. These potential sources of symptoms must be investigated. Any domestic or hygienic irritants must be removed, in combination with treatment, to break the cycle described.

On *clinical inspection,* the skin of the labia majora, labia minora, and perineal body often shows diffusely reddened areas with occasional hyperplastic or hyperpigmented plaques of red to reddish brown. One may also find occasional areas of linear hyperplasia, which show the effect of grossly hyperkeratotic ridges of epidermis. Biopsy of patients who have these characteristic findings is usually not warranted.

Empiric *treatment* to include antipruritic medications such as Benadryl (diphenhydramine hydrochloride) or Atarax (hydroxyzine hydrochloride) that inhibit nighttime, unconscious scratching, combined with a mild to moderate topical steroid cream applied to the vulva, usually provides relief. A *steroid cream* such as hydrocortisone (1% or 2%) or, for patients with significant areas of obvious hyperkeratosis, triamcinolone acetonide (0.1%; Kenalog) or betamethasone valerate (0.1%; Valisone) may be used. *If significant relief is not obtained within 3 months, diagnostic vulvar biopsy is warranted.*

The prognosis for this disorder is excellent when the offending irritating agents are removed and a topical steroid preparation is used appropriately. In most patients, these measures cure the problem and eliminate future recurrences.

Lichen Planus

Although lichen planus is usually a desquamative lesion of the vagina, occasional patients develop lesions on the vulva near the inner aspects of the labia minora and vulvar vestibule. Patients may have areas of whitish, lacy bands (Wickham's striae) of keratosis near the reddish ulcerated-like lesions characteristic of the disease. Typically, complaints include *chronic vulvar burning and/or pruritus* and *insertional* (i.e., entrance) *dyspareunia* and a *profuse vaginal discharge.* Because of the patchiness of this lesion and the concern raised by atypical appearance of the lesions, *biopsy may be warranted* to confirm the diagnosis in some patients. In lichen planus, biopsy shows no atypia. Examination of the vaginal discharge in these patients frequently reveals large numbers of acute inflammatory cells without significant numbers of bacteria. Accordingly, most often the diagnosis can be made by the typical history of vaginal/vulvar burning and/or insertional dyspareunia coupled with a physical examination that shows the bright red patchy distribution and a wet prep that shows large numbers of white cells. Histologically the epithelium is thinned, and there is a loss of the rete ridges with a lymphocytic infiltrate just beneath associated with basal cell liquefaction necrosis.

Treatment for lichen planus is topical *steroid preparations* similar to those used for LSC. This may include the use of intravaginal 1% hydrocortisone douches. Length of treatment for these patients is often shorter than that required to treat LSC, although lichen planus is more likely to recur.

Psoriasis

Psoriasis, an autosomal, dominant, inherited disorder, may involve the vulvar skin as part of a generalized dermatologic process. With approximately 2% of the general population suffering from psoriasis, the physician should be alert to its prevalence and likelihood of vulvar manifestation, moreover, because it may appear at menarche, pregnancy, and menopause.

The *lesions* are typically slightly raised round or ovoid patches with a silver scale appearance atop an erythematous base. These lesions most often measure approximately 1×1 to 1×2 cm. Though pruritus is usually minimal, these silvery lesions will reveal punctate bleeding areas if removed (Auspitz sign). *The diagnosis is generally known because of psoriasis found elsewhere on the body, obviating the need for vulvar biopsy to confirm the diagnosis.* Histologically prominent acanthosis is seen, with distinct dermal papillae that are clubbed and demonstrate chronic inflammatory cells between them.

Treatment often occurs in conjunction with consultation by a dermatologist. Like lesions elsewhere, vulvar lesions usually respond to topical coal tar preparations, followed by exposure to ultraviolet light as well as corticosteroid medications, either topically or by intralesional injection. Coal tar preparations are extremely irritating to the vagina and labial mucous membranes and should be avoided in these areas. Because vulvar application of some of the photoactivated preparations can be somewhat awkward, topical steroids are most effective, using compounds such as betamethasone valerate 0.1% (Valisone).

Seborrheic Dermatitis

Although seborrheic dermatitis is a common problem, *isolated vulvar seborrheic dermatitis is rare.* It involves a chronic inflammation of the sebaceous glands, but the exact etiology is unknown. The diagnosis is usually made in patients complaining of vulvar pruritus who are known to have seborrheic dermatitis in the scalp or other hair-bearing areas of the body. The lesion may mimic other entities such as psoriasis, tinea cruris (jock itch), or LSC. _The lesions are pale red to a yellowish pink and may be covered by an oily appearing, scaly crust._ Because this area of the body remains continually moist, occasional exudative lesions include raw "weeping" patches, caused by skin maceration, which are exacerbated by the patient's scratching. As with psoriasis, _vulvar biopsy is usually not needed_ when the diagnosis is made in conjunction with known seborrheic dermatitis in other hair-bearing areas.

For patients with acute exudative variations of seborrheic dermatitis, initial perineal hygiene includes the use of _Burrow's solution soaks_ (5% solution of aluminum acetate). After remediation of the exudative phase, standard treatment includes _topical corticosteroid lotions or creams_ containing a mixture of an agent that penetrates well such as betamethasone valerate in conjunction with Eurax (crotamiton) to control the intense pruritus. As with LSC, the use of antipruritic agents such as Atarax or Benadryl as a bedtime dose in the first 10 days to 2 weeks of treatment frequently helps break the sleep/scratch cycle and allows the lesions to heal.

Vestibulitis

Vulvar vestibulitis is a condition without known etiology. It involves the acute and chronic inflammation of the vestibular glands, which lie just inside the vaginal introitus near the hymeneal ring. The involved glands may be circumferential to include areas near the urethra, but this condition most commonly involves posterolateral vestibular glands in the 4 and 8 o'clock positions (Figure 43.1). The diagnosis should be suspected in all patients who present with _new onset insertional dyspareunia_. Patients with this condition frequently complain of progressive insertional dyspareunia to the point where they are unable to have intercourse. The history may go on a few weeks, but most typically involves progressive worsening over the course of 3 or 4 months. Patients also complain of pain on

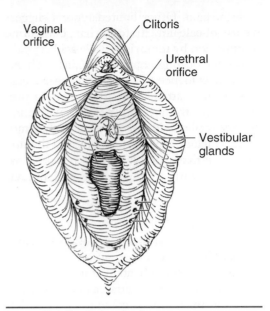

Figure 43.1. Vestibular glands.

tampon insertion and at times during washing or bathing the perineal area.

Physical examination is the key to diagnosis. Because the vestibular glands lie between the folds of the hymenal ring and the medial aspect of the vulvar vestibule, diagnosis is frequently missed when inspection of the perineum does not include these areas. Once the speculum has been placed in the vagina, the vestibular gland area becomes impossible to identify. After carefully inspecting the proper anatomic area, light touch with a moistened cotton applicator recreates the pain exactly and allows for quantification of the pain. In addition, the regions affected are most often evident as small, reddened, patchy areas.

Because the cause of vestibulitis is unknown, treatments are varied and range from changing or eliminating environmental factors, temporary sexual abstinence, and application of cortisone ointments and topical Xylocaine jelly to more radical treatments such as surgical excision of the vestibular glands. No single treatment has proved highly efficacious, and treatment must be individualized based on the severity of patient symptoms and the sexual disability that is present.

Some patients may benefit from low-dose tricyclic medication (amitriptyline and imipramine) or fluoxetine to help break the cycle of pain. Other limited reports suggest the use of calcium citrate to change the urine composition by removing oxalic acid crystals. Those advocating changing the urine chemistry cite evidence to suggest that oxalic acid crystals are particularly irritating when precipitated in the urine of patients with high urinary oxalic acid composition. Other modalities include biofeedback, physical therapy with electrical stimulation or intralesional injections with triamcinolone and bupivicaine.

Benign Vulvar Lesions

Sebaceous or inclusion cysts are caused by inflammatory blockage of the sebaceous gland ducts and are small, smooth, nodular masses, usually arising from the inner surfaces of the labia minora and majora, that contain cheesy, sebaceous material. They may be easily excised if their size or position is troublesome.

The round ligament inserts into the labium majus, carrying an investment of peritoneum. On occasion, peritoneal fluid may accumulate therein, causing a *cyst of the canal of Nuck or hydrocele*. If such cysts reach symptomatic size, excision is usually required.

Fibromas (fibromyomas) arise from the connective tissue and smooth muscle elements of vulva and vagina and are usually small and asymptomatic. Sarcomatous change is extremely uncommon, although edema and degenerative changes may make such lesions suspicious for malignancy. Of historical interest is the almost unbelievable 268-lb pedunculated vulvar fibroma reported by Buckner in 1851. Treatment is, of course, surgical excision when the lesions are symptomatic or with concerns about malignancy. *Lipomas* appear much like fibromas, are rare, and are also treated by excision if symptomatic.

Hidradenoma is a rare lesion arising from the sweat glands of the vulva. It is almost always benign, is usually found on the inner surface of the labia majora, and is treated with excision.

Nevi are benign, usually asymptomatic, pigmented lesions whose importance is that they must be distinguished from malignant melanoma, 3% to 4% of which occur on the external genitalia in females. Biopsy of pigmented vulvar lesions may be warranted, depending on clinical suspicion.

Vulvar Neoplasia

The classification of vulvar disease used descriptive terminology based on gross morphologic appearance: leukoplakia, kraurosis vulvae, and vulvar dystrophy. Standardization of nomenclature and classification by symptoms, gross appearance, and histology were lacking. To improve standardization and thus treatment of these disorders, the International Society for the Study of Vulvar Disease (ISSVD) established a modified classification in 1987 based on both gross and microscopic morphology (Table 43.2).

Vulvar dermatoses have been described previously. The following discussion includes a description of squamous cell hyperplasia (formerly hyperplastic dystrophy) and lichen sclerosis.

Squamous Cell Hyperplasia (Hyperplastic Dystrophy)

In considering the various types of vulvar neoplasia, the clinician should be aware that gross appearance may not be consistent with underlying cellular architecture and that often atrophic lesions, such as lichen sclerosis, may appear grossly to be hyperplastic. Furthermore, *within the group of true hyperplastic lesions, the clinician needs to confirm whether the hyperplasia is accompanied by atypia.* As a result *liberal use of vulvar biopsy is encouraged to provide definitive diagnosis and ensure rational treatment.*

The microscopic appearance confirms the diagnosis. *Squamous cell hyperplasia without atypia* characteristically shows hyperkeratosis as well as acanthosis without mitotic figures. These lesions are usually treated as described in the previous discussion of LSC, using various types of *topical, highly penetrating corti-*

Table 43.2.	ISSVD Classification of Vulvar Disease

Description	
I	Squamous cell hyperplasia
II	Lichen sclerosis
III	Other dermatoses
ISSVD = International Society for the Study of Vulvar Disease.	

costeroid creams. The patient can be reassured that these lesions usually respond to treatment with complete resolution and do not predispose to further premalignant or malignant vulvar disease.

Lichen Sclerosis

Lichen sclerosis, previously called lichen sclerosis et atrophicus, has confused clinicians and pathologists because of inconsistent terminology and because it is associated with other types of vulvar pathology, including those of the hyperplastic variety. As with the other disorders, *chronic vulvar pruritus* occurs in most patients. Typically, *the vulva is diffusely involved with very thin, whitish epithelial areas* termed "onion skin" epithelium. The epithelium has been termed "onion skin" or "cigarette paper" skin and described as "parchment-like." Most patients have involvement on both sides of the vulva, with the most common sites being the labia majora, labia minora, the clitoral and periclitoral epithelium, and the perineal body. The lesion may extend to include a perianal "halo" of atrophic, whitish epithelium. In severe cases, many normal anatomic landmarks are lost, including obliteration of labial and periclitoral architecture as well as severe stenosis of the vaginal introitus. Some patients have areas of cracked skin, which are prone to bleeding with minimal trauma. Patients with these severe anatomic changes complain of difficulty in having normal coital function.

The etiology of lichen sclerosis is unknown, but a familial association has been noted as well as disorders of the immune system, including thyroid disorders and Class II HLA antigens. However, the response to topical steroids further indicates the underlying inflammatory process and the role of prostaglandins, leukotrienes in the hallmark symptom of pruritus.

Microscopic confirmation of lichen sclerosis is often necessary and useful because it allows specific therapy. The histologic features are pathognomonic and include areas of hyperkeratosis, despite epithelial thinning; a zone of homogeneous, pink-staining collagenous-like material directly under the epithelial layer; and a band of chronic inflammatory cells, consisting mostly of lymphocytes. In addition to the hyperkeratosis, flattened rete pegs are also seen.

It is important to remember that associated areas of hyperplasia may be mixed throughout or adjacent to these typically atrophic-appearing areas. In patients with this so-called *mixed dystrophy,* both components need to be treated to effect resolution of symptoms. Patients with histologic confirmation of a large hyperplastic component should initially be treated with well-penetrating corticosteroid creams. With improvement of these areas (usually 2 to 3 weeks), therapy can then be directed to the lichen sclerosis component.

The treatment of choice for lichen sclerosis includes the use of topical steroid (clobetasol) preparations in an effort to ameliorate symptoms. The lesion is unlikely to resolve totally. Intermittent treatment may be needed indefinitely. This is in marked contrast to the hyperplastic lesions without atypia, which usually totally resolve within 6 months.

Neither lichen sclerosis nor hyperplastic dystrophy without atypia significantly increases the patient's risk of developing cancer. It has been estimated that this risk is in the 2% to 3% range when no preexisting atypical hyperplasia are present. However, because patients who have had these disorders are more likely to eventually develop atypical hyperplasia, they need to be followed carefully and have a rebiopsy performed frequently if a return of vulvar symptoms or new lesions occurs.

Vulvar Intraepithelial Neoplasia

Vulvar intraepithelial neoplasia (VIN) may be classified as VIN I, mild dysplasia; VIN II, moderate dysplasia; or VIN III, severe dysplasia, carcinoma in situ. Also included in the category of intraepithelial neoplasia lesions are vulvar condylomata. Other lesions represented include Paget's disease and level I melanomas. Condylomata are discussed in the section on inflammatory vulvar lesions, and Paget's disease and level I melanomas are mentioned briefly later in this section.

VIN I and VIN II

Early vulvar intraepithelial neoplasia (VIN I and VIN II) represents *true neoplastic lesions* that, as with their counterparts in the cervix, are thought to have a *high predilection for progression* to severe intraepithelial lesions and eventually carcinoma if left unattended. Almost 60% of women with vaginal intraepithelial neoplasia (VAIN) III or vulvar intraepithelial neoplasia (VIN) III will also have cervical intraepithelial neoplasia (CIN) lesions. Furthermore 10% of women with CIN III will have either VAIN or VIN.

Presenting complaints include *vulvar pruritus, chronic irritation, and a development of raised mass lesions.* Normally, the lesions are localized, fairly well isolated, and raised above the normal epithelial surface to include a slightly rough texture. These lesions are usually found along the posterior vulva and in the perineal body, although they may occur anywhere on the vulva. They typically have a whitish cast or hue. As with other vulvar lesions, diagnosis by biopsy is mandatory.

Microscopically, these lesions mimic intraepithelial neoplasia elsewhere, including mitotic figures and nuclear pleomorphism, with loss of normal differentiation in the lower one third to one half of the epithelial layer. Changes consistent with human papillomavirus (HPV) infection are occasionally seen with these lesions and suggest an association between certain types of HPV and the occurrence of VIN. Lesions that are typically condyloma in origin do not have features of attenuated maturation and have no pleomorphism and atypical mitotic figures.

VIN III (Carcinoma in Situ)

Common presenting complaints include *intractable pruritus and nonspecific vulvar irritation with gross lesions that are similar to earlier grades of VIN* occurring in patchy, fairly well-isolated areas. Occasional patients may have extensive vulvar involvement. Smoking or secondhand smoke is a common social history finding in patients with VIN. The color changes in these lesions range from white, hyperplastic areas to reddened or dusky patch-like involvement, depending on whether associated hyperkeratosis is present.

Full-thickness loss of maturation indicates lesions that are at least severely dysplastic, including areas that may represent true carcinoma in situ.

As with the other vulvar disorders, *diagnosis of VIN is made by biopsy.* In patients without obvious raised or isolated lesions, careful inspection of the vulva is warranted using a colposcope. Applying a 3% to 5% solution of acetic acid to the vulva for 2 to 5 minutes often accentuates the white lesions and may also help in revealing abnormal vascular patterns. When present, these areas should have selective biopsies performed in multiple sites to thoroughly investigate the grade of VIN and reliably exclude invasive carcinoma.

The goal in treating VIN is to quickly and completely remove all involved areas of skin. These lesions can be removed after appropriate biopsies confirm the absence of invasive cancer. Removal options include wide local excision (using electro-cautery or scalpel), laser vaporization, ablation, or topical therapy. Topical therapies that may be useful include 5-FU, immunotherapy, immiquimod, or retinoic acid compounds. It must be stressed that careful evaluation to exclude invasive disease is of paramount importance, as up to 20% of patients with VIN III will have an underlying invasive malignancy. Therefore, excision is recommended for patients with VIN III.

Paget's Disease

Paget's disease is characterized by extensive intraepithelial disease whose gross appearance is described as a fiery red background mottled with whitish hyperkeratotic areas. The histology of these lesions is similar to that of the breast lesions, with large pale cells of apocrine origin below the surface epithelium (Figure 43.2). Although not common, Paget's disease of the vulva may be associated with carcinoma of the skin. Similarly, patients with Paget's disease of the vulva have a higher incidence of underlying internal carcinoma, particularly of the colon and breast.

The treatment for vulvar Paget's disease is wide local excision or simple vulvectomy, depending on the amount of involvement. Recurrences are more common with this disorder than with VIN, necessitating wider margins when local excision or vulvectomy is performed.

Melanoma

Melanoma is the most common nonsquamous cell malignancy of the vulva.

Vulvar melanoma usually presents with *a raised, irritated, pruritic, pigmented lesion.* Most

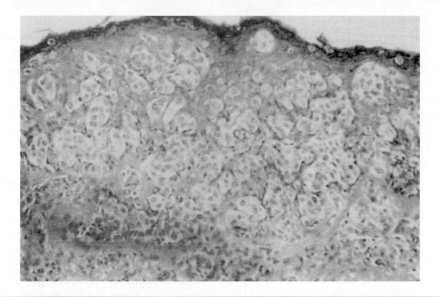

Figure 43.2. Paget's disease. Large, pale cells of apocrine origin involving the surface epithelium. From Scott JR, Di Saia PJ, Hammond CB, et al. *Danforth's Obstetrics and Gynecology,* 8th ed. Philadelphia: Lippincott Williams & Wilkins, 1999, p. 794.

commonly, melanotic lesions are located on the labia minora or the clitoris. Melanoma accounts for only 5% of all vulvar malignancies, and when suspected, *wide local excision* is necessary for diagnosis and staging. Survival approaches 100% when the lesions are confined to the intrapapillary ridges, decreasing rapidly as involvement includes the papillary dermis, reticular dermis, and finally subcutaneous tissues. In the latter instance, survival is generally < 20% because of substantial incidence of nodal involvement. Because early diagnosis and treatment by wide excision are so crucial, it is important to recognize that *irritated, pigmented, vulvar lesions mandate excisional biopsy for definitive treatment.*

Vulvar Cancer

Vulvar carcinoma accounts for approximately 5% of all gynecologic malignances, with 90% of these carcinomas being of the *squamous cell* variety. The typical clinical profile includes women in their *postmenopausal years,* most commonly between the ages of 65 and 70. About 10% of these malignancies are, however, discovered in the third and fourth decades of life. *Vulvar pruritus* is the most

common presenting complaint. In addition, patients may notice a red or white ulcerative or exophytic lesion arising most commonly on the posterior two thirds of either labium majus. An exophytic ulcerative lesion need not be present, further underscoring the need for thorough biopsy in patients of the age group who complain of vulvar symptoms. *Patients in this age group are often reluctant to present to their physicians, and physicians are further reluctant to investigate the symptoms and findings thoroughly via vulvar biopsy, which often results in a delay in treatment.*

Although a *specific etiology* for vulvar cancer is not known, progression has been shown from prior intraepithelial lesions, including those that are associated with certain types of HPV. Smokers have a high preponderance in this population of patients.

Natural History

Squamous cell carcinoma of the vulva generally *remains localized for long periods of time and then spreads in a predictable fashion to the regional lymph nodes,* including those of the inguinal and femoral chain. Lesions > 2 cm wide and 0.5 cm deep have an increased chance of nodal metastases. The overall incidence of lymph node metastasis is approximately 30%. Lesions arising in the anterior one third of the vulva may spread to the deep pelvic nodes, bypassing regional inguinal and femoral lymphatics.

Evaluation

The *staging classification* was altered by the Federation of Gynecology and Obstetrics (FIGO) in 1988 (Table 43.3). Prior to 1988, vulvar cancers were staged clinically. However, noted discrepancies in regard to predicting nodal metastasis led to a change from clinical to surgical staging. This staging convention uses the analysis of the removed vulvar tumor and microscopic assessment of the regional lymph nodes as its basis.

Treatment

Although the mainstay for the treatment of invasive vulvar cancer is surgical, many advances have been made to help individualize patients into treatment categories in an effort to reduce the amount of radical surgery while not compromising survival. Accordingly, not all patients undergo radical vulvectomy with bilateral nodal dissections. Individualized approaches include the following.

- Conservative vulvar operations for patients with unifocal lesions
- Elimination of routine pelvic lymphadenectomy
- Avoidance of groin dissection in patients with unilateral lesions < 1 mm deep
- Elimination of contralateral groin dissection in patients with unilateral T1 lesions who have negative ipsilateral nodes and are > 1 cm from the vulvar midline
- Separate groin incisions for those patients with indicated bilateral groin dissection
- Use of postoperative radiation therapy to decrease incidence of groin recurrence in patients with two or more positive groin nodes

Concomitant use of radiation and chemotherapy (5-fluorouracil plus cisplatin or mitomycin or cisplatin alone) is gaining favor for treatment of vulvar cancers that require radiation therapy. Treatment with chemotherapy in cases of recurrent vulvar cancer has only limited value.

Prognosis

The corrected 5-year survival rate for all vulvar carcinoma is approximately 70%. Five-year survival rates are 80% to 90% for stage I and II disease. Survival rates for patients with stage III disease are 60%, and those with stage IV have rates of 5% to 15%.

Carcinoma of Bartholin's Gland

Carcinoma of the Bartholin's gland is uncommon (1% to 2% of all vulvar carcinomas). Malignancies that arise from the Bartholin's gland include adenocarcinomas, squamous cell carcinomas, adenosquamous carcinomas, adenoid cystic, and transitional-cell carcinomas. These arise mainly as a result of changes occuring within the different histologic areas of the gland and ducts leading from it. Bartholin's carcinoma on average occurs in women over the age of 50; however, any new Bartholin's mass in a woman over the age of 40 should be excised. Treatment of diagnosed Bartholin's cancers is radical vulvectomy and bilateral lymphadenectomy. Recurrence is a disappointingly common event, and a 5-year overall survival rate of 50% to 60% is noted.

Vaginal Disease

Benign Vaginal Masses

Gartner duct cysts arise from vestigial remnants of the wolffian or mesonephric system that course along the outer anterior aspect of the vaginal canal. These cystic structures are usually small and asymptomatic, but on occasion they may be larger and symptomatic so that excision is required.

Inclusion cysts are usually seen on the posterior lower vaginal surface, resulting from imperfect approximation of childbirth lacerations or episiotomy. They are lined with stratified squamous epithelium, their content is usually cheesy, and they may be excised if symptomatic.

Vaginal Neoplasia

Carcinoma in situ of the vagina and invasive vaginal cancer are among the rarest of gynecologic neoplasms. They are often multifocal,

Table 43.3. Staging for Carcinoma of the Vulva

FIGO surgical staging:

Stage 0

| Tis | Carcinoma in situ; intraepithelial carcinoma |

Stage I

| T1 N0 M0 | Tumor confined to the vulva and/or perineum; <2 cm in greatest dimension; nodes are not palpable |

Stage II

| T2 N0 M0 | Tumor confined to the vulva and/or perineum; >2 cm in greatest dimension; nodes are not palpable |

Stage III

T3 N0 M0	Tumor of any size with:
T3 N1 M0	1. Adjacent spread to the lower urethra and/or the vagina, or the anus, and/or
T1 N1 M0	2. Unilateral regional lymph node metastasis
T2 N1 M0	

Stage IVA

T1 N2 M0	Tumor invades any of the following: upper urethra, bladder mucosa, rectal mucosa, pelvic and/or bilateral regional node metastasis
T2 N2 M0	
T3 N2 M0	
T4 any N M0	

Stage IVB

| Any T | Any distant metastasis, including pelvic lymph nodes |
| Any N, M1 | |

TNM clinical staging (rules for staging are similar to those for carcinoma of the cervix).

T	Primary tumor
Tis	Preinvasive carcinoma (carcinoma in situ)
T1	Tumor confined to the vulva and/or perineum; <2 cm in greatest dimension
T2	Tumor confined to the vulva and/or perineum; >2 cm in greatest dimension
T3	Tumor of any size with adjacent spread to the urethra and/or vagina and/or to the anus
T4	Tumor of any size infiltrating the bladder mucosa and/or the rectal mucosa, including the upper part of the urethral mucosa and/or fixed to the bone
N	Regional lymph nodes
N0	No lymph node metastasis
N1	Unilateral regional lymph node metastasis
N2	Bilateral regional lymph node metastasis
M	Distant metastasis
M0	No clinical metastasis
M1	Distant metastasis (including pelvic lymph node metastasis)

FIGO = Federation of Gynecology and Obstetrics; TNM = tumor, node, metastasis.

associated with other lower genital tract intraepithelial or invasive neoplasms. Vaginal intraepithelial neoplasia is similar histologically to CIN; however, it is represented in the vagina.

Carcinoma in Situ of the Vagina or Vaginal Intraepithelial Neoplasia Grade III (VAIN III)

VAIN III appears to occur more commonly in the third decade of life onward, although its exact incidence is unknown. One half to two thirds of patients with VAIN III have an antecedent or coexistent neoplasm of the lower genital tract. Approximately 1% to 2% of patients who undergo hysterectomy for CIN III and many patients who undergo radiation therapy for other gynecologic malignancy ultimately develop VAIN III. This is one of the arguments for yearly pap smears after hysterectomy. The importance of VAIN III is its potential for progression to invasive vaginal carcinoma, as the lesions themselves are usually asymptomatic and have no intrinsic morbidity.

VAIN III must be differentiated from other causes of red ulcerated or white hyperplastic lesions of the vagina such as herpes, traumatic lesions, hyperkeratosis associated with chronic irritation (e.g., from a poorly fitting diaphragm), or adenosis. Inspection and palpation of the vagina are the mainstays of diagnosis, but unfortunately, this is often done in a cursory fashion during the routine pelvic examination. *Pap smears of the vaginal mucosa are sometimes rewarding,* although *colposcopy with directed biopsy is the definitive method of diagnosis,* just as it is with cervical intraepithelial neoplasia.

The goals of treatment of VAIN III are ablation of the intraepithelial lesion while preserving vaginal depth, caliber, and sexual function. Laser ablation, local excision, and chemical treatment with 5-fluorouracil cream are all used for limited lesions; total or partial vaginectomy with application of a split thickness skin graft is usually reserved for failure of the previously described treatments. Cure rates of 80% to 95% may be expected.

Invasive Vaginal Cancer

Invasive vaginal cancer accounts for approximately 1% to 2% of gynecologic malignancies. *Squamous cell carcinoma* makes up approximately 80% to 90% of these malignancies, occurring primarily in women over 55 years old. The remainder of vaginal carcinomas consists of *adenocarcinoma of the vagina (clear cell adenocarcinoma, usually related to diethylstilbestrol [DES] exposure before 18 weeks' gestation while in utero) and vaginal melanoma.*

The staging of vaginal carcinoma is nonsurgical (Table 43.4). Radiation therapy is the mainstay of treatment for squamous cell carcinoma of the vagina. Radical hysterectomy combined with upper vaginectomy and pelvic lymphadenectomy are used for selected patients. Upper vaginal lesions and pelvic exenteration and radical vulvectomy are used for selected patients with lower vaginal lesions involving the vulva. Most young women with clear cell carcinoma have lesions located in the upper one half of the vagina and wish to maintain ovarian and vaginal function. Radical hysterectomy with upper vaginectomy combined with pelvic lymphadenectomy is often the primary treatment for these patients, with radiation therapy following. The overall 5-year survival rate for squamous cell carcinoma of the vagina is 50% and for clear cell adenocarcinoma of the vagina, 80%, with stage I and II patients having the best prognosis. Melanoma is treated with radical surgery; radiation and chemotherapy have little efficacy.

Sarcoma botryoides (or embryonal rhabdomyosarcoma) presents as a mass of grapelike

Table 43.4. Clinical Staging of Vaginal Carcinoma	
Stage	**Description**
0	Carcinoma in situ
I	Carcinoma limited to the vaginal mucosa
II	Carcinoma involving the subvaginal tissue but not extending onto the pelvic wall
III	Carcinoma extending onto the pelvic wall
IV	Carcinoma extending into the mucosa of the bladder or rectum or distant metastases

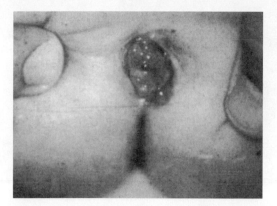

Figure 43.3. Sarcoma botryoides in a 6-month-old child. The grapelike polypoid tumors protruding through the vaginal introitus are asymptomatic, except for a slight bloody discharge.

polyps arising from the undifferentiated mesenchyme of the lamina propria of the anterior vaginal wall and protrudes from the introitus of young girls and infants (Figure 43.3). Bloody discharge is an associated symptom in these frightening tumors. The tumor spreads locally, although it may have distant hematogenous metastases. This tumor was treated in the past with pelvic exenteration, but because this procedure was so unpalatable in this age group, wide excision combined with chemotherapy or chemotherapy and radiation is often used in an attempt to salvage as much bowel and bladder function as possible.

CHAPTER 44

CERVICAL NEOPLASIA AND CARCINOMA

This chapter deals primarily with APGO Educational Topic:

Topic 52: Cervical Disease and Neoplasia

The student should understand how detection and treatment of preinvasive lesions reduces medical and social costs of, as well as mortality from, carcinoma of the cervix.

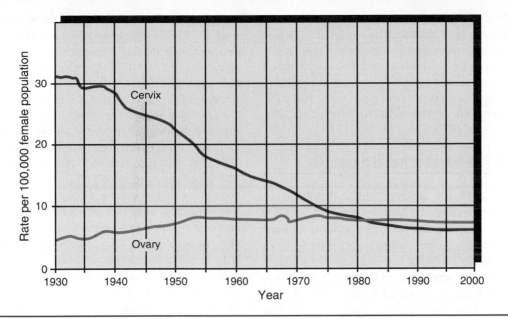

Figure 44.1. Age-adjusted death rate for cervical cancer in the United States, 1930–1996.

Cervical carcinoma serves as the model of a "controllable" cancer, controllable in the sense of (a) an identifiable precursor lesion (cervical intraepithelial neoplasia, CIN) with a natural history of usually slow progression to frank cervical cancer, (b) an inexpensive and noninvasive screening test (Pap smear) that may be augmented with adjunctive tests such as HPV DNA typing and a follow-up diagnostic procedure (colposcopy) for diagnosis, and (c) simple and effective treatments of the precursor lesion (cryotherapy, laser ablation, loop electrosurgical excision procedure [LEEP], and cold knife cone biopsy) with high cure rates.

Because it is possible to identify and treat the asymptomatic precursor lesion thereby preventing progression to actual cancer of the cervix, cervical cancer is now the second rather than the first most common malignancy in women in developed countries. Improved treatment of cervical cancer has gone beyond the precursor lesions. Cure rates of up to 90% are seen in early stage disease (stages IA1 and IA2), and increased life expectancy is seen in advanced stage disease. The gratifying effect of these interventions is graphically seen in the fall of the mortality rate for cervical cancer compared with that of ovarian carcinoma, for which no treatable precursor lesion can be easily identified (Figure 44.1).

Certain *epidemiologic factors* relating to cervical neoplasia are significant (Table 44.1). Of the factors listed, special note should be made

Table 44.1. Potential Factors in Cervical Neoplasia

Epidemiologic characteristics
    Early intercourse
    Multiple sex partners
    Early childbearing
    Male factors: "high-risk" consort
    Socioeconomic status, race
    Venereal infection
Other factors
    Immune status
    Oral contraceptives
    Cigarette smoking
    Intrauterine DES exposure
Viral relations
    Papillomavirus

DES = diethylstilbestrol.

of those relating to early sexual intercourse with multiple partners; the role of cigarette smoking; male factors, including the "high-risk" consort; immunologically compromised patients (those receiving immunosuppressive therapy and those infected with the HIV virus); and exposure to the human papillomavirus (HPV).

Cervical Intraepithelial Neoplasia

Pathology: The Squamocolumnar Junction

Understanding the pathophysiology of CIN and its association with the *squamocolumnar junction* (SCJ) and *transformation zone* (TZ) of the cervix provides the rationale for cervical Pap smear screening, diagnostic colposcopy, and the treatment of CIN. As the uterus and cervix grow during puberty and adolescence, the original SCJ "rolls out," or everts, from its position just inside the cervical os to a position on the enlarged cervical surface. In this process, original columnar endocervical tissue is also rolled to the cervical surface. This area is exposed to vaginal secretions, irritants, and a changing hormonal milieu. The process of squamous metaplasia begins at the new SCJ.

The area between the old and new SCJs, where squamous metaplasia occurs, is called the transformation zone. In the menopausal years, the uterus and cervix again decrease in size, and the new SCJ comes to lie upward into the endocervical canal, often out of direct visual contact (Figure 44.2). Approximately 95% of squamous intraepithelial neoplasia occurs within the transformation zone.

The most important risk factor for the development of cervical neoplasia and cancer is the human papillomavirus (HPV). Of the approximately 80 types, about 30 may infect the anogenital tract, and about 15 are associated with cervical neoplasia and cancer. HPV high-risk types 16, 18, 31, 33, and 45 are the most important in this regard, with low-risk types 6 and 11 associated with genital warts (condylomata accuminata) and low-grade cervical intraepithelial neoplasia. When the double-stranded DNA HPV virus infects the reproducing cells of the basal cell layer and are not integrated into the host genome, entire encapsulated virions are produced that are expressed morphologically as "koilocytes." When, however, the HPV is integrated into the DNA, the expression of the cell's regulatory genes may be altered, leading to the transformation of the cells to intraepithelial lesions or carcinoma. Because HPV infection is much more common than cervical intraepithelial neoplasia or carcinoma, it is likely that several as yet not fully identified host or environmental factors act as cofactors. A higher incidence of HPV infection and progression of intraepithelial neoplasia is seen in immunosuppressed patients, including those infected with HIV as well as those who are organ transplant recipients, who have chronic renal failure or a history of Hodgkin's lymphoma or immunosuppressive therapy for other reasons. Another factor is cigarette smoking, which is associated with a 50% higher risk for developing cervical carcinoma.

HPV DNA testing is now being used with increasing frequency, with more accurate and encompassing tests being introduced regularly. The test may be used as an adjunctive test in the Atypical Squamous Cells of Undetermined Significance (ASC-US) group. Patients who have ASC-US Paps and are HPV DNA negative for high-risk types of HPV may be followed routinely, whereas those positive for high-risk types of HPV are referred for colposcopy. Patients with low-grade squamous intraepithelial lesion (LSIL) and high-grade squamous intrapeithelial lesion (HSIL) Paps do not benefit from HPV DNA testing because 83% of LSIL patients are positive for HPV, and greater than 90% of HSIL patients are positive for HPV. The development of effective *papillomavirus vaccine* is currently under study. The FDA is currently evaluating a vaccine for HPV 16, 18, 6, and 11.

Screening: The Pap Smear

In the early 1940s and before, cervical cancer was usually diagnosed at an advanced stage with substantial morbidity and mortality compared to what might be obtained from earlier diagnosis. The diagnosis was made by biopsy of a symptomatic patient (histological sample; symptoms such as bleeding, pain, cervical mass). The Greek physician George Papanicolaou reasoned that diagnosis in the relatively long asymptomatic interval before the lesions

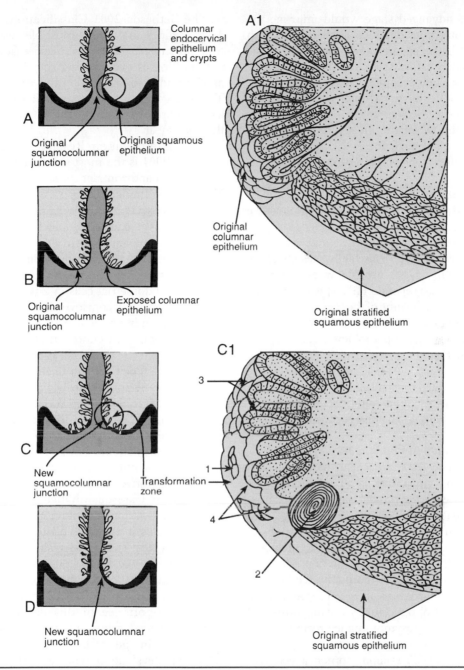

Figure 44.2. Squamocolumnar junction (SCJ) and transformation zone. (**A**) Before puberty and adolescence, the original SCJ is at or just above the external os, with the original squamous epithelium being outside and the original columnar endocervical epithelium, inside. (**A1**) Three-dimensional representation of the original SCJ. (**B**) As the cervix matures and grows, the original SCJ rolls outward, followed by endocervical columnar epithelium, which is now exposed to the vagina and its contents. (**C**) As the endocervical tissue is exposed and comes under the influence of mature hormone levels, the process of squamous metaplasia occurs, with a new SCJ forming inward from the old one. The area in between is the transformation zone, the site of this squamous metaplasia. (**C1**) Three-dimensional representation of mature SCJ, showing islets of columnar epithelium (**1**), nabothian cyst (**2**), gland openings (**3**), and metaplastic epithelium (**4**). (**D**) In menopause, the process reverses, and the new SCJ rolls inward to lie at or above the cervical os, often out of direct visual observation.

reached advanced stage would improve the dismal outcomes common at that time. With great insight, Papanicolaou proposed that the examination of cells scraped from the cervix might facilitate accurate and earlier diagnosis. This use of exfolative cytology as a screening test became the Pap smear. The Pap smear represents one of the most dramatic success stories in all of medicine.

Cells are scraped from the exocervix and endocervix with spatulae and various brushes. These cells are then either spread on a glass slide and fixed with a spray cytologic fixative agent or swirled into a liquid medium from which the cells are separated and evaluated. Liquid-based cytology also allows testing of the fluid for HPV DNA up to 3 weeks after the study, whereas separate HPV specimens must be obtained at the time of the Pap smear if a Pap slide is used. The cytologic specimens are read and reported by cytopathologists. Recently, automated Pap smear assessment devices have been introduced. At present their use is not for primary Pap smear evaluation, but rather for rescreening of large numbers of previously screened slides as a quality control measure.

Classification of Pap Smears

Through the years, Pap smears have been classified with various systems. The Bethesda 2001 classification is the present recommended classification and includes revised management suggestions. (See Tables 44.2, 44.3, and 44.4.) The basis of all the classifications, including Bethesea 2001, is the likelihood of progression of precursor lesions to more advanced lesions and eventually to cervical carcinoma and hence the window of opportunity for diagnosis and treatment in the asymptomatic precursor stage when outcomes are good.

More than 50 million women a year undergo Papanicolaou testing in the United States. Approximately 7% of these women will be diagnosed with an abnormal Pap smear. The most recent Bethesda classification system was incorportated into guidelines developed by 121 experts in the diagnosis and management of cervical cancer precursors and was published by the American Society for Colposcopy and Cervical Pathology (ASCCP) by Wright et al. in *JAMA* 2002.

The Bethesda 2001 Classification (Table 44.2) outlines the various possible results of the Pap smear. The table specifies accepted methodologies of reporting the Pap results and provides for interpretation of findings. This categorization allows for defined management options regarding the initial results of the Pap smear.

The Interpretation/Results section of Bethesda 2001 is the most substantial section of the report and contains three sections: First, Negative for Intraepithelial Lesion or Malignancy. This section also contains discussions of findings associated with infectious diseases (the Organisms subsection) and other findings (the Other nonneoplastic findings subsection). The second is Other, which includes the finding of endometrial cells in a woman over 40 years of age. It is controversial whether further evaluation is advisable because of a possible association with endometrial carcinoma, tubal carcinoma, and ovarian carcinoma. The third is the crucial section dealing with Epithelial Cell Abnormalities. Squamous cells comprise 90% to 95% of epithelial cell abnormalities and are reported in the Squamous Cell section in four categories. *Atypical squamous cells (ASC)* should comprise about 5% or less of smears and are defined as cytological changes suggestive of a squamous intraepithelial lesion that are quantitatively or qualitatively insufficient for a definitive interpretation. The ASC classification is divided into two groups; atypical squamous cells of undetermined significance (ASC-US) and the latter, atypical squamous cells, cannot exclude high-grade squamous intraepithelial lesion (ASC-H). The importance of this division is in how much evaluation and management is warranted. In general, ASC-H warrants colposcopic evaluation, whereas ASC-US has several appropriate managements.

The Interpretation/Results section of Bethesda 2001 continues with three sections that deal with more clearly identified cell abnormalities. The first is LSIL, which generally encompasses cells from lesions that will prove on histological evaluation to be HPV associated lesions, mild dysplasia, or cervical intrapeithelial neoplasia–1. The second is HSIL, which generally encompasses cells from

Table 44.2. The PAP Smear Report: Bethesda 2001	
Specimen Type	
Indicate conventional smear (Pap smear) vs. liquid-based study vs. other	
General Categorization	
(optional; information also in Interpretation/Results) Negative for intraepithelial Lesion or Malignancy	
Epithelial Cell Abnormality Other	
SPECIMEN ADEQUACY	
Satisfactory for evaluation	Includes whether endocervical/transformation zone components are present or absent.
	Includes other quality indicators (for example, inflammation, partially obscuring blood, etc.)
Unsatisfactory for evaluation	Indicates reason smear classified unsatisfactory (either without processing or after processing)
Interpretation/Result	
Negative for intraepithelial lesion or malignancy	No cellular evidence of neoplasia
Organisms	
Trichomonas vaginalis	
Fungal organisms morphologically consistent with *Candida sp.*	
Sift in floral suggestive of bacterial vaginosis Bacteria morphologically consistent with *Actinomyces sp.*	
Cellular changes associated with herpes simplex virus	
Other nonneoplastic findings	
Reactive cellular changes associated with inflammation, Radiation, or intrauterine contraceptive device	
Glandular cells status posthysterectomy Atrophy	
Other	
Endometrial cells in a woman $\geq$40 years of age, specify if negative for squamous intraepithelial lesion	
Epithelial cell abnormalities	
SQUAMOUS CELL	
Atypical squamous cells	
—of undetermined significance (ASC-US) (encompassing cells "suggestive" of SIL)	
—cannot exclude HSIL (ASC-H)	
Low-grade squamous intraepithelial lesion (LSIL)	
Encompassing: HPV/mild dysplasia/CIN-I	
High-grade squamous intraepithelial lesion (HSIL)	

(continued)

Table 44.2. continued

Encompassing: moderate and severe dysplasia, CIS/CIN-2, and CIN-3	
—with features suspicious for invasion	
Squamous cell carcinoma	
GLANDULAR CELL	
Atypical	
—endocervical cells (NOS or specify in comments)	
—endometrial cells (NOS or specify in comments)	
—glandular cells (NOS or specify in comments)	
Atypical	
—endocervical cells, favor neoplastic	
—glandular cells, favor neoplastic	
Endocervical adenocarcinoma in situ	
Adenocarcinoma	
—endocervical	
—endometrial	
—extrauterine	
—not otherwise specified (NOS)	
Other malignant neoplasms (specify)	
Automated Review	If case examined by automatic device, specify device and result
Ancillary Testing	Brief description of test methods and results to be easily understood by clinician
Educational Notes and Suggestions	Suggestions for patient education should be consistent with other standard guidelines

lesions that prove on histological evaluation to be moderate to severe dysplasia, cervical intraepithelial neoplasia–2 or –3, or carcinoma in situ. A subclassification is also provided, HSIL with features suspicious for invasion. The final group is squamous cell carcinoma, with cells consistent with exfoliation from frank cervical carcinoma.

The Interpretation/Results section of Bethesda 2001 concludes with a section addressing the 5% to 10% of epithelial cell abnormalities that are glandular cell. The importance of Pap smears with these abnormalities is disproportionate to their number because about 40% are found on evaluation to be associated with squamous intraepithelial lesions, 6% with adenocarcinoma in situ, and another 6% with frank carcinoma. This classification harbors

special importance for women over 35 years of age, as most cancers in this age group are endometrial in origin. There are four subsections. The first consists of atypical endocervical cells (either not otherwise specified or favor neoplastic), atypical endometrial cells, or atypical glandular cells (either not otherwise specified or favor neoplastic, or probably AIS [adenocarcimoma in situ]). The second is endocervical adenocarcinoma in situ (AIS). The third is adenocarcinoma, either endocervical, endometrial, extrauterine (tubal, ovarian, other), or not otherwise specified (NOS). The fourth is other, which encompases cells that may be of tubal or ovarian origin. At present, HPV DNA typing has not been found to be of similar value as in ASC, although this may change with the acquisition of further information.

Table 44.3. Comparison of Pap Smear Descriptive Conventions

Descriptive Convention						
Class system	Class I (normal)	Class II inflammation	Class III Mild dysplasia	or Moderate dysplasia	Class IV severe dysplasia CIS	Class V suggestive of cancer or CIS
CIN system	Normal	Inflammatory	CIN I	or CIN II	CIN III	Suggestive of cancer
Bethesda II system	Within normal limits	a. Without atypia b. With atypia or cellular changes associated with HPV	LSIL	HSIL	HSIL	Squamous cell cancer
Bethesda 2001	Negative for intraepithelial lesion or malignancy	ASC-US | ASC-H	LSIL	HSIL		Squamous cell Carcinoma
Histology	Basal cells	WBCs	Basement membrane			Invasive cervical cancer

CIN = cervical intraepithelial neoplasia; CIS = carcinoma in situ; HPV = human papillomavirus; WBCs = white blood cells.
ASC-US = atypical squamous cells of undetermined significance; ASC-H = atypical squamous cells, cannot exclude HSIL;
LSIL = low-grade squamous intraepithelial lesion; HSIL = high-grade squamous intraepithelial lesion

Evaluation of Abnormal Pap Smears (See Table 44.4)

The evaluation of atypical squamous cells is challenging because of the imprecision with which they are classified and the often-conflicting information about their appropriate evaluation and treatment. ASC-US Paps have a 3% to 10% chance of harboring a higher-grade lesion and are associated with a substantial lack of reproducibility of the classification itself. ASC-US can be managed either by repeat cytology in 4 to 6 months, immediate colposcopy, or HPV testing. The last method is the preferred method as it will avoid colposcopy in over 40% of the patients and allow for follow-up in 1 year if HPV testing is negative. Menopausal women with these Pap results may have an atrophic component, even if on systemic estrogen replacement therapy, so that

intravaginal estrogen therapy and a repeat Pap smear may be an appropriate management. Likewise, inflammation associated with intravaginal infection may be appropriately managed by treatment and repeat Pap smear. Immunosuppressed women with ASC-US are best evaluated with colposcopy. ASC-H is evaluated by colposcopy because of the higher likelihood of underlying CIN 2–3 lesions (variously reported at an incidence of 24% to 94% of cases) or worse, compared to ASC-US.

About 1.6% to 7.7% of Pap smears are reproducibly classified as LSIL. About 15% to 30% of these will be found to have a CIN 2–3 on biopsy. Approximately 50% of patients with CIN 1 will regress to negative, 30% will persist as CIN 1, and only 10% will progress to higher-grade CIN. Also, even if the CIN 1 does progress to a higher-grade CIN, the

Table 44.4. Evaluation of Epithelial Cell Abnormalities—Bethesda 2001 Classification

Classification	Evaluation
SQUAMOUS CELL	
ASC-US	HPV DNA testing
	If positive for high-risk HPV DNA, colposcopy
	If negative, may repeat Pap in 12 months
	Colposcopy
	Repeat Pap is acceptable but not preferred
	Repeat Pap every 3–4 months until three consecutive "negative for squamous intraepithelial lesions/malignancy" Pap smears
	Special Circumstances
	Menopausal woman: intravaginal estrogen cream nightly for 3–6 weeks, then repeat Pap; if negative, repeat in 3–4 months and if again negative, may return to routine Pap sequence; if positive, colposcopy
	Infections/severe inflammation; acceptable to treat infection and repeat Pap in 4–6 weeks; if negative, repeat in 3–4 months and if again negative, may return to routine Pap sequence; if positive, colposcopy
	Immunosuppressed woman: colposcopy
ASC-H	Colposcopy
LSIL	Colposcopy
	With follow-up Pap smears
	With treatment and then follow-up Pap smears
	Colposcopy is recommended if:
	Prior high-grade lesion/dysplasia/CIN 2 or 3/CIS (treated or untreated)
	Prior ACS-US, LSIL/HSIL, Pap without history of therapy
	Inability to follow up patient
	Postmenopausal patient without atrophy
	Strong family history of cervical or lower genital carcinoma
	Heavy smoking history
	Repeat Pap smear (if colposcopy not general scheme and none of the indications for colposcopy present)
	Repeat Pap smears every 4–6 months with return to routine screening after 3 consecutive repeat smears without evidence of intraepithelial neoplasia or carcinoma and referral for colposcopy if any repeat smear shows evidence of these abnormalities
HSIL	Colposcopy with ECC and directed biopsy of most abnormal lesion(s) as determined colposcopically;
HSIL with features suspicious for invasion	Colposcopy with ECC and directed biopsy of most abnormal lesion(s) as determined colposcopically;
Squamous cell	Colposcopy with ECC and directed biopsy of most abnormal lesion(s) as determined colposcopically;

(continued)

Table 44.4. continued

Classification	Evaluation
Atypical -endocervical cells (NOS or specify in comments) -endometrial cells (NOS or specify in comments) -glandular cells (NOS or specify in comments)	Colposcopy, endocervical sampling
Atypical -endocervical cells, favor neoplastic -glandular cells, favor neoplastic	Colposcopy, endocervical sampling, and diagnostic excisional cervical procedure (conization, preferably CKC); exception: if initial histology shows invasive carcinoma, conization should be deferred with individualized treatment by a gynecologic oncologist.
Endocervical adenocarcinoma in situ	As above
Adenocarcinoma -endocervical -endometrial -extrauterine -not otherwise specified (NOS)	As above
Special circumstances	
AGC (any kind) Women over 35 years of age with unexplained vaginal bleeding Postmenopausal women not on estrogen replacement therapy	Endometrial sampling (Pipelle endometrial sampling, D&C)
Repeat AGC, AGC "favor neoplasia," and atypical endocervical cells "suggestive of AIS" where colposcopy, cervical biopsy, endocervical sampling, and cervical excisional procedure fail to elicit the source of the cellular abnormality	Pelvic ultrasound, abdominopelvic CT scan to evaluate for nongynecologic sources of abnormal cells. Women over 35 years of age should also have hysteroscopic evaluation to reduce the risk of missed endometrial lesions. Before proceeding with this extensive evaluation, a review of all slides is recommended
Other	Colposcopy and endocervical evaluation followed by appropriate procedures to evaluate the suggested site of origin (e.g., ovary, fallopian tube, etc.)

treatment and cure rates for low-grade and higher-grade CIN are similar. ASCCP guidelines recommend colposcopy with directed biopsies as deemed appropriate for management of LSIL. The evaluation of squamous cell epithelial cell abnormalities reported as HSIL and carcinoma is relatively straightforward, involving colposcopy and directed biopsy or conization, endocervical sampling, and in some cases, endometrial sampling. This is because the likelihood of a more severe lesion or the progression of extant lesions is high. The goal of evaluation is to determine whether there is invasive cancer or a high-grade preinvasive lesion. With evidence of invasion, conization is generally indicated if the depth of invasion is <3 mm or if the depth of the invasion cannot be determined, whereas treatment for invasive cancer is pursued if the depth of invasion is determined to be >3 mm.

Glandular cell abnormalities comprise <0.5% of epithelial cell abnormalities. Their appropriate evaluation is especially important because of their association with squamous and glandular precursor lesions and carcinoma. AGC is now divided into three separate qualifier groups: AGC not otherwise specified (endocervical, endometrial, or glandular cells), AGC favor neoplasia, and AIS (endocervical adenocarcinoma in situ). All women with AGC of any variety should have colposcopy and endocervical sampling regardless of qualification. Colposcopy and endocervical curettage is recommended for all types of AGC. Biopsy-confirmed CIN II-III, AIS, or invasive cancer have been found in 9% to 41% of women with AGC NOS cytology compared to 27% to 96% of women with AGC favor neoplasia cytology. AIS cytology is associated with a high risk of women having either AIS (48% to 69%) or invasive cervical adenocarcinoma (38%). Colposcopy and ECC is recommended for women with all subcategories of AGC with the caveat that women with atypical endometrial cells should have an endometrial biopsy. Endometrial biopsy should be performed in conjunction with colposcopy in women older than 35 with AGC and in younger women with AGC with unexplained bleeding or AIS. Data is insufficient to allow an assessment of HPV DNA testing in the treatment of women with AGC or AIS.

The recommended treatment for AGC favor neoplasia or AIS is an excisional conization. The choice of which type of conization is controversial, but the preponderance of evidence supports cold conization over loop electrosurgical excision because of thermal distortion of possible glandular cell abnormalities. The exception to the cervical excisional procedure recommendation is for women with the diagnosis of invasive carcinoma on biopsy or endocervical sampling. These patients require individualized treatment by a gynecologic oncologist.

Colposcopy and Cervical Conization

Colposcopy is the most common management approach when histological evaluation is required. A colposcope is a binocular stereomicroscope with variable magnification (usually H 1 to 14) and a light source with green filters to aid in the identification of abnormal appearing blood vessels that may be associated with intraepithelial neoplasia. With colposcopy, areas with changes consistent with dysplasia are identified, allowing directed biopsy (i.e., biopsy of the area where dysplasia is most likely). Colposcopic criteria such as white epithelium, abnormal vascular patterns, and punctate lesions help identify such areas. To facilitate the examination, the cervix is washed with a 3% to 4% acetic acid solution, which acts as an epithelial desiccant of intracellular protein, enhancing visualization of dysplastic lesions. Lesions usually appear with relatively discrete borders near the SCJ. *Visualization of the entire SCJ is required for a colposcopy to be considered a satisfactory colposcopic examination.* If the SCJ is not visualized in its entirety or if the margins of abnormal areas are not seen in their entirety, the colposcopic assessment is termed *unsatisfactory,* and other evaluation such as cervical conization is indicated. This is the *first reason to perform conization: unsatisfactory colposcopy.*

The number of colposcopically directed biopsies obtained will vary depending on the number and severity of abnormal areas found. After sampling the identified lesions, an *endocervical curettage* (ECC), using a small curette, is performed, often followed by the use of an endocervical brush to retrieve additional cells dislodged but not trapped in the curette specimen.

This endocervical sample is obtained so that potential disease farther inside the cervical canal, which is not visualized by the colposcope, may be detected. The cervical biopsies and ECC are then submitted separately for pathologic assessment. ECC is positive for dysplasia in 5% to 10% of women with abnormal Pap smears. Because of the lack of tissue orientation from endocervical curettings, the degree of dysplasia determined from them is difficult to assess. This is the *second reason for cervical conization: positive ECC.*

In approximately 10% of colposcopies with directed biopsies and ECC, a substantial discrepancy is seen between the screening Pap smear and the histologic data from biopsy and ECC (i.e., the biopsy does not explain the source of the abnormal Pap). If this occurs, more tissue needs to be obtained by cervical conization so that the most severe abnormality can be explained histologically. This is the *third indication for cervical conization: a substantial discrepancy between Pap smear and biopsy results.*

Cervical conization, or cone biopsy of the cervix, is a minor surgical procedure performed under general or regional anesthesia. Usually performed with scalpel and scissors (*cold knife conization, CKC*), conization is now also performed with a laser or with a heated wire loop, the *LLETZ (large loop excision of the transformation zone)*, also known as *LEEP (loop electrosurgical excision procedure)*. As seen in Figure 33.9 a cone-shaped specimen is removed from the cervix, which encompasses the SCJ, all identified lesions on the ectocervix, and a portion of the endocervical canal, the extent of which depends on whether the ECC was positive or negative. Because LEEP uses an electrically heated wire, concern is often raised about thermal damage at the margins of the specimen obscuring the histology. This is usually not considered a problem in the evaluation of squamous epithelial abnormalities, but it may be a substantial issue in the evaluation of glandular epithelial lesions, where abnormal cells in the bottom of glandular crypts may be altered. In cases of glandular abnormalities, CKC may be more appropriate.

If the margins of the biopsy are not free of disease, the patient should have either repeat conization or close follow-up because of the possibility that disease remains. If the margins

are positive for a high-grade epithelial lesion or carcinoma in situ, the most appropriate treatment may be hysterectomy depending on her desire for future fertility and/or her views about the value of maintaining her cervix and uterus. In addition to the usual risks of any surgery (bleeding, infection, and anesthetic risks), conization has the additional risks of cervical incompetence (if the internal cervical os is compromised), and reduced cervical capacity to facilitate sperm transport because of the loss of mucous-secreting glands. Both complications may contribute to future fertility problems. Conversely, in some women the issue is not cervical incompetence, but rather cervical stenosis because of scarring, which may hinder menstrual flow and/or lead to protraction disorders of labor.

Treatment

The underlying concept in the treatment of CIN is that excision or ablation of the precursor lesion avoids progression to carcinoma. Because these lesions are superficial and usually confined to the visible and easily accessible SCJ, simple office techniques usually suffice. In general, the therapy for CIN 1 is either observation with follow-up cytology or local ablation. For preinvasive high-grade lesions (HSIL, CIN 2 and 3, CIS), ablation or excision is generally recommended because a substantial portion of these are likely to progress to invasive carcinoma of the cervix if left untreated. Ablative procedures should be used only with an adequate colposcopy and appropriate correlation between Pap smear and colposcopically directed biopsy.

Cryotherapy is a popular outpatient method used to treat low-grade CIN (Figure 33.7) The procedure involves covering the SCJ and all identified lesions with a stainless steel probe, which is then supercooled with liquid nitrogen or compressed gas (carbon dioxide or nitrous oxide). The size and shape of the probe depends on the size and shape of the cervix and the lesion to be treated. The most common technique involves a 3-minute freeze followed by a 5-minute thaw, with a repeat 3-minute freeze (Figure 44.3). The thaw period between the two freezing episodes allows the damaged tissue from the first freeze to become edematous and swell with intracellular fluid. With the second

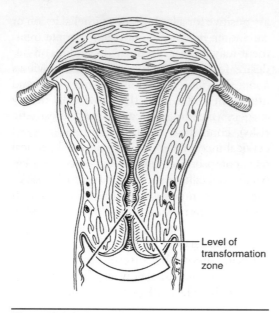

Figure 44.3. Cervical conization.

freeze, the edematous cellular architecture is re-frozen and extends the damaged area slightly deeper into the tissue. Healing after cryotherapy may take up to 4 or 5 weeks because the damaged tissue slowly sloughs and is replaced by new cervical epithelium. This process is associated with profuse watery discharge often mixed with necrotic cellular debris. It can be assumed that the entire healing process has been completed within 2 months, and usually the next follow-up Pap smear is done 12 weeks following the freezing to ascertain the effectiveness of the procedure. The cure rate for low-grade CIN using this technique approaches 90%.

Colposcopically directed *laser therapy* may be used to ablate lesions involving CIN. Because of the precision imparted by the colposcopic direction of the fine laser beam as well as the precise control of depth of ablation available, many physicians prefer laser ablation to "less-precise" techniques. Each lesion can be treated individually, and in addition, ablation of the entire SCJ is often performed (see Figure 44.3). Although laser treatment is more sophisticated than cryocautery, long-term cure rates are similar. An advantage of laser therapy is that it can be used for high-grade intraepithelial lesions because the depth of ablation can be adjusted to accommodate the extent of the lesion.

Conization, either "cold knife" or by LEEP, may be used as a therapeutic modality as well as for diagnosis and, indeed, often may serve both goals simultaneously. Hysterectomy may be indicated as an excisional modality in the case of high-grade noninvasive lesions when further fetility is not desired and the patient is fully aware of the risks and benefits of this procedure as compared to less-morbid excisional or ablative alternatives.

Follow-up to Treatment

After treatment for noninvasive epithelial cell abnormalities, either by ablation or excision, a period of follow-up Pap smears every 4 to 6 months for about 2 years is generally recommended, with variations depending on the specifics of the case. Most patients may return to a yearly evaluation thereafter. If a repeat Pap smear is abnormal, it is evaluated in the same manner as a new abnormal Pap smear. The importance of follow-up should be stressed to the patient because of the greater risk of recurrent abnormalities.

Cervical Carcinoma

Until approximately 20 years ago, cervical cancer was the most common gynecologic malignancy, with a ratio of 2:1 over endometrial carcinoma. Now the cervical carcinoma:endometrial carcinoma ratio has almost reversed; endometrial carcinoma rates are twice that for invasive cervical carcinoma. Approximately 10,000 new cases of invasive cervical carcinoma are diagnosed annually.

The average age at diagnosis for invasive cervical cancer is approximately 50 years, although the disease may occur in the very young as well as the very old patient. In studies following patients with advanced CIN, this precursor lesion precedes invasive carcinoma by approximately 10 years. In some patients, however, this time of progression may be considerably less.

The *etiology* of cervical cancer is HPV in >90% of cases. A few cervical cancers, however, are not related to HPV. There is ample evidence that advanced *CIN* arising in the squamous epithelium of the cervical transformation zone often progresses to invasive squamous cell cervical carcinoma. Studies involving genetic probes have identified papillomavirus DNA fragments within areas of invasive cervical carcinoma. Other etiologic associations are also similar to those for CIN, including *factors related to the male ejaculate, the immature transformation zone, the number of different sexual partners, and cigarette smoking. Immunocompromised patients* (e.g., transplant patients or patients with human immunodeficiency virus [HIV] infection) are a special group who seem more susceptible to this disease.

Approximately 80% of cervical cancer is of the squamous cell variety, most of the remaining cases being adenocarcinomas arising from the endocervical glands. *Three rare types of cervical cancer* are also encountered: *clear cell carcinoma* associated with diethylstilbestrol (DES) exposure in utero, *sarcoma,* and *lymphoma.* In general, the evaluation and treatment of squamous cell and adenocarcinoma of the cervix are similar. The discussions that follow reflect this similarity and apply to these two most common cervical carcinomas.

Survival *rates* for cervical carcinoma reflect the extent of disease at the time of diagnosis. Stage I has >85% 5-year survival, whereas 5-year survival for stages II, III, and IV are 50% to 60%, 30%, and 5%, respectively.

Clinical Evaluation

No classic historical presentation exists for cervical cancer. Two symptoms are often associated with cervical carcinoma, although both have other more common causes: *postcoital bleeding* and *abnormal uterine bleeding.* Other symptoms are determined by the organs involved as the cancer spreads by direct invasion to contiguous structures and by lymphatics to distant sites of metastasis.

Visible lesions on the cervix should have a biopsy taken. Lesions that should be considered for immediate biopsy include all new exophytic, friable, or bleeding lesions. These are readily differentiated from more common, normal variations of cervical anatomy such as nabothian cysts or condylomata. Pap smears are sometimes negative in this situation because exfoliative cells from frank cancer may be so distorted that they are uninterpretable. *When a visible lesion is present, colposcopic assessment need not be done unless the results of the direct biopsy do not confirm cancer.*

Staging is based on the International Federation of Gynecology and Obstetrics (FIGO) Staging Classification of 1985 (Table 44.5). This

Table 44.5.	Clinical Stages of Carcinoma of the Cervix Uteri
Stage	**Characteristics**
I	Carcinoma is strictly confined to cervix (extension to corpus should be disregarded)
IA	Preclinical carcinoma
IA1	Minimal microscopically evident stromal invasion
IA2	Microscopic lesions no more than 5 mm deep measured from base of epithelium surface or glandular from which it originates; horizontal spread not to exceed 7 mm
IB	All other cases of state I: Occult cancer should be marked "occ"
II	Carcinoma extends beyond cervix but has not extended to pelvic wall; involves vagina but not as far as lower third
IIA	No obvious parametrial involvement
IIB	Obvious parametrial involvement
III	Carcinoma has extended to pelvic wall; on rectal examination there is no cancer-free space between tumor and pelvic wall; tumor involves lower third of vagina; all cases with hydronephrosis or nonfunctioning kidney should be included, unless they are known to have another cause
IIIA	No extension to pelvic wall, but involvement of lower third of vagina
IIIB	Extension to pelvic wall, hydronephrosis, or nonfunctioning kidney caused by tumor
IV	Carcinoma has extended beyond true pelvis or has clinically involved mucosa of bladder or rectum
IVA	Spread of growth to adjacent pelvic organs
IVB	Spread to distant organs

International Federation of Gynecology and Obstetrics (FIGO) Staging Classification, revised 1985

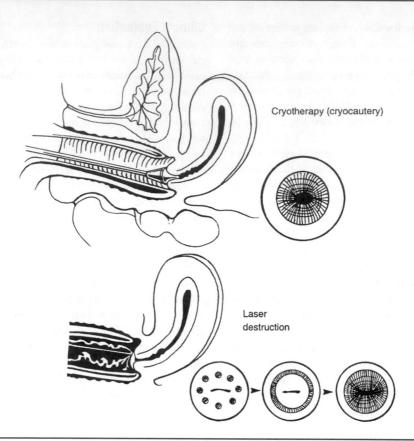

Cryotherapy (cryocautery)

Laser
destruction

Figure 44.4. Ablation of cervical intraepithelial neoplasia: cryotherapy and laser ablation. Laser ablation is a more precise technique and can be used to treat individual lesions. In this illustration, the laser is used to: define the border of the area to be treated, then circumscribe the area by "connecting the dots," then ablate the tissue within the defined area.

is a convention based both on the histologic assessment of the tumor sample and on physical and laboratory examination to ascertain the extent of disease. It is useful because of the predictable manner in which *cervical carcinoma spreads by direct invasion and by lymphatic metastasis* (Figure 44.4). The FIGO staging is based on clinical evaluation with the benefit of findings from roentgenographic examination of the chest, kidneys, and bones as well as colposcopy, cystoscopy, and proctoscopy with respective biopsies to confirm cervical cancer spread. PET scans, CT scans, lymphangiograms, arteriovenograms, laparoscopy or laparotomy findings, and radiographically directed biopsies are not used in FIGO clinical staging.

Management
Once histologic confirmation has been made of invasive cervical carcinoma, it is imperative to

refer the patient to a gynecologic oncologist for appropriate surgical and/or radiation therapy.

The mainstays of treatment for invasive cervical carcinoma include *radical surgical therapy and/or pelvic irradiation*. In general, surgical therapy is indicated for most patients with stage I disease and selected patients with stage II disease because of the limited yet predictable extent of spread in these early stages. *Radical surgical therapy* includes radical hysterectomy aimed at removing all the central disease (i.e., disease not only in the cervix itself but also in all the adjacent paracervical, parametrial, and vaginal tissue). In addition, surgical eradication of the local and regional lymph nodes is an important part of radical surgical therapy (pelvic lymphadenectomy). Whether or not a tumor is in the lymph nodes sampled defines, in part, the extent of disease and the need for further therapy, either radiation therapy or perhaps chemotherapy. It should be emphasized that simple hysterectomy with removal of the cervix is inadequate treatment for invasive cervical carcinoma. Patients with stage IA1 cancer may be treated with cCKC or simple hysterectomy with no evidence of lymphovascular space invasion. Stage IA1 with lymphovascular space invasion up to patients with stage IB1 disease may be considered for radical trachelectomy or radical hysterectomy. Some patients with Stage IB2 and IIA disease may be considered for radical hysterectomy, though this practice is losing favor in the era of chemoradiation combined therapy for more advanced stages of cervical cancer. In young women who are treated surgically, ovarian preservation is usually advisable to provide the patient with the long-term benefits from endogenous estrogen secretion. Ovarian retention presents minimal risk to the patient because squamous cervical carcinoma rarely spreads to the adnexal structures and is not estrogen dependent.

Radiation therapy is reserved for patients with stage IB or IIA disease who are poor surgical candidates and for all patients with more advanced disease. Radiation therapy is now given concurrently with either cisplatin or cisplatin with 5-Fluorouracil chemotherapy. The basis for radiation therapy in more advanced disease is the likelihood for more extensive regional nodal involvement. Even with stage III disease extending to the lateral pelvic wall, approximately one third of patients are cured with primary radiation therapy. Both high-dose external beam therapy and intracavitary irradiation are used for most patients. Intrauterine and intravaginal applicators containing radioactive materials are placed to direct treatment of the uterus, cervix, and vagina as needed, and external beam radiation is applied primarily along the paths of lymphatic extension of cervical carcinoma (Figure 44.5).

Fortunately, the adjacent nongynecologic structures, such as the bladder and distal colon, tolerate radiation fairly well. Radiation therapy

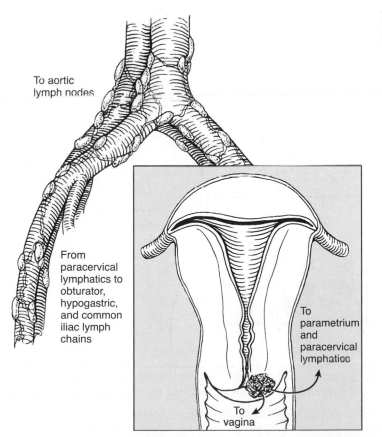

Figure 44.5. Spread patterns of cervical carcinoma.

To aortic lymph nodes

From paracervical lymphatics to obturator, hypogastric, and common iliac lymph chains

To parametrium and paracervical lymphatics

To vagina

doses are calculated by individual patient needs to maximize radiation to the tumor sites and potential spread areas, while minimizing the amount of radiation to adjacent uninvolved tissues. *Complications of radiation therapy* include radiation cystitis and proctitis, which are usually relatively easy to manage. Other more unusual complications include intestinal or vaginal fistulae, small bowel obstruction, or difficult-to-manage hemorrhagic proctitis or cystitis. It should be remembered that the tissue damage and fibrosis incurred by radiation therapy progresses over many years, and

that these effects may complicate long-term management Figure 44.6a and b).

Most authorities believe that radical surgical excision and pelvic lymphadenectomy offer distinct advantages over radiation therapy for earlier stage disease. These include the potential for preservation of ovarian function in young women, preservation of sexual function, and avoidance of long-term radiation effects. On the other hand, certain operative complications such as hemorrhage, damage to local nerves supplying the bladder, and urinary vaginal fistulae may develop from radical pelvic

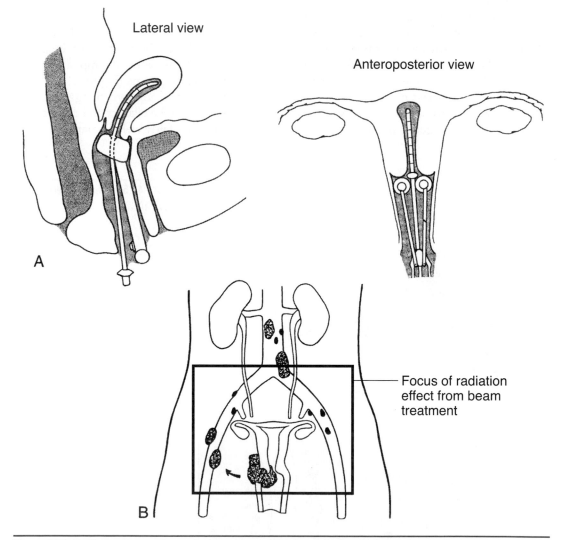

Figure 44.6. Radiation therapy for cervical carcinoma. (**A**) Intravaginal and intrauterine applicators are inserted to irradiate the cervix, vagina, and uterus. (**B**) External beam radiation is used along the paths of lymphatic spread of the tumor.

surgery. It is important for the risks and benefits of each form of therapy to be explained to
the patient, and treatment should be performed based on individual patient selection.

Follow-up of patients with cervical carcinoma is
best done by gynecologic oncologists who use
established protocols. Generally patients are
evaluated every 3 months with a Pap smear and
physical examination with a pelvic examination. Some authors recommend chest radi-
graphs every 6 months and CA-125 levels on
patients with advanced disease with known elevated levels at the time of initial diagnosis.
Most oncology centers follow patients in a specialized clinic for at least 5 years. With recurrence, 90% recurs within this time period. The
5-year survival rates for various stages of cervical carcinoma are shown in Table 44.6.

Treatment for recurrent disease is associated
with poor cure rates. Most chemotherapeutic
protocols have only limited usefulness and are
reserved for palliative efforts. Likewise, specific
"spot" radiation to areas of recurrence also
provides only limited benefit. Occasional

Table 44.6. Five-Year Survival for Treated Cervical Carcinoma			
FIGO Stage	5-Year Survival (%)	FIGO Stage	5-Year Survival (%)
0	100	IIIA	45
IA	99	IIIB	36
IB	85–90	IVA	15
IIA	73–80	IVB	2
IIB	68		

FIGO = International Federation of Gynecology and Obstetrics

patients with central recurrence (i.e., recurrence of disease in the upper vagina or the
residual cervix and uterus in radiation patients)
may benefit from ultraradical surgery with
partial or total pelvic exenteration. These candidates are few, but when properly selected,
may benefit from this aggressive therapy.

CHAPTER 45

UTERINE LEIOMYOMA AND NEOPLASIA

This chapter deals primarily with APGO Educational Topic:

Topic 53: Uterine leiomyomas

The student should understand how to diagnose and, if necessary, treat the most common gynecologic neoplasm.

Introduction

Uterine leiomyomas represent *localized prolif-eration of smooth muscle cells surrounded by a pseudocapsule of compressed muscle fibers. Uterine enlargement as a result of leiomyoma* (fibroids, myomas) is *common* in clinical practice. Up to *30% of American women have these benign tumors,* although most do not present with significant symptoms that require therapy. However, leiomyomata are the most common indication for hysterectomy, accounting for approximately 30% of all such cases. Additionally, they account for a large number of more conservative operations, including myomectomy, uterine curettage, operative hysteroscopy, and uterine artery embolization.

They are considered *hormonally responsive* benign tumors because estrogen usually induces their rapid growth in high estrogen states such as pregnancy. In contrast, menopause generally brings about cessation of tumor growth and even some atrophy. Estrogen may work by stimulation of the production of progesterone receptors in the myometrium. In turn, progesterone binding to these sites stimulates the production of several growth factors causing the growth of myomas. Although exact mechanisms are unknown, chromosomal transloca-tions/deletions, peptide growth factor, and epidermal growth factor are implicated as potential pathogenic factors of leiomyomata. Sensitive DNA studies suggest that each myoma arises from a single smooth muscle cell and that, in many cases, the smooth muscle cell is vascular in origin.

The uterine smooth muscle may also develop a rare cancer such as *leiomyosarcoma.* These are not thought to represent "degeneration" of a fibroid but, rather, a new neoplasm. Uterine malignancy is more typical in postmenopausal patients who present with rapidly enlarging uterine masses, postmenopausal bleeding, unusual vaginal discharge, and pelvic pain. An enlarging uterine mass in a postmenopausal patient should be evaluated with considerably more concern for malignancy than one in a younger woman. Other cell types may be involved in this form of malignancy. These *heterologous* mixed tumors contain other sarcomatous tissue ele-ments not necessarily found only in the uterus.

Three rare variants of apparently benign uterine myomas have been identified. All are generally thought to be benign and somewhat estrogen dependent. *Intravenous leiomyomatosis* is described as invasion of the pelvic veins and even vena cava with histologically mature and benign smooth muscle tumor. *Benign metasta-sizing leiomyoma* has been reported in cardiac, lymphatic, and pulmonary nodules, presumed to be the result of either intravenous or lymphatic embolization. *Leiomyomatosis peritonealis disseminata* involves implants on peritoneal surfaces identical to uterine myomas.

Symptoms

Bleeding is the most common presenting symptom in uterine fibroids. Although the kind of abnormal bleeding may vary, the most common presentation includes the development of progressively heavier menstrual flow that lasts longer than the normal duration (*menorrhagia,* defined as menstrual blood loss of <80 mL). This bleeding may result from significant distortion of the endometrial cavity by the underlying tumor. Three generally accepted but unproved *mechanisms for increased bleeding* include

1. Alteration of normal myometrial contractile function in the small artery and arteriolar blood supply underlying the endometrium
2. Inability of the overlying endometrium to respond to the normal estrogen/progesterone menstrual phases, which contributes to efficient sloughing of the endometrium
3. Pressure necrosis of the overlying endometrial bed, which exposes vascular surfaces that bleed in excess of that normally found with endometrial sloughing

Characteristically, the best example of a type of leiomyoma contributing to this bleeding pattern is the so-called submucous leiomyoma. In this variant, most of the distortion created by the smooth muscle tumor projects toward the endometrial cavity rather than toward the serosal surface of the uterus. Enlarging intramural fibroids likewise may contribute

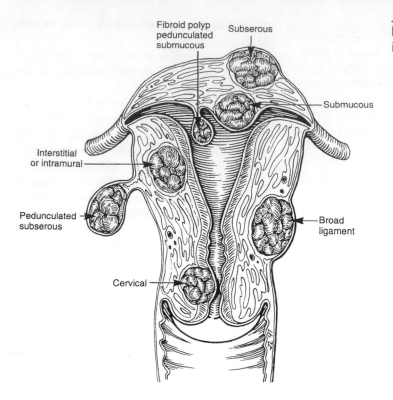

Figure 45.1. Common types of uterine fibroids.

to excessive bleeding if they become large enough to significantly distort the endometrial cavity.

Blood loss from this type of menstrual bleeding may be heavy enough to contribute to chronic iron-deficiency anemia and, rarely, to profound acute blood loss. The occurrence of isolated submucous (subendometrial) leiomyomata is unusual. Commonly, these are found in association with other types of leiomyomata (see Figure 45.1).

Another common symptom is a *progressive increase in "pelvic pressure."* This may be a sense of progressive pelvic fullness, "something pressing down," and/or the sensation of a pelvic mass. Most commonly, this is caused by slowly enlarging intramural or subserous myomas, which on occasion may attain a massive size (Figure 45.2). This type of leiomyoma is the most easily palpated on bimanual or abdominal examination and contributes to a characteristic "lumpy-bumpy," or cobblestone, sensation when multiple myomas are present. Occasionally, these large myomas present as a large asymptomatic pelvic or even abdominopelvic mass. Such

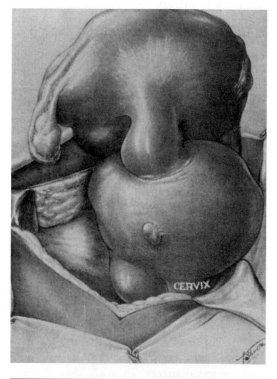

Figure 45.2. Multiple uterine fibroids. From Berek JS. *Novak's Gynecology.* 13th ed. Philadelphia: Lippincott Williams & Wilkins, 2002.

large leiomyomas may cause an uncommon but significant clinical problem: pressure on the ureters as they traverse the pelvic brim leading to *hydroureter and possibly hydronephrosis*. This can also occur if fibroids lower within the pelvis grow laterally between the leaves of the broad ligament.

Another presentation is progressively worsening *pelvic pain*. This pain is commonly manifest by the onset of secondary dysmenorrhea. Other pain symptoms, although rare, may be the result of rapid enlargement of a leiomyoma. This can result in areas of tissue necrosis or areas of subnecrotic vascular ischemia, which contribute to alteration in myometrial response to prostaglandins similar to the mechanism described for primary dysmenorrhea. Occasionally, torsion of a pedunculated myoma can occur, resulting in acute pain. Dull, intermittent low midline cramping pain is the clinical presentation when a submucous (subendometrial) myoma becomes pedunculated and progressively prolapses through the internal os of the cervix.

Diagnosis

The *diagnosis* is usually made by physical examination and imaging studies. Occasionally, irregularities of the uterine cavity are detected during endometrial sampling. Often the diagnosis is made incidentally by pathologic assessment of a uterine specimen removed for other indications. On *abdominopelvic examination*, uterine leiomyomata usually present as a large, midline, irregular-contoured mobile pelvic mass with a characteristic "hard feel" or solid quality. The degree of enlargement is usually stated in terms (weeks' size) that are used to estimate equivalent gestational size. The fibroid uterus is described separate from any adnexal disease, although on *occasion a subserosal pedunculated myoma may be difficult to distinguish from a solid adnexal mass*.

Of the *imaging studies, pelvic ultrasound* is the most commonly used for confirmation of uterine myomas. The ultrasonographer can demonstrate areas of acoustic shadow hypoechogenicity amid otherwise normal myometrial patterns and can see a distorted endometrial stripe. Occasionally cystic components may be seen as hypoechogenic areas and are

consistent in appearance with myomas undergoing degeneration. Adnexal structures, including the ovaries, are usually identifiable separate from these masses. This is reassuring information, i.e., the pathology is uterine in nature and not adnexal, which has an associated higher risk of malignancy. Neither *computerized axial tomography* nor *magnetic resonance imaging* is cost effective in diagnosing uterine myomas except in cases of extremely large myomas, because ultrasound may not image a large myoma well.

Endometrial biopsy, through either office sampling or dilation and curettage, should not be relied on to provide additional diagnostic information, because most of the sampling devices only scratch the surface of the endometrial cavity, not sampling the myomatous elements; however, an indirect appreciation for uterine enlargement may be gained by uterine sounding, which is part of this procedure. If a patient has irregular uterine bleeding and endometrial carcinoma is a consideration, endometrial sampling is useful to evaluate for this possibility independent of the myomas.

Hysteroscopy may be used to evaluate the enlarged uterus by directly visualizing the endometrial cavity. The increased size of the cavity can be documented, and submucous fibroids can be visualized and removed. Although the efficacy of hysteroscopic removal (resection) of submucous myomas has been documented, long-term follow-up suggests that up to 20% of patients require additional treatment when reexamined 10 years later.

Laparoscopy may be used in cases in which physical examination and ultrasound cannot differentiate whether the patient has a leiomyomata or other potentially more serious disease such as adnexal neoplasia. Laparoscopic resection of subserosal or intramural myoma has gained in popularity, although the long-term benefit of this procedure has not been well established.

Treatment of Uterine Fibroids

Most patients with uterine myomas do not require (surgical or medical) treatment. For example, if a patient presents with menstrual aberrations, the endometrial cavity is sampled to rule out endometrial hyperplasia or cancer. This is of particular importance for patients in the late reproductive or perimenopausal years. If the patient's bleeding is not heavy enough to cause significant alteration in hygiene or lifestyle and is not contributing to iron-deficiency anemia, reassurance and observation may be all that are necessary. Assessment of further uterine growth may be done by repeat pelvic examinations and/or serial pelvic ultrasounds.

An attempt may be made to minimize uterine bleeding by using intermittent progestin supplementation and/or prostaglandin synthetase inhibitors, which decrease the amount of secondary dysmenorrhea and in some cases the amount of menstrual flow. If significant endometrial cavity distortion is caused by intramural or submucous myomas, hormonal supplementation is of minimal benefit, because the excessive bleeding is usually related to pro-

found anatomic and vascular distortion. If effective, this conservative approach can potentially be used until the time of menopause.

Of the surgical options available, *myomectomy* is warranted in patients who desire to retain childbearing potential or whose fertility is compromised by the myomas, creating significant intracavitary distortion. Potential complications of myomectomy include excessive intraoperative blood loss; postoperative hemorrhage, infection and pelvic adhesions; and even the need for emergent hysterectomy.

Although *hysterectomy* is commonly performed for uterine myomas, it should be considered as definitive treatment only in symptomatic women who have completed childbearing. *Indications* should be specific and well documented (Table 45.1). Depending on the size of the fibroids and the skill of

---

Table 45.1. Criteria for Hysterectomy for Leiomyomata*

Indication

Leiomyomata

Confirmation of indication (1, 2, or 3)

1. Asymptomatic leiomyomata of such size that they are palpable abdominally and are a concern to the patient

2. Excessive uterine bleeding evidenced by either of the following:
   a. Profuse bleeding with flooding or clots or repetitive periods lasting >8 days
   b. Anemia caused by acute or chronic blood loss

3. Pelvic discomfort caused by myomata (a, b, or c):
   a. Acute and severe
   b. Chronic lower abdominal or low back pressure
   c. Bladder pressure with urinary frequency not caused by urinary tract infection

Actions before procedure

1. Confirm no cervical malignancy

2. Eliminate anovulation and other causes of abnormal bleeding

3. When abnormal bleeding is present, confirm no endometrial malignancy

4. Assess surgical risk from anemia and need for treatment

5. Consider patient's medical and psychological risks concerning hysterectomy

Contraindications

1. Desire to maintain fertility, in which case myomectomy should be considered

2. Asymptomatic leiomyomata of size <12 weeks' gestation determined by physical examination or ultrasound examination

Modified from the American College of Obstetricians and Gynecologists. *Quality assessment and improvement in obstetrics and gynecology.* Washington, DC, 1994.

the surgeon, both myomectomy and hysterectomy can potentially be performed via laparoscopy.

Besides surgery, *pharmacologic inhibition of estrogen secretion* has been used to treat fibroids. This is particularly applicable in the perimenopausal years when women are more likely anovulatory with relatively more endogenous estrogen. Pharmacologic removal of the ovarian estrogen source can be achieved by suppression of the hypothalamic-pituitary-ovarian axis through the use of *gonadotropin-releasing hormone agonists (GnRH analogs)*, which can reduce fibroid size by as much as 40% to 60%. This treatment is commonly used before planned hysterectomy to reduce blood loss as well as the difficulty of the procedure. It can also be used as a temporizing medical therapy until natural menopause occurs.

In patients with an adequate endogenous estrogen source, this treatment does not permanently reduce the size of uterine myomas, as withdrawal of the medication predictably results in regrowth of the myomas. Although less successful, other pharmacologic agents such as danazol have also been used as medical treatment for myomas by reducing endogenous production of ovarian estrogen.

Other therapeutic modalities have been used in clinical practice, although their efficacy is yet to be demonstrated. Included in these are myolysis and arterial embolization. The safety and efficacy of uterine artery embolization (UAE) have been studied to the point that it is now considered a viable alternative to hysterectomy and myomectomy. The procedure involves selective uterine artery catheterization with embolization using polyvinyl alcohol particles, which creates acute infarction of the target myomas. For maximal efficacy, bilateral uterine artery cannulation and embolization is necessary. In assessing outcomes data, the three most common symptoms of myomas, bleeding, pressure, and pain, are ameliorated in over 85% of patients. Acute postembolization pain requiring hospitalization occurs in approximately 10% to 15% of patients. Other complications include delayed infection and/or passage of necrotic fibroids through the cervix up to 30 days after the procedure. It is currently not recommended as a procedure to consider in patients who desire future childbearing.

The ultimate decision to perform a hysterectomy or not should include an assessment of the patient's future reproductive plans as well as careful assessment of clinical factors, including the amount and timing of bleeding, the degree of enlargement of the tumors, and the associated disability for the individual patient. Uterine myomas alone do not necessarily warrant hysterectomy.

Although leiomyomas are equivocally associated with infertility, patients with leiomyoma do become pregnant. *Pregnancy with leiomyoma* is usually unremarkable, with a normal antepartum course, labor, and delivery. Myomas may sometimes cause pain as they can outgrow their blood supply during pregnancy, resulting in *red or carneous degeneration*. Bed rest and strong analgesics are usually sufficient as treatment, although on occasion myomectomy may be needed. The risk of abortion or preterm labor following myomectomy is relatively high, so that prophylactic β-adrenergic tocolytics are sometimes used. *Vaginal birth after myomectomy* is controversial and must be decided on a case-by-case basis. Rarely, myomas are located below the fetus, in the lower uterine segment or cervix, causing a soft tissue dystocia, leading to a need for cesarean birth.

Leiomyosarcoma

Uterine sarcomas represent an *unusual gynecologic malignancy* accounting for approximately *3% of cancers involving the body of the uterus.* Progressive uterine enlargement occurring in the postmenopausal years should not be assumed to be the result of simple uterine leiomyomata, because appreciable endogenous ovarian estrogen secretion is absent, thereby minimizing this as a potential cause for progressive uterine enlargement. In addition, postmenopausal women on low-dose hormone-replacement therapy are not at risk for stimulation of uterine enlargement. In this situation, uterine sarcoma (leiomyosarcoma) should be considered. Other symptoms of uterine sarcoma include postmenopausal bleeding, unusual pelvic pain coupled with uterine enlargement, and an increase in unusual vaginal discharge. Surgical removal is the method of most reliable diagnosis. Accordingly, hysterectomy is usually indicated in patients with documented, and especially progressive, uterine enlargement.

The *virulence of uterine sarcoma* is directly related to the number of mitotic figures and cellular atypia as defined histologically. In addition, these tumors are more likely to spread hematogenously than endometrial adenocarcinoma. When uterine sarcoma is suspected, patients should undergo typical tumor survey to include assessment for distant metastatic disease. At the time of hysterectomy, it is necessary to thoroughly explore the abdomen and sample commonly affected node chains, including the iliac and periaortic areas. The staging for uterine sarcoma is surgical and identical to that for endometrial adenocarcinoma.

Unfortunately the 5-year survival of patients with a uterine sarcoma is only 50%. Radiation and chemotherapy provide little benefit as adjuvant therapy to hysterectomy.

CHAPTER 46

ENDOMETRIAL HYPERPLASIA AND CANCER

This chapter deals primarily with APGO Educational Topic:

Topic 54: Endometrial Carcinoma

The student should be familiar with the risk factors as well as the diagnosis and treatment of the most common gynecologic malignancy.

Table 46.1. Risk Factors for Endometrial Hyperplasia and Carcinoma

Factor	Observations	Relative Risk
Menopause	2.4 times more likely for women undergoing menopause after age 52 than between 49 and 52	2–3
Unopposed estrogen therapy	Estrogen replacement without progestins; risk increased with dosage and duration of use	4–8
Nulliparity		2–3
Obesity	3 times more likely at 20–50 pounds overweight, up to 10 times if >50 pounds overweight; associated with aromatization of adrenally produced androstenedione to estrone in fat cells	3–10
Tamoxifen therapy		2–3
Diabetes mellitus		3

Endometrial carcinoma is the most common genital tract malignancy and the fourth most common cancer after breast, bowel, and lung carcinoma. Approximately 34,000 new cases of endometrial carcinoma are diagnosed annually in the United States, resulting in over 6,000 deaths. Most *women develop endometrial carcinoma in their perimenopausal or postmenopausal years.* Fortunately, patients with this disease usually present early in the disease course with some form of abnormal uterine bleeding, particularly postmenopausal bleeding. Accordingly, *women older than 35 years old with irregular menstrual bleeding may need endometrial biopsy.* With early diagnosis, survival rates are excellent.

Pathogenesis and Risk Factors

Two kinds of endometrial hyperplasia/carcinoma have been identified. The first is *"estrogen-dependent" endometrial carcinoma,* common to younger perimenopausal women with a history of unopposed endogenous or exogenous estrogen stimulation. In these women, endometrial hyperplasia develops, progressing in some women through atypical forms to endometrial carcinoma, which is usually well differentiated and hence has a more favorable prognosis. The second type, *"estrogen-independent" endometrial carcinoma,* occurs spontaneously, characteristically in thin, older postmenopausal women without unopposed estrogen excess, arising in an atrophic endometrium rather than a hyperplastic one. These cancers tend to be less well differentiated with a poorer prognosis. The estrogen-independent cancer is less common than the estrogen-dependent one.

Many of the risk factors for endometrial carcinoma and hyperplasia are identified, are related to prolonged hyperestrogenism, and identify women who require endometrial biopsy (Table 46.1). When an endometrial

Table 46.2. Estrogen Sources

Endogenous
  Glandular
    Estradiol (ovary)
    Estrone (ovary)
  Peripheral
    Estrone (fat, conversion of androstenedione)
  Tumor
    Granulosa cell of ovary (an uncommon tumor and source)
Exogenous
  Medications
    Conjugated estrogen (mostly estrone)
    Lyophilized estradiol
    Cutaneous patches
    Vaginal creams

biopsy shows atypical endometrial hyperplasia, the risk of a coincident cancer is approximately 30%.

Estrogen-Dependent Endometrial Hyperplasia/Carcinoma

The *underlying pathophysiologic process* in the development of endometrial hyperplasia and endometrial cancer is overgrowth of the endometrium in response to excess estrogen. Sources of estrogen may be endogenous (ovarian; peripheral conversion of androgenic precursors) or exogenous (Table 46.2).

This relationship between estrogen and endometrial growth (proliferation) is clear. Endometrial proliferation represents a normal part of the menstrual cycle and occurs during the follicular or estrogen-dominant phase of

the cycle. With continued estrogen stimulation through either endogenous mechanisms or by exogenous administration, simple endometrial proliferation will become endometrial hyperplasia (Figure 46.1). *Endometrial hyperplasia is the "abnormal proliferation of both glandular and stromal elements showing altered histologic architecture."* True endometrial proliferation is a simple overabundance of normal endometrium, whereas endometrial hyperplasia involves histologic features with cellular architectural abnormalities. When proliferation becomes hyperplasia is not clear, although studies showing sequential change suggest it requires 6 months or longer of "unopposed estrogen" stimulation.

Endometrial hyperplasia is classified based on the amount of endometrium, density of

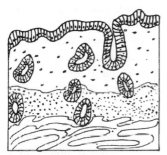 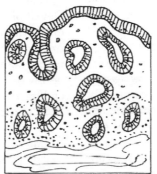 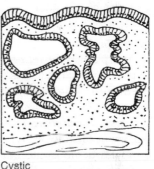

Proliferative endometrium

Simple hyperplasia

Cystic hyperplasia (simple hyperplasia)

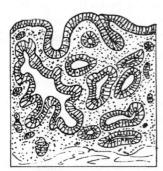 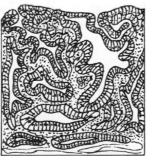 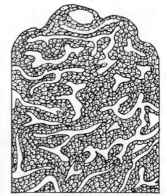

Adenomatous hyperplasia (complex hyperplasia)

Atypical adenomatous hyperplasia (atypical hyperplasia with cellular atypia)

Cancer of the endometrium

Figure 46.1. Endometrial histology: hyperplasia to carcinoma (International Society of Gynecologic Pathologists Terminology).

Table 46.3. Classifications of Endometrial Hyperplasia

Types	Risk progressing to cancer (%)
Simple hyperplasia without atypia	1
Complex hyperplasia without atypia	3
Simple hyperplasia with atypia	8
Complex hyperplasia with atypia	29

glands, structural abnormalities of glands, and cytologic features of glandular epithelium. Table 46.3 shows the most recent classification with the likelihood of each type to progress to carcinoma if left untreated.

Simple Hyperplasia

Simple hyperplasia is the *least-significant form* of endometrial hyperplasia and is not commonly associated with progression to endometrial carcinoma. *In this variety of hyperplasia, both glandular elements and stromal cell elements proliferate excessively.* Histologically, glands that are simple tubules demonstrate marked variation in size, from small to cystically dilated and enlarged glands (the hallmark of this hyperplasia). Cystic glandular hyperplasia should not be confused with a normal postmenopausal variant—cystic involution of the endometrium—which is histologically not a hyperplastic condition.

Complex Hyperplasia

This hyperplasia represents an *abnormal proliferation of primarily glandular elements without concomitant proliferation of stromal elements.* This increased gland:stroma ratio gives the endometrium a "crowded" picture, frequently with glands appearing almost back to back. As the severity of the hyperplasia increases, the glands become more crowded and more structurally bizarre. It is thought that complex hyperplasia represents a true intraepithelial neoplastic process, and it is occasionally found coexisting with areas of endometrial adenocarcinoma; however, it may also be found microscopically in small areas within normal proliferative endometrium.

Hyperplasia (Simple or Complex) with Cytologic Atypia

Hyperplasia, which *contains significant numbers of glandular elements that exhibit cytologic atypia and disordered maturation (loss of cellular polarity, nuclear enlargement with increased nucleus-to-cytoplasmic ratio, dense chromatin, and prominent nucleoli)*, is considered particularly important as a precursor lesion to endometrial carcinoma. This so-called carcinoma in situ of the endometrium has at least a 20% to 30% risk for malignant transformation.

Estrogen-Independent Endometrial Carcinoma

Developing from seemingly atrophic endometrium, *estrogen-independent endometrial carcinoma* is more common in older, postmenopausal, thin women and is often more poorly differentiated than estrogen-dependent endometrial carcinoma. It follows, then, that it has a poorer prognosis.

Evaluation

The diagnosis of endometrial hyperplasia or carcinoma is made by taking a sample of the endometrium for histologic evaluation. This is most easily accomplished by any of a number of different atraumatic aspiration devices used in the office (e.g., Pipelle) (Figure 33.6). The diagnostic accuracy of office endometrial biopsy is 90% to 98% when compared with dilation and curettage (D&C) or hysterectomy. The routine *Pap smear is not reliable* in diagnosing endometrial hyperplasia or cancer, as only 30% to 40% of patients with endometrial carcinoma have abnormal Pap test results. On the other hand, endometrial carcinoma must be considered and endometrial sampling obtained when atypical endometrial cells or atypical glandular cells of undetermined significance (AGUS) are found on the Pap smear.

The most common *indication for endometrial sampling is abnormal bleeding,* with liberal consideration given to obtaining a specimen *in patients older than 35 years of age who present with abnormal uterine bleeding*. After ruling out pregnancy with a urine pregnancy test in premenopausal women, patients can be adequately sampled with relatively little discomfort. Further management is usually dictated by the results of the biopsy specimen. D&C or hysteroscopy with directed endometrial biopsy may be undertaken when outpatient sampling is not possible (e.g., a stenotic cervical os or a patient cannot tolerate the outpatient procedure) or when the outpatient sampling has been nondiagnostic.

Sometimes the office endometrial biopsy will be reported as "insufficient tissue for diagnosis." In a postmenopausal woman not on estrogen replacement, these data may be sufficient, because they are compatible with the suspected atrophic condition of the endometrium. In other cases, the clinical suspicion of a possible hyperplastic endometrial process may be high enough to warrant hysteroscopic evaluation with directed sampling, which allows more complete evaluation of the endometrium as well as direct diagnosis of polyps, myomas, and structural abnormalities. Although more expensive and inconvenient for the patient, it offers advantages over a blind biopsy, especially because traditional endometrial biopsy techniques sample only a small part of the surface area of the endometrial cavity.

Transvaginal ultrasound (with or without the installation of fluid for contrast, *ultrasonohysterography*) is used as an adjunctive means of evaluation for endometrial hyperplasia as well as polyps, myomas, and structural abnormalities of the uterus. An endometrial thickness of greater than 5 mm in a menopausal patient, a polypoid mass, or fluid collection is often considered indication for further evaluation to obtain histologic samples. It is also useful to help determine if, for patients with multiple medical problems, the risks of endometrial sampling are less than the risk of not sampling. However, an endometrial stripe of <5 mm, although consistent with menopause and endometrial atrophy, does not exclude the possibility of a nonestrogen-dependent carcinoma of the atrophic endometrium.

In women whose breast cancer treatment includes tamoxifen (which acts as a weak estrogen and is associated with increased risk of endometrial hyperplasia and carcinoma) the optimal manner of monitoring the endometrium is unclear. Endometrial biopsy is indicated with any abnormal bleeding, but some recommend regular transvaginal ultrasound and/or endometrial sampling, perhaps yearly, whereas others recommend that neither ultrasound nor sampling is needed on a routine basis.

Management

If endometrial hyperplasia without atypia is found on tissue sample, medical treatment is usually offered because the therapy has low risk and some of these hyperplasias may progress to cancer (Table 46.3). The mean duration of progression from endometrial hyperplasia to carcinoma in those that do progress is relatively long, perhaps 10 years for those without atypia and 4 years for those with atypia. In most cases, *medical treatment* involves the administration of a form of synthetic progesterone (progestin) in doses that inhibit and eventually reverse the hyperplastic response evoked by estrogen stimulation. Probably the most common regimen is Provera (medroxyprogesterone acetate), 10 to 20 mg/day for 10 to 14 days each month, although a continuous regimen using megestrol acetate (Megace) 20 to 40 mg daily is also often used and likewise effective. Progestin therapy works to alter the enzymatic pathways, which eventually convert endogenous estradiol to weaker estrogens, as well as to decrease the number of estrogen receptors in the endometrial glandular cells. Progestins have a net effect of decreasing endometrial glandular proliferation and, when administered for sufficient periods of time or in high enough doses, actually render the endometrium atrophic. In addition, with progestin withdrawal, the endometrium is sloughed (the so-called chemical D&C), analogous to corpus luteum progesterone withdrawal in a normal menstrual cycle.

Hyperplasia with atypia is usually treated surgically by hysterectomy because it is much more likely to become endometrial carcinoma. This treatment decision is usually fairly clear, because most patients with this disorder are in their late reproductive or perimenopausal years. In selected patients (e.g., younger women who may wish to become pregnant), longer-term, high-dose progestin management may be used in an attempt to avoid a hysterectomy. Patients who are treated medically for atypical hyperplasia should also be followed with periodic endometrial sampling (3 months after therapy and then once to twice per year) so that treatment response can be gauged.

Endometrial Polyps

Most endometrial polyps represent focal accentuated benign hyperplastic processes. Their histologic architecture is characteristic and may commonly be found in association with other types of endometrial hyperplasia or even carcinoma. Polyps occur most frequently in perimenopausal or immediately postmenopausal women, when the ovary is characterized by unopposed estrogen production because of chronic anovulation. The most common presenting symptom is abnormal bleeding. Small polyps often may be incidentally found as part of endometrial sampling or curettage done for evaluation of the bleeding problem. Rarely, a large polyp may begin to protrude through the cervical canal, and the patient presents not only with bleeding irregularities but also with low, dull, midline pain as the cervix is slowly dilated and effaced. In these cases, surgical removal is necessary to reduce the amount of bleeding and to prevent infection developing within the exposed endometrial surface. *Less than 5% of polyps show malignant change,* and when they do, they may represent any endometrial histologic variant. Polyps in postmenopausal women are more likely to be associated with endometrial carcinoma than are those found in reproductive-age women.

Endometrial Carcinoma

Endometrial carcinoma is typically a disease of the postmenopausal woman. Approximately 75% of patients with endometrial carcinoma are postmenopausal, whereas 15% to 20% are perimenopausal and only 5% to 10% are premenopausal. Between 15% and 25% of postmenopausal women with bleeding have uterine malignancy.

Most primary endometrial carcinomas are adenocarcinomas. Because squamous epithelium may coexist with the glandular elements in an adenocarcinoma, descriptive terms that include the squamous element may be used. In cases where the squamous element is benign and makes up >10% of the histologic picture, the term *adenoacanthoma* is used. Uncommonly, the squamous element may appear malignant on histologic assessment, and this is referred to as *adenosquamous carcinoma*. Other descriptions such as clear cell carcinoma and papillary serous adenocarcinoma may be applied, depending on the histologic architecture. All these carcinomas are considered under the general category of adenocarcinoma of the endometrium.

The diagnosis of endometrial cancer is most frequently made by endometrial sampling after a patient presents with abnormal uterine bleeding. Indeed, vaginal bleeding or discharge is the only presenting complaint in 80% to 90% of women with endometrial carcinoma. In some, often older patients, cervical stenosis may sequester the blood in the uterus with the presentation being hematometra or pyometra and a purulent vaginal discharge. In more advanced disease, pelvic discomfort or an associated sensation of pressure caused by uterine enlargement or extrauterine disease spread may accompany the complaint of vaginal bleeding or even be the presenting complaint. Less than 5% of women found to have endometrial carcinoma are actually asymptomatic. Thus, special consideration should be given to the patient who presents with postmenopausal bleeding (i.e., bleeding that occurs after 6 months of amenorrhea in a patient who has been diagnosed as menopausal). In this group of patients, it is mandatory to assess the endometrium histologically because the chance of having an endometrial carcinoma is approximately 10% to 15%, although other causes are more common (Table 46.4). Other gynecologic assessments should also be made, including careful physical and pelvic examination as well as a screening Pap smear.

Because the current International Federation of Gynecology and Obstetrics (FIGO) staging of endometrial carcinoma (Table 46.5)

Table 46.4. Causes of Postmenopausal Uterine Bleeding

Cause	Frequency (%)
Atrophy of the endometrium	60–80
Hormone replacement therapy	15–25
Endometrial carcinoma	10–15
Endometrial polyps	2–12
Endometrial hyperplasia	5–10

is surgical rather than clinical, differential sampling of the endocervical canal and endometrial cavity (i.e., "fractional curettage") before therapy is no longer necessary. Fractional curettage should, however, be considered for staging purposes in patients who are not surgical candidates.

Route of Spread and Histologic Types of Endometrial Carcinoma

Endometrial carcinoma usually spreads throughout the endometrial cavity first and then begins to invade the myometrium, endocervical canal, and eventually, lymphatics. Hematogenous spread occurs with endometrial carcinoma more readily than in cervical cancer or ovarian cancer. Invasion of adnexal structures may occur through lymphatics or direct implantation through the fallopian tubes. After extrauterine spread to the peritoneal cavity, cancer cells may spread widely in a fashion similar to that of ovarian cancer.

Unusual histologic subtypes, including *papillary serous adenocarcinoma and clear cell adenocarcinoma* of the endometrium, tend to be more aggressive than the more common adenocarcinoma (Table 46.6). Microscopic spread may also be present despite no gross abdominal pelvic lesions. Accordingly, cytologic assessment of peritoneal washings is important at the outset of surgical treatment for endometrial carcinoma. The current FIGO guidelines for the staging of endometrial carcinoma emphasize the need for thorough surgical assessment of the abdominopelvic cavity, including sampling of both periaortic and pelvic lymph nodes when depth of invasion is more than one-third of the myometrial thickness and in cases of obvious peritoneal foci of tumor.

Table 46.5. FIGO Surgical Staging of Endometrial Carcinoma (1988)

Stage	Description
IB G123	Invasion to less than one-half of the myometrium
IC G123	Invasion to more than one-half of the myometrium
IIA G123	Endocervical glandular involvement only
IIB G123	Cervical stromal invasion
IIIA G123	Tumor invading serosa, adnexa, or both and/or positive peritoneal cytology
IIIB G123	Vaginal metastases
IIIC G123	Metastases to pelvic and/or periaortic lymph nodes
IVA G123	Tumor invades bladder, bowel mucosa, or both
IVB	Distant metastases, including intra-abdominal and/or inguinal lymph node

Rules related to staging

1. Because corpus cancer is now surgically staged, procedures previously used for differentiation of stages are no longer applicable (e.g., the findings of dilation and curettage to differentiate between stage I and stage II). It is appreciated that a small number of patients with corpus cancer may be treated primarily with radiation therapy. If that is the case, the clinical staging adopted by FIGO in 1971 would still apply, but use of that staging system would be noted.

2. Ideally, the width of the myometrium is measured along with the width of tumor invasion.

Table 46.6. Histologic Types of Endometrial Carcinoma

Histologic Type	Discussion	Percentage of Endometrial Carcinomas
Endometrioid	Composed of glands that *resemble* normal endometrial glands but that contain more solid areas, less glandular formation, and more cytologic atypia as they become less well differentiated	80–85
Endometrial carcinoma with squamous differentiation	Encompasses tumors with benign-appearing squamous areas (also called adenoacanthomas) and those with malignant-looking squamous elements (also called adenosquamous carcinomas)	15–25
Villoglandular	Endometrial cells with characteristics of endometrioid cells, arranged in papillary fibrovascular stalks, always well differentiated	2
		1
Secretory endometrial carcinoma		
Mucinous	50% of cells have intracytoplasmic mucin; most behave like well-differentiated endometrioid carcinoma; good prognosis	5
Papillary serous	Endometrial carcinoma that resembles serous carcinoma of the ovary and fallopian tube; very aggressive, poorer prognosis	3–4
Clear cell	Mixed histologic pattern; more common in older women; very aggressive, poor prognosis	<5
Squamous	Generally pure cell type, some with glands; associated with older women and cervical stenosis; very poor prognosis	<1
		<1

Prognostic Factors

The single most important prognostic factor for endometrial carcinoma is histologic grade. Histologically, poorly differentiated or undifferentiated tumors are associated with a considerably poorer prognosis because of the likelihood of extrauterine spread through adjacent lymphatics and peritoneal fluid. This is true even of relatively limited lesions. Therefore, this finding is important in the initial surgical management of the patient and is of significance in deciding on adjunctive therapy with radiation or chemotherapy.

The grading system of the *FIGO adopted in 1988 lists three grades of endometrial carcinoma:* G1 is highly differentiated adenomatous carcinoma (<5% of the tumor shows a solid growth pattern), G2 is moderately differentiated adenomatous carcinoma with partly solid areas (6% to 50% of the tumor shows a solid growth pattern), and G3 is predominantly solid or entirely undifferentiated carcinoma (>50% of the tumor shows a solid growth pattern). Most patients with endometrial carcinoma have G1 or G2 lesions by this classification, with 15% to 20% having undifferentiated or poorly differentiated G3 lesions.

Depth of myometrial invasion is the second most important prognostic factor. When the tumor has invaded greater than one-third of the thickness of the myometrium, the prognosis is significantly worsened. Worsening grade of tumor closely parallels depth of myometrial invasion and lymph node metastasis. Other factors that have prognostic value include the original tumor volume both within the uterus and defined by extrauterine spread, lymphatic involvement, and hematogenous spread.

Survival rates vary widely, depending on the grade of tumor and depth of penetration into the myometrium. A patient with a G1 tumor that does not invade the myometrium has a 95% 5-year survival rate, whereas a patient with a poorly differentiated (G3) tumor with deep myometrial invasion may have a 5-year survival rate of only 20%.

Treatment

Because endometrial carcinoma is a surgically staged disease, *primary surgical treatment is the cornerstone of management.* After opening the abdomen, peritoneal washings are obtained. The abdominopelvic cavity is manually and visually explored, and then a *total abdominal hysterectomy with bilateral salpingo-oophorectomy* is performed. The decision to include pelvic and/or periaortic nodes is determined by the depth of myometrial invasion. *Vaginal hysterectomy* has been used successfully in the treatment of stage I disease in selected patients and may be especially useful in patients for whom the stress of abdominal surgery may be problematic. *Vaginal apex recurrence* occurs 5% to 10% of the time after simple hysterectomy for endometrial carcinoma, probably because of paravaginal lymphatic involvement in most cases. Postoperative adjuvant radiation reduces the apex recurrence but does not change the overall survival rate.

Many gynecologic oncologists advise routine *sampling of the common iliac nodes,* regardless of depth of penetration or histologic grade, citing as their reason the inherent inaccuracies of gross myometrial inspection and frozen-section assessment of the histologic grade and depth of penetration. In addition, they cite the incidence of pelvic nodal metastasis as between 2% and 10% for all stage I lesions, G1–3.

Adjunctive therapy after hysterectomy, which may include external-beam radiation, has been shown to significantly reduce the risk of pelvic and vaginal recurrence. *Postoperative radiation* therapy may be especially valuable in patients with deeply invasive cancers, those with cervical involvement, and those with poorly differentiated tumors. *Preoperative radiation* may be useful to those patients with obvious endocervical involvement and/or may be important in reducing a bulky endometrial tumor.

Recurrent Endometrial Carcinoma

Recurrent endometrial carcinoma occurs in about one-fourth of patients treated for early disease, one half of these within 2 years and three-fourths within 3 to 4 years. In general, those with recurrent vaginal disease have a better prognosis than those with pelvic recurrence, who in turn fare better than those with distant metastatic disease (lung, abdomen, lymph nodes, liver, brain, and bone).

The first line of *treatment for recurrent disease with estrogen/progestin receptor (usually well-differentiated histology)* is high-dose *progestin.* A major advantage of high-dose progestin therapy is its minimal complication rate. *Chemotherapy* with drugs, including Adriamycin (doxorubicin) and cisplatin, produces occasional favorable short-term results, but long-term remissions with these therapies are rare.

Hormone Replacement Therapy After Treatment for Endometrial Carcinoma

The use of *estrogen replacement therapy* in patients previously treated for endometrial carcinoma is controversial. Retrospective studies suggest minimal harm. Whether or not to include progestational agents is not clear from present data, although intuitively it would seem appropriate to do so. Cautious individualized assessment of risks and benefits should be accorded on a case-by-case basis.

CHAPTER 47

OVARIAN AND ADNEXAL DISEASE

This chapter addresses APGO Educational Topic:

Topic 55: Ovarian Neoplasms

The student should understand the physiologic and pathologic origins of both symptomatic and asymptomatic adnexal masses as well as the relevant diagnostic and therapeutic options.

The structures occupying the area between the lateral pelvic wall and the cornu of the uterus are referred to as the *adnexa*. These include the ovaries, fallopian tubes, upper portion of the broad ligament and mesosalpinx, and remnants of the embryonic müllerian duct. Of these, the organs most commonly affected by disease processes are the ovaries and fallopian tubes.

Adnexal Space and Associated Nongynecologic Disease

In addition to the reproductive organs, parts of the urinary and gastrointestinal tracts are located near the adnexal space. The most common urologic disorders are upper and lower *urinary tract infection* and the less common *renal and ureteral calculi*. Even rarer are anatomic abnormalities such as a *ptotic kidney*, which may present as a solid pelvic mass. An isolated pelvic kidney may likewise present as an asymptomatic, solid, cul-de-sac mass. Right adnexal signs and symptoms are associated with acute *appendicitis*, which should be considered in the differential diagnosis of acute right lower quadrant pain, usually preceded by anorexia. Less commonly, symptoms in the right adnexa may be related to intrinsic *inflammatory bowel disease* involving the ileocecal junction. Left-sided bowel disease involving the rectosigmoid is seen more often in older patients, as in acute or chronic diverticular disease. Because of the age of these patients and the proximity of the left ovary to the sigmoid, *sigmoid diverticular disease* is included in the differential diagnosis of a left-sided adnexal mass. Finally, left-sided pelvic pain or a mass may be related to *rectosigmoid carcinoma*. Midline disease can sometimes be related to a process involving a meckel's diverticulum, or a sacral tumor.

The Ovaries

A thorough pelvic examination is essential for evaluation of the ovary. Symptoms that may arise from physiologic and pathologic processes of the ovary must be correlated with physical examination findings. Also, because some ovarian conditions are asymptomatic, incidental physical examination findings may be the only information available when an evaluation begins. Interpretation of examination findings requires knowledge of the physical characteristics of the ovary during the stages of the life cycle.

In the *premenarchal age group*, the ovary *should not be palpable*. If it is, a pathologic condition is presumed, and further evaluation is necessary.

In the *reproductive age group*, the normal *ovary is palpable about half the time*. Important considerations include ovarian size, shape, consistency (firm or cystic), and mobility. In reproductive-age women taking oral contraceptives, the ovaries are palpable less frequently and are smaller and more symmetric than in women who are not using contraceptives.

In the *postmenopausal* patient, the ovaries are functionally different because they are less responsive to gonadotropin secretion, and therefore their surface follicular activity diminishes over time, disappearing in most women within 3 years of the onset of natural menopause. Women who are close to natural menopause are more likely to have residual functional cysts. In general, palpable ovarian enlargement in a postmenopausal patient should be assessed more critically than in a younger woman, because the incidence of ovarian malignant neoplasm is increased in this group.

One quarter of all ovarian tumors in postmenopausal women are malignant, whereas in reproductive-age women only about 10% of ovarian tumors are malignant. Indeed, this risk was considered so great in the past that any ovarian enlargement in a postmenopausal woman was an indication for surgical investigation, the so-called palpable postmenopausal ovary (PPO) syndrome. With the advent of more sensitive pelvic imaging techniques to assist in diagnosis, routine removal of minimally enlarged postmenopausal ovaries is no longer recommended. If the patient is within 3 years of natural menopause and transvaginal ultrasonography confirms a simple, unilocular cyst of <5 cm wide, the management may be serial pelvic and transvaginal ultrasound examinations. Masses that are larger or have a complex or solid appearance are more likely best managed with surgery.

Functional Ovarian Cysts

Functional ovarian cysts are not neoplasms but rather anatomic variations, arising as a result of normal ovarian function. They may present as an asymptomatic adnexal mass or become symptomatic, requiring evaluation and possibly treatment.

When an ovarian follicle fails to rupture during follicular maturation, ovulation does not occur, and a *follicular cyst* may develop. This, by definition, involves a lengthening of the follicular phase of the cycle with resultant secondary amenorrhea. Follicular cysts are lined by normal granulosa cells, and the fluid contained in them is rich in estrogen.

A follicular cyst becomes clinically significant if it is large enough to cause pain or if it persists beyond one menstrual interval. For poorly understood reasons, the granulosa cells lining the follicular cyst persist through the time when ovulation should have occurred and continue to enlarge through the second half of the cycle. A cyst may enlarge beyond 5 cm and continue to fill with estrogen-rich follicular fluid from the thickened granulosa cell layer. Symptoms associated with a follicular cyst may include mild to moderate unilateral lower abdominal pain and alteration of the menstrual interval. The latter may be the result of both failed subsequent ovulation and bleeding stimulated by the large amount of estradiol produced in the follicle. This estrogen-rich environment along with the lack of ovulation overstimulates the endometrium and causes irregular bleeding. Pelvic examination findings may include unilateral tenderness with a palpable, mobile, cystic adnexal mass.

Given a patient with these findings, the physician must decide whether further diagnostic assessment and treatment are necessary. Pelvic ultrasonography is often warranted in reproductive-age patients who have cysts larger than 5 cm wide. Ultrasound characteristics include a unilocular simple cyst without evidence of blood, soft tissue elements, or evidence of external excrescences. For many patients, however, ultrasound confirmation is not required. Instead, the patient may be reassured and followed with a repeat pelvic examination in about 6 weeks, once pregnancy has been ruled out.

Most follicular cysts spontaneously resolve during this time. Alternatively, an estrogen- and progesterone-containing oral contraceptive may be given to suppress gonadotropin stimulation of the cyst. Although this practice has not been shown to "shrink" the existing follicle cyst, it may suppress the development of a new cyst and permit resolution of the existing problem. If the cyst persists despite expectant management, another type of cyst or neoplasm should be suspected and further evaluated by imaging studies and/or surgery.

On occasion, *rupture of a follicular cyst* may cause acute pelvic pain. Because release of follicular fluid into the peritoneum produces only transient symptoms, surgical intervention is rarely necessary.

A *corpus luteum cyst* is the other common type of functional ovarian cyst, designated a cyst rather than simply a corpus luteum when its diameter exceeds about 3 cm. It is related to the postovulatory (i.e., progesterone-dominant) phase of the menstrual cycle. Two variations of corpus luteum cysts are encountered. The first is a slightly enlarged corpus luteum, which may continue to produce progesterone for longer than the usual 14 days. Menstruation is delayed from a few days to several weeks, although it usually occurs within 2 weeks of the missed period. Persistent corpus luteum cysts are often associated with dull lower quadrant pain. This pain and a missed menstrual period are the most common complaints associated with *persistent corpus luteum cysts*. Pelvic examination usually discloses an enlarged, tender, cystic or solid adnexal mass. Because of the triad of missed menstrual period, unilateral lower quadrant pain, and adnexal enlargement, ectopic pregnancy is often considered in the differential diagnosis. A negative pregnancy test eliminates this possibility, whereas a positive pregnancy test mandates further evaluation regarding the location of the pregnancy. Patients with recurrent persistent corpus luteum cysts may benefit from cyclic oral contraceptive therapy.

The second less-common type of corpus luteum cyst is the rapidly enlarging luteal-phase cyst into which there is spontaneous hemorrhage. Sometimes called the *corpus hemorrhagicum,* this hemorrhagic corpus luteum cyst may rupture late in the luteal phase, resulting in the following clinical picture: a patient not using oral contraceptives, with regular periods, who presents with acute pain late in the luteal phase. Some patients present with evidence of hemoperitoneum as well as hypovolemia and require surgical resection of the bleeding cyst. In others, the acute pain and blood loss are self-limited. These patients may be managed with mild analgesics and reassurance. Patients at risk for repetitive hemorrhagic corpus luteum cysts include those that are receiving anticoagulation medication and those that have inherent bleeding disorders. This process may be the hallmark to initiate an investigation for an inherent bleeding disorder.

The least common functional cyst is the *theca lutein cyst,* associated with pregnancy and usually bilateral. They are more common in multiple gestation, trophoblastic disease and also with ovulation induction with clomiphene and human menopausal gonadotropin/human chorionic gonadotropin. They may become large and are multicystic, but also regress spontaneously in most cases without intervention.

Benign Ovarian Neoplasms

Although most ovarian enlargements in the reproductive age group are functional cysts, about 25% prove to be nonfunctional ovarian neoplasms. In the reproductive age group, 90% of these neoplasms are benign, whereas the risk of malignancy rises to approximately 25% when postmenopausal patients are also included. Thus, ovarian masses in older patients and in reproductive patients with no response to oral contraceptives are of special concern. Unfortunately, unless the mass is particularly large or becomes symptomatic, these masses may remain undetected for some time. Many ovarian neoplasms are first discovered at the time of routine pelvic examination.

Ovarian neoplasms are usually categorized by the cell type of origin: (a) epithelial cell tumors, the largest class of ovarian neoplasm; *(b) germ cell tumors,* which include the most common ovarian neoplasm in reproductive-age women, the benign cystic teratoma or dermoid; and *(c) stromal cell tumors.* The classification of ovarian tumors by cell line of origin is presented in Table 47.1.

Table 47.1. Histologic Classification of All Ovarian Neoplasms
From coelomic epithelium (epithelial)
Serous
Mucinous
Endometrioid
Brenner
From gonadal stroma
Granulosa theca
Sertoli–Leydig (arrhenoblastoma)
Lipid cell fibroma
From germ cell
Dysgerminoma
Teratoma
Endodermal sinus (yolk sac)
Choriocarcinoma
Miscellaneous cell line sources
Lymphoma
Sarcoma
Metastatic
Colorectal
Breast
Endometrial

Benign Epithelial Cell Neoplasms

The exact cell source for the development of epithelial cell tumors of the ovary is unclear; however, the cells are characteristic of typical glandular epithelial cells. Evidence exists to suggest that these cells are derived from mesothelial cells lining the peritoneal cavity. Because the müllerian duct-derived tissue becomes the female genital tract by differentiation of the mesothelium from the gonadal ridge, it is hypothesized that these tissues are also capable of differentiating into glandular tissue. The more common epithelial tumors of the ovary are grouped into serous, mucinous, and endometrioid neoplasms, as shown in Table 47.2.

The most common epithelial cell neoplasm is the *serous cystadenoma.* Seventy percent of serous tumors are benign; approximately 10% have intraepithelial cellular characteristics, which suggest that they are of low malignant potential; and the remaining 20% are frankly

Table 47.2. Histologic Classification of the Common Epithelial Tumors of the Ovary

Serous tumors

Serous cystadenomas

Serous cystadenomas with proliferating activity of the epithelial cells and nuclear abnormalities but with no infiltrative destructive growth (low potential malignancy)

Serous cystadenocarcinoma

Mucinous tumors

Mucinous cystadenomas

Mucinous cystadenomas with proliferating activity of the epithelial cells and nuclear abnormalities but with no infiltrative destructive growth (low potential malignancy)

Mucinous cystadenocarcinoma

Endometrioid tumors (similar to adenocarcinomas in the endometrium)

Endometrioid benign cysts

Endometrioid tumors with proliferating activity of the epithelial cells and nuclear abnormalities but with no infiltrative destructive growth (low potential malignancy)

Adenocarcinoma

Brenner tumor

Unclassified carcinoma

malignant by both histologic criteria and clinical behavior. These tumors may occur in any age group, although they are more common in the perimenopausal and postmenopausal patient. On ultrasonography, these cysts tend to appear multilocular, are bilateral 15% of the time, and can be large. The *treatment of serous tumors* is surgical because of the relatively high rate of malignancy. In the younger patient with smaller tumors, an attempt can be made to perform an ovarian cystectomy to try to minimize the amount of ovarian tissue removed. For large, unilateral serous tumors in young patients, unilateral oophorectomy with preservation of the contralateral ovary is indicated to maintain fertility. In patients past the reproductive age, bilateral oophorectomy along with hysterectomy may be indicated, not only because of the chance of future malignancy but because of the increased risk of a similar occurrence in the contralateral ovary.

The *mucinous cystadenoma* is the second most common epithelial cell tumor of the ovary. The malignancy rate of 15% is lower than that for serous tumor, as is the 5% rate of bilaterality. These cystic tumors can become large, sometimes filling the entire pelvis and extending into the abdominal cavity. Ultrasound assessment will often reveal multilocular septations. Surgery is the treatment of choice.

A third type of benign epithelial neoplasm is the *endometrioid tumor*. Most benign endometrioid tumors take the form of endometriomas, which are cysts lined by well-differentiated, endometrial-like glandular tissue. For further discussion of this neoplasm, see "Malignant Ovarian Neoplasms," later in the chapter.

The *Brenner cell tumor* is an uncommon benign epithelial cell tumor of the ovary. This tumor is usually described as a solid ovarian tumor because of the large amount of stroma and fibrotic tissue that surrounds the epithelial cells. It is more common in older women and occasionally occurs in association with mucinous tumors of the ovary. When discovered as an isolated tumor of the ovary, it is relatively small compared with the large size often attained by the serous and especially by the mucinous cystadenomas. It is rarely malignant.

Benign Germ Cell Neoplasms

Germ cell tumors are derived from the primary germ cells. The tumors arise in the ovary and may contain relatively differentiated structures such as hair or bone. The most common tumor found in women of all ages is the *benign cystic teratoma*, also called a *dermoid cyst* or *dermoid*. Eighty percent occur during the reproductive years, with a median age of occurrence of 30 years. However, in children and adolescents, mature cystic teratomas account for about one-half of benign ovarian neoplasms. Dermoids may contain differentiated tissue from all three embryonic germ layers (ectoderm, mesoderm, and endoderm). The most common elements found are of ectodermal origin, primarily squamous cell tissue such as skin appendages (sweat, sebaceous glands) with associated hair follicles and sebum. It is because of this predominance of dermoid derivatives that the term *dermoid* is used. Other constituents of dermoids include central nervous system tissue, cartilage, bone, teeth, and intestinal glandular elements, most of which are found in well-differentiated form. One unusual variant is the *struma ovarii,* in which functioning thyroid tissue is found.

A dermoid cyst is frequently encountered as an asymptomatic, unilateral cystic adnexal mass that is mobile and nontender. This tumor often has a high fat content that makes it more readily identified by CT evaluation, as well as giving it a more buoyant tendency in the pelvis, resulting in a relatively high rate of ovarian torsion (15%), in comparison to other types of neoplasms.

Treatment of benign cystic teratomas is necessarily surgical, even though the rate of malignancy is <1%. Surgical removal is required because of the possibility of ovarian torsion and rupture, resulting in intense chemical peritonitis and a potential surgical emergency. Between 10% and 20% of these cysts are bilateral, underscoring the need for examination of the contralateral ovary at the time of surgery.

Benign Stromal Cell Neoplasms

Stromal cell tumors of the ovary are usually considered solid tumors and are derived from specialized sex cord stroma of the developing gonad. These tumors may develop along a primarily female cell type into *granulosa theca cell tumors* or into a primarily male gonadal type of tissue, known as *Sertoli–Leydig cell tumors.* Both of these tumors are referred to as functioning tumors because of their hormone production. *Granulosa theca cell tumors primarily produce estrogenic components* and may be manifest in patients through feminizing characteristics, and *Sertoli–Leydig cell tumors produce androgenic components,* which may contribute to hirsutism or virilizing symptoms. These neoplasms occur with approximately equal frequency in all age groups, including pediatric patients. When the granulosa cell tumor occurs in the pediatric age group, it

may contribute to signs and symptoms of precocious puberty, including precocious thelarche and vaginal bleeding. Vaginal bleeding may also occur when this tumor develops in the postmenopausal years. Both the granulosa cell tumor and the Sertoli–Leydig cell tumor have malignant potential, as discussed later.

The *ovarian fibroma* is the result of collagen production by spindle cells. These tumors account for 4% of ovarian tumors and are most common during middle age. It is unlike other stromal cell tumors in that it does not secrete sex steroids. It is usually a small, solid tumor with a smooth surface and occasionally is clinically misleading because ascites are present. The combination of benign ovarian fibroma coupled with ascites and right pleural effusion has historically been referred to as *Meigs syndrome.*

In summary, the following points regarding benign ovarian neoplasms can be made: (a) they are more common than malignant tumors of the ovary in all age groups, (b) the chance for malignant transformation increases with increasing age, (c) they warrant surgical treatment because of their potential for malignancy or torsion, (d) preoperative assessment may be assisted by the use of pelvic imaging techniques such as ultrasound, and (e) surgical treatment may be conservative for benign tumors, especially if future reproduction is desired.

Malignant Ovarian Neoplasms

Ovarian cancer is the *fifth most common of all cancers in women* in the United States and the *second most common gynecologic malignancy,* having a frequency of approximately one-fourth that of endometrial carcinoma. Yet the *mortality rate of this disease is the highest of all the gynecologic malignancies,* primarily because of the difficulty in detecting the disease before widespread dissemination. Symptoms of ovarian cancer are often confused with benign conditions or interpreted as part of the aging process with the final diagnosis often delayed. The most common symptoms in order from highest percentage to lowest are: abdominal fullness or distension, abdominal or back pain, decreased energy or lethargy, and urinary frequency. Because no clinically applicable screening test is available, approximately two-thirds of patients with ovarian cancer have advanced disease at the time of diagnosis. Of the 25,000 to 30,000 new cases of ovarian cancer yearly, some 60% will die within 5 years.

The most important demographic observation regarding ovarian cancer is that it *presents most commonly (90%) in the fifth and sixth decades of life.* The incidence of ovarian cancer in Western European countries and in the United States is higher, with a five- to seven-fold greater incidence than age-matched populations in East Asia. Whites are 50% more likely to develop ovarian cancer than blacks living in the United States.

A woman's risk for development of ovarian cancer during her lifetime is approximately 1%. The risk increases with age until approximately 70 years, at which time it declines modestly. The certain epidemiologic factors associated with development of ovarian cancer include low parity, decreased fertility, and delayed child-bearing. In addition, the *BRCA-1* gene has been found to be associated with ovarian cancers in approximately 5% to 10% of cases. A woman with a mutation of BRCA-1 or BRCA-2 has a lifetime risk of 15% to 45% of developing ovarian cancer. Currently, routine testing for this gene has limited clinical value. Similarly, mutations in the tumor suppressor gene, *P53,* have been shown to have some association with epithelial cell carcinomas, but are not useful in patient management as yet.

Long-term suppression of ovulation may protect against the development of ovarian cancer, at least for epithelial cell tumors. It has been suggested that so-called incessant ovulation may predispose to neoplastic transformation of the epithelial cell surfaces of the ovary. Oral contraceptives that prevent ovulation appear to provide significant protection against the occurrence of ovarian cancer. Five years' cumulative use of oral contraceptives decreases the lifetime risk by one-half. No evidence exists to implicate the use of postmenopausal hormone replacement therapy in the development of ovarian cancer.

Pathogenesis and Diagnosis

Malignant ovarian epithelial cell tumors spread primarily by direct extension within the peritoneal cavity as a result of direct cell sloughing from the ovarian surface. This process explains widespread peritoneal dissemination at the time of diagnosis, even with relatively small primary ovarian lesions. Although epithelial cell ovarian cancers also spread by lymphatic and blood-borne routes, it is the direct extension into the virtually unlimited space of the peritoneal cavity that is the primary basis for their late clinical presentation.

The early diagnosis of ovarian cancer is made even more difficult by the *lack of effective screening tests.* CA-125 is a tumor assay that should not be routinely used to screen for ovarian cancer, but, instead, should be used to follow response to therapy and evaluate for recurrent disease. Its use in selected cases can increase suspicion for ovarian cancer in a previously undiagnosed patient. This antigenic determinant is recognized by the monoclonal antibody OC-125. CA-125 is not expressed by either normal fetal or adult ovaries. Generally in adults CA-125 is increased with any inflammation of the pleura, pericardium or peritoneum. A serum value of 35 U/mL is considered the upper limit of normal. Both false–positive and false–negative results limit its use as a screening tool.

Histologic Classification

Malignant ovarian neoplasms are usually categorized by the cell type of origin, similar to their benign counterparts: *(a) malignant epithelial cell tumors,* which are the most common type; *(b) malignant germ cell tumors;* and *(c) malignant stromal cell tumors* (see Table 47.1). Most malignant ovarian tumors have histologically similar but benign counterparts. The relationship between a benign ovarian neoplasm and its malignant counterpart is clinically important. If the benign counterpart is found in a patient, removal of both ovaries is strongly considered because of the possibility of future malignant transformation in the remaining ovary. The decision regarding removal of one or both ovaries, however, must be individualized based on age, type of tumor, and future risks.

Staging

The staging of ovarian carcinoma is based on extent of spread of tumor and histologic evaluation of the tumor. The International

Federation of Gynecology and Obstetrics (FIGO) classification of ovarian cancer is presented in Table 47.3.

Borderline Ovarian Tumors

Approximately 10% of seemingly benign epithelial cell tumors may contain histologic evidence of intraepithelial neoplasia, commonly referred to as borderline malignancies, or "tumors of low malignant potential." These tumors generally remain confined to the ovary, are more common in premenopausal women (between 30 and 50 years of age), and have good prognoses. About 20% of such tumors show spread beyond the ovary. They require carefully individualized therapy following the initial surgical resection of the primary tumor. If frozen section pathology demonstrates borderline histology, unilateral

oophorectomy with a staging procedure and follow-up is appropriate, assuming the woman wishes to retain ovarian function and/or fertility and understands the risks of such conservative management.

Epithelial Cell Ovarian Carcinoma

Approximately 90% of all ovarian malignancies are of the epithelial cell type, derived from mesothelial cells. The ovary contains these cells as part of an ovarian capsule just overlying the actual stroma of the ovary. When these mesothelial cell elements are situated over developing follicles, they go through metaplastic transformation whenever ovulation occurs. Repeated ovulation is, therefore, associated with the histologic change in these cells derived from coelomic epithelium.

Table 47.3. FIGO Staging for Primary Carcinoma of the Ovary

Stage	Description
I	Growth limited to the ovaries
Ia	Growth limited to one ovary; no ascites containing malignant cells; no tumor on the external surface; capsule intact
Ib	Growth limited to both ovaries; no ascites containing malignant cells; no tumor on the external surface; capsule intact
Ic	Tumor either stage Ia or Ib but with tumor on the surface of one or both ovaries; or with capsule ruptured, or with ascites present containing malignant cells, or with positive peritoneal washings
II	Growth involving one or both ovaries with pelvic extension
IIa	Extension and/or metastases to the uterus and/or tubes
IIb	Extension to other pelvic tissues
IIc	Tumor either stage IIa or IIb but with tumor on the surface of one or both ovaries; or with capsule(s) ruptured, or with ascites present containing malignant cells, or with positive peritoneal washings
III	Tumor involving one or both ovaries with peritoneal implants outside the pelvis and/or positive retroperitoneal or inguinal nodes; superficial liver metastasis equals stage III; tumor is limited to the true pelvis, but histologically proven malignant extension is to small bowel or omentum
IIIa	Tumor grossly limited to the true pelvis with negative nodes but with histologically confirmed microscopic seeding of abdominal peritoneal surfaces
IIIb	Tumor of one or both ovaries with histologically confirmed implants of abdominal peritoneal surface; none exceeding 2 cm wide; nodes negative
IIIc	Abdominal implants >2 cm wide and/or positive retroperitoneal or inguinal nodes
IV	Growth involving one or both ovaries with distant metastasis; if pleural effusion is present, positive cytologic test results must deem a case stage IV; parenchymal liver metastasis equals stage IV

Malignant epithelial serous tumors (serous cystadenocarcinoma) are the most common malignant epithelial cell tumors. Approximately 50% of these cancers are thought to be derived from their benign precursors (serous cystadenoma), and as many as 30% of these tumors are bilateral at the time of clinical presentation. They are typically multiloculated and often have external excrescences on an otherwise smooth capsular surface. Calcified, laminated structures, *psammoma bodies,* are found in more than one-half of serous carcinomas.

Another epithelial cell variant that contains cells reminiscent of endocervical glandular mucous-secreting cells is the *malignant mucinous epithelial tumor (the mucinous cystadenocarcinoma).* They make up 36% of all epithelial tumors, with 80% being benign, 15% estimated to be of low malignant potential, and 5% cancerous. These tumors have a lower rate of bilaterality (10% to 15%) and can be among the largest of ovarian tumors, often measuring greater than 20 cm. They may be associated with widespread peritoneal extension with thick, mucinous ascites, termed *pseudomyxomatous peritonei.*

Although most epithelial carcinomas occur sporadically, a small percentage (5% to 10%) occurs in familial or hereditary patterns involving first- or second-degree relatives with a history of epithelial ovarian cancer. Having a first-degree relative (i.e., mother, sister, daughter) with an epithelial carcinoma gives a 5% lifetime risk for ovarian cancer, whereas having two first-degree relatives increases this risk to 20% to 30%. Such hereditary ovarian cancers generally occur earlier than nonhereditary tumors.

Breast/ovarian familial cancer syndrome, a combination of epithelial ovarian and breast cancers in first- and second-degree family members, are at two to three times the risk of these cancers as the general population. Women with this syndrome have an increased risk of bilaterality of breast cancer and developing ovarian tumors at a younger age. This syndrome has been associated with the BRCA-1 gene, a locus on the 17q chromosome. Women with this gene mutation have a cumulative lifetime risk of 85% to 90% for breast cancer and 50% for ovarian cancer. Women of Ashkenazi Jewish extraction have a 1% chance of carrying this gene, a 10-fold risk over the general population.

Lynch II syndrome occurs in families with first- and second-degree members with combinations of colon, ovarian, endometrial, and breast cancers. Women in families with this syndrome may have a threefold increased risk of cancer over the general population. Women in families with these syndromes should have more frequent screening tests and may benefit from prophylactic surgery in some cases.

Endometrioid Tumors Endometrioid tumors account for 8% of epithelial tumors, with 80% being malignant. These tumors contain histologic features similar to those of endometrial carcinoma. Up to 40% of these tumors are found in association with endometriosis, and 10% are found to coincide with endometrial cancer of the uterus.

Other Epithelial Cell Ovarian Carcinomas Of the remaining epithelial cell carcinomas of the ovary, *clear cell carcinomas* are thought to arise from mesonephric elements, and Brenner tumors are thought to arise uncommonly (<5%) from their benign counterpart. Interestingly, Brenner tumors occur approximately 10% of the time in the same ovary that contains mucinous cystadenoma; the reason for this is unclear.

Germ Cell Tumors

Germ cell tumors constitute *<5% of all ovarian malignancies.* However, they are the *most common ovarian cancers in women younger than 20 years of age,* making up 60% of the malignant tumors discovered in this age group. Germ cell tumors may be functional, producing human chorionic gonadotropin (hCG) or α-fetoprotein (AFP), both of which can be used as tumor markers. The most common germ cell malignancies are *dysgerminoma* and *immature teratoma.* Other tumors are recognized as *mixed germ cell tumors, endodermal sinus tumors, and embryonal tumors.* Improved chemotherapeutic and radiation protocols have resulted in greatly improved 5-year survival rates.

Dysgerminomas are unilateral in approximately 90% of patients. They are the *most common type of germ cell tumor seen in patients with gonadal dysgenesis.* These tumors often arise in benign counterparts called the gonadoblastoma. The tumors are particularly *radiosensitive and chemosensitive,* rendering adjunctive therapy efficacious.

Because of the young age of patients with dysgerminomas, removal of only the involved ovary with preservation of the uterus and contralateral tube and ovary may be considered if the tumor is less than approximately 10 cm and if no evidence of extraovarian spread is found. Unlike the epithelial cell tumors, these malignancies are more likely to spread by lymphatic channels, and therefore the pelvic and periaortic lymph nodes must be assessed carefully at the time of surgery. If disease has spread outside the ovaries, conventional hysterectomy and bilateral salpingo-oophorectomy are necessary, usually followed by cisplatin-based chemotherapy that is in combination with bleomycin and etoposide. The prognosis of these tumors is generally excellent. The overall 5-year survival rate for patients with dysgerminoma is 90% to 95% when the disease is limited to one ovary that is <10 cm wide.

Immature teratomas are the malignant counterpart of benign cystic teratomas (dermoids). These are the *second most common germ cell cancer and are most often found in women younger than 25 years of age.* They are usually unilateral, although on occasion a benign counterpart may be found in the contralateral ovary. Because these tumors are rapidly growing, they may produce painful symptomatology relatively early, because of hemorrhage and necrosis during the rapid growth process. As a result, the diagnosis is made when the disease is limited to one ovary in two-thirds of these young women. As with dysgerminoma, if an immature teratoma is limited to one ovary, unilateral oophorectomy is sufficient. Dramatic progress has been made in the treatment of these tumors in the past 15 years, with a 5-year survival rate greater than 80% for patients with well-differentiated tumors.

Rare Germ Cell Tumors

Endodermal sinus tumors and embryonal cell carcinomas are uncommon malignant ovarian tumors that have had a remarkable improvement in cure rate. Before about 10 years ago, these tumors were almost uniformly fatal. New chemotherapeutic protocols have resulted in an overall 5-year survival rate of greater than 60%. These tumors typically occur in childhood and adolescence, with the primary treatment being surgical resection of the involved ovary followed by combination chemotherapy. The endodermal sinus tumor produces α-fetoprotein, whereas the embryonal cell carcinoma produces both α-fetoprotein and β-hCG.

Gonadal Stromal Cell Tumors

The gonadal stromal cell tumors make up an unusual group of tumors characterized by hormone production; hence, these tumors are called *functioning tumors.* The hormonal output from these tumors is usually in the form of female or male sex steroids, or on occasion, adrenal steroid hormones.

The *granulosa cell tumor* is the *most common in this group.* These tumors occur in all ages, although in older patients they are more likely to be benign. Granulosa cell tumors may *secrete large amounts of estrogen, which in 15% to 20% of older women may cause endometrial hyperplasia or endometrial carcinoma.* Thus, endometrial sampling is especially important when ovarian tumors such as the granulosa tumor are estrogen producing. Surgical treatment should include removal of the uterus and both ovaries in postmenopausal women as well as in women of reproductive age who no longer wish to remain fertile. In a young woman with the lesion limited to one ovary with an intact capsule, unilateral oophorectomy with careful surgical staging may be adequate. This tumor may demonstrate recurrences up to 10 years later. This is especially true with large tumors, which have a 20% to 30% chance of late recurrence.

Sertoli–Leydig cell tumors (arrhenoblastoma) are the rare, testosterone-secreting counterparts to granulosa cell tumors. They usually occur in older patients and should be suspected in the differential diagnosis of perimenopausal or postmenopausal patients with hirsutism or virilization and an adnexal mass. Treatment of these tumors is similar to that for other ovarian malignancies in this age group and is based on extirpation of uterus and ovaries.

Other stromal cell tumors include *fibromas* and *thecomas,* which rarely demonstrate malignant counterparts, the *fibrosarcoma* and *malignant thecoma.*

Other Ovarian Malignancies

Rarely, the ovary may be the site of initial manifestation of *lymphoma.* These are usually found in association with lymphoma elsewhere, although cases have been reported of primary ovarian lymphoma. Once the diagnosis has been made, management is similar to that for lymphoma of other origin.

Malignant mesodermal sarcomas (carcinosarcomas) are another rare type of ovarian tumor that usually show aggressive behavior and are diagnosed at late stages. The survival rate is poor, and clinical experience with these tumors is limited.

Cancer Metastatic to the Ovary

Classically, the term *Krukenberg tumor* describes an ovarian tumor that is metastatic from other sites such as the gastrointestinal tract (80% from stomach, remainder from colon), breast, and endometrium. They account for 30% to 40% of cancers metastatic to the ovary. Most of these tumors are characterized as infiltrative, mucinous carcinoma of predominantly signet-ring cell type and as bilateral and associated with widespread metastatic disease. On occasion, these tumors are associated with abnormal uterine bleeding or virilization, leading to the supposition that some may produce estrogens or androgens. Breast cancer metastatic to the ovary is common, with autopsy data suggesting ovarian metastasis in one quarter of cases.

In 10% of patients with cancer metastatic to the ovary, an extraovarian primary site cannot be demonstrated. In this regard, it is important to consider ovarian preservation versus prophylactic oophorectomy at the time of hysterectomy in patients who have a strong family history (first-degree relatives) of epithelial ovarian cancer, primary gastrointestinal tract cancer, or breast cancer. In patients previously treated for breast cancer or gastrointestinal cancer, consideration should be given to the incidental removal of the ovaries at the time of hysterectomy, because these patients have a high predilection for development of ovarian cancer.

The prognosis for most patients with carcinoma metastatic to the ovary is dismal, with 5% to 10% 5-year survival rates being quoted.

Fallopian Tubes

Normal fallopian tubes cannot be palpated and usually are not considered in the differential diagnosis of adnexal disease *in the asymptomatic patient.* Common problems involving the fallopian tubes include ectopic pregnancy, salpingitis/hydrosalpinx/tubo-ovarian abscess, and endometriosis (which can present as masses or be symptomatic). These conditions are discussed in other chapters.

Benign Disease of the Fallopian Tube and Mesosalpinx

Paraovarian cysts develop in the mesosalpinx from vestigial wolffian duct structures, tubal epithelium, and peritoneum inclusions. These are differentiated from *paratubal cysts,* which are found near the fimbriated end of the fallopian tube, are common, and are called *hydatid cysts of Morgagni.* Both are usually small and symptomatic, although rarely they can reach large proportions.

Carcinoma of the Fallopian Tube

Primary fallopian tube carcinoma is usually an adenocarcinoma, although other cell types, including adenosquamous carcinoma and sarcoma, are rarely reported. About two-thirds of patients with this rare gynecologic malignancy (<1% of gynecologic malignancies) are postmenopausal. Grossly, these tumors are often rather large, resembling a hydrosalpinx, with a normal contralateral tube in 95% of cases. Microscopically, most are typical papillary serous cystadenocarcinomas of the ovary. The symptoms of this tumor are so slight that the tumor is often advanced before recognition of a problem. The most common complaint associated with fallopian tube carcinoma is postmenopausal bleeding followed by abnormal vaginal discharge. If such a discharge is profuse and serosanguineous, it is termed *hydrotubae profluens,* sometimes considered diagnostic of this tumor; however, the classic triad of symptoms associated with fallopian tube carcinoma (watery vaginal discharge, pain, and pelvic mass) is

Table 47.4. Surgical Staging for Primary Tubal Carcinoma

Stage	Description
I	
IA	Disease confined to one tube with no ascites
IB	Disease confined to both tubes with no ascites
IC	Disease confined to one or both tubes but ascites present with malignant cells in the fluid
II	
IIA	Extension to the uterus or ovaries or both
IIB	Extension to the uterus or ovaries and to other intraperitoneal organs or tissues beyond the true pelvis
III	Extension to the uterus or ovaries and to other intraperitoneal organs and tissues beyond the true pelvis
IV	Metastases present in organs or tissues outside the peritoneal cavity

noted in <15% of cases. Staging is surgical, *similar to that for ovarian carcinoma* (Table 47.4); progression is similar to that of ovarian carcinoma, with intraperitoneal metastases and ascites. Because the fallopian tubes are richly permeated with lymphatic channels, para-aortic and pelvic lymph node spread is common, the former in perhaps one-third of all cases. Unlike ovarian cancer, 70% of fallopian tube cancer presents as stage I or II disease. The overall 5-year survival rate is 35% to 45%, with stage I having the best rate, approaching 70%. Too few data are available to ascertain whether adjunctive therapy is useful, and this management must be made on a case-by-case basis; however, initial management with staging and debulking is the the same as for ovarian cancer treatment.

Carcinoma metastatic to the fallopian tube, coming mainly from the uterus and ovary, is far more common than primary fallopian tube carcinoma. A few cases of *other, rare tumors of the fallopian tube are reported,* including malignant mixed müllerian tumors, primary choriocarcinoma, fibroma, and adenomatoid tumors.

General Principles in the Surgical Management of Ovarian and Fallopian Tube Malignancy

Primary surgical therapy is indicated in most of the ovarian malignancies, using the principle of *cytoreductive surgery, or "tumor debulking."* The rationale for cytoreductive surgery is that adjunctive radiation therapy and chemotherapy are more effective when all tumor masses are reduced to <1 cm in size (see Chapter 41). Because direct peritoneal seeding is the primary method of intraperitoneal spread, multiple adjacent structures commonly contain tumor, resulting in cytoreductive procedures that are often extensive. Each procedure includes the following.

1. Peritoneal cytology is obtained on entering the abdomen to assess microscopic spread of tumor. Gross ascites is aspirated and submitted for cytologic analysis, or if no ascites are found, saline irrigation is used to "wash" the peritoneal cavity in an attempt to find microscopic disease.
2. Inspection and palpation of the entire peritoneal cavity is done to determine the extent of disease. This includes the pelvis, both pericolic gutters, omentum, and upper abdomen, including the liver, spleen, and undersurface of the diaphragm.
3. Omentectomy is usually performed, whether or not tumor involvement is evident.
4. Sampling of the pelvic and periaortic lymph nodes is performed. Without gross disease, biopsies are obtained from the anterior and posterior cul-de-sac, right and left pelvic sidewalls, right and left pericolic gutters, and diaphragm.

Because most ovarian cancer presents at an advanced stage, *adjunctive treatment* using chemotherapy is usually necessary. First-line chemotherapy is with *paclitaxel (Taxol)* combined with *carboplatin.*

With *recurrence of disease,* other chemotherapeutic agents may be used, including ifosfamide, hexamethylmelamine, doxorubicin, topotecan, gemcytabine, etoposide, vinorelbine, and tamoxifen. *Radiation therapy* has only a limited role in the management of ovarian cancer.

Follow-up consists of clinical history and examination, various imaging studies (ultrasound and/or computed tomography), and in epithelial cell tumors, the use of serum tumor markers such as CA-125.

UNIT VI

HUMAN SEXUALITY

CHAPTER 48

HUMAN SEXUALITY

This chapter deals primarily with APGO Educational Topic:

Topic 56: Sexuality and Modes of Sexual Expression

The student should understand how to address a patient's sexual concerns as well as health-care issues that may be related to her modes of sexual expression.

In the United States the topic of female sexual dysfunction is receiving increased attention in both the professional and popular media. Estimates of sexual complaints, symptoms, or concerns vary dramatically, with one recent national survey finding that between 35 and 45 percent of women report some type of sexual complaint. The problem cited most frequently in that study was low sexual desire.

Determinants of healthy sexuality are complex and multifactorial. Intrapersonal factors include the sense of one's self as a sexual being, one's overall health status, a general perception of well-being, and the quality of an individual's previous sexual experiences. For partnered individuals, this same list applies to the partner. Interpersonal aspects include the duration and overall quality of the relationship, communication styles, and the number and type of ongoing life events and stressors. Examples of generally "positive" life events, which can contribute to sexual dysfunctions, include the birth of a child and retirement.

The perceived importance of physical intimacy for a given couple depends largely on whether or not they are satisfied with that aspect of their relationship. Among couples who are not experiencing sexual dysfunctions, each partner will estimate that the sexual component of their relationship accounts for approximately 10% of their overall happiness. In couples experiencing sexual difficulties, however, the sexual aspects are estimated as accounting for approximately 60% of the overall relationship quality. This dramatic shift in perception underscores the importance that physical intimacy holds within the context of the overall relationship.

Health-care providers play an important role in the identification, evaluation, and management of sexual dysfunctions. By demonstrating a supportive and nonjudgmental attitude, the physician creates a sense that it is permissible to discuss sexual matters and problems. Several existing classification systems and medical interview tools are available to help guide clinicians and patients through this process.

Developmental Aspects of Sexuality

At the most basic level, the experience of sexuality begins with an individual's genotype and phenotype. From this basic biologic underpinning, children develop a gender identity during early childhood. Eventually, each individual develops a sense of self as a sexual being and a sexual orientation. Each of these latter components is fluid and can vary over time and with particular circumstances. For example, many individuals who consider themselves heterosexual periodically engage in sexual encounters with same-sex partners.

Physiologic Models of Human Sexual Response Cycles

The human sexual response cycle has been conceptualized in various ways. The work of Masters and Johnson, which documented the physiologic responses of orgasmic couples, is perhaps the best-known paradigm. They used their data to characterize the sequence of physiologic response into four phases: excitement, plateau, orgasm, and resolution. An important modification of the model was introduced by Kaplan, who conceptualized a desire phase preceding the excitement phase.

Systemically, the physiologic components of the female sexual response (Table 48.1) are mediated by increased activity of the autonomic nervous system and include tachycardia and skin flushing. Several neurotransmitters have been linked to the sexual response cycle. Norepinephrine, dopamine, and oxytocin are thought to have positive sexual effects; prolactin and gamma-amino butyric acid are thought to affect the cycle negatively. Serotonin has mixed effects, depending on the particular serotonin receptor being activated.

Within the pelvis, changes in uterine muscle tone (myotonic activity) and changes in blood flow (vasocongestion) are noted. The latter can be demonstrated by measured increases in the pulse amplitude of vaginal blood flow. The upper portion of the vagina dilates via a mechanism that is poorly understood. Figures 48.1 through 48.4 demonstrate some of the physiologic changes seen in these phases. The duration of each phase varies with each individual and for a given individual at different times in her life. The value of these classifications lies in their use in identifying the physiologic events that occur during intimate

Table 48.1. Physiologic Reactions of Women During the Orgasmic Sexual Response Cycles (as documented by Masters and Johnson)

Phase	Sex-Organ Response	General Body Response
Excitement	Vaginal lubrication Thickening of vaginal walls and labia Expansion of inner vagina Elevation of cervix and corpus Tumescence of clitoris	Nipple erection Sex-tension flush
Plateau	Orgasmic platform in outer vagina Full expansion of inner vagina Secretion of mucus by Bartholin's gland Withdrawal of clitoris	Sex-tension flush Carpopedal spasm Generalized skeletal muscle tension Hyperventilation Tachycardia
Orgasm	Contractions of orgasmic platform at 0.8-sec intervals External rectal sphincter contractions at 0.8-sec intervals External urethral sphincter contractions at irregular intervals	Special skeletal muscle contractions Hyperventilation Tachycardia
Resolution	Ready return to orgasm with retarded loss of pelvic vasocongestion Return of normal color and orgasmic platform in primary (rapid) stage Loss of clitoral tumescence and return to position	Sweating reaction Hyperventilation Tachycardia

encounters leading to climax. Clinically, the provider can inquire about whether or not these responses exist during the initial interview and in response to ongoing therapy.

The phases of the sexual response cycle as described by the Masters and Johnson and Kaplan models are typically depicted in a linear fashion. A limitation of this construct is the inability to automatically take previous experiences, both positive and negative, into account. More recent models, such as the intimacy-based female sexual response cycle described by Basson, are deliberately constructed in a cyclic manner. The influence of positive and

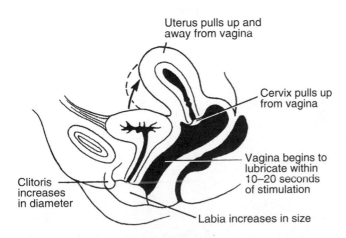

Uterus pulls up and away from vagina

Cervix pulls up from vagina

Vagina begins to lubricate within 10–20 seconds of stimulation

Labia increases in size

Clitoris increases in diameter

Figure 48.1. Excitement stage.

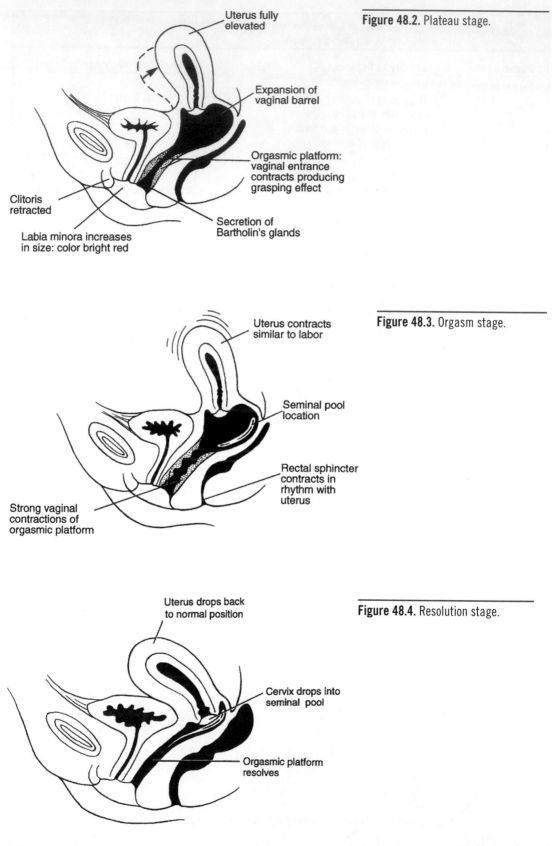

Figure 48.2. Plateau stage.

Uterus fully elevated

Expansion of vaginal barrel

Orgasmic platform: vaginal entrance contracts producing grasping effect

Clitoris retracted

Secretion of Bartholin's glands

Labia minora increases in size: color bright red

Figure 48.3. Orgasm stage.

Uterus contracts similar to labor

Seminal pool location

Rectal sphincter contracts in rhythm with uterus

Strong vaginal contractions of orgasmic platform

Figure 48.4. Resolution stage.

Uterus drops back to normal position

Cervix drops into seminal pool

Orgasmic platform resolves

negative feedback loops on current sexual function is therefore integral to the model (see Figure 48.5). In some studies, graphing a patient's symptoms onto a copy of the cycle has proven useful in the context of ongoing therapy.

Diagnostic Categories for Female Sexual Dysfunction

In 1998 the American Foundation of Urologic Disease (AFUD) sponsored a consensus committee to develop definitions and criteria for diagnosing female sexual dysfunction. Their recommendations were published in the *Journal of Urology* in 2000. They classified female sexual dysfunctions into the following four general areas.

1. Hypoactive sexual desire disorder
2. Female sexual arousal disorder
3. Female orgasmic disorder
4. Pain disorders

Most patients report symptoms in more than one category. Their partners may also manifest symptoms of sexual dysfunction.

According to the consensus definitions, hypoactive sexual desire disorder (HSDD) is defined as "the persistent or recurrent deficiency or absence of sexual fantasies, thoughts and/or desire for or receptivity to sexual activity, which causes personal distress." HSDD is the most common form of female sexual dysfunction. Several subtle, but important, concepts are built into this definition. Importantly, the person who needs to be bothered by the symptom is the patient herself. Determining this can be complicated. For example, is the patient personally distressed by her lack of interest in sexual relations with her partner, or is she distressed by the response of her partner to her lack of interest? Such distinctions are not always easy to make. A second subtlety inherent in the definition is the concept of receptivity to a partner's intimate overtures (i.e., women who do not initiate sexual contact, but are responsive to their partner's overtures do not have HSDD).

HSDD patients are further subcategorized on the basis of the duration of symptoms and the context in which the symptoms occur.

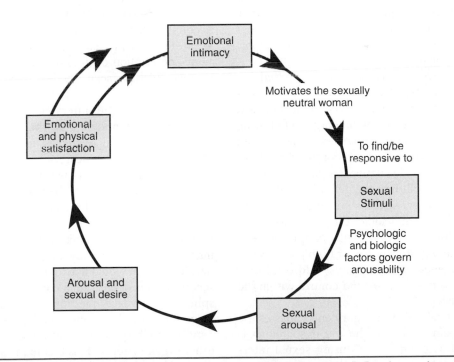

Figure 48.5. Negative and positive feedback loops on sexual function. (From Basson R. Female sexual response: the role of drugs in the management of sexual dysfunction. *Obstet Gynecol* 2001;98:350–359.)

With regard to duration, the clinician must establish whether the patient's symptoms are lifelong or acquired. If the symptoms appear to be acquired, the clinician should redirect the line of questioning to elucidate which factors seem to have contributed to the change. With regard to context, the lack of interest in sexual encounters may either be global or specific to a particular situation or partner.

The second AFUD category is labeled Female Sexual Arousal Disorder (FSAD). FSAD is defined as "the persistent or recurrent inability to attain or maintain sufficient sexual excitement, causing personal distress." This can manifest as a lack of subjective mental excitement (missed arousal disorder), a lack of physiologic response (genital arousal disorder), or both (generalized arousal disorder). In some cases, the patient reports physiologic changes in response to appropriate stimuli, but interprets these responses neutrally (anhedonic arousal) or even negatively (dysphoric arousal). Patients with either of these conditions may report sexual coercion or assault as part of their past or current medical histories. In studies measuring vaginal blood flow among patients with FSAD, missed arousal disorder is the most common finding. Once again, the clinician must determine whether the symptoms are lifelong or acquired, global or situational.

The third AFUD category is entitled Female Orgasmic Disorder (FOD). This is defined as the "persistent or recurrent difficulty, delay or absence of attaining orgasm following sufficient stimulation or arousal, which causes personal distress." Subcategories reflect both the duration and situational aspects of the disorder. Also built into the definition is the concept of sufficient sexual stimulation or arousal, which may be difficult for the patient to define. Psychologists working with couples experiencing anorgasmia in one or both partners frequently encounter and must address issues related to trust, power, and control within the relationship.

The final AFUD category encompasses the sexual pain disorders. The first, dyspareunia, is defined as genital pain during sexual intercourse. The second, vaginismus, refers to painful contraction of the musculature of the lower third of the vagina in response to vaginal penetration.

Typically, more than one dysfunction is present. Coexistent partner dysfunctions, such as erectile dysfunction or premature ejaculation, are also prevalent. A thorough history therefore helps both clinicians and patients comprehend the complexities of sexual dysfunctions.

Evaluation of Patients Reporting Sexual Dysfunction

The Medical Interview

The medical interview is the cornerstone of the initial evaluation of patients reporting sexual dysfunctions. The interview has four basic components and serves multiple purposes. The history of the present illness establishes the number of dysfunctions present in the patient and her partner, the order in which they occurred, the relationship they have to each other, and their current severity. The complete medical history helps the clinician identify medical cofactors that may be contributing to the patient's sexual symptomatology. The third portion is a brief overview of the patient's account of her sexual and romantic development. The final piece of the interview is the patient's description of the immediate backdrop against which her sexuality developed and currently functions.

Throughout the interview, the patient needs to feel confident that the clinician regards sexuality and related issues as a legitimate part of her health care. This message can be conveyed in various ways. A few, brief, open-ended questions can be readily incorporated into the standard medical interview. Examples include "Are you sexually active?" "Do you find the sexual aspect of your life satisfying?" or "Do you have any concerns of a sexual nature that you would like to discuss today?" A second means of creating a comfortable atmosphere is to weave questions about sexuality throughout the interview, moving seamlessly between such questions and those related to other organ systems. This technique serves to demystify and normalize sexual concerns. Finally, the terminology used should be accurate as well as comfortable for both the clinician and the patient. For example, masturbation can be referred to as self-stimulation or self-pleasuring. The attentive physician can help guide the patient in this regard.

The interview can be conducted in any order. One general approach is to elicit the chief complaint and then focus initially on the patient's past medical, surgical, psychiatric, and social history, followed by a complete list of the patient's current medications, use of tobacco, alcohol, and recreational drugs. This general format and line of questioning is familiar to both the patient and the clinician and allows them to establish therapeutic rapport. Information collected during this portion of the interview is often relevant when etiologies for sexual concerns are being entertained and treatments considered.

Once the background information is collected, focus can return to the history of the sexual complaint. Data is collected using the AFUD categories as a reference. The order in which various symptoms appeared in the patient and in her partner is important to elucidate. The patient should be allowed to articulate the impact her symptoms have had on her overall relationship and her concerns for the future.

One technique for obtaining the history in chronological order is based on the concept of romantic and sexual milestones. The line of questioning begins by asking the patient when she first became aware of herself as a sexual being. Follow-up questions focus on specific events in her sexual development, including the age at which she first became interested in romantic partners, when she went on her first date, experienced her first kiss, and first became active sexually either with herself or with a partner. The circumstances surrounding each of these milestones and her current understanding of those events should also be ascertained. Certainly, negative experiences and a history of assault and/or coercion should also be elicited and discussed within this framework. The chronology continues until the onset of symptoms is identified and is then traced to the present.

The patient usually alludes to her key intimate partners as this chronology unfolds.

Attention is directed toward the number of serious life partners she has had, the overall nature and quality of those relationships, and the patient's account of why previous relationships ultimately ended. The role of partnered and unpartnered sexual activity both outside and concurrent with these serious relationships can be discussed. The lack of long-term intimate partners is also notable.

As the final piece of the intake interview, a family history is taken. A family of origin genogram is a convenient tool for obtaining and organizing this portion of the patient's sexual history. Using a conventional genogram format, the clinician records basic information about the patient's parents, siblings, and children. Events such as divorces and remarriages are recorded using standard symbols. Other significant individuals, events, and influences can also be noted as the patient sees fit.

Once the basic genogram is mapped, the patient is asked to describe how various individuals and couples within the family express emotional and physical intimacy. The ways in which information of a sexual nature is typically handled within the family unit are also elucidated. For patients with current partners, this step is repeated for the partner's family. Seeing this background information displayed visually helps the patient understand her own situation in context. At the same time, the clinician may identify patterns of behavior possibly relevant to the patient's case.

Collecting this information takes time and may need to be completed over multiple visits. Although obtaining this baseline information is important, it is incumbent on the provider to refrain from acting as a sex therapist, couple's counselor, or psychotherapist without the proper training or credentials. In fact, one of the primary benefits of this exercise is for the primary care provider to help the patient recognize the role various mental health providers might play in her treatment.

The Physical Examination

A thorough abdominal and pelvic examination is an integral part of the evaluation of patients with sexual dysfunction, with specific attention directed toward the patient's complaints. For patients complaining of dryness, the overall health of the vaginal and vulvar tissues should be noted. For patients with insertional pain, signs of vestibulitis should be noted and specific lesions investigated. Patients experiencing deep dyspareunia might have normal anatomic retroversion or pelvis masses. Throughout the examination, the clinician should educate the patient about the normal anatomy of the female genital tract and mention pertinent findings that are healthy and normal.

Special Considerations

The relationship between clinical depression and sexual function is complex. Clearly, both correlate with an overall sense of personal well-being. Approximately one-third of women presenting with sexual dysfunction are clinically depressed. Patients should therefore be screened for depression during the initial interview, possibly using standard screening tools. Therapy should be initiated and referrals made as appropriate. Among individuals in whom depression has already been diagnosed, the type and progress of ongoing therapy should be noted.

The commonly prescribed selective serotonin-reuptake inhibitors, such as fluoxetine, paroxetine, sertraline, and escitalopram, can be associated with decreased sexual desire. Up to 70% of women taking these medications report decreased sexual desire. Strategies for managing this side effect include dose reduction, switching antidepressant, and periodic use of other medications, including bupropion. It should be noted, however, that all antidepressants, not just the SSRIs, have been associated with an increased incidence of sexual dysfunction. Further complicating this picture is that depression itself causes a decrease in sexual desire.

The role androgens play in the management of HSDD is an area of ongoing investigation. Difficulty establishing a direct correlation between specific androgen levels and sexual desire is related to the limitations of widely available laboratory assays. In general, most published studies on the role of androgens in female sexual desire report lower levels among women experiencing symptoms than among those without symptoms. Currently, no testosterone-containing products have been approved by the Food and Drug Administration (FDA) for the treatment of HSDD. The need for adequate estrogen levels for successful response to testosterone has been demonstrated.

Other products currently under investigation for the treatment of HSDD include melanocortin-stimulating hormone (MSH) agonists. MSH is thought to be responsible for various basic physiologic functions, including sleep response patterns and appetite.

Referrals

A wide range of professionals play important roles in treating patients and couples who are experiencing sexual dysfunction. Urologists should be consulted to address issues related to male sexual function. Physical therapists can help patients address pain-related issues with the use of vaginal dilators and biofeedback. Licensed marital therapists, sex counselors, couples counselors, and psychotherapists provide useful consultation for addressing those psychosocial issues that are contributing to or being affected by the sexual dysfunction. Working as a team will help patients and their partners tackle all aspects of this multidimensional health problem.

VII

UNIT VII

VIOLENCE AGAINST WOMEN

CHAPTER 49

SEXUAL ASSAULT AND DOMESTIC VIOLENCE

This chapter deals primarily with APGO Educational Topics:

Topic 57: Sexual Assault
Topic 58: Domestic Violence

Students should be able to define adult and child sexual assault and describe the evaluation and management of each, including age-appropriate sexual assault history and physical examination, forensic examination, as well as counseling. Students should also be able to describe the types of violence against women in domestic situations, their evaluation and management, and the psychosocial issues that they engender.

Sexual assault and domestic violence are the experience of far too many women and girls (and men and boys also) in the United States. They pose obvious immediate health and emotional risks, but in addition are associated with long-term effects on the mental and physical health of the victim and her family. The compassionate and thoughtful care of victims and their families is an important goal of everyone involved in the health care of women and girls.

Sexual Assault

Sexual assault is the nonconsensual performance of acts, which in a consensual setting would be sexual or perceived as sexual, or which involve the body in such a manner that the victim perceives a sexual intrusion. An estimated one of every four women and children in the United States are sexual assault victims. This statistic usually engenders a shocked response and, often, one of disbelief. "This just cannot be," is an understandable response; it is difficult to accept this reality, or the attendant one, the real risk of being a victim. Further, because of the stigma associated with sexual assault, only 1 of 10 victims seeks help. Unfortunately, those victims who do seek help are often as traumatized by those from whom they seek help as by those who assaulted them. Because of the complex problems caused by sexual assault, treatment by a *multidisciplinary team* using prepared protocols is best. The health-care team has three tasks:

- Care for the victim's emotional needs
- Evaluate and treat medically
- Collect forensic specimens

Caring for the Adult Sexual Assault Victim

Rape Trauma Syndrome

During sexual assault, the victim realizes that she cannot escape the situation and has lost control. This *loss of control,* which is the most serious emotional problem faced by the victim, is based in fact, because *threatened or actual violence is always an integral part of sexual assault.* Victims of sexual assault may react to the experience in various ways. The *rape trauma syndrome* is a useful descriptive and therapeutic model for these responses and has three phases. The *acute phase of rape trauma syndrome* begins with the assault, but may not be fully manifest until the time of initial disclosure, when the victim first tells someone of the assault. In this emotionally volatile time, the victim may appear calm, may be tearful and agitated, or may move from one extreme to another. *An inability to think clearly or remember things such as her past medical history, termed "cognitive dysfunction," is a particularly distressing aspect of the syndrome.* The involuntary loss of cognition may raise fears of "being crazy" or of being perceived as "crazy" by others. It is also frustrating for the health care team unless it realizes that this is an involuntary reaction to the assault and not a willful action.

After the assault and before seeking care, the victim may have performed routine tasks such as shopping or cleaning the house. This *retreat to routine activities* is an emotional attempt to regain control, which is not related to the severity of the assault. *Safety and regaining control are the victim's main emotional needs during this time.* The patient should be reassured about her immediate safety and offered as much control over events as is reasonable for her clinical situation. Discussing the sexual assault within a supportive environment facilitates a sense of control, even if the topics of discussion are themselves unpleasant.

During the *middle or "readjustment" phase,* the patient appears to resolve most issues about the assault. This resolution involves a rationalization that she should or could have prevented the assault, coupled with unrealistic plans to avoid another assault. The plans of this phase ultimately break down in the *late or "reorganization" phase,* as the victim begins to deal with the reality of her victimization. The late phase, which may be lengthy, is a difficult and painful time, often characterized by drastic changes in lifestyle, friends, and work. Ongoing counseling is important if the victim is to recover fully from the emotional traumas of the assault.

Initial Care

A team member should remain with the patient to help provide a sense of safety and security.

The patient should be encouraged, in a supportive, nonjudgmental manner, to talk about the assault and her feelings. This starts the patient's emotional care and also provides historical data. Treatment for life-threatening trauma is, of course, begun immediately. Fortunately, such trauma is uncommon, although minor trauma is seen in one-fourth of victims. Even in life-threatening situations, any sense of control that can be given the patient is helpful. Obtaining consent for treatment is not only a legal requirement but also an important aspect of the emotional care of the victim. Although patients are often reticent to do so, they should be gently encouraged to work with the police, because such cooperation is clearly associated with improved emotional outcomes for victims.

History taking about a sexual assault is uncomfortable for victims and health-care providers alike. History taking is not, however, an additional trauma. Instead, it is both a necessary activity to gain medical and forensic information and an important therapeutic activity. Recalling the details of the assault in the supportive environment of the health-care setting allows the victim to begin to gain an understanding of what has happened and to see that she and others can deal with the events. Victims of sexual assault characteristically perceive themselves as guilty of causing the assault, especially in situations in which they used poor judgment (e.g., hitchhiking). To say that any activity was acceptable when it involved poor judgment is a falsehood that destroys the patient's ultimate trust and the care provider's credibility. Reminding the patient that *"poor judgment is not a rapable offense"* helps the patient begin to place blame where it truly belongs: on the rapist.

Victims of sexual assault should be given a *complete general physical examination,* including a pelvic examination. Forensic specimens should be collected, and cultures for sexually transmitted diseases should be obtained. When collecting *forensic specimens,* it is critical that the clinician follow the directions on the forensic specimens kit. These specimens are kept in a health professional's possession or control until turned over to an appropriate legal representative. This "protective custody" of the specimens ensures that the correct specimen reaches the forensic laboratory and is called the "chain of evidence."

Initial *laboratory tests* should include cultures from the vagina, the anus, and, usually, the pharynx for gonorrhea and *Chlamydia,* rapid plasma reagin (RPR) for syphilis, hepatitis antigens, human immunodeficiency virus (HIV) if indicated (usually), urinalysis (UA) and culture and sensitivity (C&S), and a pregnancy test for menstrual-aged women (regardless of contraceptive status).

Antibiotic prophylaxis should be offered to all adult victims. The risk of infection is unknown, but it is clearly higher than for a consensual sexual experience. Recommended regimens include oral *doxycycline* (100 mg orally twice daily for 7 days) or oral *amoxicillin* (3 g orally once) plus *probenecid* (1 g orally once), followed by oral *erythromycin* base (500 mg orally twice daily for 7 days) for pregnant victims or those allergic to tetracyclines. In areas with a prevalence rate greater than 1% for antibiotic-resistant strains of *Neisseria gonorrhoeae,* ceftriaxone (Rocephin; 250 mg intramuscularly [IM]) followed by oral doxycycline (100 mg orally twice daily for 7 days) is recommended. *Tetanus toxoid* should be administered if indicated.

Emergency contraception, should be offered and is described in Chapter 25.

Within 24 to 48 hours, victims should be contacted by phone or seen for an *immediate posttreatment evaluation.* At this time, emotional or physical problems are managed and follow-up appointments arranged for 1 and 6 weeks. Potentially serious problems such as suicidal ideation, rectal bleeding, or evidence of pelvic infection may go unrecognized by the victim during this time because of fear or continued cognitive dysfunction. Gently stated but specific questions must be asked to ensure that such problems have not arisen.

Subsequent Care

At the 1-week visit, a general review of the patient's progress is made and any specific new problems addressed. The next routine visit is at 6 weeks, when a complete evaluation, including physical examination, repeat cultures for sexually transmitted diseases, and a repeat RPR, is performed. Another visit at 12 to

18 weeks may be indicated for repeat HIV titers, although the current understanding of HIV infection does not allow an estimate of the risk of exposure for sexual assault victims. Each victim should receive as much counseling and support as is necessary, with referral to a long-term counseling program if needed.

Caring for the Child Sexual Assault Victim

A total of 90% of child victimization is by parents, family members, or family friends; "stranger rape" is relatively uncommon in children. The assailants play on the child's need for love and her dependency on family. To get past this conflict, it is best to interview child victims apart from parents and other family members, if possible by interviewers skilled in child interview techniques. Although such interviewing and the interpretation of information gained are difficult, in general, a child who displays a knowledge of sexual matters, anatomy, or function beyond that expected for her years is likely a victim of sexual abuse. Expert interviewers may use such specialized techniques as anatomically correct doll play and drawing interpretation to facilitate the process.

The physical examination of a small child requires patience and much experience. Sedation should be avoided, because it cannot be done sufficiently to allay anxiety in an outpatient setting. Instead, it usually adds to the child's fear and sense of helplessness. Examination under anesthesia may be required, although nonobtrusive techniques have been developed to avoid this procedure.

Prophylactic antibiotic therapy should be offered to children if the assailant is infected, if follow-up compliance is unlikely, or if the assailant is a stranger. Otherwise, prophylactic antibiotic therapy usually is not indicated. Of course, any diagnosed infection in the child is treated as appropriate. Recommended regimens include amoxicillin (50 mg/kg body weight once) plus probenecid (25 mg/kg body weight to a maximum dose of 1 g). For penicillin-allergic children or in geographic areas with a high prevalence of penicillinase-producing gonococci, spectinomycin (40 mg/kg body

weight IM) or ceftriaxone (125 mg IM once) followed by erythromycin (50 mg/kg body weight orally for 7 days) can be given.

It is the responsibility of the care team to determine if the child may safely return home or if the risk of ongoing abuse requires foster home placement or hospitalization. *Because suspected child sexual abuse must be reported to police and child welfare authorities,* these agencies may officially help in this decision, although responsibility rests with the care team at the time of the initial disclosure.

Domestic Violence

Domestic violence is experienced by an estimated 25% to 50% of women during their life and is suggested as a significant source of illness and injury to women. Consider that one in five women who present to an emergency room has been injured by her partner; approximately 90% of domestic homicides show a history of a police call for domestic violence within the year; about 10% of adolescents are battered by a parent; and an estimated three-fourths of women indicate that they have been victims of domestic violence and would have discussed the situation with their physician if they had been asked.

What is domestic violence, and how is it recognized? *Domestic violence* may involve one or more of three presentations. *Physical abuse* such as hitting, slapping, kicking, and choking is the most obvious presentation. It is suspected with evidence of trauma, especially to the head and neck or trunk associated with a history of violence, or when an explanation of the trauma doesn't seem appropriate (Table 49.1). Unfortunately, pregnancy appears to be a period of greater risk for such episodes. *Sexual abuse* is another presentation of domestic violence. The third presentation is *emotional* or *psychological abuse* and is often traumatic. Examples include undermining of self-worth, deprivation of sleep or emotional support, repetitive unpredictability of response to life situations, threats, destruction of personal property or the killing of pets, lies, manipulation of friends, and interference in the workplace. Domestic violence is usually cyclic and repetitive, with periods of calm alternating

Table 49.1. Indicators of Physical Abuse in Domestic Violence

Area of Injury	Descriptions
Head and neck	Bruises, abrasions, strangle marks, black eye, broken nose, orbital ridge, or jaw, pulled hair, permanent hearing loss, facial lacerations
Trunk	Evidence of blunt trauma, including bruises (especially breasts and abdomen), fractured collarbones and ribs
Skin	Multiple lesions in various stages of healing, "rug rash" abrasions, burns (cigarette, lighter, liquid splash), bites
Extremities	Evidence of restraint, including muscle strains, spiral fractures, rope or restraint burns, "crescent moon" shape fingernail marks or bruises in the shape of a hand or blunt instrument

with periods of rapidly increasing tensions or violence, the latter often increasing in severity with each iteration of the cycle.

Recognition is the first, most important, and most often missed issue. When domestic violence is suspected, compassionate and thoughtful discussion with the possible victim as well as attention to any physical injury is requisite. Indeed, all patients should be asked about violence in their lives as part of the routine health history.

When addressing this issue with a patient, the acronym *SAFE* is easy to remember and addresses the basic issues:

S–Does the patient feel safe? At home? At school? In the workplace? If not, whom or what does she fear, and why?

A–Has the patient felt abused in a relationship? Has she felt abused in her present relationship? How? When someone is angry in the patient's home, what is it like, and what is likely to happen?

F–Does the patient have friends or family, or clergy, who can help? Whom can the patient turn to for support?

E–Does the patient have a plan, or idea, of what she would do in an emergency? If she has children, do they know where to go for and how to get help?

Clearly, no simple rule will suffice to deal with these complex and emotionally charged situations. Each must be dealt with according to its specifics and the wishes of the patient. As in the evaluation and treatment of the sexual assault victim, the patient's consent for each stage of care is needed and facilitates the process. Similarly, if evidence exists of immediate risk to the patient or to her children or someone else, law enforcement contact is required.

Just listening and being supportive is in itself helpful. Follow-up may include referral to a battered women's hotline, shelter, or counseling center. Therefore, familiarity with these resources in the practice area is important.

STUDY QUESTIONS

Instructions for Study Questions

The Study Questions are designed to help you test how well you learned the content of each chapter, and to maximize the usefulness of the question you should:

1. Read the chapter through completely at least once.
2. Answer all of the study questions (do not check your answer after each question).
3. Reread the parts of the chapter related to the questions you answered incorrectly.

The correct answer to each question is contained in the chapter. Questions do not necessarily follow the order that the information is presented in the chapter.

The questions are in multiple choice format. Please select the single best answer.

Questions and Answers Chapter 1: Health Care for Women

1.1 The last menstrual period is dated from the
a. first day of the last normal period
b. last day of the last normal period
c. first day of the last bleeding episode
d. last day of the last bleeding episode

1.2 Postmenopausal bleeding is defined as
a. bleeding beginning 6 months after cessation of menses
b. irregular bleeding continuing for 6 months after cessation of regular menses
c. bleeding beginning 12 months after cessation of menses
d. irregular bleeding continuing for 12 months after cessation of regular menses

1.3 The passage of clots during menstruation
a. is always abnormal
b. may be either normal or abnormal
c. is always normal
d. is extremely rare

1.4 In the abbreviation of the obstetric history–G[1] P[2] [3] [4] [5]–"1" stands for the number of
a. living children
b. pregnancies
c. term pregnancies
d. preterm pregnancies
e. abortions

1.5 In the abbreviation of the obstetric history–G[1] P[2] [3] [4] [5]–"2" stands for the number of
a. living children
b. pregnancies
c. term pregnancies
d. preterm pregnancies
e. abortions

1.6 In the abbreviation of the obstetric history–G[1] P[2] [3] [4] [5]–"3" stands for the number of
a. living children
b. pregnancies
c. term pregnancies
d. preterm pregnancies
e. abortions

1.7 In the abbreviation of the obstetric history–G[1] P[2] [3] [4] [5]–"4" stands for the number of
a. living children
b. pregnancies
c. term pregnancies
d. preterm pregnancies
e. abortions

1.8 In the abbreviation of the obstetric history–G[1] P[2] [3] [4] [5]–"5" stands for the number of
a. living children
b. pregnancies
c. term pregnancies
d. preterm pregnancies
e. abortions

1.9 Inquiry concerning adult and child history of sexual abuse and assault should be included in the sexual history
a. only for a patient with whom the physician has a long-standing rapport
b. only if a specific indication is noted
c. always, even for a new patient
d. sometimes, if the length of the visit permits

1.10 Tanner's classification with respect to the breast relates to changes in the breast
a. before and after lactation
b. associated with malignancy
c. associated with maturation
d. configuration associated with galactorrhea

Answers

1.1	a	1.3	b	1.5	c	1.7	e	1.9	c
1.2	a	1.4	b	1.6	d	1.8	a	1.10	c

1.11 Breast examination is done with the patient in what position?
a. Supine
b. Sitting
c. Both supine and sitting positions
d. Neither position

1.12 Peau d'orange change in the breast is associated with
a. edema of the lymphatic glands
b. jaundice
c. too vigorous breast feeding
d. galactorrhea

1.13 Which kind of speculum is often most suitable for examination of the nulliparous patient?
a. Graves speculum
b. Pederson speculum
c. Mogans speculum
d. Ling speculum

1.14 Vaginal lubricant is most useful for
a. obtaining cervical cytology
b. obtaining cervical cultures
c. completing wet preparation
d. inserting the speculum

1.15 Which uterine configuration is most difficult to assess for size, shape, configuration, and mobility?
a. Anteverted
b. Anteverted, anteflexed
c. Midposition
d. Retroverted
e. Retroverted, retroflexed

1.16 Pap smears using slide technology should be fixed no more than how many seconds after preparation?
a. 1
b. 10
c. 30
d. 60

1.17 The rectovaginal examination should be performed
a. only when there are symptoms of pelvic relaxation or fecal incontinence
b. only at the initial patient visit, except when symptoms are present
c. at intervals of 5 years
d. at the initial patient visit and all annual visits

1.18 The thyroid-stimulating hormone screening test for thyroid disease should be performed at what interval?
a. Every 5 years from age 19, every 3 to 4 years after age 65
b. Every other year from age 40, yearly after age 50
c. Every 3 to 5 years after age 65
d. Annually from puberty or from the onset of sexual activity
e. Every 3 to 5 years after age 40

1.19 The Pap smear for cervical dysplasia should be performed at what interval?
a. Every 5 years from age 19, then every 3 to 4 years after age 65
b. Every other year from age 40, then yearly after age 50
c. Every 3 to 5 years after age 65
d. Every 2 to 3 years after age 30 if 3 consecutive tests are negative
e. Every 3 to 5 years after age 40

1.20 A cholesterol/lipid profile should be performed at what interval?
a. Every 5 years from age 19, then every 3 to 4 years after age 65
b. Every other year from age 40, then yearly after age 50
c. Every 3 to 5 years after age 65
d. Annually from puberty or from the onset of sexual activity
e. Every 3 to 5 years after age 40

Answers

1.11 c	1.13 b	1.15 e	1.17 d	1.19 d
1.12 a	1.14 d	1.16 b	1.18 c	1.20 a

1.21 A mammmography to detect breast cancer should be performed at what interval?
a. Every 5 years from age 19, then every 3 to 4 years after age 65
b. Every other year from age 40, then yearly after age 50
c. Every 3 to 5 years after age 65
d. Annually from puberty or from the onset of sexual activity
e. Every 3 to 5 years after age 40

1.22 A sigmoidoscopy to detect bowel cancer should be performed at what interval?
a. Every 5 years from age 19, then every 3 to 4 years after age 65
b. Every other year from age 40, then yearly after age 50
c. Every 3 to 5 years after age 65
d. Annually from puberty or from the onset of sexual activity
e. Every 3 to 5 years after age 40

1.23 What is the appropriate interval for the tetanus-diphtheria booster?
a. Every 10 years from age 19 to 64 when at risk
b. Once between ages 14 and 16
c. Once for at-risk groups
d. Every 10 years between ages 19 and 64 when at risk, then yearly after age 65

1.24 What is the appropriate interval for the administration of influenza vaccine?
a. Every 10 years from age 19 to 64 when at risk
b. Once between ages 14 and 16
c. Once for at-risk groups
d. Every 10 years between ages 19–64 when at risk; then yearly after age 65

1.25 What is the appropriate interval for administration of pneumococcal vaccine?
a. Every 10 years from age 19 to 64 when at risk
b. Once between ages 14 and 16
c. Once for at-risk groups
d. Every 10 years between ages 19 and 64 when at risk, then yearly after age 65

1.26 What is the appropriate interval for administration of Hepatitis B vaccine?
a. Every 10 years from age 19 to 64 when at risk
b. Once between ages 14 and 16
c. Once for at-risk groups
d. Every 10 years between ages 19 and 64 when at risk, then yearly after age 65

1.27 The MMR (measles, mumps, rubella) vaccine should be administered
a. every 10 years from age 19 to 64 when at risk
b. once between ages 14 and 16
c. for women of childbearing age lacking evidence of immunity
d. every 10 years between ages 19 and 64 when at risk, then yearly after age 65

1.28 Which of the following is a significant cause of morbidity for women who are 12–18 years of age?
a. Hearing and vision impairment
b. Orthopaedic conditions
c. Urinary incontinence
d. Accidental injury

1.29 Which of the following is a significant cause of morbidity for women who are 19–39 years of age?
a. Sexual abuse
b. Hypertension
c. Acute urinary conditions
d. Heart disease

Answers

| 1.21 | b | 1.23 | b | 1.25 | a | 1.27 | c | 1.29 | c |
| 1.22 | e | 1.24 | d | 1.26 | c | 1.28 | d | | |

1.30 Which of the following is a significant cause of morbidity for women who are 40–64 years of age?
a. Upper respiratory conditions
b. Sexual abuse
c. Accidental injury
d. Digestive tract conditions

1.31 Which of the following is a significant cause of morbidity for women who are more than 65 years of age?
a. Infection (viral, parasites, bacterial)
b. Accidental injury
c. Sexual abuse
d. Digestive tract conditions

1.32 Which of the following is NOT a significant cause of mortality for women between 15 and 34 years of age?
a. Homicide
b. Diabetes
c. Suicide
d. Motor vehicle accidents

1.33 Which of the following is the most significant cause of mortality for women between 35 and 54 years of age?
a. Heart disease
b. HIV
c. Diabetes
d. Cancer

1.34 Of the following, which is the most significant cause of mortality for women between 55 and 74 years of age?
a. Uterine cancer
b. Suicide
c. Cerebrovascular accident
d. Pneumonia/influenza

1.35 Of the following, which is the LEAST significant cause of mortality for women more than 75 years of age?
a. Cardiovascular disease
b. Accidents
c. Alzheimer's disease
d. Chronic obstructive pulmonary disease

1.36 Which of the following is the most appropriate screening mechanism for cervical dysplasia?
a. Yearly physical examination
b. Hemogram
c. Physical examination of suspicious lesions
d. Pap smear

1.37 Which of the following is the most appropriate screeining mechanism for skin cancer?
a. Physical examination of suspicious lesions
b. Hemogram
c. Self-examination
d. Black-light evaluation

1.38 Which of the following is the most appropriate screening mechanism for anemia?
a. Fecal occult blood test
b. Hemogram
c. Yearly physical examination
d. Chest radiograph

1.39 Which of the following is the most appropriate screening mechanism for hypercholesterolemia/coronary artery disease?
a. Cholesterol/lipid profile
b. Hemogram
c. Yearly examination by physician
d. Auscultation

1.40 Which of the following is NOT an appropriate screening mechanism for breast cancer?
a. Yearly examination by physician
b. Self-examination
c. Screening mammogram
d. Physical examination of suspicious lesions

Answers

1.30	a	1.32	b	1.34	c	1.36	d	1.38	b
1.31	b	1.33	d	1.35	c	1.37	a	1.39	a

1.40	d

1.41 Which of the following is the most appropriate screening mechanism for colorectal cancer?
  a. Computed tomographic scan
  b. Hemogram
  c. Physical examination of suspicious lesions
  d. Colonoscopy

1.42 Which of the following is the most appropriate screening mechanism for thyroid disease?
  a. Thyroid-stimulating hormone
  b. Free thyroxine
  c. Yearly examination by physician
  d. Thyroid-binding globulin

1.43 Which of the following is NOT usually a task for the physician at the time of the initial patient evaluation?
  a. Establishing and developing a professional relationship of mutual trust and respect with the patient
  b. Gathering historical information
  c. Gathering physical information
  d. Making a differential diagnosis
  e. Making a definitive diagnosis

1.44 If a patient becomes uncomfortable with a topic during a history-taking session, the best response of the physician is to
  a. ignore the discomfort and proceed with questioning
  b. discontinue discussion of the topic to avoid further patient discomfort and damage to the patient–physician relationship
  c. address the patient's discomfort in a positive and supportive manner
  d. make a joke about the patient's evident discomfort to relieve tension

1.45 Inquiry about pelvic pain, which interferes with daily activities or requires more analgesia than provided by plain aspirin or acetaminophen, should include questions about
  a. the duration and quality of pain
  b. the timing of the pain in relation to menses
  c. the radiation of pain to areas outside of the pelvis
  d. the association of pain with body position
  e. all of the above items

1.46 In the gynecologic history, it is often possible to distinguish between vaginitis and pelvic inflammatory disease by inquiring about
  a. the association of pain with body position
  b. the symptoms present (fever/chills, itching)
  c. the duration of the pain
  d. the timing of pain in relation to menses

1.47 Which of the following should be included in the history of a patient with infertility?
  a. Previous fertility in only the female partner
  b. Previous fertility in only the male partner
  c. Previous disease in only the female partner
  d. Previous disease in both the female and male partners

1.48 Which of the following should be included in the history about breast disease and breast cancer?
  a. Use of diethylstilbestrol by the patient's mother
  b. Use of self-medications
  c. Family history of breast cancer
  d. History of maternal uterine cancer

Answers

1.41	d	1.43	e	1.45	e	1.47	d
1.42	a	1.44	c	1.46	b	1.48	c

1.49 Which of the following statements about fibrocystic disorder is correct?
a. The incidence increases with age
b. The breast lump(s) have limited mobility
c. There typically are only one or two cysts
d. The cysts are well circumscribed

1.50 The most cost-effective and reliable means of early detection of breast cancer is a yearly
a. mammogram alone
b. breast examination alone
c. breast examination, combined with appropriately scheduled mammography
d. breast examination and instruction in self-breast examination, combined with appropriately scheduled mammography

1.51 Which of the following statements about the steps in the breast examination is correct?
a. Palpation is done first
b. Inspection is done first
c. Palpation is only done if inspection is abnormal
d. Palpation and inspection are done simultaneously

1.52 Elevating the head of the examining table approximately 30° facilitates the
a. ability of the patient to comfortably look around to distract her from the examination
b. contraction of the abdominal wall muscle groups, making examination easier
c. observation of the patient's responses
d. physician not being distracted by eye contact with the patient

1.53 Which type of speculum is most appropriate for the examination of a parous menstrual woman?
a. Graves speculum
b. Pederson speculum
c. Mogans speculum
d. Ling speculum

1.54 Normal ovaries are palpable in the menstrual-aged woman what percent of the time?
a. 10%
b. 25%
c. 50%
d. 75%
e. 100%

1.55 Which of the following is characteristic of fibroadenoma?
a. The incidence increases with age
b. There typically are multiple lumps
c. There is axillary involvement
d. The cysts are mobile

1.56 Which of the following is characteristic of breast carcinoma?
a. The lumps typically are mobile
b. The incidence peaks at age 25 to menopause
c. The lumps are irregular and poorly delineated from other tissue
d. There typically are multiple lumps

1.57 Which of the following characteristics of the breast lumps distinguishes fibrocystic disorder from carcinoma?
a. The presence of nipple discharge
b. The mobility of the lumps
c. The number of lumps
d. All of the above

Answers

1.49	d	1.51	b	1.53	a	1.55	d	1.57	d
1.50	d	1.52	c	1.54	c	1.56	c		

Questions and Answers Chapter 2: Ethics in Obstetrics and Gynecology

2.1 The principle that the patient should be given what is "due" most closely matches the principle of
a. beneficence
b. nonmalificence
c. autonomy
d. justice

2.2 The principle that there should be respect for the patient's right of self-determination best matches the principle of
a. beneficence
b. nonmalificence
c. autonomy
d. justice

2.3 The principle that there is a duty not to inflict harm or injury bext matches the principle of
a. beneficence
b. nonmalificence
c. autonomy
d. justice

2.4 The principle that there is a duty to promote the good of the patient best matches the principle of
a. beneficence
b. nonmalificence
c. autonomy
d. justice

2.5 A 32-year-old patient has delivered at 25 weeks of gestation, 3 days after premature rupture of the membranes. She has discussed the circumstances with her obstetrician and requests that no attempts at resuscitation should be made. At delivery there are rare gasping, breathing movements. The pediatrician demands that intubation be done. The individual with the clearest primary responsibility for this decision is the
a. mother
b. pediatrician
c. obstetrician
d. hospital attorney

2.6 Quality of life issues primarily concern the
a. physician's estimate of outcome
b. patient's experience of outcome
c. population-based evaluation of outcome
d. patient's choice of outcome

2.7 Respect for patient wishes (autonomy) primarily requires that there be assessment of which of the following?
a. Cost of the proposed treatment
b. Patient's ability to consider information
c. Physician's concurrence with the patient's wishes
d. The legal risk to the physician and hospital

2.8 A 62-year-old woman with newly diagnosed stage III ovarian cancer refuses chemotherapy. She wants to "go home to die." The next step in evaluating this patient is to
a. assess the patient's comprehension and look for evidence of depression
b. accept the patient's wishes and discharge her from the hospital
c. call the hospital attorney to assess risk of malpractice
d. call the family for a conference

2.9 A 90-year-old woman is found to have a 20-cm pelvic/abdominal mass. Her CA-125 is 90. Your recommendation for care should be based on the ethical principle of
a. beneficence–nonmaleficence
b. statutory law
c. autonomy
d. justice

Answers

2.1	d	2.3	b	2.5	a	2.7	b	2.9	a
2.2	c	2.4	a	2.6	b	2.8	a		

2.10 A 33-year-old physician sees a 21-year-old primigravid woman in the emergency room for a urinary tract infection. She discovers the patient is going to give the child up for adoption and gives the patient her lawyer's phone number. She states she has been looking for a child to adopt and goes over all the advantages she can offer the child. Her actions fall into the ethical principle of
a. beneficence–nonmaleficence
b. statutory law
c. autonomy
d. conflict of interest

2.11 A 28-year-old woman with metastatic breast cancer wants to try a bone marrow transplant supported treatment. Her insurance company refuses. The ethical principle involved is
a. futility
b. autonomy
c. justice
d. quality of life

2.12 Which of the following illustrative questions best matches the medical indication?
a. What does the patient want?
b. What are the needs of society?
c. What impact will the proposed treatment or lack of it have on the patient's life?
d. What is the best treatment? Best alternatives?

2.13 Which of the following illustrative questions best matches the patient preference?
a. What does the patient want?
b. What are the needs of society?
c. What impact will the proposed treatment or lack of it have on the patient's life?
d. What is the best treatment? Best alternatives?

2.14 Which of the following illustrative questions best matches the issue of quality of life?
a. What does the patient want?
b. What are the needs of society?
c. What impact will the proposed treatment or lack of it have on the patient's life?
d. What is the best treatment? Best alternatives?

2.15 Which of the following illustrative questions best matches contextual issues?
a. What does the patient want?
b. What are the needs of society?
c. What impact will the proposed treatment or lack of it have on the patient's life?
d. What is the best treatment? Best alternatives?

2.16 Which of the following ethical principles best relates to the issue of medical indications?
a. Beneficence
b. Nonmaleficence
c. Autonomy
d. Justice

2.17 Which of the following ethical principles best relates to the issue of patient preferences?
a. Beneficence
b. Nonmaleficence
c. Autonomy
d. Justice

2.18 Which of the following ethical principles best relates to the issue of quality of life?
a. Beneficence
b. Nonmaleficence
c. Autonomy
d. Justice

Answers

2.10	d	2.12	d	2.14	c	2.16	a	2.18	b
2.11	c	2.13	a	2.15	b	2.17	c		

2.19 Which of the following ethical principles best relates to contextual issues?
   a. Beneficence
   b. Nonmaleficence
   c. Autonomy
   d. Justice

2.20 Which of the following best characterizes professionalism?
   a. The desire to uphold the law
   b. The desire to put the interests of
      the health care system above the
      physician's interests
   c. The desire to put the interests of
      the patient above the physician's
      interests
   d. The desire to bring about social
      change

Answers

2.19	d	**2.20**	c

Questions and Answers Chapter 3: Embryology, Anatomy, and Reproductive Genetics

3.1 The genital system develops from embryonic
   a. ectoderm
   b. mesoderm
   c. endoderm

3.2 The urogenital ridges give rise to elements of the
   a. cardiovascular system
   b. reproductive system
   c. muscular system
   d. skeletal system

3.3 What part of the ovary comes to contain the developing follicles?
   a. Cortex
   b. Medulla
   c. Both

3.4 The first indication of the sex of the embryo is the
   a. entry of primordial germ cells
   b. formation of the tunica albuginea
   c. formation of primordial follicles
   d. degeneration of the genital ducts

3.5 The primordial germ cells can be identified during the fourth week of development in the
   a. yolk sac
   b. gonadal ridge
   c. urogenital sinus
   d. cortical cords

3.6 In the female, which of the following persists to form the major parts of the reproductive tract?
   a. Paramesonephric (müllerian) ducts
   b. Mesonephric (wolffian) ducts
   c. Both
   d. Neither

3.7 The formation of the uterus and fallopian tubes
   a. depends on the presence of ovaries
   b. does not depend on the presence of ovaries
   c. depends on the persistence of the mesonephric ducts

3.8 Absence of the ovaries
   a. is the most common anomaly of the female reproductive tract
   b. typically occurs in association with other anomalies
   c. results from the failure of the paramesonephric ducts to fuse
   d. is caused by the absence of primordial germ cells

3.9 Which of the following results in the absence of the uterus?
   a. Inferior parts of the paramesonephric ducts do not fuse
   b. Paramesonephric ducts degenerate
   c. Primordial germ cells do not migrate
   d. Mesonephric ducts degenerate

3.10 Which of the following results in the formation of a double uterus (uterus didelphys)?
   a. Inferior parts of the paramesonephric ducts do not fuse
   b. Paramesonephric ducts degenerate
   c. Primordial germ cells do not migrate
   d. Mesonephric ducts degenerate

3.11 Which of the following results in the absence of the vagina?
   a. Vaginal plate does not canalize
   b. Vaginal plate does not develop
   c. Paramesonephric ducts degenerate early
   d. The genital tubercle does not develop

Answers

3.1	b	3.3	a	3.5	a	3.7	b	3.9	b	3.11	b
3.2	b	3.4	b	3.6	a	3.8	b	3.10	a		

3.12 Which of the following results in vaginal atresia?
  a. Vaginal plate does not canalize
  b. Vaginal plate does not develop
  c. Paramesonephric ducts degenerate early
  d. The genital tubercle does not develop

3.13 Which of the following arises from the urogenital sinus?
  a. Urethra
  b. Clitoris
  c. Uterus
  d. Rectum

3.14 Which of the following passes through an indifferent (undifferentiated) stage during development?
  a. Genital ducts
  b. Gonads
  c. External genitalia
  d. All of the above

3.15 The labia minora develop from the
  a. genital tubercle
  b. urogenital folds
  c. labioscrotal swellings
  d. urogenital sinus

3.16 The labia majora develop from the
  a. genital tubercle
  b. urogenital folds
  c. labioscrotal swellings
  d. urogenital sinus

3.17 The clitoris develops from the
  a. genital tubercle
  b. urogenital folds
  c. labioscrotal swellings
  d. urogenital sinus

3.18 The fallopian tube is derived from the
  a. wolffian (mesonephric) ducts
  b. metanephric ducts
  c. müllerian (paramesonephric) ducts
  d. urogenital sinus

3.19 The vagina originates from the
  a. urogenital sinus and müllerian ducts
  b. müllerian ducts and wolffian ducts
  c. mesonephric ducts and metanephric ducts
  d. urogenital sinus and wolffian ducts

3.20 In the female, the embryologic homolog of the penis is the
  a. labia majora
  b. frenulum
  c. clitoris
  d. labia minora

3.21 The innominate bones are composed of the fused ileum, ischium and
  a. sacrum
  b. pubis
  c. coccyx
  d. acetabulum

3.22 The false pelvis and true pelvis are separated by the
  a. acetabulum
  b. sacrospinous ligament
  c. linea terminalis
  d. obturator membrane
  e. obturator foramen

3.23 The dimensions of which pelvis must be adequate to permit passage of the fetus during labor?
  a. True pelvis
  b. False pelvis

3.24 The false pelvis is separated from the true pelvis by the plane of the
  a. pelvic inlet
  b. greatest diameter
  c. least diameter
  d. pelvic outlet

3.25 Arrest of fetal descent occurs most commonly at the plane of the
  a. pelvic inlet
  b. greatest diameter
  c. least diameter
  d. pelvic outlet

Answers

3.12	a	3.15	b	3.18	c	3.21	b	3.24	a
3.13	a	3.16	c	3.19	a	3.22	c	3.25	c
3.14	d	3.17	a	3.20	c	3.23	a		

3.26 Which is the value of the obstetric conjugate?
  a. 10.0–11.0
  b. 10.0
  c. 12.5
  d. 13.5

3.27 Which is the value of the transverse diameter of the pelvic inlet?
  a. 10.0–11.0
  b. 10.0
  c. 12.5
  d. 13.5

3.28 Which is the value of the bispinous diameter of pelvic midplane?
  a. 10.0–11.0
  b. 10.0
  c. 12.5
  d. 13.5

3.29 Which is the transverse diameter of greatest diameter?
  a. 10.0–11.0
  b. 10.0
  c. 12.5
  d. 13.5

3.30 Based on the Caldwell and Moloy classification, the most common pelvic type is the
  a. gynecoid
  b. android
  c. anthropoid
  d. platypelloid

3.31 Which of the following are found in the labia majora?
  a. Sebaceous glands
  b. Sweat glands
  c. Hair follicles
  d. All of the above

3.32 Which of the following is NOT found in the labia minora?
  a. Sebaceous glands
  b. Sweat glands
  c. Hair follicles

3.33 Bartholin duct is lined with what type of epithelium?
  a. Squamous
  b. Columnar
  c. Transitional

3.34 Skene duct is lined with what type of epithelium?
  a. Squamous
  b. Columnar
  c. Transitional

3.35 The urethra is lined with what type of epithelium?
  a. Squamous
  b. Columnar
  c. Transitional

3.36 The vagina is lined with what type of epithelium?
  a. Squamous
  b. Columnar
  c. Transitional

3.37 The endocervical canal is lined with what type of epithelium?
  a. Squamous
  b. Columnar
  c. Transitional

3.38 Compared with the posterior wall, the anterior wall of the vagina is
  a. longer
  b. the same length
  c. shorter

3.39 The uterine (fallopian) tubes enter into which part of the uterus?
  a. Fundus
  b. Cornu
  c. Mesosalpinx
  d. Cardinal ligament
  e. Lower uterine segment

3.40 The two main anatomic divisions of the uterus are the
  a. corpus and fundus
  b. cornu and fundus
  c. corpus and cervix
  d. cervix and isthmus

Answers

3.26	a	3.29	c	3.32	c	3.35	c	3.38	c
3.27	d	3.30	a	3.33	c	3.36	a	3.39	b
3.28	b	3.31	d	3.34	c	3.37	b	3.40	c

3.41 In addition to the uterine artery, the uterus is supplied by the
   a. vaginal artery
   b. ovarian artery
   c. hypogastric artery

3.42 The uterine veins enter the
   a. common iliac veins
   b. internal iliac veins
   c. inferior vena cava
   d. femoral veins
   e. external iliac veins

3.43 The portion of the fallopian tube that borders the ovary is the
   a. isthmus
   b. ampulla
   c. infundibulum

3.44 Which of the following ligaments DOES NOT support the uterus?
   a. Cardinal ligament
   b. Infundibulopelvic (suspensory) ligament
   c. Broad ligament
   d. Round ligament
   e. Uterosacral ligament

3.45 Which of the following ligaments supports the ovary?
   a. Cardinal ligament
   b. Broad ligament
   c. Round ligament
   d. Uterosacral ligament

3.46 Before puberty, the ratio of the length of the body of the uterus to the length of the cervix is approximately
   a. 1:1
   b. 2:1
   c. 3:1
   d. 4:1

3.47 The portion of the broad ligament between the ovaries and the fallopian tube is called the
   a. round ligament
   b. ligament of Jacobs
   c. cardinal ligament
   d. mesosalpinx

3.48 The uterosacral ligaments
   a. arise from the lateral wall of the uterus
   b. attach to the sacrum at S3–4
   c. prevent prolapse of the uterus into the vagina
   d. exert tension on the cervix ventrally

3.49 Oogonia cease to form after
   a. the tenth week of development
   b. the sixth month of development
   c. birth
   d. puberty

3.50 The blood supply to the fallopian tubes is from
   a. the ovarian arteries only
   b. the uterine arteries only
   c. both the ovarian and uterine arteries

3.51 Compared with the reproductive years, the size of the ovary of a menopausal woman is
   a. increased
   b. unchanged
   c. decreased

3.52 The diploid number of chromosomes in humans is
   a. 23
   b. 32
   c. 46
   d. 48
   e. 92

3.53 At least what percent of first-trimester spontaneous abortions have a structural or numerical chromosomal anomaly?
   a. 5%
   b. 10%
   c. 25%
   d. 50%

3.54 Overall, what percent of live births have a chromosome abnormality?
   a. 0.06%
   b. 0.6%
   c. 1.0%
   d. 2.6%

Answers

3.41	b	3.44	b	3.47	d	3.50	c	3.53	d
3.42	b	3.45	b	3.48	c	3.51	c	3.54	b
3.43	c	3.46	a	3.49	c	3.52	c		

3.55 Which of the following chromosome abnormalities is the most common among live-born infants?
a. Trisomy 21
b. Trisomy 18
c. Trisomy 13
d. Turner syndrome
e. Cri-du-chat (del 5p) syndrome

3.56 Chorionic villus sampling can be used for the detection of
a. neural tube defects
b. fetal omphalocele
c. trisomy 18
d. achondroplasia
e. Marfan syndrome

3.57 The most common chromosomal abnormality reliably diagnosed by amniocentesis is
a. trisomy 13
b. 21/22 translocation
c. 13–15/21 translocation
d. trisomy 18
e. trisomy 21

3.58 Which of the following is a characteristic feature of del(5) (cri-du-chat) syndrome?
a. No live births
b. Multiple organic abnormalities
c. Tall, eunuchoid habitus
d. Microcephaly, distinctive facial features

3.59 Which of the following is a characteristic feature of Klinefelter syndrome?
a. Severe mental retardation
b. Multiple organic abnormalities
c. Tall, eunuchoid habitus
d. Microcephaly, distinctive facial features

3.60 Which of the following is a characteristic of trisomy 16?
a. Severe mental retardation
b. No live births
c. Multiple organic abnormalities
d. Tall, eunuchoid habitus

3.61 Which of the following is a characteristic of trisomy 18 (Edwards syndrome)?
a. Severe mental retardation
b. No live births
c. Tall, eunuchoid habitus
d. Microcephaly, distinctive facial features

3.62 Which of the following is a characteristic of trisomy 13 (Patau syndrome)?
a. No live births
b. Multiple organic abnormalities
c. Tall, eunuchoid habitus
d. Microcephaly, distinctive facial features

3.63 In autosonal dominant inheritance,
a. male offspring are twice as likely to be affected as females
b. the inheritance is a result of a pair of mutant genes situated on an autosomal chromosome
c. one half of the children born to an affected person are affected
d. one quarter of the siblings of an affected person are affected

3.64 If there is complete failure of testicular development following the formation of an XY zygote,
a. the individual will develop as a female with uterus, tubes, vagina, and vulva
b. the individual will develop as a male with undescended testes and hypospadias
c. the external genitalia will be normal
d. the external genitalia will be ambiguous and there will be an absence of vagina, uterus, and tubes
e. the individual will become a transsexual

Answers

3.55	a	3.57	e	3.59	c	3.61	a	3.63	c
3.56	c	3.58	d	3.60	b	3.62	b	3.64	a

3.65 The level of α-fetoprotein is normal in amniotic fluid in which of the following conditions?
a. Spina bifida
b. Anencephaly
c. Omphalocele
d. Gastroschisis
e. Postmaturity

3.66 In which of the following will an afflicted individual typically live to at least 10 years of age?
a. Trisomy 21
b. Trisomy 18
c. Trisomy 16
d. Trisomy 13
e. All of the above

3.67 Advanced maternal age as a screening test question fails to detect pregnancies with Down syndrome in what percent of cases?
a. 20%
b. 40%
c. 60%
d. 80%

3.68 Triple screen detects about what percent of fetal Down syndrome?
a. 20%
b. 40%
c. 60%
d. 80%

3.69 Finding a fetal cardiac malformation on antepartum obstetric ultrasound examinations is associated with what percent chance of the fetus having a chromosomal abnormality?
a. 20%
b. 40%
c. 60%
d. 80%

3.70 The most commonly used maternal serum screening test involves measurement of
a. maternal α-fetoprotein, human chorionic gonadotropin, and unconjugated estriol
b. maternal progesterone, human chorionic gonadotropin, and unconjugated estriol
c. maternal α-fetoprotein, human chorionic gonadotropin, and maternal progesterone
d. maternal α-fetoprotein, maternal progesterone, and unconjugated estriol

3.71 The most common genetic cause of mental retardation is
a. fragile-X
b. Down syndrome
c. intrauterine growth restriction
d. cystic fibrosis

3.72 In a woman who has a child with a neural tube defect, in subsequent pregnancies she should take a prenatal vitamin that contains how much folic acid?
a. 0.04 mg
b. 0.4 mg
c. 4 mg
d. 40 mg

3.73 Prenatal ingestion of an appropriate dose of folic acid daily acts to prevent
a. the occurrence of neural tube defects
b. the recurrence of neural tube defects
c. both the occurrence and recurrence of neural tube defects
d. neither the occurrence nor the recurrence of neural tube defects

3.74 The developing brain is most susceptible to teratogens during what specific period?
a. 3 to 6 weeks
b. 3 to 16 weeks
c. 2 to 4 weeks
d. 3 to 4 months

Answers

3.65	e	3.67	d	3.69	b	3.71	a	3.73	c
3.66	a	3.68	c	3.70	a	3.72	c	3.74	b

3.75 The developing neural tube is most susceptible to teratogens during what specific period?
   a. 3 to 6 weeks
   b. 3 to 16 weeks
   c. 2 to 4 weeks
   d. 3 to 4 months

3.76 The developing heart is most susceptible to teratogens during what specific period?
   a. 3 to 6 weeks
   b. 3 to 16 weeks
   c. 2 to 4 weeks
   d. 3 to 4 months

3.77 Angiotensin-converting enzyme inhibitors have which of the following teratogenic effects?
   a. Limb reduction, phocomelia, ventricular septal defect, gastrointestinal atresia
   b. Staining of primary dentition
   c. Intrauterine growth retardation, fetal hypotension, pulmonary hypoplasia
   d. Nasal hypoplasia, vertebral abnormalities, CNS malformations
   e. Vaginal and cervical carcinoma, genital tract abnormalities
   f. Skeletal defects, cleft palate
   g. CNS and ear defects, cleft lip/palate, cardiac and great vessel defects

3.78 The antiepileptic drugs have which of the following teratogenic effects?
   a. Limb reduction, phocomelia, ventricular septal defect, gastrointestinal atresia
   b. Staining of primary dentition
   c. Intrauterine growth retardation, fetal hypotension, pulmonary hypoplasia
   d. Nasal hypoplasia, vertebral abnormalities, CNS malformations
   e. Vaginal and cervical carcinoma, genital tract abnormalities
   f. Skeletal defects, cleft palate
   g. CNS and ear defects, cleft lip/palate, cardiac and great vessel defects

3.79 Cyclophosphamide has which of the following teratogenic effects?
   a. Limb reduction, phocomelia ventricular septal defect, gastrointestinal atresia
   b. Staining of primary dentition
   c. Intrauterine growth retardation, fetal hypotension, pulmonary hypoplasia
   d. Nasal hypoplasia, vertebral abnormalities, CNS malformations
   e. Vaginal and cervical carcinoma, genital tract abnormalities
   f. Skeletal defects, cleft palate
   g. CNS and ear defects, cleft lip/palate, cardiac and great vessel defects

3.80 Warfarin has which of the following teratogenic effects?
   a. Limb reduction, phocomelia, ventricular septal defect, gastrointestinal atresia
   b. Staining of primary dentition
   c. Intrauterine growth retardation, fetal hypotension, pulmonary hypoplasia
   d. Nasal hypoplasia, vertebral abnormalities, CNS malformations
   e. Vaginal and cervical carcinoma, genital tract abnormalities
   f. Skeletal defects, cleft palate
   g. CNS and ear defects, cleft lip/palate, cardiac and great vessel defects

3.81 Accutane has which of the following teratogenic effects?
   a. Limb reduction, phocomelia, ventricular septal defect, gastrointestinal atresia
   b. Staining of primary dentition
   c. Intrauterine growth retardation, fetal hypotension, pulmonary hypoplasia
   d. Nasal hypoplasia, vertebral abnormalities, CNS malformations
   e. Vaginal and cervical carcinoma, genital tract abnormalities
   f. Skeletal defects, cleft palate
   g. CNS and ear defects, cleft lip/palate, cardiac and great vessel defects

Answers

3.75 c	3.77 c	3.79 g	3.81 g
3.76 a	3.78 f	3.80 d	

3.82 Thalidomide has which of the following teratogenic effects?

a. Limb reduction, phocomelia, ventricular septal defect, gastrointestinal atresia
b. Staining of primary dentition
c. Intrauterine growth retardation, fetal hypotension, pulmonary hypoplasia
d. Nasal hypoplasia, vertebral abnormalities, CNS malformations
e. Vaginal and cervical carcinoma, genital tract abnormalities
f. Skeletal defects, cleft palate
g. CNS and ear defects, cleft lip/palate, cardiac and great vessel defects

3.83 Diethylstilbestrol has which of the following teratogenic effects?

a. Limb reduction, phocomelia, ventricular septal defect, gastrointestinal atresia
b. Staining of primary dentition
c. Intrauterine growth retardation, fetal hypotension, pulmonary hypoplasia
d. Nasal hypoplasia, vertebral abnormalities, CNS malformations
e. Vaginal and cervical carcinoma, genital tract abnormalities
f. Skeletal defects, cleft palate
g. CNS and ear defects, cleft lip/palate, cardiac and great vessel defects

3.84 Tetracycline has which of the following teratogenic effects?

a. Limb reduction, phocomelia, ventricular septal defect, gastrointestinal atresia
b. Staining of primary dentition
c. Intrauterine growth retardation, fetal hypotension, pulmonary hypoplasia
d. Nasal hypoplasia, vertebral abnormalities, CNS malformations
e. Vaginal and cervical carcinoma, genital tract abnormalities
f. Skeletal defects, cleft palate
g. CNS and ear defects, cleft lip/palate, cardiac and great vessel defects

Answers

3.82   a   3.83   e   3.84   b

Questions and Answers Chapter 4: Maternal–Fetal Physiology

4.1 Which of the following statements about dental care during pregnancy is correct?
  a. Dental care is not advisable throughout pregnancy, except in situations where the mother's health is placed in extreme risk by delaying care
  b. Dental care is permissible in the second and third, but not first, trimesters
  c. Dental care is permissible in pregnancy, but anesthesia and radiographs must be avoided because of fetal risks
  d. Dental care is permissible during pregnancy

4.2 In pregnancy, the incidence of dental caries
  a. increases
  b. remains the same
  e. decreases

4.3 In pregnancy, the incidence of gingival disease
  a. increases
  b. remains the same
  c. decreases

4.4 Oxygen crosses the placenta by
  a. simple diffusion
  b. facilitated diffusion
  c. active transport
  d. pinocytosis

4.5 Glucose crosses the placenta by
  a. simple diffusion
  b. facilitated diffusion
  c. active transport
  d. pinocytosis

4.6 Amino acids cross the placenta by
  a. simple diffusion
  b. facilitated diffusion
  c. active transport
  d. pinocytosis

4.7 Pregnancy has what effect on appetite?
  a. The appetite typically increases.
  b. The appetite typically decreases.
  c. The appetite typically remains the same.
  d. The effect on appetite is unpredictable.

4.8 Pregnancy has what effect on gastric motility?
  a. Gastric motility typically increases.
  b. Gastric motility typically decreases.
  c. Gastric motility typically remains the same.
  d. The effect on gastric motility is unpredictable.

4.9 Pregnancy has what effect on intestinal transit time?
  a. Intestinal transit time increases.
  b. Intestinal transit time decreases.
  c. Intestinal transit time remains the same.
  d. The effect on intestinal transit time is unpredictable.

4.10 Pregnancy has what effect on the timing of gallbladder emptying?
  a. Emptying is faster.
  b. Emptying is delayed.
  c. Emptying remains the same.
  d. The timing of emptying is unpredictable.

4.11 Pregnancy has what effect on liver enzyme (such as alkaline phosphatase) production?
  a. Levels are increased.
  b. Levels are decreased.
  c. Levels remain the same.
  d. The effect is unpredictable.

4.12 During pregnancy, gastric reflux
  a. increases
  b. decreases
  c. remains the same
  d. is unpredictable

Answers

4.1	d	4.3	a	4.5	b	4.7	a	4.9	a	4.11	a
4.2	b	4.4	a	4.6	c	4.8	b	4.10	b	4.12	a

4.13 "Morning sickness" typically begins during which weeks of pregnancy?
a. 1 to 3
b. 4 to 8
c. 10 to 12
d. 14 to 18

4.14 Treatment of typical morning sickness includes all of the following EXCEPT
a. reassurance
b. frequent small meals
c. three large meals with antacids
d. inclusion of bland foods

4.15 Ptyalism is caused by
a. excess production of saliva
b. excess production of gastric acid
c. inability of the patient to swallow normal amounts of saliva
d. allergic reactions to various foods during pregnancy

4.16 Decreased gastrointestinal motility during pregnancy is related to increased levels of
a. progesterone
b. human chorionic gonadotropin
c. estrogen
d. androstenedione
e. thyrotropin-releasing factor

4.17 The recommended dietary allowance in pregnancy is how many additional calories per day?
a. 100
b. 300
c. 500
d. 700
e. 900

4.18 Transit time in the stomach and small bowel increase by what percent in the second and third trimesters of pregnancy?
a. 1 to 15%
b. 15 to 30%
c. 30 to 45%
d. 45 to 60%

4.19 During pregnancy the tone of the sphincter at the gastroesophageal junction
a. increases
b. is unchanged
c. decreases
d. varies with the fetus' gestational age

4.20 Which of the following is NOT contributory to constipation in pregnancy?
a. Mechanical obstruction of the colon by the enlarging bowel
b. Reduced motility of the colon
c. Increased gastrointestinal motility elsewhere than the colon
d. Increased water absorption

4.21 Pica can include craving for which of the following?
a. Ice
b. Laundry starch
c. Clay
d. All of the above

4.22 Epulis is a pregnancy-related vascular swelling of the
a. gums
b. nares
c. epiglottis
d. nail beds
e. larynx

4.23 Which of the following pulmonary measurements is decreased in pregnancy?
a. Oxygen requirement
b. Carbon dioxide pressure
c. Oxygen pressure
d. Tidal volume

4.24 Which of the following measures of pulmonary function decreases in late pregnancy?
a. Functional reserve capacity
b. Tidal volume
c. Respiratory rate
d. Inspiratory capacity

Answers

4.13	b	4.15	c	4.17	b	4.19	c	4.21	d	4.23	b
4.14	c	4.16	a	4.18	b	4.20	c	4.22	a	4.24	a

4.25 Which of the following pulmonary measurements is increased in pregnancy?
a. Inspiratory capacity
b. Vital capacity
c. Minute volume
d. All of the above

4.26 The increased nasal stuffiness and perception of increased nasal secretions during pregnancy are associated with
a. mucosal hyperemia
b. increased immunoglobulin production
c. increased interluminal production of mast cell toxins
d. all of the above

4.27 The maternal acid–base balance in pregnancy is characterized by
a. mild respiratory alkalosis
b. mild metabolic alkalosis
c. mild respiratory acidosis
d. mild metabolic acidosis

4.28 The tidal volume in pregnancy increases by what percent?
a. 10 to 20%
b. 30 to 40%
c. 50 to 60%
d. 70 to 80%

4.29 In a normal singleton pregnancy, maternal blood volume
a. increases by 10 to 15%
b. increases by 45%
c. decreases by 10 to 15%
d. decreases by 45%

4.30 Which of the following is NOT characteristic of a normal pregnancy?
a. The cardiac volume increases by 10%
b. The electrocardiogram shows deviation to the left
c. Arterial blood pressure and vascular resistance increase
d. The rest pulse rate increases by approximately 10 to 15 beats per minute
e. The heart is displaced upward and to the left

4.31 During pregnancy, maternal arterial pH is
a. increased from normal prepregnancy levels
b. maintained at normal prepregnancy levels
c. decreased from normal prepregnancy levels

4.32 Measured blood pressure in a pregnant woman is highest when she is
a. seated
b. supine
c. supine on her side

4.33 In the lateral recumbent position, maternal blood pressure in the inferior arm is
a. higher than in the superior arm
b. the same as in the superior arm
c. lower than in the superior arm

4.34 Pregnancy-associated systolic ejection murmurs are best heard over the
a. left upper sternal border
b. left midclavicular line
c. cardiac apex
d. inferior aspect of the sternum

Answers

4.25	d	4.27	a	4.29	b	4.31	b	4.33	a
4.26	a	4.28	b	4.30	c	4.32	a	4.34	a

4.35 Compensation for the occlusion of the inferior vena cava by the pregnant uterus is accomplished by shunting blood through
a. the uterine venous plexus
b. the sacral plexus
c. the paraverterbral collateral circulation
d. the renal venous plexus

4.36 Blood flow to which of the following organs is NOT increased during pregnancy?
a. Kidney
b. Breast
c. Skin
d. Brain

4.37 Inferior vena cava syndrome is caused by
a. baroreceptor changes in cardiac function associated with changes in position
b. transient release of epinephrine associated with uterine displacement caused by fetal movement
c. transient cardiac arrhythmias secondary to positional changes in the mother
d. spasm of the inferior vena cava secondary to fetal movement
e. compression of the inferior vena cava by the gravid uterine corpus

4.38 The peripheral vascular resistance decreases during pregnancy because of increased levels of
a. estrogen
b. progesterone
c. androstenedione
d. estrone

4.39 Which of the following normal physical findings during pregnancy is a result of a hyperdynamic state of the cardiovascular system?
a. Distended neck veins
b. Low-grade systolic ejection murmur
c. Diastolic murmurs
d. All of the above

4.40 On chest radiography, the heart appears to demonstrate cardiomegaly during pregnancy because it is displaced
a. upward and to the left
b. upward and to the right
c. downward and to the left
d. downward and to the right

4.41 Plasma volume begins to increase at the sixth week of pregnancy and reaches its maximum at approximately
a. 20 to 24 weeks
b. 25 to 29 weeks
c. 30 to 34 weeks
d. 35 to 39 weeks
e. term

4.42 Which of the following hematologic parameters is decreased in pregnancy?
a. Mean cell volume
b. Total erythrocyte volume
c. Hematocrit
d. All of the above

4.43 Which of the following hematologic parameters is increased during pregnancy?
a. Serum iron
b. Total iron-binding capacity
c. Hemoglobin concentration
d. All of the above

4.44 During pregnancy, the risk for thromboembolism
a. increases
b. decreases
c. remains the same
d. increases for the first month, then decreases toward term

Answers

4.35	c	4.37	e	4.39	b	4.41	c	4.43	b
4.36	d	4.38	b	4.40	a	4.42	c	4.44	a

4.45 A lack of maternal iron ingestion during pregnancy may result in
a. fetal anemia
b. fetal anomalies
c. maternal anemia
d. all of the above

4.46 Which of the following renal parameters is increased during pregnancy?
a. Renal plasma flow
b. Glomerular filtration rate
c. Renin
d. All of the above

4.47 Which of the following renal parameters is NOT increased in pregnancy?
a. Angiotensin I
b. Angiotensin II
c. Renin substrate
d. 24-hour protein excretion

4.48 During pregnancy, what is the normal effect of progesterone on the ureters?
a. There is more dilation of the left ureter than of the right
b. There is more dilation of the right ureter than of the left
c. Both ureters dilate equally
d. Both ureters constrict equally

4.49 The decreased bladder tone in pregnancy caused by progesterone is associated with which of the following?
a. Increased residual volume
b. Dilated collecting systems
c. Urinary stasis
d. All of the above

4.50 In normal pregnancy, which of the following renal parameters is decreased?
a. Creatinine
b. Uric acid
c. Blood urea nitrogen
d. All of the above

4.51 Striae gravidarum in which anatomic sites are affected by weight control?
a. Abdominal wall
b. Breasts
c. Thighs
d. All of the above
e. None of the above

4.52 Chloasma is the
a. increased hair growth seen in early pregnancy
b. loss of hair that occurs soon after delivery
c. physiologic nipple discharge during late pregnancy
d. change in facial pigmentation during pregnancy
e. transient depression encountered after delivery

4.53 Which of the following statements accurately reflects the description of the normal effects of pregnancy on bone?
a. Bone density decreases as pregnancy progresses
b. Bone density increases as pregnancy progresses
c. The rate of bone turnover increases during pregnancy
d. Bone turnover is inversely proportional to calcium intake

4.54 Blurred vision during pregnancy is a result of
a. swelling of the lens
b. aging of the patient
c. reduced blood flow to the eye
d. increased retinal glucose metabolism

4.55 What percent of total cardiac output is channeled to the uterus at term?
a. 5%
b. 10%
c. 20%
d. 30%
e. 40%

Answers

4.45	c	4.47	d	4.49	d	4.51	e	4.53	c	4.55	c
4.46	d	4.48	b	4.50	d	4.52	d	4.54	a		

4.56 Which of the following is characteristic of normal pregnancy?
a. Hyperglycemia
b. Hypoinsulinemia
c. Hypotriglyceridemia
d. All of the above

4.57 The "hemorrhoids" that develop in late pregnancy are caused by
a. a response to infection
b. increased pelvic venous outflow
c. loose stools
d. irritation from increased vaginal secretions
e. elevated pelvic venous pressure

4.58 The net effects of the normal thyroid changes of pregnancy will result in patients typically being
a. moderately hypothyroid
b. mildly hypothyroid
c. euthyroid
d. mildly hyperthyroid
e. moderately hyperthyroid

4.59 Diastasis recti is the
a. dilation of the rectum
b. constipation that occurs during pregnancy
c. linear stretch marks found on the abdomen
d. midline separation of the rectus muscles
e. fatigue syndrome of early pregnancy

4.60 In the later half of pregnancy, the CO_2 gradient between fetus and mother
a. increases
b. remains the same
c. decreases

4.61 The blood urea nitrogen falls about what percent in the first trimester of pregnancy?
a. 10%
b. 25%
c. 40%
d. 55%

4.62 Urinary protein loss in pregnancy is approximately
a. 0 to 200 mg/24 hours
b. 100 to 300 mg/24 hours
c. 200 to 400 mg/24 hours
d. 300 to 500 mg/24 hours

4.63 The hair loss commonly encountered in the second to fourth month postpartum will return to the prepregnant state approximately how many months after delivery?
a. 3 to 6 months
b. 6 to 12 months
c. 12 to 18 months
d. 18 to 24 months

4.64 The breast enlargement associated with pregnancy typically is seen starting in which trimester?
a. First
b. Second
c. Third

4.65 The vision changes in pregnancy associated with increased thickness of the cornea typically regress within the first
a. few days postpartum
b. 1 to 3 weeks postpartum
c. 6 to 8 weeks postpartum
d. 6 months postpartum
e. 1 year postpartum

4.66 The common practice of giving supplemental vitamin K to newborns is a response to
a. the relative deficiency of maternal vitamin K
b. maternal liver dysfunction in pregnancy
c. fetal liver immaturity in the immediate newborn period
d. lack of vitamin K absorption

Answers

4.56	a	4.58	c	4.60	a	4.62	b	4.64	a	4.66	c
4.57	e	4.59	d	4.61	b	4.63	b	4.85	c		

4.67 As compared to nonpregnant normal values, serum bicarbonate levels in normal pregnancy are
   a. significantly lower
   b. somewhat lower
   c. equivalent to
   d. somewhat higher
   e. significantly higher

4.68 The umbilical blood flow represents about what percent of the combined output of both fetal ventricles?
   a. 20%
   b. 40%
   c. 60%
   d. 80%

4.69 The fetal kidney forms urine at what rate?
   a. 50 to 100 mL/day
   b. 100 to 300 mL/day
   c. 400 to 1,200 mL/day
   d. 1,500 to 2,000 mL/day

4.70 The output of the fetal kidney provides what contribution to amniotic fluid?
   a. The primary source of amniotic fluid
   b. A secondary source of amniotic fluid
   c. No contribution to amniotoc fluid

4.71 In the latter half of pregnancy, umbilical blood flow is approximately
   a. 100 mL/mg per minute
   b. 300 mL/mg per minute
   c. 500 mL/mg per minute
   d. 700 mL/mg per minute

4.72 The fetal cardiac output remains relatively constant at a fetal heart rate range of
   a. 80 to 120 beats per minute
   b. 120 to 180 beats per minute
   c. 80 to 180 beats per minute
   d. >40 but <200 beats per minute

4.73 Maternal diastolic blood pressure and mean arterial volume nadir at approximately
   a. 8 to 12 weeks
   b. 12 to 16 weeks
   c. 16 to 20 weeks
   d. 20 to 24 weeks

4.74 An increase in breast volume of what percent is common in pregnancy?
   a. 10 to 25%
   b. 25 to 50%
   c. 50 to 75%
   d. 75 to 90%

Answers

4.67	a	**4.69**	c	**4.71**	b	**4.73**	c
4.68	b	**4.70**	a	**4.72**	b	**4.74**	b

Questions and Answers Chapter 5: Antepartum Care

5.1 Which of the following is NOT an early sign of pregnancy?
    a. Fatigue
    b. Urinary retention
    c. Nausea
    d. Breast tenderness
    e. Bloating

5.2 Quickening is generally first felt by how many weeks of gestation?
    a. 12
    b. 16
    c. 20
    d. 24

5.3 A positive pregnancy test may be associated with
    a. spontaneous abortion
    b. intrauterine pregnancy
    c. ectopic pregnancy
    d. trophoblastic disease
    e. all of the above

5.4 Congestion and a bluish color of the vagina is called
    a. Chadwick sign
    b. Hegar sign
    c. Newman sign
    d. Smith sign
    e. Stoppard sign

5.5 A softening of the cervix on physical examination is referred to as
    a. Chadwick sign
    b. Hegar sign
    c. Newman sign
    d. Smith sign
    e. Stoppard sign

5.6 Fetal heart tones in a normal, viable pregnancy may routinely be heard by simple auscultation at or beyond how many weeks' gestational age?
    a. 12 to 14
    b. 15 to 17
    c. 18 to 20
    d. 21 to 23

5.7 Commonly used electronic Doppler devices will detect fetal heart tones at approximately how many weeks of gestation?
    a. 8
    b. 10
    c. 12
    d. 14
    e. 16

5.8 Most home urine pregnancy tests typically become positive approximately how many weeks following the first day of the last normal menstrual period?
    a. 3
    b. 4
    c. 5
    d. 6
    e. 8

5.9 A serum progesterone level of >25 ng/mL is usually consistent with
    a. incomplete abortion
    b. nonviable intrauterine pregnancy
    c. ectopic pregnancy
    d. viable intrauterine pregnancy

5.10 Intrauterine pregnancy is generally detectable by transvaginal ultrasonography when the β human chorionic gonadotropin concentration is greater than
    a. 500 to 750 mIU/mL
    b. 1 000 to 2,000 mIU/mL
    c. 3,000 to 4000 mIU/mL
    d. 5,000 to 6000 mIU/mL

5.11 Which of the following tests is done as part of routine prenatal care?
    a. Blood group/Rh
    b. Antibody screen
    c. Complete blood count
    d. All of the above

Answers

5.1	b	5.3	e	5.5	b	5.7	c	5.9	d	5.11	d
5.2	c	5.4	a	5.6	c	5.8	b	5.10	b		

5.12 In approximately what percent of pregnant women is the rubella titer positive?
a. 55%
b. 65%
c. 75%
d. 85%
e. 95%

5.13 Specific screening for treponema is required following a positive
a. sickle cell test
b. rubella titer
c. hepatitis B surface antigen
d. rapid plasma reagin
e. maternal serum α-fetoprotein

5.14 Maternal serum α-fetoprotein testing is best done at
a. 7 to 10 weeks
b. 11 to 14 weeks
c. 15 to 18 weeks
d. 19 to 22 weeks

5.15 "Normal" pregnancy lasts 40 weeks from the first day of the last menstrual period with a margin of error of how many weeks?
a. 1
b. 2
c. 3
d. 4

5.16 The fertilization age or conception age is how many weeks less than the menstrual or gestational age?
a. 1
b. 2
c. 3
d. 4

5.17 Data from which of the following is NOT used in the final determination of the expected date of delivery?
a. Determination of last menstrual period
b. Date of quickening
c. Maternal α-protein level
d. Date when fundus is at the level of the umbilicus

5.18 In a normal singleton pregnancy, from approximately 16 to 18 weeks' gestation until approximately 36 weeks' gestation, the fundal height in centimeters is roughly equal to
a. one half the number of weeks' gestational age
b. the number of weeks' gestational age
c. the number of weeks' gestational age minus 5
d. twice the number of weeks' gestational age

5.19 The generally prescribed recommendation for weight gain during pregnancy is
a. 15 to 20 pounds
b. 25 to 35 pounds
c. 40 to 45 pounds
d. 50 to 55 pounds

5.20 Which of the following is a direct result of "lightening"?
a. Rupture of the membranes
b. Expulsion of cervical mucous plug
c. Urinary retention
d. Decreased fundal height
e. Appearance of bloody show

5.21 A cephalic presentation occurs in what percentage of deliveries?
a. 1%
b. 3.5%
c. 15%
d. 95%

5.22 A breech presentation occurs in what percentage of deliveries?
a. 1%
b. 3.5%
c. 15%
d. 95%

5.23 A shoulder presentation occurs in what percentage of deliveries?
a. 1%
b. 3.5%
c. 15%
d. 95%

Answers

5.12	d	5.14	c	5.16	b	5.18	b	5.20	d	5.22	b
5.13	d	5.15	b	5.17	c	5.19	b	5.21	d	5.23	a

5.24 Estimation of gestational age by ultrasound is least accurate at which of the following times during pregnancy?
a. 4 to 6 weeks
b. 16 to 18 weeks
c. 26 to 28 weeks
d. 36 to 38 weeks

5.25 The normal fetal heart rate at term is
a. 50 to 75 bpm
b. 80 to 100 bpm
c. 120 to 160 bpm
d. 175 to 190 bpm

5.26 A reactive nonstress test is characterized by a fetal heart rate increase of how many beats per minute?
a. 50
b. 25
c. 15
d. 5

5.27 Which of the following statements correctly describes an abnormal contraction stress test?
a. Fetal heart rate decreases in response to a uterine contraction
b. Fetal heart rate increases in response to fetal movement
c. Maternal heart rate decreases in response to a uterine contraction
d. Maternal blood pressure increases in response to fetal movement

5.28 The number of contractions in a 10-minute window that must occur for a contraction stress test to be measurable is
a. 1
b. 2
c. 3
d. 4
e. 5

5.29 A biophysical profile in which there is one or more episodes of fetal breathing in 30 minutes, three or more discrete movements in 30 minutes, opening/closing of the fetal hand, a nonreactive nonstress test, and no pockets of amniotic fluid greater than 1 cm would have a total score of
a. 2
b. 4
c. 6
d. 8

5.30 Exclusive of the fetal heart rate reactivity, which of the following elements of the biophysical profile is generally considered most important?
a. Fetal breathing
b. Gross body movement
c. Fetal tone
d. Qualitative amniotic fluid volume

5.31 Repetitive decelerations following each contraction when three contractions occur in a 10-minute window is generally an indication of
a. increased placental blood flow
b. nonreassuring fetal status
c. reduced amniotic fluid
d. fetal well-being

5.32 Further evaluation of fetal well-being should follow which answer to the question, "Is your baby moving more, less, or the same this week compared to last week?"
a. Moving more
b. Moving the same
c. Moving less

5.33 Tests of fetal lung maturity are generally used when delivery of a fetus is contemplated at a gestational age of less than how many weeks?
a. 30
b. 32
c. 34
d. 36
e. 38

Answers

5.24	d	5.26	c	5.28	c	5.30	d	5.32	c
5.25	c	5.27	a	5.29	c	5.31	b	5.33	d

5.34 At how many weeks' gestational age does phospholipid production increase, resulting in a positive phosphatidyl-glycerol test?
- a. 27 to 29
- b. 30 to 31
- c. 32 to 33
- d. 34 to 35
- e. 36 to 37

5.35 What percent of correctly performed positive tests of fetal lung maturity are associated with a subsequent development of respiratory distress syndrome?
- a. 0%
- b. 2%
- c. 4%
- d. 6%
- e. 8%

5.36 Which of the following activities is CONTRAINDICATED during pregnancy?
- a. Regular, non-weight-bearing activity on a three-times-per-week schedule
- b. Supine exercises
- c. Bathtub bathing
- d. Air travel after 28 weeks

5.37 During a normal pregnancy, the patient should be encouraged to engage in non-weight-bearing activity at what interval?
- a. Weekly
- b. Three times a week
- c. Twice daily
- d. Not at all

5.38 Which of the following information is NOT included in antepartum infant feeding (breast feeding, bottle feeding) counseling?
- a. Breast feeding may contribute to a "natural child spacing"
- b. Breast feeding promotes more rapid uterine involution postpartum
- c. Breast feeding is inferior in nutritional value to other methods
- d. Breast feeding helps provide immunologic protection for the infant in the immediate newborn period

5.39 Which of the following is NOT included in the list of "high risk" situations for which sexual activity is generally proscribed?
- a. Uterine leiomyoma
- b. History of preterm labor and/or delivery
- c. Placenta previa
- d. Premature rupture of the membranes

5.40 "Physiologic" constipation in pregnancy is NOT associated with
- a. increased transit time
- b. increased water absorption
- c. decreased blood flow to the gut
- d. decreased bulk in the maternal diet

5.41 Which of the following statements about low back pain in pregnancy is INCORRECT?
- a. Low back pain is associated with an altered center of gravity
- b. Platform shoes can readjust the center of gravity reducing the severity of low back pain
- c. Maternity girdles can readjust the center of gravity reducing the severity of low back pain
- d. Heat and focused massage can reduce the severity of low back pain

Answers

5.34	c	5.36	b	5.38	c	5.40	c
5.35	b	5.37	b	5.39	a	5.41	b

5.42 In pregnancy, *psyllium hydrophilic mucilloid* is useful in the management of
  a. heartburn
  b. constipation
  c. low back pain
  d. headache

5.43 Because of the position of the fetus, round ligament pain is often more pronounced
  a. on the right side
  b. in the center
  c. on the left side
  d. in the fundus

5.44 The neonatal mortality rate is
  a. synonymous with the stillbirth rate
  b. the number of neonatal deaths per 1,000 births
  c. the number of neonatal deaths per 1,000 live births
  d. the number of neonatal deaths per 1,000 population
  e. the number of neonatal deaths in the first 7 days of life

5.45 The maternal mortality rate is
  a. the number of deaths in pregnant women per 1,000 population
  b. the number of deaths in pregnant women
  c. the number of deaths in pregnant women per 100,000 live births
  d. the number of deaths in pregnant women per 1,000 pregnant women

5.46 PRF (pregnancy risk factor) A suggests that the risk of fetal harm is
  a. certain
  b. probable
  c. possible
  d. remote

5.47 PRF B indicates that human controlled studies
  a. do not exist
  b. appear comparable to animal studies
  c. focus on the third trimester only
  d. are in process

5.48 PRF C means that
  a. animal studies show clear danger to humans
  b. animal studies show no risk to humans
  c. the drug is shown to be safe in humans
  d. the drug should only be given if the potential benefits outweigh the risks

5.49 PRF D suggests what type of evidence exists for human fetal risk?
  a. Nonexistent evidence
  b. Rare evidence
  c. Positive evidence
  d. Uncertain evidence

5.50 PRF X carries what important clinical implication?
  a. Controlled human studies demonstrate no evidence of risk in pregnancy in any trimester
  b. Animal-reproduction studies have not demonstrated fetal risk and there are no controlled human studies
  c. Animal-reproduction studies have demonstrated an adverse fetal effect and there are no controlled human studies
  d. Positive evidence of human fetal risk exists
  e. Animal-reproduction and human studies demonstrate fetal abnormalities such that the risk of use of drugs in this PRF in pregnant women clearly outweighs any possible benefit

Answers

5.42	b	5.44	c	5.46	d	5.48	d	5.50	e
5.43	a	5.45	c	5.47	a	5.49	c		

5.51 Factors to be considered in the selection of medications during pregnancy include
a. whether the drug is contraindicated in pregnancy
b. drug interactions
c. physiologic parameters such as renal or hepatic function
d. serious or uncomfortable side effects and their frequency
e. all of the above

5.52 Which pregnancy risk factor category is characterized by the presence of human studies where there is no demonstrable fetal risk during pregnancy?
a. A
b. B
c. C
d. D
e. X

Answers
5.51 e   **5.52** a

Questions and Answers Chapter 6: Intrapartum Care

6.1 Which of the following is NOT required for a diagnosis of true labor?
   a. Rhythmic contractions
   b. Cervical dilatation
   c. Cervical effacement
   d. Bloody show

6.2 At term, bloody show is associated with
   a. marginal placental separation as labor ensues
   b. spiral artery breakdown under labor-associated progesterone influence
   c. extrusion of endocervical gland mucus
   d. altered maternal coagulation mechanisms

6.3 Low back pain is commonly associated with
   a. active labor
   b. false labor
   c. both active and false labor
   d. neither active nor false labor

6.4 Uterine contractions of increasing intensity are commonly associated with
   a. active labor
   b. false labor
   c. both active and false labor
   d. neither active nor false labor

6.5 Spontaneous onset of uterine activity is commonly associated with
   a. active labor
   b. false labor
   c. both active and false labor
   d. neither active nor false labor

6.6 Progressive cervical dilation is commonly associated with
   a. active labor
   b. false labor
   c. both active and false labor
   d. neither active nor false labor

6.7 Lower abdomen and groin pain are commonly associated with
   a. active labor
   b. false labor
   c. both active and false labor
   d. neither active nor false labor

6.8 Waxing and waning intensity of uterine contractions is commonly associated with
   a. active labor
   b. false labor
   c. both active and false labor
   d. neither active nor false labor

6.9 Progressive cervical effacement is commonly associated with
   a. active labor
   b. false labor
   c. both active and false labor
   d. neither active nor false labor

6.10 Which of the following is characteristic of "Braxton Hicks" contractions?
   a. Rhythmic contractions
   b. No cervical change on serial examinations
   c. Lower abdominal discomfort
   d. All of the above

6.11 The descent of the fetal head into the pelvis and the changing contour of the abdomen late in pregnancy is termed
   a. false descent
   b. lightening
   c. Braxton Hicks labor
   d. effacement

6.12 Frequent urination found in late pregnancy is the result of
   a. increased clearance of free water
   b. fluid shifts from diminishing amniotic fluid volume
   c. decreased pressure on the maternal diaphragm
   d. pressure on the bladder from the enlarging gravid uterus

Answers

6.1	d	6.3	c	6.5	c	6.7	b	6.9	a	6.11	b
6.2	c	6.4	a	6.6	a	6.8	b	6.10	d	6.12	d

6.13 With lightening, a patient may notice
    a. increased urinary frequency
    b. increased ease of respiratory effort
    c. a flatter upper abdomen
    d. all of the above

6.14 Which of the following is NOT an indication that a patient in late pregnancy should come to the hospital for evaluation?
    a. Regular contractions 15 to 20 minutes apart
    b. Sudden gush of fluid
    c. Continuing gradual leakage of fluid
    d. Vaginal bleeding
    e. Decreased fetal movement

6.15 The term "fetal lie" is defined as the
    a. relationship of the fetal presenting part to the right and left side of the maternal pelvis
    b. relationship of the long axis of the fetus with the maternal long axis
    c. portion of the fetus lowest in the birth canal
    d. part of the fetus that is most easily palpable on abdominal examination

6.16 Presentation is determined by the
    a. relationship of the fetal presenting part to the right and left side of the maternal pelvis
    b. relationship of the long axis of the fetus with the maternal long axis
    c. portion of the fetus lowest in the birth canal
    d. part of the fetus that is most easily palpable on abdominal examination

6.17 Position is defined as the
    a. relationship of the fetal presenting part to the right and left side of the maternal pelvis
    b. relationship of the long axis of the fetus with the maternal long axis
    c. portion of the fetus lowest in the birth canal
    d. part of the fetus that is most easily palpable on abdominal examination

6.18 Leopold maneuvers are used to establish all of the following EXCEPT
    a. fetal gender
    b. fetal lie
    c. fetal presentation
    d. fetal position

6.19 The descent of the presenting part is identified by which Leopold maneuver?
    a. First maneuver
    b. Second maneuver
    c. Third maneuver
    d. Fourth maneuver

6.20 The location of small parts is determined by which Leopold maneuver?
    a. First maneuver
    b. Second maneuver
    c. Third maneuver
    d. Fourth maneuver

6.21 Determining what occupies the fundus is accomplished by what Leopold maneuver?
    a. First maneuver
    b. Second maneuver
    c. Third maneuver
    d. Fourth maneuver

6.22 Identifying the cephalic prominence is accomplished by what Leopold maneuver?
    a. First maneuver
    b. Second maneuver
    c. Third maneuver
    d. Fourth maneuver

6.23 The most common fetal lie found during early labor is
    a. oblique
    b. transverse
    c. vertex
    d. longitudinal

Answers

6.13 d	6.15 b	6.17 a	6.19 c	6.21 a	6.23 d
6.14 a	6.16 c	6.18 a	6.20 b	6.22 d	

6.24 The most common fetal presentation found in early labor is
a. oblique
b. transverse
c. vertex
d. longitudinal

6.25 The effacement of a patient in early labor with the cervix approximately 1 cm in length and 1 cm dilated is
a. 10%
b. 25%
c. 50%
d. 75%
e. 100%

6.26 The turning of the fetal head toward the sacrum is termed
a. transverse lie
b. anterior asynclitism
c. left side position
d. occipital presentation

6.27 The station of a patient in labor with the presenting part (vertex) at the level of the ischial spines is
a. +2
b. +1
c. 0
d. −1
e. −2

6.28 At 0 station, where is the biparietal diameter of the fetal head in relation to the pelvic inlet?
a. It has not yet reached the pelvic inlet
b. It is at the pelvic inlet
c. It has passed below the pelvic inlet

6.29 The clinical significance of the fetal head presenting at 0 station is that the biparietal diameter of the fetal head has negotiated the
a. pelvic inlet
b. pelvic midplane
c. pelvic outlet

6.30 Cervical effacement relates to
a. how far the cervix is opened
b. the degree of cervical thinning
c. the relation of the presenting part to the cervix
d. the softness of the cervix

6.31 The first stage of labor is best described as the
a. complete dilation of the cervix to delivery of the infant
b. delivery of infant to the delivery of the placenta
c. onset of labor to full cervical dilation
d. period extending up to 2 hours after delivery of the placenta

6.32 The second stage of labor is best described as the
a. complete dilation of the cervix to delivery of the infant
b. delivery of infant to the delivery of the placenta
c. onset of labor to full cervical dilation
d. period extending up to 2 hours after delivery of the placenta

6.33 The third stage of labor is best described as the
a. complete dilation of the cervix to delivery of the infant
b. delivery of infant to the delivery of the placenta
c. onset of labor to full cervical dilation
d. period extending up to 2 hours after delivery of the placenta

6.34 The fourth stage of labor is best described as the
a. complete dilation of the cervix to delivery of the infant
b. delivery of infant to the delivery of the placenta
c. onset of labor to full cervical dilation
d. period extending up to 2 hours after delivery of the placenta

Answers

6.24	c	6.26	b	6.28	c	6.30	b	6.32	a	6.34	d
6.25	c	6.27	c	6.29	a	6.31	c	6.33	b	

6.35 The active phase of the first stage of labor is generally defined to begin when the cervix is how dilated?
   a. 2 cm
   b. 3 cm
   c. 4 cm
   d. 5 cm
   e. 6 cm

6.36 The vertex presentation occurs in approximately what percent of term labors?
   a. 65%
   b. 75%
   c. 85%
   d. 95%

6.37 Which of the following terms describes the cardinal movement of labor that allows the smaller diameter of the fetal head to present to the maternal pelvis?
   a. Engagement
   b. Flexion
   c. Descent of the presenting part
   d. Extension of the fetal head

6.38 Which of the following terms describes the movement of the fetal head as it reaches the introitus?
   a. Engagement
   b. Flexion
   c. Descent of the presenting part
   d. Extension of the fetal head

6.39 Which of the following describes the movement of the fetal head to "face forward" relative to the shoulders?
   a. Flexion
   b. Internal rotation
   c. External rotation
   d. Extension

6.40 Descent is a fetal movement in labor best defined as
   a. movement of the presenting part through the birth canal
   b. the smaller diameter of the head presenting to the maternal pelvis
   c. the fetal head reaching the introitus
   d. the delivery of the head

6.41 The latent phase of stage one labor in nulliparas has a mean duration of
   a. 1.0 hours
   b. 2.5 hours
   c. 4.5 hours
   d. 6.5 hours

6.42 The active phase of stage one labor in nulliparas has a mean duration of
   a. 1.0 hours
   b. 2.5 hours
   c. 4.5 hours
   d. 6.5 hours

6.43 The second stage of labor in nulliparas has a mean duration of
   a. 1.0 hours
   b. 2.5 hours
   c. 4.5 hours
   d. 6.5 hours

6.44 The latent phase of stage one labor in multiparas has a mean duration of
   a. 0.5 hours
   b. 2.5 hours
   c. 4.5 hours
   d. 5.0 hours

6.45 The active phase of stage one in multiparas has a mean duration of
   a. 0.5 hours
   b. 2.5 hours
   c. 4.5 hours
   d. 6.5 hours

Answers

6.35 c	**6.37** b	**6.39** c	**6.41** d	**6.43** a	**6.45** b
6.36 d	**6.38** d	**6.40** a	**6.42** c	**6.44** d	

6.46 The second stage of labor in multiparas has a mean duration of
   a. 0.5 hours
   b. 2.5 hours
   c. 4.5 hours
   d. 6.5 hours

6.47 All of the following are part of the examination after spontaneous rupture of the membranes EXCEPT
   a. examination of the fluid for blood
   b. examination of the fluid for meconium
   c. auscultation or measurement of the fetal heart rate
   d. measurement of the pH of the fluid

6.48 During the active phase of labor, if electronic fetal monitoring is not used, the fetal heart rate should be auscultated every
   a. 5 minutes
   b. 10 minutes
   c. 15 minutes
   d. 20 minutes
   e. 25 minutes

6.49 During the second stage of labor in the absence of electronic fetal monitoring, fetal heart rate auscultation should be performed after
   a. each uterine contraction
   b. every other uterine contraction
   c. every third uterine contraction
   d. every contraction generating >15 to 20 mm Hg pressure

6.50 An external tocodynamometer provides information about
   a. contraction frequency
   b. fetal heart rate variability
   c. contraction strength
   d. baseline uterine pressure

6.51 The sensory nerves from the lower birth canal and perineum enter the spinal cord at
   a. T1 through T2
   b. T6 through T8
   c. T9
   d. L1 through L3
   e. S2 through S4

6.52 Epidural anesthesia is best used to provide
   a. perineal anesthesia for vaginal delivery
   b. anesthesia for the active phase of labor and delivery
   c. short-term anesthesia for vaginal or abdominal delivery
   d. anesthesia for the latent phase of labor

6.53 Spinal anesthesia is best used to provide
   a. perineal anesthesia for vaginal delivery
   b. anesthesia for the active phase of labor and delivery
   c. short-term anesthesia for vaginal or abdominal delivery
   d. anesthesia for the latent phase of labor

6.54 Pudendal anesthesia or block is best used to provide
   a. perineal anesthesia for vaginal delivery
   b. anesthesia for the active phase of labor and delivery
   c. short-term anesthesia for vaginal or abdominal delivery
   d. anesthesia for the latent phase of labor

6.55 Which of the following anesthetic techniques is associated with maternal aspiration?
   a. General anesthesia
   b. Spinal anesthesia
   c. Epidural anesthesia
   d. Pudendal anesthesia

Answers

6.46	a	6.48	c	6.50	a	6.52	b	6.54	a
6.47	d	6.49	a	6.51	e	6.53	c	6.55	a

6.56 Which of the following is an associated maternal risk when spinal anesthesia is used?
  a. Hypotension
  b. Loss of desire to push
  c. Headache
  d. All of the above

6.57 Maternal aspiration syndrome is a particularly significant risk of general anesthesia in obstetric cases because
  a. of the high alkaline content of the maternal gut during pregnancy
  b. of decreased gastrointestinal function during labor
  c. of the picalike eating habits of women just before labor
  d. most general anesthetics cause reflex spasm of the stomach

6.58 The major cause of maternal mortality from obstetrical anesthesia is
  a. cardiac arrest
  b. aspiration of vomitus
  c. hemorrhage and shock
  d. fatal reaction to local anesthetic
  e. respiratory failure from excessive concentration

6.59 The most common result of compression of the fetal head during labor is
  a. mental retardation
  b. epilepsy
  c. cerebral palsy
  d. cleft lip
  e. molding

6.60 Outlet forceps during delivery should best be used when
  a. the fetal head is engaged and the leading edge of the skull is above +2 station
  b. the fetal skull at perineal floor, scalp visible, anteroposterior, right occiput anterior to left occiput anterior (45°)
  c. the leading edge of the skull is beyond +2 station
  d. there is a complete breech presentation

6.61 A low forceps delivery should best be used when
  a. the fetal head is engaged and the leading edge of the skull is above +2 station
  b. the fetal skull at perineal floor, scalp visible, anteroposterior, right occiput anterior to left occiput anterior (45°)
  c. the leading edge of the skull is beyond +2 station
  d. there is a complete breech presentation

6.62 A midforceps delivery should best be used when
  a. the fetal head is engaged and the leading edge of the skull is above +2 station
  b. the fetal skull at perineal floor, scalp visible, anteroposterior, right occiput anterior to left occiput anterior (45°)
  c. the leading edge of the skull is beyond +2 station
  d. there is a complete breech presentation

6.63 Forceps may be used to
  a. rotate the fetal head
  b. augment maternal voluntary pushing efforts
  c. control delivery of fetal head
  d. all of the above

6.64 The usual postpartum blood loss in a vaginal delivery is
  a. 100 mL
  b. 300 mL
  c. 500 mL
  d. 700 mL
  e. 900 mL

6.65 What percent of patients will undergo spontaneous labor and delivery between 37 and 42 weeks?
  a. 80%
  b. 85%
  c. 90%
  d. 95%
  e. Greater than 99%

Answers

6.56 d	**6.58** b	**6.60** b	**6.62** a	**6.64** c
6.57 b	**6.59** e	**6.61** c	**6.63** d	**6.65** b

6.66 First-degree vaginal laceration at birth
a. involves underlying fascia or muscle but not rectal sphincter or rectal mucosa
b. extends through the rectal sphincter but not into the rectum
c. extends into the rectal mucosa
d. involves the vaginal mucosa and perineal skin

6.67 Second-degree vaginal laceration at birth
a. involves underlying fascia or muscle but not rectal sphincter or rectal mucosa
b. extends through the rectal sphincter but not into the rectum
c. extends into the rectal mucosa
d. involves the vaginal mucosa and perineal skin

6.68 Third-degree vaginal laceration at birth
a. involves underlying fascia or muscle but not rectal sphincter or rectal mucosa
b. extends through the rectal sphincter but not into the rectum
c. extends into the rectal mucosa
d. involves the vaginal mucosa and perineal skin

6.69 Fourth-degree vaginal laceration at birth
a. involves underlying fascia or muscle but not rectal sphincter or rectal mucosa
b. extends through the rectal sphincter but not into the rectum
c. extends into the rectal mucosa
d. involves the vaginal mucosa and perineal skin

6.70 Compared with extension of a mediolateral episiotomy, what is the risk of extension of a midline episiotomy?
a. Greater risk
b. Same risk
c. Less risk

6.71 During delivery of the fetal head, the likelihood of laceration or extension of episiotomy is decreased by performance of
a. Spinelli maneuver
b. Leopold maneuver
c. Ritgen maneuver
d. Marceaus maneuver

6.72 Which of the following is NOT a sign of placental separation?
a. The uterus rises in abdomen to become globular in shape
b. There is a decreased sensation of pressure
c. There is a gush of blood
d. There is an apparent "lengthening" of the umbilical cord

6.73 It is customary to wait approximately how many minutes for spontaneous extrusion of the placenta?
a. 10
b. 20
c. 30
d. 40
e. 50

6.74 Obstetric cervical lacerations are most commonly discovered at what "o-clock" during postpartum cervical inspection?
a. 12
b. 12 and 6
c. 3 and 9
d. 6

6.75 The maternal mortality rate associated with cesarean delivery is how many times that of a vaginal birth?
a. One to two
b. Two to four
c. Four to eight
d. Eight to twelve

Answers

6.66 d	6.68 b	6.70 a	6.72 b	6.74 c
6.67 a	6.69 c	6.71 c	6.73 c	6.75 b

6.76 Postpartum uterine hemorrhage occurs in approximately what percent of patients?

a. 1%
b. 3%
c. 5%
d. 7%

6.77 Vaginal examination of a patient in early labor finds the presenting part (vertex) to be at the level of the ischial spines. The station is reported as

a. +4
b. +2
c. 0
d. −2
e. −4

Answers

6.76   a   6.77   c

Questions and Answers Chapter 7: Abnormal Labor

7.1 Which of the following statements about prolapse of the umbilical cord is INCORRECT?
- a. It occurs in approximately 0.5% of patients
- b. It occurs more frequently in patients of high parity
- c. It most frequently occurs in breech presentation, with twins, and in the presence of polyhydramnios
- d. It is associated with an increased perinatal mortality
- e. Manual replacement of the cord is indicated when the presenting part is not engaged in the pelvis

7.2 Which of the following is NOT associated with uterine rupture?
- a. Amniocentesis
- b. Previous cesarean section
- c. Myomectomy
- d. Administration of oxytocin
- e. Difficult forceps delivery

7.3 Older gravidas have an increased incidence of
- a. uterine inertia
- b. malpresentation
- c. hypertension
- d. all of the above

7.4 The breech hydrocephalus is best managed by
- a. cesarean delivery
- b. destructive procedure
- c. decompression of the head transvaginally
- d. decompression of the head transabdominally

7.5 Abnormal labor, or dystocia, can result from
- a. anatomic anomalies of the fetus
- b. anatomic anomalies of the maternal bony pelvis
- c. anatomic anomalies of the uterus
- d. functional abnormalities of the uterus
- e. all of the above

7.6 No progress from the latent to the active stage of labor in a nullipara is defined as prolonged latent phase if it lasts more than how many hours?
- a. 10 hours
- b. 15 hours
- c. 20 hours
- d. 24 hours

7.7 Protraction disorder is an abnormal labor pattern related to
- a. lack of progress from the latent to the active phase of labor
- b. secondary arrest of dilatation
- c. prolonged active phase of labor
- d. absence of engagement of the fetal head

7.8 Arrest disorder is an abnormal labor pattern related to
- a. slow progress from the latent to the active phase of labor
- b. secondary arrest of dilatation
- c. prolonged active phase of labor
- d. absence of engagement of the fetal head

7.9 Cervical dilation that proceeds at less than 1.2 cm/hr (for a nulligravida) would be classified as
- a. a prolonged latent phase
- b. a protraction disorder
- c. an arrest disorder
- d. a normal labor

Answers

7.1	e	7.3	d	7.5	e	7.7	c	7.9	b
7.2	a	7.4	a	7.6	c	7.8	b		

7.10 A situation where there has been no descent of the presenting part for over 1 hour during the second stage of labor would be classified as
a. a prolonged latent phase
b. a protraction disorder
c. an arrest disorder
d. a normal labor

7.11 Which of the following provides a quantitative measurement of the strength of uterine contractions?
a. Manual palpation of maternal abdomen
b. Intrauterine pressure catheter
c. "Indentation" of uterus on palpation during contraction
d. Tocodynamometer

7.12 For a labor pattern to be considered optimal, contractions must generate a maximum intrauterine pressure of approximately how many mm Hg?
a. 10 to 20
b. 30 to 40
c. 50 to 60
d. 70 to 80

7.13 The incidence of shoulder dystocia and the need for cesarean delivery increase markedly if the fetus has an estimated weight of at least
a. 2,500 g
b. 3,500 g
c. 4,500 g
d. 5,500 g

7.14 Which of the following typically converts to either a vertex or face presentation?
a. Brow
b. Compound
c. Breech
d. Shoulder

7.15 What is the frequency of brow presentation?
a. 1 in 30
b. 1 in 300
c. 1 in 3,000
d. 1 in 30,000

7.16 What is the frequency of face presentation?
a. 1 in 60
b. 1 in 600
c. 1 in 6,000
d. 1 in 10,000

7.17 Which of the following usually resolves spontaneously as labor continues?
a. Compound presentation
b. Breech presentation
c. Shoulder presentation
d. Vertex presentation

7.18 Causes of dystocia may include
a. a contracted bony maternal pelvis
b. a distended bladder or colon
c. an adnexal mass
d. uterine leiomyomata
e. all of the above

7.19 Which of the following is appropriate to use for the augmentation of labor?
a. Oxytocin
b. Prostaglandin gel
c. Laminaria
d. All of the above

7.20 In a primigravid patient, the active phase of labor is defined as prolonged if it lasts longer than
a. 10 hours
b. 12 hours
c. 14 hours
d. 16 hours
e. 18 hours

Answers

7.10	c	7.12	c	7.14	a	7.16	b	7.18	e	7.20	b
7.11	b	7.13	c	7.15	c	7.17	a	7.19	a		

7.21 In multiparous patients, the active phase is defined as prolonged if it lasts more than
   a. 2 hours
   b. 4 hours
   c. 6 hours
   d. 8 hours
   e. 10 hours

7.22 There has been secondary arrest of dilation when cervical dilation during the active phase of labor stops for at least
   a. 1 hour
   b. 2 hours
   c. 3 hours
   d. 4 hours

7.23 What is the Bishop's score for the following findings: a dilation of 1 to 2 cm, 60% effacement, a cephalic part of −1 station, and a soft cervix that is midposition?
   a. 9
   b. 7
   c. 5
   d. 3

7.24 There is a significant likelihood that induction has failed if the Bishop's score falls below
   a. 2 points
   b. 4 points
   c. 6 points
   d. 8 points
   e. 10 points

7.25 The prolonged latent phase in labor may be managed by
   a. rest
   b. augmentation with pitocin
   c. amniotomy
   d. all of the above

7.26 Which of the following is NOT a risk to the fetus from prolonged labor?
   a. Sepsis
   b. Subdural hematoma
   c. Delivery associated trauma
   d. Hemorrhage

7.27 Meconium aspiration syndrome is associated with
   a. prolonged labor
   b. postdates pregnancy
   c. intrauterine growth restriction
   d. chronic maternal hypertension
   e. all of the above

7.28 What percent of singleton term deliveries are breech presentations?
   a. 1%
   b. 3%
   c. 5%
   d. 7%
   e. 9%

7.29 Vaginal delivery of the term breech is generally avoided when the fetus weighs less than
   a. 1,000 g
   b. 1,500 g
   c. 2,000 g
   d. 2,500 g
   e. 3,000 g

7.30 Which of the following is NOT a selection criterion for external cephalic version?
   a. Normal fetus
   b. Reassuring fetal heart rate tracing
   c. No uterine surgical scars
   d. Presenting part in the pelvis
   e. Adequate amniotic fluid

7.31 All of the following are risks of external cephalic version EXCEPT
   a. uterine rupture
   b. sepsis
   c. cord accident
   d. placental abruption
   e. premature rupture of the membranes

Answers

7.21	c	**7.23**	b	**7.25**	d	**7.27**	e	**7.29**	c	**7.31**	b
7.22	b	**7.24**	b	**7.26**	d	**7.28**	b	**7.30**	d		

7.32 Cesarean delivery is required in what percent of term breeches because of hyperextension of the fetal head?
a. 5%
b. 10%
c. 15%
d. 20%
e. 25%

7.33 Outlet forceps-assisted vaginal delivery is appropriately considered with the fetus at what station?
a. At the +2 station
b. At the perineal floor
c. Above the +2 station

7.34 Low forceps-assisted vaginal delivery occurs with the fetus at what station?
a. At the +2 station
b. At the perineal floor
c. Above the +2 station

7.35 Midforceps-assisted vaginal delivery is defined with the fetus at what station?
a. At the +2 station
b. At the perineal floor
c. Above the +2 station

7.36 Uterine contractions occurring at irregular intervals is characteristic of
a. true labor
b. false labor
c. both true and false labor
d. neither true nor false labor

7.37 Sedation provides relief from discomfort of uterine contractions in
a. true labor
b. false labor
c. both true and false labor
d. neither true nor false labor

7.38 Uterine contractions of unchanging intensity are characteristic of
a. true labor
b. false labor
c. both true and false labor
d. neither true nor false labor

7.39 Abdominal but not back discomfort with contractions is characteristic of
a. true labor
b. false labor
c. both true and false labor
d. neither true nor false labor

7.40 Vasa previa is a(n)
a. indication for induction of labor
b. contraindication to induction of labor
c. indication of fetal anomalies
d. cause of pre-eclampsia

7.41 Prior classic uterine incision is a(n)
a. indication for induction of labor
b. contraindication to induction of labor
c. transverse uterine incision
d. risk factor for preterm labor in future pregnancies

7.42 Premature rupture of membranes at term is a(n)
a. indication for induction of labor
b. contraindication to induction of labor
c. finding associated with third trimester bleeding
d. risk factor for postpartum hemmorhage

7.43 Intrauterine fetal demise is a(n)
a. indication for induction of labor
b. contraindication to induction of labor
c. risk factor for ruptured uterus
d. cause of uterine atony

7.44 Cord presentation is a(n)
a. indication for induction of labor
b. contraindication to induction of labor
c. cause of polyhydramnios
d. result of placental abruption

Answers

7.32	a	7.35	c	7.38	b	7.41	b	7.44	b
7.33	b	7.36	b	7.39	b	7.42	a		
7.34	a	7.37	b	7.40	b	7.43	a		

7.45 Abnormal fetal lie is a(n)
  a. indication for induction of labor
  b. contraindication to induction of labor
  c. risk for postpartum hemorrhage
  d. cause of shoulder dystocia

7.46 Chorioamnionitis is a(n)
  a. indication for induction of labor
  b. contraindication to induction of labor
  c. result of coitus in the third trimester
  d. cause of congenital blindness in the newborn

7.47 Active genital herpes infection is a(n)
  a. indication for induction of labor
  b. contraindication to induction of labor
  c. cause of postpartum hemorrhage
  d. result of inadequate prenatal care

7.48 The delivery of the fetal head in the assisted breech delivery is often facilitated with what type of forceps?
  a. Simpson
  b. Piper
  c. Kielland
  d. Elliott

Answers

7.45 b	**7.46** a	**7.47** b	**7.48** c

Questions and Answers Chapter 8: Intrapartum Fetal Surveillance

8.1 Nonreassuring fetal status during labor occurs in approximately what percent of pregnancies?
  a. Less than 1%
  b. 5 to 10%
  c. 15 to 20%
  d. 25 to 30%

8.2 Which of the following is NOT a criterion suggestive of fetal asphyxia?
  a. Metabolic or mixed acidemia
  b. Persistent Apgar scores of 3 or below
  c. Evidence of neonatal neurologic sequelae
  d. Heart rate acceleration

8.3 If a fetus experiences progressive and sustained hypoxia, the mixed metabolic and respiratory acidosis that may ensue typically results from
  a. aerobic glycolysis
  b. anaerobic glycolysis
  c. aerobic gluconeogenesis
  d. anaerobic gluconeogenesis

8.4 The 1-minute Apgar for a newborn with a heart rate of less than 100, slow respiratory rate, flaccid muscle tone, a grimace, and blue color is
  a. 1
  b. 2
  c. 3
  d. 4
  e. 5

8.5 The 1-minute Apgar for a newborn with a heart rate of more than 100, good respiratory effort, active muscular activity, a good grimace, and pink color is
  a. 6
  b. 7
  c. 8
  d. 9
  e. 10

8.6 Intermittent fetal heart rate auscultation to monitor fetal well-being should be employed at least how often during the active phase of labor?
  a. Every 1 minute
  b. Every 5 minutes
  c. Every 10 minutes
  d. Every 15 minutes
  e. Every 20 minutes

8.7 Intermittent fetal heart rate auscultation to monitor fetal well-being should be employed at least how often in the second stage of labor?
  a. Every 1 minute
  b. Every 5 minutes
  c. Every 10 minutes
  d. Every 15 minutes
  e. Every 20 minutes

8.8 Baseline fetal tachycardia is defined as a heart rate greater than how many beats per minute?
  a. 150
  b. 160
  c. 170
  d. 180
  e. 190

8.9 The common cause of fetal tachycardia is
  a. fetal anemia
  b. maternal anemia
  c. maternal hypothermia
  d. maternal hyperthermia

8.10 Baseline fetal bradycardia is defined as a heart rate of less than how many beats per minute?
  a. 90
  b. 100
  c. 110
  d. 120
  e. 130

Answers

8.1	b	8.3	b	8.5	d	8.7	b	8.9	d
8.2	d	8.4	c	8.6	d	8.8	b	8.10	d

8.11 A sinusoidal fetal heart rate pattern is frequently associated with
    a. Rh isoimmunization
    b. umbilical cord prolapse
    c. placental abruption
    d. preeclampsia

8.12 Fetal arrhythmias are seen in what percent of monitored labors?
    a. Less than 1%
    b. 5%
    c. 10%
    d. 15%

8.13 During fetal sleep, the fetal heart rate variability is
    a. increased
    b. unchanged
    c. decreased

8.14 Which of the following was considered characteristic of the old term short-term variability?
    a. Variation in amplitude seen on a beat-to-beat basis
    b. Ampliude of 3 to 8 bpm
    c. Normally encountered after approximately 28 weeks' gestation
    d. All of the above

8.15 The term "long-term fetal heart rate variability" was associated with an amplitude of
    a. 1 to 3 bpm
    b. 5 to 16 bpm
    c. 15 to 20 bpm
    d. 60 to 80 bpm

8.16 Accelerations of the fetal heart rate (FHR) are defined as an increase in the FHR above the baseline of at least how many bpm, usually of 15- to 20-second duration?
    a. 5
    b. 10
    c. 15
    d. 20
    e. 25

8.17 Accelerations of the FHR are associated with an intact fetal mechanism that is
    a. mildly stressed by hypoxia and acidemia
    b. moderately stressed by hypoxia and acidemia
    c. severely stressed by hypoxia and acidemia
    d. unstressed by hypoxia and acidemia

8.18 If an observed FHR pattern is a mixture of two more patterns and variations of baseline values, it is usually prudent to manage the obstetric situation based on
    a. the most reassuring pattern present
    b. an equal weighting of both patterns observed
    c. the most substantially nonreassuring pattern
    d. fetal scalp sampling for pH

8.19 Fetal tachycardia is associated with all of the following EXCEPT
    a. maternal fever and infection
    b. maternal treatment with β-blockers
    c. fetal immaturity
    d. fetal hypoxia

8.20 Which of the following is a cause of fetal tachycardia?
    a. Maternal thyrotoxicosis
    b. Fetal anemia
    c. Fetal infection
    d. All of the above

8.21 All of the following are associated with fetal bradycardia EXCEPT
    a. maternal treatment with β-blockers
    b. maternal treatment with atropine
    c. fetal anoxia
    d. fetal congenital heart block

8.22 Early FHR decelerations are associated with
    a. umbilical cord compression
    b. pressure on the fetal head
    c. uteroplacental insufficiency
    d. maternal tachycardia

Answers

8.11	a	8.13	c	8.15	b	8.17	d	8.19	b	8.21	b
8.12	a	8.14	d	8.16	c	8.18	c	8.20	d	8.22	b

8.23 Variable FHR decelerations are associated with
a. umbilical cord compression
b. pressure on the fetal head
c. uteroplacental insufficiency
d. maternal tachycardia

8.24 Late FHR decelerations are associated with
a. umbilical cord compression
b. pressure on the fetal head
c. uteroplacental insufficiency
d. maternal tachycardia

8.25 The presence of persistent late decelerations and decreased beat-to-beat variability should lead to which of the following?
a. Direct measurement of fetal acid-base status
b. Monitoring the frequency of fetal movement
c. Measurement of maternal blood pressure
d. Measurement of amniotic volume

8.26 Which of the following best describes a late FHR deceleration?
a. Deceleration starts after uterine contraction begins, reaches nadir after peak of uterine contraction, resolves to baseline after uterine contraction is over
b. Deceleration begins with uterine contraction, reaches nadir at peak of uterine contraction, returns to baseline at end of uterine contraction
c. Deceleration may start before or after the start of the uterine contraction

8.27 Repetitive late FHR decelerations are considered particularly ominous with respect to fetal well-being if associated with
a. variable decelerations
b. early decelerations
c. increased FHR variability
d. decreased FHR variability

8.28 In the face of evidence of intrauterine fetal compromise, which drug may relax uterine tone and slow contraction rate?
a. Atropine
b. Meperidine
c. Terbutaline
d. Succinylcholine
e. Morphine

8.29 The single most reliable indicator of fetal status using electronic fetal monitoring is
a. variability
b. baseline
c. accelerations
d. periodic decelerations

8.30 Uteroplacental insufficiency should be suspected in the presence of
a. maternal hypertension
b. diabetes mellitus
c. toxemia
d. all of the above

8.31 A normal fetal scalp blood gas pH is in the range of
a. 6.80 to 6.95
b. 7.00 to 7.15
c. 7.25 to 7.40
d. 7.50 to 7.65

8.32 Fetal compromise is strongly expected with a scalp pH less than
a. 7.26
b. 7.24
c. 7.22
d. 7.20
e. 7.18

8.33 Which of the following patterns of FHR is most ominous?
a. early decelerations
b. variable decelerations
c. late decelerations
d. late decelerations with loss of variability
e. tachycardia

Answers

8.23	a	8.25	a	8.27	d	8.29	a	8.31	c	8.33	d
8.24	c	8.26	a	8.28	c	8.30	d	8.32	d		

8.34 Transient loss of fetal sino-atrial node function is noted when the FHR falls below
a. 60
b. 80
c. 100
d. 120
e. 140

8.35 Which of the following is likely to result from acute intrapartum blood flow disruption?
a. Dyskinetic cerebral palsy
b. Spastic quadriplegia
c. Ataxic cerebral palsy
d. Mental retardation
e. Attention-deficit hyperactivity disorder

8.36 What is the association between neonatal encephalopathy and permanent neonatal neurologic impairment?
a. They are always associated if the encephalopathy occurs at any stage of fetal development
b. They are always associated only if the encephalopathy occurs after 42 weeks of gestational age
c. They are not always associated

8.37 What is the incidence of neonatal encephalopathy caused by intrapartum hypoxia (absent other coincident preconceptual or antepartum abnormalities)?
a. 1.6/100,000
b. 3.2/100,000
c. 6.4/100,000
d. 12.8/100,000
e. 25.6/100,000

8.38 A fetal scalp pH of 7.24 is
a. reassuring
b. nonreassuring

8.39 Which of the following medications would be most useful in an attempted intrauterine resuscitation?
a. terbutaline
b. oxytocin
c. methergine
d. dexamethasone

8.40 Which of the following maneuvers is potentially useful in an attempt to resuscitate the fetus in utero?
a. change the maternal position to left lateral
b. increase oxytocin administration rate
c. reduce the rate of intravenous infusion of fluids
d. stimulate the fetal scalp

8.41 Moderate variability is best characterized by an amplitude range that is
a. undetectable
b. detectable but at 5 bpm or less
c. 6 to 25 bpm
d. >25 bpm

8.42 Marked variability is best characterized by an amplitude range that is
a. undetectable
b. detectable but at 5 bpm or less
c. 6 to 25 bpm
d. >25 bpm

8.43 Minimal variability is best characterized by an amplitude range that is
a. undetectable
b. detectable but at 5 bpm or less
c. 6 to 25 bpm
d. >25 bpm

8.44 Absent variability is best characterized by an amplitude range that is
a. undetectable
b. detectable but at 5 bpm or less
c. 6 to 25 bpm
d. >25 bpm

Answers

8.34	a	8.36	c	8.38	a	8.40	a	8.42	d	8.44	a
8.35	b	8.37	a	8.39	a	8.41	c	8.43	b		

8.45 Accelerations are considered to be present at or after 32 weeks of gestation when an acceleration has an acme of
   a. 10 bpm and a duration of >15 seconds but <2 minutes
   b. 15 bpm and a duration of >15 seconds but <2 minutes
   c. 10 bpm and a duration of >10 seconds but <2 minutes
   d. 10 bpm and a duration of >10 seconds but <2 minutes

8.46 Accelerations are considered to be present before 32 weeks of gestation when an acceleration has an acme of
   a. 10 bpm and a duration of >15 seconds but <2 minutes
   b. 15 bpm and a duration of >15 seconds but <2 minutes
   c. bpm and a duration of >10 seconds but <2 minutes
   d. 10 bpm and a duration of >10 seconds but <2 minutes

8.47 Fetal heart decelerations are defined as
   a. visually apparent and gradual
   b. visually apparent and rapid
   c. auditorily apparent and gradual
   d. auditorily apparent and rapid

8.48 Early FHR decelerations are considered
   a. physiologic and not a cause for concern
   b. physiologic and a cause for concern
   c. pathophysiologic and not a cause for concern
   d. pathophysiologic and a cause for concern

Answers
8.45   b   8.46   a   8.47   a   8.48   a

Questions and Answers Chapter 9: Immediate Care of the Newborn

9.1 Which of the following clinical circumstances has a higher-than-usual risk of
the need for neonatal resuscitation?
  a. Cesarean delivery
  b. Suspected fetal anomaly
  c. Maternal fever
  d. Multiple gestation
  e. All of the above

9.2 Approximately what percent of cesarean deliveries may require the need
for neonatal resuscitation personnel?
  a. Less than 1%
  b. 5%
  c. 10%
  d. 50%

9.3 In what position is the infant placed in
the warming unit?
  a. Supine, with the head lowered,
     turned to one side
  b. Supine, with the head up
  c. In the sitting position
  d. In the prone position with the head
     lowered

9.4 Which of the following are examples of
mild stimulation to the newborn?
  a. Suctioning
  b. Rubbing the back
  c. Slapping the feet
  d. All of the above

9.5 Which of the following statements regarding the Apgar score is an accurate
reflection of its proper use?
  a. It is used to define birth asphyxia
  b. It indicates the cause of the
     newborn's depression
  c. The 1-minute Apgar score identifies
     newborns requiring special attention
  d. The 5-minute Apgar score predicts
     neurologic injury

9.6 Mild-to-moderate depression of the
newborn is defined as Apgar scores of
  a. less than 2
  b. 2 to 4
  c. 4 to 7
  d. 8 to 9

9.7 Causes of neonatal asphyxia may
include
  a. trauma
  b. severe maternal disease
  c. decreased uteroplacental blood flow
  d. all of the above

9.8 The management of a term infant
born by vaginal delivery almost immediately on arrival in the labor unit who
is covered with meconium fluid, is
limp with a heart rate of 100, and has
only a grimace, should include which
of the following?
  a. Oxygen by face mask
  b. Blood gas sampling
  c. External cardiac massage
  d. Intubation

9.9 In the neonate, scalp hair that is coarse
suggests an estimated gestational age
greater than how many weeks?
  a. 33
  b. 35
  c. 37
  d. 39

9.10 A neonate's ear lobe that lacks cartilage
suggests a gestational age below how
many weeks?
  a. 34
  b. 36
  c. 38
  d. 40

Answers

9.1	e	**9.3**	a	**9.5**	c	**9.7**	d	**9.9**	d
9.2	b	**9.4**	d	**9.6**	c	**9.8**	d	**9.10**	b

9.11 At 37 to 38 weeks' gestation, a neonate's breast nodule is expected to be about how many millimeters?
   a. 2
   b. 4
   c. 6
   d. 8

9.12 Which of the following describes the sole creases on the feet of a 39-week neonate?
   a. There are no sole creases
   b. There is a single anterior transverse crease
   c. Creases cover two thirds of the foot
   d. There are extensive creases covering the entire sole

9.13 Which of the following is the correct management of the umbilical cord stump in a newborn?
   a. Keep it covered with Vaseline
   b. Apply antiseptic solution daily
   c. Keep uncovered to expose it to air
   d. Excise it after 24 hours of life

9.14 What percent of newborns will pass stool within the first 24 hours of life?
   a. 60%
   b. 70%
   c. 80%
   d. 90%

9.15 Which of the following are characteristics of normal stool in the first 2 to 3 days of life?
   a. Greenish-brown in color
   b. Sterile
   c. Odorless
   d. All of the above

9.16 Which of the following statements regarding newborn weight loss is correct?
   a. Preterm newborns lose relatively more weight than their term counterparts
   b. Preterm newborns regain their weight faster than their term counterparts
   c. Term infants do not lose weight in the newborn period until one week of life
   d. Newborn weight loss in preterm newborns is regained in the first 4 days of life

9.17 Application of silver nitrate is designed to prevent
   a. conjunctivitis
   b. optic neuritis
   c. corneal scarring
   d. all of the above

9.18 Physiologic jaundice of the newborn occurs in what proportion of all newborns?
   a. 1 in 10
   b. 1 in 3
   c. 1 in 2
   d. 2 in 3

9.19 Jaundice becomes clinically apparent in the newborn when bilirubin levels reach what level?
   a. 1 mg/dL
   b. 3 mg/dL
   c. 5 mg/dL
   d. 10 mg/dL

9.20 Meconium-stained amniotic fluid is encountered in what percent of gestations?
   a. 0 to 5%
   b. 10 to 15%
   c. 20 to 25%
   d. 30 to 35%
   e. 40 to 45%

Answers

9.11 b	9.13 c	9.15 d	9.17 a	9.19 c
9.12 d	9.14 d	9.16 a	9.18 b	9.20 b

9.21 The most meaningful assessment of metabolic status of the baby at the time of delivery is through analysis of blood gases from the
  a. umbilical artery
  b. umbilical vein
  c. both the umbilical artery and the umbilical vein

9.22 About what proportion of infants born with meconium in the amniotic fluid will have meconium in the lungs?
  a. 1/3
  b. 2/3
  c. all

9.23 About what proportion of infants born with meconium in the amniotic fluid will develop significant respiratory distress?
  a. 1/10
  b. 3/10
  c. 1/2
  d. 7/10

9.24 Immediate intubation and suctioning should be performed under what circumstances when there is thin meconium-stained amniotic fluid?
  a. At all times
  b. Only if a neonatologist is present at delivery
  c. For all postdates neonates
  d. Only when warranted by the clinical judgment of the delivering clinician or physician and/or pediatrician attending the delivery.

9.25 The scrotum of newborn males of >39 weeks' gestational age is characterized by
  a. few rugae
  b. intermediate numbers of rugae
  c. extensive rugae

9.26 In the fetal circulation, the highest PO_2 is contained in the
  a. umbilical vein
  b. umbilical arteries
  c. fetal aorta
  d. fetal pulmonary artery
  e. pulmonary vena cava

9.27 Fetal cord blood gases most closely represent the condition in the baby at the
  a. end of the first stage of labor
  b. end of the second stage of labor
  c. first minute of extrauterine life
  d. fifth minute of extrauterine life

9.28 Which of the following is the most useful initial arterial cord blood value to manage the acidotic newborn?
  a. pH
  b. PCO_2
  c. PO_2
  d. Base deficit

9.29 When is the gastrointestinal tract of the newborn first colorized by normal bacterial flora?
  a. During labor after rupture of membranes
  b. At the time of delivery
  c. At 1 hour of life
  d. At 12 hours of life
  e. At 72 hours of life

9.30 Currently, the most effective newborn prophylaxis to prevent ophthalmia neonatorum is
  a. penicillin
  b. erythromycin
  c. tetracycline
  d. silver nitrate
  e. cephalosporin

9.31 Ioterus neonatorum is most often caused by
  a. temporary hepatic obstruction
  b. billary atresia
  c. reabsorption of free bilirubin from the fetal intestine
  d. increased erythrocyte destruction of fetal hemoglobin

Answers

9.21	a	9.23	a	9.25	c	9.27	b	9.29	d
9.22	a	9.24	d	9.26	a	9.28	d	9.30	d

9.31 c

Questions and Answers Chapter 10: Postpartum Care

10.1 The puerperium, which is the period following birth during which the reproductive tract returns to its normal, nonpregnant state, lasts approximately
a. 4 weeks
b. 6 weeks
c. 8 weeks
d. 10 weeks
e. 12 weeks

10.2 Uterine involution is a result of a decrease in the
a. number of cells in the uterine myometrium
b. size of cells in the uterine myometrium
c. size of the intercellular spaces in the uterine myometrium
d. number of intercellular spaces in the uterine myometrium

10.3 How many weeks does it take for the uterus to return to its prepregnancy position in the true pelvis?
a. 1
b. 2
c. 3
d. 4
e. 5

10.4 How many weeks does it take for the uterus to return to its prepregnancy size?
a. 2
b. 3
c. 4
d. 5
e. 6

10.5 Immediate postpartum uterine hemostasis is maintained by
a. primary clotting of blood in the uterine artery
b. contraction of the uterine smooth muscle
c. scar formation within the uterine cavity
d. tamponade effect of clots

10.6 The remnants of the hymen in the postpartum woman appear as fleshy tags at the introitus that are called
a. the hymenal ring
b. myrtiform caruncles
c. inclusion bodies
d. hyperplastic nodes of Smith

10.7 The mean time to ovulation in the nonlactating postpartum woman is approximately
a. 2 weeks
b. 4 weeks
c. 6 weeks
d. 8 weeks
e. 10 weeks

10.8 Fifty percent of women ovulate within how many days of delivery?
a. 30
b. 60
c. 90
d. 120
e. 150

10.9 The elevated pulse rate characteristic of pregnancy
a. decreases at the end of the third stage of labor
b. decreases approximately 1 hour after delivery
c. persists for approximately 3 weeks postpartum
d. is a reflection of the fetal heart rate

10.10 Transitory urinary retention in the postpartum period following vaginal delivery is primarily related to
a. sympathomimetic discharge
b. peripartum cystitis
c. periurethral edema
d. progesterone-associated loss of bladder contractility

Answers

10.1	b	10.3	b	10.5	b	10.7	e	10.9	b
10.2	b	10.4	e	10.6	b	10.8	c	10.10	c

10.11 Immediately after delivery, how much does a normal uterus weigh?
a. 500 g
b. 1,000 g
c. 1,500 g
d. 2,000 g

10.12 Postpartum uterine contractile pain is greater in breast-feeding women because suckling releases
a. progesterone
b. prostaglandins
c. oxytocin
d. estrogen

10.13 Breast engorgement in non–breast-feeding women typically occurs how many days postpartum?
a. 1
b. 3
c. 5
d. 7
e. 9

10.14 Postpartum breast engorgement in a non–breast-feeding mother is best managed with
a. local heat
b. breast binder
c. nipple stimulation
d. broad-spectrum antibiotics
e. bromocriptine

10.15 Which of the following best describes breast engorgement?
a. Unilateral location, localized swelling, intense localized pain, patient generally feels ill
b. Unilateral location, localized swelling, localized pain, patient generally feels well
c. Bilateral location, generalized swelling, generalized pain, patient generally feels well
d. Associated with fever

10.16 Which of the following best describes a plugged duct?
a. Unilateral location, localized swelling, intense localized pain, patient generally feels ill
b. Unilateral location, localized swelling, localized pain, patient generally feels well
c. Bilateral location, generalized swelling, generalized pain, patient generally feels well
d. Associated with fever

10.17 Approximately what percent of the total dosage of any medication is seen in breast milk?
a. 1%
b. 4%
c. 7%
d. 10%
e. 13%

10.18 Which of the following drugs can be safely administered to a breast-feeding mother?
a. lithium carbonate
b. tetracycline
c. bromocriptine
d. methotrexate
e. dicloxacillin

10.19 On approximately what postpartum day does milk production begin?
a. First
b. Third
c. Fifth
d. Seventh
e. Ninth

10.20 When after delivery is the endometrium reestablished in most patients?
a. First week
b. Second week
c. Third week
d. Fourth week
e. Fifth week

Answers

10.11	b	10.13	b	10.15	c	10.17	a	10.19	b
10.12	c	10.14	b	10.16	b	10.18	e	10.20	c

10.21 The silvery stripes seen on the abdomen skin postpartum are called
a. diastasis recti
b. tunica albuginea
c. striae
d. myrtiform caruncles

10.22 In a normal patient immediately after delivery, what is the weight of fluid lost through diuresis and loss of extravascular fluid?
a. 1 kg
b. 3 kg
c. 5 kg
d. 7 kg
e. 9 kg

10.23 Infection of the episiotomy site occurs in what percent of patients?
a. 0.1%
b. 1%
c. 10%
d. 25%

10.24 Which vitamin is not found in human breast milk?
a. A
b. D
c. C
d. K
e. E

10.25 The likelihood that a woman who had a previous postpartum mood disorder will have another episode is
a. 100%
b. 75%
c. 50%
d. 25%
e. 5%

10.26 Secretion of colostrum usually lasts
a. 2 days
b. 5 days
c. 2 weeks
d. 1 month
e. 6 weeks

10.27 Which of the following is the LEAST involved in stimulating milk production and secretion?
a. Testosterone
b. Progesterone
c. Human placental lactogen
d. Prolactin
e. Cortisol

10.28 A patient who asks about weight loss after delivery should be counseled that her weight should return to its prepregnancy level in about
a. 1 month
b. 6 weeks
c. 2 months
d. 3 months
e. 6 months

10.29 Postpartum depression is more severe in cases of
a. spontaneous abortion
b. fetal demise in the second trimester
c. perinatal loss at term
d. liveborn twins
e. liveborn preterm delivery

10.30 Mastitis followed by breast abscess is most frequently casued by
a. bacterial vaginosis
b. *Pneumococcus*
c. *Escherichia coli*
d. *Streptococcus pyogenes*
e. *Staphylococcus aureus*

10.31 The return of normal tone to the pelvic floor muscles postpartum may be enhanced by
a. exogenous estrogen supplementation
b. exogenous progesterone supplementation
c. Kegel exercises
d. avoiding coitus for 3 to 6 months

Answers

10.21	c	10.23	a	10.25	d	10.27	a	10.29	c	10.31	c
10.22	c	10.24	d	10.26	b	10.28	e	10.30	e		

10.32 Heavy postpartum bleeding associated with separation and passage of the placental eschar most commonly begins between what days postpartum?
a. 2 and 8
b. 5 and 11
c. 8 and 14
d. 11 and 17
e. 14 and 20

10.33 What percent of patients with excessive postpartum bleeding will have a diagnosis of delayed postpartum hemorrhage?
a. 1
b. 3
c. 5
d. 7
e. 9

10.34 The heavier postpartum bleeding associated with placental escar passage is best managed by
a. suction curettage
b. oxytocic administration
c. hysteroscopic surgery
d. reassurance
e. hypogastric artery ligation

10.35 Delayed postpartum hemorrhage is associated with retained placental tissues in about what percent of cases?
a. 10
b. 30
c. 50
d. 70
e. 90

10.36 Surgical management of postpartum hemorrhoids may be considered how soon postpartum?
a. Immediately
b. 3 months
c. 6 months
d. 9 months
e. 12 months

10.37 What is the expulsion rate for intrauterine devices inserted immediately postpartum?
a. 0 to 10%
b. 10 to 20%
c. 20 to 30%
d. 30 to 40%
e. 40 to 50%

10.38 Which of the following forms of postpartum contraception is most likely to adversely affect milk production?
a. Intrauterine contraceptive device
b. Depot-medroxyprogesterone acetate
c. Estrogen-progestin oral contraceptives
d. Progestin-only oral contraceptives
e. Natural family planning

10.39 A 22-year-old primiparous patient, 6 weeks postpartum, has recently attempted coitus for the first time since delivery and describes pain on penetration. The best treatment is
a. topical estrogen
b. oral estrogen
c. antidepressant
d. analgesic
e. topical anesthetic

10.40 A 30 year-old patient complains of stress incontinence at the time of her first postpartum visit 4 weeks after giving birth. The best treatment is
a. anticholinergic medication
b. tricyclic antidepressant medication
c. topical estrogen medication
d. retropubic urethropexy
e. reassurance and reevaluation in 2 months

Answers

| 10.32 | c | 10.34 | d | 10.36 | c | 10.38 | c | 10.40 | e |
| 10.33 | a | 10.35 | b | 10.26 | b | 10.39 | a | | |

Questions and Answers Chapter 11: Isoimmunization

11.1 When the father is homozygous Rh+ and the mother is Rh−, what is the probability that the fetus will be Rh+?
a. 25%
b. 50%
c. 75%
d. 100%

11.2 Which of the following statements about isoimmunization is INCORRECT?
a. It involves the development of fetal antibodies in response to maternal red blood cells
b. The antibodies involved in isoimmunization cross the placental barrier
c. The ability of the fetus to produce red blood cells can to some degree counter the isoimmunization process
d. The father must be Rh+ and the mother Rh− for Rh isoimmunization to occur

11.3 The major class of antibody responsible for Rh isoimmunization is
a. immunoglobulin G (IgG)
b. IgM
c. IgE
d. IgA

11.4 In the case of an Rh+ fetus and an Rh− mother, complications will typically first appear in which pregnancy?
a. First
b. Second
c. Third
d. Fourth

11.5 Pregnancies with severely affected Rh-immunized fetuses may be complicated by
a. polyhydramnios
b. fetal hydrops
c. fetal cardiac failure
d. fetal anemia
e. all of the above

11.6 Which of the following is the precipitating cause of hydrops fetalis?
a. Severe fluid retention caused by renal failure in the fetus
b. Irreversible carbohydrate metabolic failure
c. Decreased fetal aldosterone secretion
d. The ability of the fetal hematopoietic tissue to compensate for anemia resulting from red cell destruction

11.7 Which of the following is NOT associated with hydrops fetalis?
a. Fetal ascites
b. Low-output cardiac failure
c. Anemia
d. Decreased oncotic pressure in the fetal intravascular space

11.8 The risk of Rh sensitization from a mismatched blood transfusion is
a. <1%
b. 3 to 4%
c. 5 to 6%
d. 15%
e. 90%

11.9 The risk of Rh sensitization from a spontaneous abortion is
a. <1%
b. 3 to 4%
c. 5 to 6%
d. 15%
e. 90%

11.10 The risk of Rh sensitization from an ectopic pregnancy is
a. <1%
b. 3 to 4%
c. 5 to 6%
d. 15%
e. 90%

Answers

11.1	d	11.3	a	11.5	e	11.7	b	11.9	b
11.2	a	11.4	b	11.6	d	11.8	e	11.10	a

11.11 The risk of Rh sensitization from a full-term delivery is
a. <1%
b. 3 to 4%
c. 5 to 6%
d. 15%
e. 90%

11.12 The risk of Rh sensitization from an induced abortion is
a. <1%
b. 3 to 4%
c. 5 to 6%
d. 15%
e. 90%

11.13 In cases of fetal Rh isoimmunization, which statement reflects the relationship between the degree of fetal hypoproteinemia and fetal hepatic red cell production?
a. They are positively correlated
b. They are negatively correlated
c. They are unrelated

11.14 Antibody development will occur in approximately what percent of index pregnancies involving an Rh− mother and an Rh+ fetus?
a. 5%
b. 15%
c. 25%
d. 35%
e. 45%

11.15 The spectrophotometric curve used in the evaluation of hemolytic disease of the newborn is based on the measurement of what component in the amniotic fluid?
a. Whole red blood cells
b. Hemoglobin
c. Rh-D antigen
d. Bilirubin
e. Albumin

11.16 The major cause of fetal erythrocytes entering the maternal circulation is
a. labor and delivery
b. normal placental circulation
c. spontaneous abortion
d. premature rupture of membranes
e. low-level placental abruption

11.17 Rh immune globulin (RhoGAM) is effective against which antigen of the Rh system?
a. A
b. B
c. C
d. D
e. E

11.18 Rh immune globulin should be administered to an Rh− patient at all of the following times EXCEPT
a. at 28 weeks' gestation
b. within 3 days of delivery of an Rh+ infant
c. at the time of amniocentesis
d. at the onset of labor

11.19 When is administration of RhoGAM appropriate for an Rh−patient?
a. After an ectopic pregnancy
b. After a spontaneous abortion
c. After an elective abortion
d. In all of the above circumstances

11.20 Human RhoGAM
a. prevents the transfer of incompatible fetal cells to the mother
b. attaches to the fetal Rh+ cells in the maternal circulation and obscures the antigen sites
c. prevents antibody production in the maternal hematopoietic system
d. destroys fetal Rh+ cells in the maternal circulation

Answers

11.11 d	11.13 a	11.15 d	11.17 d	11.19 d
11.12 c	11.14 b	11.16 a	11.18 d	11.20 b

11.21 The administration of a 300-mg dose of RhoGAM to Rh− patients at 28 weeks' gestation is found to reduce the risk of sensitization to approximately what level?
  a. 0.2%
  b. 0.5%
  c. 1.0%
  d. 5.0%
  e. 10.0%

11.22 The standard 300-mg dose of RhoGAM will effectively neutralize how many milliliters of fetal red blood cells?
  a. 5
  b. 10
  c. 15
  d. 20
  e. 25

11.23 Direct fetal transfusion into the umbilical cord under ultrasound guidance carries with it a risk of fetal death of up to
  a. 1%
  b. 3%
  c. 5%
  d. 7%
  e. 15%

11.24 The volume of fetal red cells required to elicit an antibody response is estimated to be
  a. 0.001 mL
  b. 0.01 mL
  c. 0.1 mL
  d. 1.0 mL
  e. 10.0 mL

11.25 Which of the following statements about the Kleihauer-Betke test is INCORRECT?
  a. It is used to detect feto-maternal hemorrhage
  b. A negative result is an indication to administer RhoGAM
  c. It identifies fetal cells in the maternal circulation
  d. The ratio of fetal to maternal cells is assessed microscopically

11.26 The relative proportion of patients with ABO hemolytic disease and non-Rh D/non-ABO hemolytic disease, as compared with patients with Rh isoimmunization has
  a. increased
  b. remained the same
  c. decreased

11.27 Which of the following statements about ABO hemolytic disease is INCORRECT?
  a. It results in milder fetal kernicterus than Rh hemolytic disease
  b. It is rarely associated with hydrops fetalis
  c. The disease severity is probably related to the relatively smaller number of A and B antigenic sites on fetal red blood cells
  d. It usually occurs in the second trimester

11.28 What is the appropriate next management step for patients with a positive screen for Kell–K?
  a. Test the father for presence of antigen
  b. No further management is required
  c. Perform amniocentesis

11.29 What is the appropriate next management step for patients with a positive screen for Duffy–Fy^b?
  a. Test the father for presence of antigen
  b. No further management is required
  c. Perform amniocentesis

11.30 What is the appropriate next management step for patients with a positive screen for Lutheran–Lu^a, Lu^b?
  a. Test the father for presence of antigen
  b. No further management is required
  c. Perform amniocentesis

Answers

11.21 a	11.23 b	11.25 b	11.27 d	11.29 b
11.22 c	11.24 b	11.26 a	11.28 a	11.30 b

11.31 What is the appropriate next management step for patients with a positive screen for Kidd–Jk^a, Jk^b?

   a. Test the father for presence of antigen

   b. No further management is required

   c. Perform amniocentesis

11.32 What is the appropriate next management step for patients with a positive screen for non-D Rh–c, C, e, E?

   a. Test the father for presence of antigen

   b. No further management is required

   c. Perform amniocentesis

11.32 What at is the appropriate next management step for patients with a positive screen for I, P?

   a. Test the father for presence of antigen

   b. No further management is required

   c. Perform amniocentesis

11.33 What at is the appropriate next management step for patients with a positive screen for Duffy–Fy^a?

   a. Test the father for presence of antigen

   b. No further management is required

   c. Perform amniocentesis

11.34 What at is the appropriate next management step for patients with a positive screen for Lewis–Le^a, Le^b?

   a. Test father for presence of antigen

   b. No further management is required

   c. Perform amniocentesis

11.35 A 22-year-old G1 P0 presents for prenatal care at 28 weeks by dates and size. On review of her initial laboratory work, you note that her blood type is O−. She does not know the blood type of the father. Which of the following should be your management of this patient?

   a. Do not bring up the issue of Rh status.

   b. Do not offer RhoGAM until the father's status is known.

   c. Offer RhoGAM on the possibility that the father is Rh+.

11.36 A 28-year-old gravida presents for prenatal care at 7 weeks of gestation. Her antibody screen is positive for anti-Kell. What is the first step in management of this patient?

   a. Order a level II obstetric ultrasound

   b. Order an amniocentesis

   c. Order a cordocentesis

   d. Take no action until the status of the father is obtained

Answers

11.31 a	**11.33** a	**11.35** c
11.32 a	**11.34** b	**11.36** d

Review

Questions and Answers Chapter 12: Postpartum Hemorrhage

12.1 The traditional definition of postpartum hemorrhage is blood loss in excess of
   a. 250 mL
   b. 500 mL
   c. 750 mL
   d. 1000 mL

12.2 The most common cause of postpartum hemorrhage is
   a. uterine laceration
   b. uterine atony
   c. cervical laceration
   d. retained uterine tissue
   e. vaginal laceration

12.3 Excessive postpartum bleeding from the placental implantation site is primarily prevented by
   a. muscular contraction of the uterus
   b. coagulation of the uterine vascular bed
   c. mechanical obstruction of vessels
   d. sludging effect of the postpartum state

12.4 Which of the following characteristics of labor is associated with uterine atony?
   a. Prolonged labor
   b. Augmentation of labor
   c. Precipitous delivery
   d. All of the above

12.5 Which of the following medications may interfere with uterine contractility resulting in uterine atony?
   a. Magnesium sulfate
   b. Ampicillin
   c. Demerol
   d. All of the above

12.6 Following prolonged induction of labor in a 25-year-old G1 P0, a 9.5-lb boy is born by forceps-assisted delivery at 42 weeks of gestational age. Shortly after delivery of the placenta, the patient develops vaginal bleeding caused by uterine atony. Which of the following is NOT a risk factor for the uterine atony in this case?
   a. Forceps delivery
   b. Prolonged pregnancy
   c. Oxytocin induction
   d. Prolonged labor
   e. Large infant

12.7 Which of the following is appropriate for the initial treatment of uterine atony?
   a. Rapid infusion of oxytocin
   b. Uterine massage
   c. Administration of methergine
   d. Administration of prostaglandin
   e. All of the above are appropriate

12.8 Persistent uterine atony is treated with which of the following invasive modalities?
   a. Uterine artery ligation
   b. Hypogastric artery ligation
   c. Hysterectomy
   d. Selective arterial embolization
   e. All of the above

12.9 Which of the following is NOT a predisposing factor to lower genital tract laceration?
   a. Forceps delivery
   b. Breech delivery
   c. Delivery of a macrosomic infant
   d. Precipitous delivery
   e. Premature rupture of the membranes

Answers

12.1	b	12.3	a	12.5	a	12.7	e	12.9	e
12.2	b	12.4	d	12.6	a	12.8	e		

12.10 Which of the following statements about vulvar hematomas is INCORRECT?
a. They usually are associated with exquisite pain
b. They usually are associated with shock
c. If less than 5 cm and stable in size, they may be managed expectantly
d. If the size is increasing, surgical management usually is required

12.11 The site of postpartum hematoma associated with the greatest morbidity is the
a. vulva
b. lower vagina
c. upper vagina
d. cervix

12.12 Placenta accreta is characterized by penetration
a. into the uterine muscle
b. into the superficial lining of the uterus
c. involving the full thickness of the muscular uterine wall

12.13 Placenta increta is characterized by penetration
a. into the uterine muscle
b. into the superficial lining of the uterus
c. involving the full thickness of the muscular uterine wall

12.14 Placenta percreta is characterized by penetration
a. into the uterine muscle
b. into the superficial lining of the uterus
c. involving the full thickness of the muscular uterine wall

12.15 Which of the following is NOT a predisposing factor to retention of parts of the placenta?
a. Uterine leiomyomas
b. Previous cesarean delivery
c. Multiple gestation
d. Prior uterine curettage
e. Succenturiate lobe

12.16 Patients treated intrapartum and postpartum with intravenous magnesium sulfate are predisposed to
a. uterine atony
b. retained placenta
c. uterine inversion
d. placental infarction

12.17 The presence of retained placental tissue can be identified by
a. external palpation of the abdomen
b. ultrasound examination of the uterus
c. measurement of progesterone levels
d. hysteroscopy

12.18 The most common cause of death in amniotic fluid embolism is
a. cardiorespiratory collapse
b. afibrinogenemia
c. massive hemorrhage
d. acute renal failure
e. cerebral infarction

2.19 Which laceration can be directly related to the postpartum placement of a Foley catheter?
a. Second-degree vaginal
b. Third-degree vaginal
c. Fourth-degree vaginal
d. Periurethral
e. Cervical

Answers

12.10 b	12.12 b	12.14 c	12.16 a	12.18 a
12.11 c	12.13 a	12.15 c	12.17 b	12.19 d

12.20 Which of the following is the most common sequence of events associated with amniotic fluid embolis?
a. Respiratory distress, cardiovascular collapse, cyanosis, hemorrhage, coma
b. Cyanosis, cardiovascular collapse, respiratory distress, hemorrhage, coma
c. Respiratory distress, cyanosis, cardiovascular collapse, hemorrhage, coma
d. Cardiovascular collapse, respiratory distress, cyanosis, coma, hemorrhage

12.21 What is the maternal mortality in amniotic fluid embolism?
a. 10 to 30%
b. 30 to 50%
c. 50 to 70%
d. 70 to 90%

12.22 The initial management of a patient with immediate postpartum hemorrhage should include all of the following EXCEPT
a. careful but rapid inspection for lacerations
b. administration of oxytocin
c. inspection of the placenta
d. uterine artery ligation
e. uterine massage

12.23 A 32-year-old G2 P1001 undergoes a spontaneous vaginal delivery of a healthy 8-lb girl after an unremarkable spontaneous delivery. After 10 minutes without spontaneous delivery of the placenta, traction is applied to the umbilical cord. Placental tissue is expelled with the umbilical cord, followed immediately by vaginal hemorrhage. The placenta is not intact. Repeated attempts to dislodge placental tissue in the uterus are not successful and no cleavage plain is apparent between the uterine wall and the placental tissue. The most likely diagnosis is
a. placenta previa
b. placental abruption
c. placenta accreta
d. uterine inversion

Answers

| 12.20 c | 12.21 b | 12.22 d | 12.23 c |

Questions and Answers Chapter 13: Postpartum Infection

13.1 The definition of puerperal febrile morbidity includes a temperature greater than
a. 37.5°C
b. 38°C
c. 38.5°C
d. 39°C

13.2 Which of the following factors does NOT predispose to postpartum infection?
a. Maternal obesity
b. Anemia
c. Prolonged labor
d. Postdates pregnancy
e. Premature rupture of the membranes

13.3 Infection of the urinary tract (cystitis, pyelonephritis) is most likely to occur on which postpartum day?
a. Day 1
b. Day 2
c. Day 3
d. Day 4

13.4 Infection of the lungs (atelectasis, pneumonia) is most likely to occur on which postpartum day?
a. Day 1
b. Day 2
c. Day 3
d. Day 4

13.5 Wound infection (superficial infection, necrotizing fasciitis) is most likely to occur on which postpartum day?
a. Day 1
b. Day 2
c. Day 3
d. Day 4

13.6 Infection of the extremities (thrombophlebitis) is most likely to occur on which postpartum day?
a. Day 1
b. Day 2
c. Day 3
d. Day 4

13.7 The most common infection following cesarean delivery is
a. metritis
b. pneumonia
c. pyelonephritis
d. pelvic abscess
e. wound infection

13.8 The cause of postpartum pelvic infection is most commonly
a. Gram-positive aerobes
b. Gram-negative aerobes
c. Gram-positive anaerobes
d. Gram-negative anaerobes
e. polymicrobial

13.9 All of the following are Gram-positive aerobes EXCEPT
a. *Enterococcus*
b. *Staphylococcus*
c. *Streptococcus*
d. *Peptostreptococcus*

13.10 All of the following are Gram-negative aerobes EXCEPT
a. *Proteus*
b. *Escherichia coli*
c. *Klebsiella*
d. *Clostridium*

13.11 Which of the following is a Gram-negative anaerobe?
a. *Bacteroides*
b. *Clostridium*
c. *Klebsiella*
d. *Proteus*

Answers

13.1	b	13.3	b	13.5	c	13.7	a	13.9	d	13.11	a
13.2	d	13.4	a	13.6	d	13.8	e	13.10	d		

13.12 Which of the following is NOT a feature that can accompany metritis?
a. Fever
b. Uterine tenderness
c. Diminished or absent bowel sounds
d. Leukocytosis in the range of 15,000 to 30,000 cells/mL
e. Calf tenderness

13.13 Intravenous antibiotic therapy for metritis is continued until the patient
a. is asymptomatic
b. has normal bowel function
c. is afebrile for at least 24 hours
d. is all of the above

13.14 It is customary to provide additional antibiotic therapy in a patient being treated for postpartum metritis if there has been no response to the initial therapy within
a. 12 to 24 hours
b. 24 to 36 hours
c. 36 to 48 hours
d. 48 to 72 hours
e. 72 to 96 hours

13.15 A postpartum pseudomass associated with fever is most commonly the result of postcesarean
a. phlegmon
b. pelvic abscess
c. hematoma
d. urinoma

13.16 All of the following are characteristics of a pelvic abscess as a complication of postpartum metritis EXCEPT
a. persistent fever
b. paradoxical sense of well-being
c. delayed return to gastrointestinal function
d. localized pain or tenderness on abdominal examination
e. evidence of pelvic mass on imaging

13.17 Which of the following statements about the management of a pelvic abscess complicating postpartum metritis is INCORRECT?
a. Ultrasound, computed tomography, and/or magnetic resonance imaging are often useful in diagnosis
b. Initial therapy should include broad-spectrum antibiotics
c. Initial therapy should include drainage of the abscess
d. Rupture may be associated with shock and constitutes a surgical emergency

13.18 As compared with cesarean delivery, postpartum urinary tract infections after vaginal delivery are
a. less common
b. as common
c. more common

13.19 Which of the following is useful in identifying the presence of postpartum urinary tract infection?
a. Dysuria
b. Frequency of urination
c. Costovertebral tenderness
d. Urinary hesitancy

13.20 Which of the following statements concerning management of an infected incision site following cesarean delivery is INCORRECT?
a. The incision should be probed to determine the extent of infection
b. Broad-spectrum antibiotic therapy often is used
c. Culture of the wound usually is not required
d. Drainage of the wound is required

13.21 The initial treatment for an episiotomy site infection includes
a. suture removal
b. drainage
c. sitz bath
d. all of the above

Answers

13.12 e	13.14 d	13.16 b	13.18 a	13.20 c
13.13 d	13.15 a	13.17 c	13.19 c	13.21 d

13.22 Which of the following statements concerning necrotizing fascitis is correct?
   a. It is the most common postpartum infection
   b. It typically involves adjacent fascial, muscle, and subcutaneous tissue
   c. It is rarely fatal
   d. It requires surgical debridement in only rare cases

13.23 Mastitis most often first appears
   a. at the onset of nursing
   b. in the first week postpartum
   c. about 1 month postpartum
   d. about 6 months postpartum

13.24 Which of the following statements about respiratory complications following delivery is correct?
   a. Complications characteristically appear on the third postpartum day
   b. Complications are often associated with atelectasis
   c. Pneumonia is rare and typically not associated with predelivery respiratory disease
   d. General anesthesia results in fewer complications

13.25 Which of the following statements about septic pelvic thrombophlebitis is INCORRECT?
   a. It is a sequela of postpartum pelvic infection
   b. It is associated with venous stasis and bacterial colonization
   c. It may be complicated by microembolization to the lungs and other organs by way of the inferior vena cava
   d. It usually presents as residual fever and tachycardia during treatment for metritis
   e. The patient typically experiences severe uterine tenderness and absent bowel sounds

13.26 The standard treatment for septic pelvic thrombophlebitis in the postpartum period is
   a. a switch from double- to triple-antibiotic therapy
   b. placement of an inferior vena cava sieve
   c. empiric treatment with heparin
   d. administration of fever-reducing drugs and rest

13.27 In a case of necrotizing fascitis, which organism is most likely to contribute to the appearance of subcutaneous gas on radiography or computed tomography?
   a. *Bacteriodes* species
   b. *Escherichia coli*
   c. *Pseudomonas*
   d. *Clostridium*
   e. *Staphylococcus aureus*

13.28 Puerperal mastitis is most often caused by
   a. *Staphylococcus aureus*
   b. β-Hemolytic streptococcus
   c. α-Hemolytic streptococcus
   d. *Proteus* species

13.29 In cases of mastitis, the breast is colonized by a pathogen that comes from
   a. infected lochia
   b. infected skin
   c. the newborn's oral pharynx
   d. the maternal oral pharynx

13.30 Which of the following organisms is most likely to produce fulminant maternal sepsis from metritis within 24 hours following delivery?
   a. Beta-hemolytic streptococcus
   b. *Escherichia coli*
   c. *Clostridium* species
   d. *Pseudomonas*
   e. *Bacteroides* species

Answers

13.22 b	13.24 b	13.26 c	13.28 a	13.30 a
13.23 b	13.25 e	13.27 d	13.29 c	

13.31 The timing of prophylactic antibiotics at the time of cesarean delivery is based on providing maximal protection
  a. of the surgical wound
  b. from maternal pulmonary complications
  c. for the newborn
  d. for the upper urinary tract

13.32 At 9 days postpartum, a new mother complains of feeling awful and is runnjng a slight fever. She has no complaints of sore throat, dysuria,or pelvic pain (except cramping associated with breast feeding). One breast is slightly warmer to the touch and slightly more tender. Appropriate management at this time includes
  a. surgical drainage of the infected breast
  b. cannulation of the breast ducts over the affected lobules
  c. administration of an oral penicillinase-resistant antibiotic
  d. instructions to cease breast feeding until the infection clears
  e. an early mammogram to rule out carcinoma

13.33 A G1 P0 undergoes cesarean delivery at 42 weeks. Her immediate postpartum course is unremarkable, and she is bottle feeding her infant. On the third partum day, she develops a fever of 102.3°F with chills and lower quadrant abdominal pain. Examination reveals a tender uterine fundus and somewhat diminished but not absent bowel sounds. Ther cervix is tender to manipulation. A complete blood count reveals a hematocrit of 29 and a WBC count of 14,500 with a left shift. Your initial management of this patient should include
  a. single-agent intravenous antibiotic therapy
  b. multiple-agent intravenous antibiotic therapy
  c. anticoagulation with heparin
  d. diagnostic laparoscopy or laparotomy
  e. observation

Answers

13.31 c	13.32 c	13.33 a

Questions and Answers Chapter 14: Abortion

14.1 Abortion is generally defined as termination of pregnancy before what gestational age?
   a. 12 weeks
   b. 15 weeks
   c. 20 weeks
   d. 25 weeks

14.2 Abortion is generally defined as a pregnancy loss in which the fetus weighs less than
   a. 100 g
   b. 200 g
   c. 500 g
   d. 1,000 g

14.3 Approximately 80% of spontaneous abortions occur by what gestational age?
   a. 6 weeks
   b. 8 weeks
   c. 10 weeks
   d. 12 weeks

14.4 What is the incidence of clinically recognized spontaneous abortion?
   a. 5 to 10%
   b. 15 to 25%
   c. 30 to 40%
   d. 50 to 60%

14.5 What is the most common chromosomal anomaly associated with early spontaneous abortion?
   a. Trisomy
   b. Monosomy
   c. Triploidy
   d. Tetraploidy

14.6 Trisomy accounts for what percent of chromosomal abnormalities identified in early spontaneous abortion?
   a. 20 to 30%
   b. 30 to 40%
   c. 40 to 50%
   d. 50 to 60%
   e. 60 to 70%

14.7 Recurrent abortion is associated with what chance that one parent is an asymptomatic carrier of a chromosomal abnormality?
   a. 1%
   b. 3%
   c. 5%
   d. 7%

14.8 A 34-year-old patient reports that her first pregnancy ended in the spontaneous abortion of a chromosomally abnormal fetus at 10 weeks of gestation. Her risk of having another such event is
   a. increased compared with her first pregnancy
   b. decreased compared with her first pregnancy
   c. the same as in her first pregnancy
   d. indeterminate

14.9 All of the following are risk factors for spontaneous abortion EXCEPT
   a. increasing maternal age
   b. increasing paternal age
   c. increasing parity
   d. increasing maternal weight

14.10 A spontaneous abortion at which of the following gestational ages is most likely to be chromosomally abnormal?
   a. 6 weeks
   b. 10 weeks
   c. 14 weeks
   d. 20 weeks

14.11 Which of the following is the least likely cause for a second-trimester spontaneous abortion?
   a. Abnormal placentation
   b. Chromosomal abnormality
   c. Maternal systemic disease
   d. Uterine anomaly

Answers

| 14.1 | c | 14.3 | d | 14.5 | a | 14.7 | b | 14.9 | d | 14.11 | b |
| 14.2 | c | 14.4 | b | 14.6 | c | 14.8 | a | 14.10 | a | | |

14.12 Which of the following maternal infections has been associated with spontaneous abortion?
a. *Chlamydia trachomatis*
b. *Neisseria gonorrhoeae*
c. *Ureaplasma urealyticum*
d. *Herpes zoster*

14.13 How is luteal phase defect best diagnosed?
a. Timed serum progesterone
b. Timed endometrial biopsy
c. Timed serum estradiol
d. Timed serum luteinizing hormone
e. Hysterosalpingogram

14.14 Which of the following drugs is used to manage luteal phase defect?
a. Bromocriptine
b. Thyroxine
c. Estrogen
d. Clomiphene citrate

14.15 What is the effect on the rate of spontaneous abortion if the mother smokes more than one pack of cigarettes per day?
a. No documented effect on the rate
b. Twofold increase
c. Fourfold increase
d. Undetermined effect

14.16 Which location of leiomyomata is most associated with spontaneous abortion?
a. Subserosal
b. Submucosal
c. Intramural
d. Pedunculated

14.17 Pregnancies complicated by first-trimester bleeding are at higher risk for which of the following?
a. Preeclampsia
b. Preterm delivery
c. Fetal macrosomia
d. Intrauterine infection

14.18 The combination of which two tests is most valuable in the evaluation of threatened abortion?
a. Ultrasound and complete blood count (CBC)
b. Human chorionic gonadotropin (hCG) and CBC
c. Ultrasound and hCG
d. hCG and progesterone

14.19 Transabdominal ultrasonography can identify an intact gestational sac if the β-human chorionic gonadotropin level is at least
a. 1,500 mIU/mL
b. 2,500 mIU/mL
c. 5,000 mIU/mL
d. 7,500 mIU/mL

14.20 What is the appropriate therapy for a missed abortion at 10 weeks of gestation?
a. Hysterotomy
b. Suction curettage
c. Administration of Methergine (methylergonovine maleate)
d. Dilation and evacuation

14.21 Approximately what percentage of threatened abortions proceed to spontaneous abortion?
a. 10%
b. 25%
c. 50%
d. 75%

14.22 The characteristic history of incompetent cervix includes
a. pain but no bleeding
b. no pain or bleeding
c. bleeding but no pain
d. both pain and bleeding

Answers

14.12	c	**14.14**	d	**14.16**	b	**14.18**	c	**14.20**	b	**14.22**	b
14.13	b	**14.15**	b	**14.17**	b	**14.19**	c	**14.21**	c		

14.23 Cervical incompetence typically results in the expulsion of a normal sac and fetus between what weeks of gestation?
a. sixth and 20th
b. 12th and 26th
c. 18th and 32nd
d. 24th and 38th

14.24 Ultrasonographic findings associated with cervical incompetence include cervical funneling and
a. cervical shortening
b. cervical blunting
c. cervical lengthening

14.25 What is the appropriate time for placement of a McDonald cerclage?
a. Before pregnancy
b. Early in pregnancy, before dilation occurs
c. Early in pregnancy, after dilation has reached 3 cm
d. Immediately after an abortion

14.26 The Shirodkar cerclage is characterized by what placement of the suture?
a. Through and through
b. Submucosal

14.27 The presence of Asherman syndrome is confirmed by which of the following?
a. History
b. Physical examination
c. Hysteroscopy
d. Ultrasound

14.28 Treatment of Asherman syndrome involves lysis of the adhesions and treatment with
a. estrogen
b. progesterone
c. steroids
d. clomiphene citrate
e. oral contraceptives

14.29 All of the following are techniques for second trimester pregnancy termination EXCEPT
a. dilation and evacuation
b. prostaglandin vaginal suppository
c. intra-amniotic infusion of hypertonic saline
d. suction curettage

14.30 Which of the following may be present in cases of septic abortion?
a. Sepsis
b. Shock
c. Renal failure
d. Hemorrhage
e. All of the above

14.31 All of the following should be included in the management of septic abortion EXCEPT
a. intravenous fluids
b. antibiotics
c. evacuation of the uterus
d. prostaglandins

14.32 What percent of women with septate uteri have problems with fetal wastage?
a. 5%
b. 15%
c. 25%
d. 35%

14.33 The differential diagnosis of threatened abortion should include all of the following EXCEPT
a. placental abruption
b. friable cervix
c. cervical polyp
d. ectopic pregnancy

14.34 All of the following medical conditions are associated with an increased risk of first-trimester spontaneous abortion EXCEPT
a. diabetes
b. luteal phase inadequacy
c. hypothyroidism
d. hyperthyroidism

Answers

14.23	c	14.25	b	14.27	c	14.29	d	14.31	d	14.33	a
14.24	a	14.26	b	14.28	a	14.30	e	14.32	b	14.34	c

14.35 Postabortal syndrome following elective pregnancy termination results from
a. retained fetal tissue
b. uterine atony
c. inadequate surgical technique
d. the presence of a combined pregnancy

14.36 Which of the following is NOT indicated for a patient who just has been given the diagnosis of a spontaneous abortion?
a. Continued clinical observation
b. Administration of RhoGAM if the patient is Rh−
c. Transvaginal ultrasonography to rule out ectopic pregnancy
d. Discussion of caffeine and alcohol intake

14.37 A 26-year-old G3 P2002 presents to the emergency room 1 day after a first-trimester abortion complaining of abdominal pain and increasingly severe vaginal bleeding, but no fever or chills. She is normotensive and afebrile, her abdomen is mildly tender suprapubically, bowel sounds are present and normal, and there is neither guarding or rebound. Her cervix is open 1 cm, and clot and white tissue are present. The uterus is 12-week size, soft, and slightly tender. There are no adnexal masses. The most likely diagnosis is
a. missed abortion
b. uterine perforation
c. incomplete abortion
d. appendicitis

14.38 A 20-year old G1 P0 presents with a complaint of vaginal bleeding for 2 days that started 6 weeks after her last menstrual period. The patient passed some blood clots earlier in the day. The bleeding has been dark in color and associated with moderate lower abdominal cramping. Examination shows a small amount of dark blood in the vagina and the cervical os. The cervix is closed and no tissue is visible. Bimanual examination reveals a slightly softened, normal-sized uterus and normal adnexa without masses or tenderness. Her quantitative β-hCG 2 days ago was 846 mIU/mL; a repeat β-hCG today is 146 mIU/mL. The working diagnosis is
a. missed abortion
b. threatened abortion
c. incomplete abortion
d. complete abortion
e. ectopic pregnancy

14.39 The best management for a patient who comes to the emergency department and receives a diagnosis of incomplete abortion is
a. discharge home with instructions to follow up with her private physician within 24 hours
b. discharge home with prescriptions for Methergine and doxycycline and instructions to follow up with her private physician within 24 hours
c. Immediate repeat suction-curettage
d. Immediate diagnostic laparoscopy

Answers

14.35 b	14.36 c	14.37 c	14.38 d	14.39 c

Questions and Answers Chapter 15: Ectopic Pregnancy

15.1 About what percentage of women who have had an ectopic pregnancy are subsequently successful in having a full-term live birth?
   a. 10%
   b. 25%
   c. 50%
   d. 75%

15.2 Currently, the ratio of ectopic to intrauterine pregnancies in the United States is approximately
   a. 1:25
   b. 1:50
   c. 1:100
   d. 1:200

15.3 Which of the following is associated with the greatest increased risk of ectopic pregnancy?
   a. Use of oral contraceptives
   b. Intrauterine contraceptive device use
   c. Previous elective abortion
   d. Previous ectopic pregnancy

15.4 At what gestational age do women with tubal ectopic pregnancies typically first experience clinical symptoms?
   a. 2 weeks
   b. 4 weeks
   c. 6 weeks
   d. 8 weeks
   e. Varies with location of the tubal pregnancy

15.5 Which of the following symptoms is NOT associated with ectopic pregnancy?
   a. Acute pelvic pain
   b. Lower abdominal pain
   c. Vaginal bleeding
   d. Acute nausea and vomiting
   e. Amenorrhea

15.6 Which of the following physical findings can be compatible with the diagnosis of ectopic pregnancy?
   a. Abdominal tenderness
   b. Adnexal mass
   c. Uterine enlargement
   d. Normal blood pressure
   e. All of the above

15.7 What is the etiology for vaginal bleeding in cases of ectopic pregnancy?
   a. Coagulopathy
   b. Sloughing of decidua
   c. Bleeding from the fallopian tube
   d. Progesterone excess

15.8 Absence of villi on uterine curettage rules out which of the following diagnoses?
   a. Combined pregnancy
   b. Heterotropic pregnancy
   c. Tubal pregnancy
   d. None of the above diagnoses is ruled out

15.9 Most ectopic pregnancies implant in the
   a. ovary
   b. cervix
   c. peritoneal cavity
   d. fallopian tube

15.10 Of tubal ectopic pregnancies, approximately 80% implant in the
   a. isthmus
   b. fimbriae
   c. ampulla
   d. corneau

15.11 Which of the following laboratory and radiologic findings are consistent with the diagnosis of ectopic pregnancy?
   a. Empty uterine cavity on ultrasound
   b. A white blood count of 16,500
   c. A hematocrit of 37%
   d. Serum progesterone of 25 ng/mL
   e. All of the above

Answers

15.1	b	15.3	d	15.5	d	15.7	b	15.9	d	15.11	e
15.2	b	15.4	e	15.6	e	15.8	d	15.10	c		

15.12 In the diagnosis of ectopic pregnancy, a culdocentesis that obtains 3 mL of straw-colored fluid would be considered
a. negative
b. positive
c. nondiagnostic
d. unsatisfactory

15.13 Implantation in which of the following sites is likely to reach term?
a. Abdomen
b. Ovary
c. Cervix
d. Fallopian tube
e. Implantation in none of the above sites is likely to reach term

15.14 A heterotropic pregnancy is defined as
a. an ectopic pregnancy outside the fallopian tube
b. a twin ectopic pregnancy in the same site
c. coexistent intrauterine and ectopic pregnancies
d. ectopic pregnancy in two different sites outside the uterus

15.15 All of the following are included in the Spiegelberg criteria for ovarian pregnancy EXCEPT
a. an intact fallopian tube
b. an ovary in the normal position
c. ovarian tissue in the wall of the gestational sac
d. a fallopian tube connected to the uterus by the ovarian ligament

15.16 In the management of ectopic pregnancy, methotrexate may be administered
a. orally
b. intramuscularly
c. by direct injection into the ectopic gestational sac
d. through all of the above routes

15.17 All of the following are useful in the diagnosis of an ectopic pregnancy EXCEPT
a. observation of the Arias-Stella reaction on histologic examination
b. the presence of a gestational sac visualized on ultrasound examination of the fallopian tube
c. observation of an empty uterus on ultrasound accompanied by human chorionic gonadotropin level of 8500 mIU/mL
d. the laparoscopic visualization of 3-cm mass in the fallopian tube

15.18 The incidence of tubal ectopic pregnancy has been steadily rising in the United States, primarily because of increased
a. use of oral contraceptives
b. incidence of elective abortion
c. incidence of pelvic inflammatory disease
d. delay in the onset of sexual activity in couples

15.19 The mortality rate associated with ectopic pregnancy has decreased from 3.5 maternal deaths per 1,000 cases to less than one death per 1,000 cases primarily because of
a. earlier detection of the ectopic pregnancy
b. greater availability of blood for transfusion
c. modern intensive care technology to combat shock and blood loss
d. increased use of sophisticated laparoscopic surgical techniques

Answers

15.12	a	**15.14**	c	**15.16**	d	**15.18**	c
15.13	e	**15.15**	d	**15.17**	a	**15.19**	a

15.20 In which of the following situations is ectopic pregnancy NOT part of the differential diagnosis?
  a. A patient presents with lower abdominal pain and vaginal bleeding and with a positive pregnancy test
  b. A patient presents with lower abdominal pain and no vaginal bleeding and with a positive pregnancy test
  c. A patient presents with a negative pregnancy test and lower abdominal pain and vaginal bleeding

15.21 Which of the following is the most significant risk factor for ectopic pregnancy?
  a. Oral contraceptive use
  b. Current intrauterine device use
  c. Prior history of salpingitis
  d. Young maternal age
  e. Sterilization

15.22 Compared with women 15 to 23 years of age, women in the 35 to 44 years of age bracket have
  a. a decreased risk of ectopic pregnancy
  b. an equal risk of ectopic pregnancy
  c. an increased risk of ectopic pregnancy

15.23 Over half of all ectopic pregnancies occur in women who have had at least
  a. two pregnancies
  b. three pregnancies
  c. four pregnancies
  d. five pregnancies

15.24 Hemoperitoneum associated with ruptured ectopic pregnancy may result in irritation of the diaphragm and pain referred to the
  a. flank
  b. shoulder
  c. midchest
  d. arm

15.25 Which of the following statements concerning ectopic gestation is correct?
  a. Ectopic pregnancies are symptomatic from the early stages
  b. Abdominal pain, amenorrhea, and vaginal bleeding are noted in virtually all cases of ectopic pregnancy
  c. The patient feels pain on the side of the ectopic pregnancy in virtually all cases
  d. Ectopic pregnancy is more likely to be symptomatic if implantation is in the proximal portion of the tube

15.26 Syncope is reported in what proportion of patients with ruptured tubal ectopic pregnancies and hemoperitoneum?
  a. One in six
  b. One in three
  c. Two in three
  d. All

15.27 Approximately what percent of patients with tubal ectopic pregnancy present with hypovolemic shock?
  a. 5%
  b. 15%
  c. 25%
  d. 35%

15.28 In cases of ectopic pregnancy, how often are urinary pregnancy tests found to be positive?
  a. 90%
  b. 80%
  c. 70%
  d. 60%

15.29 Early in pregnancy, quantitative β-human chorionic gonadotropin levels should increase by what percent in 48 hours?
  a. 90%
  b. 75%
  c. 66%
  d. 50%

Answers

15.20	b	15.22	c	15.24	b	15.26	b	15.28	a
15.21	c	15.23	b	15.25	d	15.27	a	15.29	c

15.30 Transvaginal pelvic ultrasonography should be able to identify an intrauterine pregnancy by the time the serum β-human chorionic gonadotropin level reaches what level?
a. 500 mIU/mL
b. 1,500 mIU/mL
c. 2,500 mIU/mL
d. 3,500 mIU/mL

15.31 As a clinical cut-off, a serum progesterone below what level suggests a nonviable pregnancy?
a. 1 ng/mL
b. 5 ng/mL
c. 10 ng/mL
d. 15 ng/mL

15.32 What percent of all abnormal pregnancies, ectopic or intrauterine, are associated with serum progesterone levels of >25 ng/mL?
a. 0.5%
b. 2.5%
c. 4.5%
d. 6.5%
e. 7.5%

15.33 Survival of the intrauterine twin of a combined pregnancy has been reported in approximately what percentage of cases?
a. 20%
b. 33%
c. 50%
d. 75%

15.34 The Rubin criteria for cervical pregnancy include all of the following EXCEPT
a. cervical glands opposite the placental attachment
b. chorionic villi in the cervical canal
c. chorionic villi in the corpus uteri
d. internal cervical os closed, external cervical os open or closed

15.35 The use of assisted reproductive technology has what effect on the incidence of combined (heterotropic) pregnancy?
a. No effect on the incidence
b. A decrease in the incidence
c. An increase in the incidence

15.36 As compared with pregnancy following a "normal cycle," a combined pregnancy following the use of assisted reproductive technology is
a. more likely
b. as likely
c. less likely

15.37 Following a normal menstrual cycle, the incidence of cervical ectopic pregnancy is
a. 1 in 3,000 to 4,000
b. 1 in 7,000 to 50,000
c. 1 in 10,000 to 20,000
d. 1 in 18,000 to 25,000

15.38 Following a normal menstrual cycle, the incidence of abdominal ectopic pregnancy is
a. 1 in 3,000 to 4,000
b. 1 in 7,000 to 50,000
c. 1 in 10,000 to 20,000
d. 1 in 18,000 to 25,000

15.39 Following a normal menstrual cycle, the incidence of ovarian ectopic pregnancy is
a. 1 in 3,000 to 4,000
b. 1 in 7,000 to 50,000
c. 1 in 10,000 to 20,000
d. 1 in 18,000 to 25,000

Answers

15.30	b	15.32	b	15.34	c	15.36	a	15.38	a
15.31	b	15.33	b	15.35	c	15.37	b	15.39	c

15.40 Which of the following statements about the pelvic pain associated with tubal ectopic pregnancy is INCORRECT?
  a. The pain may be caused by peritoneal irritation from blood
  b. The pain usually is colicky
  c. The patient always feels the pain on the same side as the ectopic pregnancy
  d. The pain may be caused by distension of the fallopian tube

15.41 Which of the following situations associated with tubal ectopic pregnancy is LEAST COMMON?
  a. Tubal rupture with intraperitoneal hemorrhage
  b. Tubal abortion with or without intraperitoneal hemorrhage
  c. Tubal abortion with subsequent implantation on an intraperitoneal structure

15.42 A serum progesterone of less than 5.0 ng/mL strongly suggests a nonviable pregnancy that is
  a. intrauterine in location
  b. extrauterine in location
  c. either intrauterine or extrauterine in location

15.43 Of all tubal ectopic pregnancies, the percent that are cornual is
  a. 2%
  b. 6%
  c. 12%
  d. 80%

15.44 Of all tubal ectopic pregnancies, the percent that are fimbrial is
  a. 2%
  b. 6%
  c. 12%
  d. 80%

15.45 Of all tubal ectopic pregnancies, the percent that are isthmic is
  a. 2%
  b. 6%
  c. 12%
  d. 80%

15.46 Of all tubal ectopic pregnancies, the percent that are ampullary is
  a. 2%
  b. 6%
  c. 12%
  d. 80%

15.47 What is the most common kind of tubal ectopic pregnancy?
  a. Ampullary
  b. Isthmic
  c. Fimbrial
  d. Cornual

15.48 Cervical pregnancy is how many times more likely following the use of assisted reproductive technology?
  a. Two
  b. Four
  c. Six
  d. Eight
  e. Ten

Answers

15.40	c	**15.42**	c	**15.44**	b	**15.46**	d	**15.48**	a
15.41	c	**15.43**	a	**15.45**	c	**15.47**	a		

15.49 All of the following tests are helpful in the diagnosis of ectopic pregnancy EXCEPT
   a. transvaginal ultrasound
   b. serum β-hCG
   c. maternal serum α-fetoprotein
   d. serum progesterone

15.50 Which of the following is NOT an acceptable management option for a diagnosed ectopic pregnancy?
   a. Exploratory laparotomy
   b. Methotrexate therapy
   c. Observation
   d. Operative laparoscopy

15.51 Which of the following statements about methotrexate therapy for ectopic pregnancy is INCORRECT?
   a. Methotrexate therapy typically is used for an ectopic pregnancy less than 3.5 cm in diameter and no cardiac activity
   b. Follow-up therapy includes serial transvaginal ultrasounds
   c. Pretherapy evaluation includes β-hCG, liver function tests, creatinine, CBC, blood type, and Rh factor determination
   d. Additional methotrexate therapy or surgery is needed if trophoblastic function persists as evidenced by persistent or rising levels of β-hCG

Answers

15.49 c	**15.50** c	**15.51** b

Questions and Answers Chapter 16: Medical and Surgical Conditions of Pregnancy

16.1 Anemia in pregnancy is generally defined as a hemoglobin level of less than
   a. 6 g/dL
   b. 8 g/dL
   c. 10 g/dL
   d. 12 g/dL

16.2 The most frequent type of anemia in pregnancy is
   a. iron deficiency anemia
   b. folate deficiency anemia
   c. sickle cell anemia
   d. vitamin B_{12} deficiency anemia
   e. thalassemia anemia

16.3 During pregnancy, the serum iron usually is
   a. increased
   b. unchanged
   c. decreased

16.4 During pregnancy, the total iron-binding capacity is
   a. increased
   b. unchanged
   c. decreased

16.5 Which of the following statements accurately reflects iron deficiency anemia in pregnancy?
   a. One pregnancy can cause anemia in the next pregnancy
   b. Adequate treatment is 100 mg ferrous gluconate daily.
   c. With absent iron stores, a patient with iron deficiency anemia can be treated with 60 mg of elemental iron daily
   d. All of the above are accurate

16.6 Women with sickle cell trait (HbSA disease) have increased
   a. incidence of spontaneous abortion
   b. perinatal mortality
   c. incidence of urinary tract infections
   d. incidence of preterm births
   e. incidence of low-birth-weight babies

16.7 Patients with sickle cell disease are more likely to have
   a. asymptomatic bacteria
   b. urinary tract infections
   c. nephrolithiasis
   d. cholelithiasis
   e. all the above

16.8 Which of the following is NOT characteristic of von Willebrand disease?
   a. Decreased factor VII
   b. Decreased factor VIII
   c. Family history of the disease
   d. Prolonged bleeding time

16.9 When iron therapy is initiated during a normal pregnancy, the response is first seen as an increase in the reticulocyte count within
   a. 24 hours
   b. 48 hours
   c. 96 hours
   d. 1 week

16.10 Anemia associated with folate deficiency may be found in
   a. multiple gestation
   b. patients with a high alcohol intake
   c. patients taking Dilantin
   d. patients eating the normal adult intake of folate
   e. all of the above

16.11 Vitamin B_{12} deficiency is associated with which of the following diseases?
   a. Chronic malabsorption syndrome
   b. Pancreatic disease
   c. Crohn's disease
   d. Ulcerative colitis
   e. All of the above

Answers

| 16.1 | c | 16.3 | c | 16.5 | a | 16.7 | e | 16.9 | d | 16.11 | e |
| 16.2 | a | 16.4 | a | 16.6 | c | 16.8 | b | 16.10 | e | | |

16.12 A mixed iron and folate deficiency is characterized by
a. normocytic and normochromic anemia
b. microcytic and normochromic anemia
c. microcytic and megaloblastic anemia
d. normocytic and megaloblastic anemia

16.13 Which of the following anemias presents as microcytic and hypochromic but with a normal serum iron and total iron-binding capacity?
a. Iron deficiency anemia
b. Thalassemia trait
c. Sickle cell anemia
d. Sickle cell trait

16.14 The pH of urine in pregnancy, as compared with a nonpregnant state, is
a. increased
b. the same
c. decreased
d. dependent on gestational age

16.15 The appropriate management for a pregnant patient with asymptomatic bacteriuria is
a. no treatment
b. antibiotics
c. dietary alterations
d. recommendation for changes in sexual behavior
e. urinary alkalization

16.16 What percent of patients with asymptomatic bacteriuria during pregnancy will develop symptomatic urinary tract infections?
a. 25%
b. 50%
c. 75%
d. 100%

16.17 If a pregnant patient with pyelonephritis does not improve while taking appropriate intravenous antibiotic therapy within 48 to 72 hours, consideration would be given to
a. the possibility of urinary tract obstruction
b. reevaluation of the antibiotic used for treatment
c. the use of single-shot intravenous pyelogram or ultrasonography
d. all of the above

16.18 The most common organism cultured from the urine of pregnant patients with urinary tract symptoms is
a. *Pseudomonas*
b. *Escherichia coli*
c. *Proteus*
d. *Neisseria gonorrhoeae*

16.19 In pregnancy, the glomerular filtration rate increases by
a. 25%
b. 50%
c. 75%
d. 100%

16.20 Which of the following is NOT related to the increased incidence of symptomatic urinary tract infection in pregnancy?
a. Decreased ureteral tone
b. Compression of the ureters at the pelvic brim
c. Decreased pH of the urine
d. Pregnancy-associated mild glycosuria
e. Bladder compression

16.21 Provided other complications are absent in patients with mild renal impairment, individuals with serum creatinine levels below what figure generally have uneventful pregnancies?
a. 0.6 mg/dL
b. 1.0 mg/dL
c. 1.4 mg/dL
d. 1.8 mg/dL
e. 2.2 mg/dL

Answers

16.12	a	16.14	a	16.16	a	16.18	b	16.20	c
16.13	b	16.15	b	16.17	d	16.19	b	16.21	c

16.22 What factor in association with pre-existing renal disease results in a particularly poor prognosis for baby and mother?
a. Retinopathy
b. Hypertension
c. Atrophic skin changes
d. Obesity
e. Anemia

16.23 Bronchial asthma is encountered in approximately what percent of pregnant patients?
a. 0.01%
b. 0.1%
c. 1.0%
d. 10%

16.24 Pregnant patients who smoke have an increased risk of
a. spontaneous abortion
b. ectopic pregnancy
c. preterm labor and delivery
d. all of the above

16.25 Pneumonia occurs in approximately what percent of all pregnancies?
a. 0.01 to 0.1%
b. 0.1 to 1.0%
c. 1.0 to 5.0%
d. 5.0 to 10.0%
e. 25%

16.26 The most common bacterial pneumonia is associated with what organism?
a. *Streptococcus pneumoniae*
b. *Haemophilus influenza*
c. *Klebsiella pneumoniae*
d. *Staphylococcus aureus*
e. *Mycoplasma pneumoniae*

16.27 Pneumonia in pregnancy is associated with an overall mortality rate of
a. 1 to 2%
b. 3 to 4%
c. 5 to 6%
d. 7 to 8%
e. 9 to 10%

16.28 Acute febrile illness is associated with which of the following pneumonias in pregnancy?
a. Bacterial pneumonia
b. Mycoplasma pneumonia
c. Both bacterial and mycoplasma pneumonia
d. Neither bacterial nor mycoplasma pneumonia

16.29 A low-grade fever is associated with which of the following pneumonias in pregnancy?
a. Bacterial pneumonia
b. Mycoplasma pneumonia
c. Both bacterial and mycoplasma pneumonia
d. Neither bacterial nor mycoplasma pneumonia

16.30 A substantial leukocytosis is associated with which of the following pneumonias in pregnancy?
a. Bacterial pneumonia
b. Mycoplasma pneumonia
c. Both bacterial and mycoplasma pneumonia
d. Neither bacterial nor mycoplasma pneumonia

16.31 A lobar chest radiograph pattern is associated with which of the following pneumonias in pregnancy?
a. Bacterial pneumonia
b. Mycoplasma pneumonia
c. Both bacterial and mycoplasma pneumonia
d. Neither bacterial nor mycoplasma pneumonia

16.32 A nonproductive cough is associated with which of the following pneumonias in pregnancy?
a. Bacterial pneumonia
b. Mycoplasma pneumonia
c. Both bacterial and mycoplasma pneumonia
d. Neither bacterial nor mycoplasma pneumonia

Answers

16.22	b	**16.24**	d	**16.26**	a	**16.28**	a	**16.30**	a	**16.32**	b
16.23	c	**16.25**	b	**16.27**	b	**16.29**	b	**16.31**	a		

16.33 A productive cough is associated with which of the following pneumonias in pregnancy?
   a. Bacterial pneumonia
   b. Mycoplasma pneumonia
   c. Both bacterial and mycoplasma pneumonia
   d. Neither bacterial nor mycoplasma pneumonia

16.34 Influenza pneumonia in pregnancy is usually self-limited, with spontaneous resolution in
   a. 1 to 2 days
   b. 3 to 4 days
   c. 5 to 6 days
   d. 7 to 8 days
   e. 9 to 10 days

16.35 *Varicella* pneumonia occurs in up to what percent of women with *varicella* infection (chicken pox) in pregnancy?
   a. 10%
   b. 20%
   c. 30%
   d. 40%
   e. 50%

16.36 *Varicella* pneumonia is associated with a maternal mortality of
   a. 5 to 15%
   b. 15 to 25%
   c. 25 to 35%
   d. 35 to 45%
   e. 45 to 55%

16.37 *Varicella* pneumonia in pregnancy is usually appropriately treated with
   a. outpatient supportive therapy
   b. outpatient acyclovir oral therapy
   c. inpatient parenteral acyclovir therapy
   d. inpatient parenteral amoxicillin therapy

16.38 What percentage of pregnant women experience no change in their asthma or worsening of symptoms?
   a. 10%
   b. 20%
   c. 30%
   d. 40%
   e. 50%

16.39 What percent of pregnant women experience an improvement of their asthma symptoms?
   a. 10%
   b. 20%
   c. 30%
   d. 40%
   e. 50%

16.40 The peak expiratory flow rate (PEFR)
   a. doubles in pregnancy
   b. remains unchanged in pregnancy
   c. halves in pregnancy
   d. changes in pregnancy in proportion to the BMR

16.41 Which finding on sputum Gram's stain of a pregnant patient with an acute asthma attack is most consistent with an allergic response?
   a. Eosinophils
   b. Neutrophils
   c. Platelets
   d. Erythrocytes
   e. Hyphae

16.42 A peak flow less than approximately what percent of the predicted value in a pregnant patient with an acute asthmatic attack should be a stimulus for therapy?
   a. 80 to 90%
   b. 60 to 70%
   c. 50 to 60%
   d. 40 to 50%

Answers

16.33	a	16.35	b	16.37	c	16.39	b	16.41	a
16.34	b	16.36	c	16.38	d	16.40	b	16.42	b

16.43 Treatment for an acute asthma attack in pregnancy is centered in β_2 agonist therapy, with bronchodilation starting within
  a. 1 to 3 minutes
  b. 3 to 5 minutes
  c. 5 to 10 minutes
  d. 10 to 15 minutes
  e. 15 to 30 minutes

16.44 The management of an acute asthmatic exacerbation in pregnancy includes administration of oxygen sufficient to maintain a PO_2 of over
  a. 98 mm Hg
  b. 90 mm Hg
  c. 80 mm Hg
  d. 70 mm Hg
  e. 60 mm Hg

16.45 In chronic mild asthma in pregnancy, serial peak flow measurements are expected to remain in the range of
  a. 90 to 100%
  b. 80 to 90%
  c. 70 to 80%
  d. 60 to 70%
  e. 50 to 60%

16.46 Symptoms occurring up to how many times per week are consistent with, although not entirely diagnostic of, mild chronic asthma in pregnancy?
  a. 2
  b. 3
  c. 4
  d. 5
  e. 6

16.47 Intravenous hydrocortisone (100 mg every 8 hours) is indicated for asthmatic patients in labor who
  a. are classified as having mild asthma
  b. are classified as having moderate asthma
  c. are classified as having severe asthma
  d. have been taking two agents during pregnancy
  e. have been taking steroids during pregnancy

16.48 Albuterol is classified as a
  a. β-agonist
  b. steroid
  c. anti-inflammatory

16.49 Hydrocortisone is classified as a
  a. β-agonist
  b. steroid
  c. anti-inflammatory

16.50 Terbutaline is classified as a
  a. β-agonist
  b. steroid
  c. anti-inflammatory

16.51 Cromolyn sodium is classified as a
  a. β-agonist
  b. steroid
  c. anti-inflammatory

16.52 Newborns of women taking tuberculosis therapy should receive a purified protein derivative (PPD) at birth and again at how many months of age?
  a. 1
  b. 3
  c. 6
  d. 12
  e. 18

Answers

16.43	c	16.45	b	16.47	e	16.49	b	16.51	c
16.44	d	16.46	a	16.48	a	16.50	a	16.52	b

16.53 The appropriate regimen for conversion of PPD within 2 years and negative a chest radiograph is
  a. isoniazid, 300 mg/day for 6 to 9 months postpartum
  b. isoniazid, 300 mg/day, after first trimester, for 6 to 9 months thereafter
  c. isoniazid and rifampin for 9 months

16.54 The appropriate regimen for unknown conversion of PPD and age under 35 years of age is
  a. isoniazid, 300 mg/d for 6–9 months postpartum
  b. isoniazid, 300 mg/d, after first trimester, for 6–9 months thereafter
  c. isoniazid and rifampin for 9 months

16.55 The appropriate regimen for active tuberculosis in pregnancy is
  a. isoniazid, 300 mg/day for 6 to 9 months postpartum
  b. isoniazid, 300 mg/day, after first trimester, for 6 to 9 months thereafter
  c. isoniazid and rifampin for 9 months

16.56 Pyridoxine (Vitamin B_6) therapy is indicated for pregnant patients taking isoniazid to combat
  a. retinopathy
  b. nephropathy
  c. neuropathy
  d. cardiomyopathy
  e. dermatitis

16.57 Most pregnant patients with tuberculosis
  a. are asymptomatic
  b. have night sweats
  c. have low-grade fevers
  d. have leukocytosis on blood count
  e. have hemoptysis

16.58 Pregnant smokers or their infants are at increased risk of all of the following EXCEPT
  a. placenta previa
  b. abruptio placentae
  c. decreased birth weight
  d. intrauterine growth restriction
  e. long-term neurologic abnormalities

16.59 During pregnancy, the incidence and severity of the common cold upper respiratory infection (URI) are
  a. increased
  b. unchanged
  c. decreased

16.60 Patients with which of the following cardiac diseases are best advised not to become pregnant?
  a. Primary pulmonary hypertension
  b. Uncorrected tetralogy of Fallot
  c. Eisenmenger syndrome
  d. All of the above

16.61 In normal patients, cardiac output in pregnancy increases approximately
  a. 20%
  b. 40%
  c. 60%
  d. 80%
  e. 100%

16.62 Which of the following most closely matches the symptoms associated with New York Heart Association Class I?
  a. No symptoms of cardiac decompensation at rest; marked limitation of physical activity
  b. No cardiac decompensation or limitation of physical activity
  c. No symptoms of cardiac decompensation at rest; minor limitations of physical activity
  d. Symptoms of cardiac decompensation at rest; increased discomfort with any physical activity

Answers

16.53	c	16.55	a	16.57	a	16.59	b	16.61	b
16.54	b	16.56	c	16.58	a	16.60	b	16.62	b

16.63 Which of the following most closely matches the symptoms associated with New York Heart Association Class II?
   a. No symptoms of cardiac decompensation at rest; marked limitation of physical activity
   b. No cardiac decompensation or limitation of physical activity
   c. No symptoms of cardiac decompensation at rest; minor limitations of physical activity
   d. Symptoms of cardiac decompensation at rest; increased discomfort with any physical activity

16.64 Which of the following most closely matches the symptoms associated with New York Heart Association Class III?
   a. No symptoms of cardiac decompensation at rest; marked limitation of physical activity
   b. No cardiac decompensation or limitation of physical activity
   c. No symptoms of cardiac decompensation at rest; minor limitations of physical activity
   d. Symptoms of cardiac decompensation at rest; increased discomfort with any physical activity

16.65 Which of the following most closely matches the symptoms associated with New York Heart Association Class IV?
   a. No symptoms of cardiac decompensation at rest; marked limitation of physical activity
   b. No cardiac decompensation or limitation of physical activity
   c. No symptoms of cardiac decompensation at rest; minor limitations of physical activity
   d. Symptoms of cardiac decompensation at rest; increased discomfort with any physical activity

16.66 The fetuses of patients with functionally significant cardiac disease are at increased risk for:
   a. low birth weight
   b. sepsis
   c. congenital heart defects
   d. neural tube defects

16.67 Obstetric patients with severe cardiac disease are most likely to die during the
   a. second trimester
   b. third trimester
   c. intrapartum period
   d. postpartum period

16.68 Which of the following is characteristic of patients at increased risk for peripartum cardiomyopathy?
   a. Asian heritage
   b. History of preeclampsia
   c. Under 25 years of age
   d. First pregnancy

16.69 What percent of the offspring of pregnant patients with Marfan syndrome will inherit the disease?
   a. Less than 3%
   b. 25%
   c. 50%
   d. 100%

16.70 Which of the following best describes the onset of type I diabetes?
   a. Adult-onset glucose intolerance
   b. Glucose intolerance diagnosed in childhood
   c. Glucose intolerance identified during pregnancy

16.71 Which of the following best describes the onset of type II diabetes?
   a. Adult-onset glucose intolerance
   b. Glucose intolerance diagnosed in childhood
   c. Glucose intolerance identified during pregnancy

Answers

16.63	c	16.65	d	16.67	d	16.69	c	16.71	a
16.64	a	16.66	a	16.68	b	16.70	b		

16.72 Which of the following best describes the onset of gestational diabetes?
a. Adult-onset glucose intolerance
b. Glucose intolerance diagnosed in childhood
c. Glucose intolerance identified during pregnancy

16.73 In pregnancy, human placental lactogen results in all of the following EXCEPT
a. increased levels of free fatty acids
b. increased gluconeogenesis
c. decreased glucose uptake
d. increased lipolysis

16.74 Which of the following best describes White classification "A" of diabetes in pregnancy?
a. Onset between ages 10 and 19, duration 10 to 19 years, no vascular disease
b. Onset under age 10, duration >20 years, some vascular disease
c. Onset after 2 years of age, duration <10 years, no vascular disease
d. Gestational diabetes, onset in pregnancy

16.75 Which of the following best describes White Classification "B" of diabetes in pregnancy?
a. Onset between ages 10 and 19, duration 10–19 years, no vascular disease
b. Onset under age 10, duration greater than 20 years, some vascular disease
c. Onset after 20 years of age, duration less than 10 years, no vascular disease
d. Gestational diabetes, onset in pregnancy

16.76 Which of the following best describes White classification "C" of diabetes in pregnancy?
a. Onset between ages 10 and 19, duration 10 to 19 years, no vascular disease
b. Onset under age 10, duration >20 years, some vascular disease
c. Onset after 20 years of age, duration <10 years, no vascular disease
d. Gestational diabetes, onset in pregnancy

16.77 Which of the following best describes White classification "D" of diabetes in pregnancy?
a. Onset between ages 10 and 13, duration 10 to 19 years, no vascular disease
b. Onset under age 10, duration >20 years, some vascular disease
c. Onset after 2 years of age, duration <10 years, no vascular disease
d. Gestational diabetes, onset in pregnancy

16.78 Which of the following best describes White classification "E" of diabetes in pregnancy?
a. Pelvic arteriosclerosis by radiography
b. Transplantation
c. Proliferative retinopathy
d. Vascular nephritis

16.79 Which of the following best describes White classification "F" of diabetes in pregnancy?
a. Pelvic arteriosclerosis by radiography
b. Transplantation
c. Proliferative retinopathy
d. Vascular nephritis

Answers

16.72	c	**16.74**	d	**16.76**	a	**16.78**	a
16.73	b	**16.75**	c	**16.77**	b	**16.79**	d

16.80 Which of the following best describes White classification "R" of diabetes in pregnancy?
   a. Pelvic arteriosclerosis by radiography
   b. Transplantation
   c. Proliferative retinopathy
   d. Vascular nephritis

16.81 Which of the following best describes White classification "T" of diabetes in pregnancy?
   a. Pelvic arteriosclerosis by radiography
   b. Transplantation
   c. Proliferative retinopathy
   d. Vascular nephritis

16.82 During normal pregnancy, how many milligrams of glucose are spilled per day in the urine?
   a. 10
   b. 100
   c. 300
   d. 500
   e. 700

16.83 Infants of diabetic mothers are at an increased risk for which of the following congenital anomalies?
   a. Cardiac deformities
   b. Craniofacial deformities
   c. Reproductive tract deformities
   d. Situs inversus

16.84 Infants born to mothers with insulin-dependent diabetes are at higher risk for
   a. neonatal hyperbilirubinemia
   b. neonatal hypoglycemia
   c. hypocalcemia
   d. polycythemia
   e. all of the above

16.85 Which of the following are known risk factors for gestational diabetes?
   a. History of giving birth to an infant weighing >4,000 g
   b. History of repeated spontaneous abortion
   c. History of unexplained stillbirth
   d. Family history of diabetes
   e. All of the above

16.86 Beginning at approximately 30 to 32 weeks' gestation in pregnant women with diabetes, which of the following measures of fetal well-being is commonly employed?
   a. Daily fetal kick counts
   b. Serial nonstress testing
   c. Serial biophysical profile testing
   d. Serial ultrasonography
   e. All of the above

16.87 Most pregnant women with diabetes are maintained on a daily caloric intake of approximately
   a. 1,600 to 1,700
   b. 2,300 to 2,400
   c. 2,800 to 2,900
   d. 3,300 to 3,400

16.88 For a patient with diabetes taking a mixed regimen of neutral protamine Hagedom (NPH) and regular insulin in the morning and evening, the fasting glucose reflects the
   a. regular insulin given in the morning
   b. NPH insulin given in the morning
   c. NPH insulin given the previous evening
   d. regular insulin given in the evening

16.89 In the well-controlled diabetic patient with no complications, induction of labor is often undertaken at how many weeks' gestation?
   a. 40 to 42
   b. 38 to 40
   c. 36 to 38
   d. 34 to 36
   e. 32 to 34

Answers

16.80	c	16.82	c	16.84	e	16.86	e	16.88	c
16.81	b	16.83	a	16.85	e	16.87	b	16.89	b

16.90 What percent of gestational diabetic patients return to a normal glucose status postpartum?
a. Over 95%
b. 85 to 95%
c. 75 to 85%
d. 65 to 75%
e. 55 to 65%

16.91 What is the currently recognized upper normal limit for the 1-hour 50-g glucose challenge test?
a. 120 mg/dL
b. 140 mg/dL
c. 160 mg/dL
d. 180 mg/dL
e. 200 mg/dL

16.92 Of the patients screened by the 1-hour 50-g glucose challenge test between 24 and 28 weeks' gestation, approximately 15% will be found to have an abnormal glucose value. Of these, approximately how many will be found to have gestational diabetes using a 3-hour glucose tolerance test?
a. 5%
b. 15%
c. 30%
d. 45%
e. 60%

16.93 "Ideal" control for a pregnant diabetic patient would be maintaining a fasting plasma glucose measurement in the range of
a. 60 to 70 mg/mL
b. 90 to 100 mg/mL
c. 100 to 110 mg/mL
d. 110 to 120 mg/mL

16.94 What percent of pregnancies are complicated by hyperthyroidism?
a. .2%
b. 2%
c. 5%
d. 10%

16.95 Which of the following is a symptom of hyperthyroidism in pregnancy?
a. Weakness
b. Palpitations
c. Tremor
d. Heat intolerance
e. All of the above

16.96 Which of the following is a potential side effect of propylthiouracil when used as treatment for hyperthyroidism during pregnancy?
a. Neonatal hypothyroidism
b. Neonatal hyperbilirubinemia
c. Neonatal seizures
d. Placental abruption
e. Intrauterine growth restriction

16.97 How many weeks does it take for thyroid-stimulating hormone levels to return to normal after initiation of appropriate therapy for hypothyroidism?
a. 2
b. 4
c. 6
d. 8
e. 10

Instructions for items 16.98–16.103. Match the thyroid function test with the effect of pregnancy on its normal value.

16.98 In pregnancy, the results of a total thyroxine (T_4) test will be
a. elevated
b. lowered
c. unchanged

16.99 In pregnancy, the results of a $3,5,3^1$-tri-iodothyronine (T_3) test will be
a. elevated
b. lowered
c. unchanged

Answers

16.90	a	**16.92**	b	**16.94**	a	**16.96**	a	**16.98**	a
16.91	b	**16.93**	b	**16.95**	e	**16.97**	d	**16.99**	a

16.100 In pregnancy, the results of a T_3 resin uptake (T_3RU) test will be
a. elevated
b. lowered
c. unchanged

16.101 In pregnancy, the results of a thyroxine-binding globin test will be
a. elevated
b. lowered
c. unchanged

16.102 In pregnancy, the results of the free T_4 test will be
a. elevated
b. lowered
c. unchanged

16.103 In pregnancy, the results of a free T_3 test will be
a. elevated
b. lowered
c. unchanged

16.104 To avoid toxoplasma infection, pregnant women should be advised to
a. eat only well-cooked meat
b. avoid exposure to cats
c. avoid exposure to cat feces
d. do all of the above

16.105 Microcephaly, chorioretinitis, deafness, and mental retardation are the characteristic results of which intrauterine infection?
a. Cytomegalovirus
b. Coxsackie B
c. Mumps
d. Rubcola
e. Rubella

16.106 Which of the following antibiotics, when given to a mother during pregnancy, may produce enamel defects and yellowing of the teeth in her infant?
a. Cephaloridine
b. Colistimethate sodium
c. Penicillin
d. Tetracycline
e. Chloramphenicol

16.107 T_4 and T_3 serum concentrations are lowered during pregnancy primarily because of
a. estrogen-induced alterations of thyroid gland production
b. progesterone-induced alterations of thyroid gland production
c. estrogen-induced increases in thyroxin-binding globulin
d. progesterone-induced increases in thyroxin-binding globulin

16.108 Approximately what percent of pregnant women have asymptomatic cervical colonization by β-hemolytic streptococci?
a. 10%
b. 30%
c. 50%
d. 70%
e. 90%

16.109 Hutchinson teeth, mulberry molars, saddle nose, and saber shins are characteristic of congenital
a. rubella
b. syphilis
c. toxoplasmosis
d. bacterial vaginosis

16.110 *Treponema pallidum* reaches the fetus by
a. direct contact through the chorion
b. transplacental circulation
c. the amniotic fluid
d. lymphatic glands

16.111 Which of the following is associated with congenital syphilis?
a. Cutaneous lesions
b. Osteochondritis of the long bones
c. Pseudoparalysis
d. Hepatosplenomegaly
e. All of the above

Answers

16.100	b	**16.102**	c	**16.104**	d	**16.106**	d	**16.108**	b	**16.110**	b
16.101	a	**16.103**	c	**16.105**	a	**16.107**	c	**16.109**	b	**16.111**	e

16.112 What increase in the serologic titer for syphilis indicates either inadequate treatment or reinfection and is an indication for further therapy?
a. Twofold
b. Fourfold
c. Sixfold
d. Eightfold
e. 10-fold

16.113 Which of the following is successful in preventing neonatal gonococcal ophthalmia in the newborn of a woman with *Neisseria gonorrhoeae* infection?
a. Penicillin
b. Tetracycline
c. Ampicillin
d. All of the above

16.114 Bacterial vaginosis in the antepartum period has been associated with an increased incidence of
a. postpartum metritis
b. premature rupture of membranes
c. amniotic fluid infection
d. preterm labor
e. all of the above

16.115 Approximately what percent of women with bacterial vaginosis in pregnancy are asymptomatic?
a. 10%
b. 25%
c. 50%
d. 75%
e. 100%

16.116 Clue cells are the single most reliable diagnostic criterion for bacterial vaginosis when they account for greater than what percent of the cells seen?
a. 10%
b. 20%
c. 30%
d. 40%
e. 50%

16.117 Delivery of an infant through a birth canal with primary herpes infection is associated with a neonatal infection rate of
a. 10%
b. 20%
c. 30%
d. 40%
e. 50%

16.118 The risk of congenital rubella syndrome is greatest if the woman contracts the infection during which trimester?
a. First
b. Second
c. Third

16.119 Congenital rubella syndrome following vaccination during an undiagnosed pregnancy occurs in
a. approximately 1% of cases
b. approximately 0.5% of cases
c. approximately 0.1% of cases
d. approximately 0.01% of cases
e. no known cases (has not been reported)

16.120 Which of the following is NOT a neonatal abnormality associated with congenital rubella infection?
a. Cataracts and/or retinopathy
b. Patent ductus arteriosus or pulmonary artery hyperplasia
c. Musculoskeletal anomalies, including phocomelia
d. Deafness or impaired hearing
e. Hepatosplenomegaly

16.121 The most classic eye finding in fetal congenital rubella is
a. retinopathy
b. cataracts
c. glaucoma
d. microphthalmia
e. myopia

Answers									
16.112	b	16.114	e	16.116	b	16.118	a	16.120	c
16.113	b	16.115	c	16.117	e	16.119	e	16.121	b

16.122 Approximately what percent of Americans infected with HIV are women?
a. 20%
b. 40%
c. 60%
d. 80%

16.123 What percent of pediatric HIV infection is caused by vertical transmission from mother to fetus?
a. 20%
b. 40%
c. 60%
d. 80%
e. 100%

16.124 The sensitivity and specificity of the combined use of enzyme-linked immunoabsorbent assay and Western blot tests for HIV infection is
a. 59%
b. 69%
c. 79%
d. 89%
e. 99%

16.125 The management of labor for an HIV-infected woman should include all the following EXCEPT
a. avoiding the use of fetal scalp electrodes
b. avoiding fetal scalp blood sampling
c. intrapartum administration of zidovudine as part of an intrapartum–antepartum–postpartum regimen
d. cesarean section to avoid infection

16.126 The risk of deep vein thrombosis during pregnancy as compared with in the immediate postpartum period is
a. higher
b. the same
c. lower
d. unpredictable

16.127 The goal of heparin anticoagulation for deep thrombophlebitis during pregnancy is to maintain a partial thromboplastin time that is how many times greater than baseline?
a. Twofold
b. Threefold
c. Fourfold
d. Fivefold

16.128 Recurrent pulmonary embolization from pelvic thrombophlebitis is best treated with
a. anticoagulation
b. ligation of femoral veins
c. ligation of inferior vena cava
d. paravertebral block of sympathetic chain

16.129 In pregnanct women with epilepsy, the risk of bearing children with congenital anomalies is increased
a. twofold
b. fourfold
c. sixfold
d. eightfold

16.130 During an epileptic seizure, the immediate risk to the fetus includes
a. abruptio placentae
b. placenta previa
c. vasa previa
d. all of the above

16.131 Because of concerns about teratogenesis, which is the most commonly used anticonvulsant drug during pregnancy?
a. Phenytoin
b. Dilantin
c. Carbamazepine
d. Phenobarbital

Answers

16.122	a	16.124	e	16.126	c	16.128	c	16.130	a
16.123	d	16.125	d	16.127	a	16.129	b	16.131	c

16.132 Hyperemesis gravidarum is characterized by all of the following EXCEPT
  a. weight loss
  b. increased appetite
  c. dehydration
  d. ketosis

16.133 Which of the following is a cause of gastroesophageal reflux in pregnancy?
  a. Decrease of intra-abdominal space
  b. Increased pressure from the enlarging uterus
  c. Progesterone effect decreasing esophageal sphincter tone
  d. All of the above

16.134 The most common perinatal complication associated with appendicitis in pregnancy is
  a. premature rupture of membranes
  b. premature labor
  c. placenta previa
  d. abruptio placentae

16.135 The morbidity of regional enteritis in pregnancy is primarily related to
  a. intestinal obstruction
  b. toxic megacolon
  c. colonic perforation
  d. colonic stricture

16.136 Which of the following characterizes hepatitis A?
  a. Often associated with fulminant hepatitis
  b. Represents 50% of cases of hepatitis in pregnancy
  c. Spread by water, food, or fecal contamination
  d. Spread primarily by blood or blood product transfusion
  e. Associated with unexpected high maternal mortality

16.137 Which of the following characterizes hepatitis B?
  a. Often associated with fulminant hepatitis
  b. Represents 50% of cases of hepatitis in pregnancy
  c. Spread by water, food, or fecal contamination
  d. Spread primarily by blood or blood product transfusion
  e. Associated with unexpected high maternal mortality

16.138 Which of the following characterizes hepatitis C?
  a. Often associated with fulminant hepatitis
  b. Represents 50% of cases of hepatitis in pregnancy
  c. Spread by water, food, or fecal contamination
  d. Spread primarily by blood or blood product transfusion
  e. Associated with unexpected high maternal mortality

16.139 Which of the following characterizes hepatitis D?
  a. Often associated with fulminant hepatitis
  b. Represents 50% of cases of hepatitis in pregnancy
  c. Spread by water, food, or fecal contamination
  d. Spread primarily by blood or blood product transfusion
  e. Associated with unexpected high maternal mortality

Answers

16.132	b	16.134	b	16.136	c	16.138	d
16.133	d	16.135	a	16.137	b	16.139	a

16.140 Which of the following characterizes hepatitis E?
- a. Often associated with fulminant hepatitis
- b. Represents 50% of cases of hepatitis in pregnancy
- c. Spread by water, food, or fecal contamination
- d. Spread primarily by blood or blood product transfusion
- e. Associated with unexpected high maternal mortality

16.141 Acute fatty liver of pregnancy is associated with a fetal mortality rate of
- a. 90%
- b. 75%
- c. 60%
- d. 45%
- e. 30%

16.142 Patients with cholestasis of pregnancy present with which of the following?
- a. Pruritus
- b. Fatigue
- c. Jaundice
- d. All of the above

16.143 Cholelithiasis and cholecystitis complicate about what percent of pregnancies?
- a. 1%
- b. 3%
- c. 5%
- d. 7%
- e. 9%

16.144 Cholecystectomy during pregnancy is associated with a fetal loss rate of
- a. 1%
- b. 3%
- c. 5%
- d. 7%
- e. 9%

16.145 If pancreatitis is present at the time of cholecystectomy during pregnancy, the fetal loss rate approaches
- a. 50%
- b. 60%
- c. 70%
- d. 80%
- e. 90%

16.146 The most important obstetric consideration involving blunt abdominal trauma to the abdomen is
- a. uterine perforation
- b. abruptio placentae
- c. premature rupture of the membranes
- d. uterine rupture

16.147 Newborn narcotic withdrawal syndrome is seen in up to what proportion of infants born to mothers who use opiates?
- a. 1 in 6
- b. 1 in 3
- c. 2 in 3
- d. 3 in 4
- e. 9 in 10

16.148 At least how many beers, glasses of wine, or standard mixed drinks daily during pregnancy is highly associated with fetal alcohol syndrome in the newborn?
- a. 2
- b. 4
- c. 6
- d. 8
- e. 10

16.149 Fetal alcohol syndrome is associated with
- a. mental retardation
- b. prenatal and postnatal growth deficiency
- c. cardiovascular and central nervous system anomalies
- d. craniofacial anomalies
- e. all of the above

Answers

16.140	e	16.142	d	16.144	c	16.146	b	16.148	b
16.141	c	16.143	b	16.145	b	16.147	c	16.149	e

16.150 Segmental intestinal atresia, limb-reduction defects, disruptive brain anomalies, congenital heart defects, and prune belly syndrome are associated with the ingestion of
a. marijuana
b. cocaine
c. alcohol
d. caffeine

16.151 In a woman with immune thrombocytopenic purpura (ITP), a platelet count of less than what level on percutaneous umbilical sampling may be considered an indication for cesarean delivery?
a. $10,000/mm^3$
b. $50,000/mm^3$
c. $100,000/mm^3$
d. $150,000/mm^3$
e. $200,000/mm^3$

16.152 Immune thrombocytopenic purpura occurs in what proportion of pregnancies?
a. 8 to 10 per 1,000
b. 6 to 7 per 1,000
c. 4 to 5 per 1,000
d. 1 to 2 per 1,000

16.153 Thrombocytopenia-associated spontaneous bleeding during pregnancy usually occurs with a platelet concentration of less than
a. $100,000/mm^3$
b. $80,000/mm^3$
c. $60,000/mm^3$
d. $40,000/mm^3$
e. $20,000/mm^3$

16.154 The initial treatment of ITP in pregnancy is
a. administration of γ-globulin
b. splenectomy
c. administration of corticosteroids
d. transfusion of platelets

16.155 Patients with lupus anticoagulant have a rate of reproductive wastage in excess of
a. 30%
b. 50%
c. 70%
d. 90%

16.156 Other than genetic causes, what is the most common cause of mental retardation?
a. Cocaine use in pregnancy
b. Marijuana use in pregnancy
c. Alcohol use in pregnancy
d. Opiate use during labor
e. Fetal asphyxia during labor

16.157 The stage-for-stage survival rates for breast cancer in pregnancy is
a. one-half that in the absence of pregnancy
b. one-fourth that in the absence of pregnancy
c. the same as that in the absence of pregnancy
d. twice that in the absence of pregnancy

16.158 Colorectal carcinoma is encountered in what proportion of pregnancies?
a. 1 in 1,000
b. 1 in 10,000
c. 1 in 100,000
d. 1 in 1,000,000

16.159 The need for folate during pregnancy for maternal and fetal growth is approximately
a. 200 mcg/day
b 500 mcg/day
c. 800 mcg/day
d. 1,100 mcg/day
e. 1,400 mcg/day

Answers

| 16.150 | b | 16.152 | d | 16.154 | c | 16.156 | c | 16.158 | c |
| 16.151 | b | 16.153 | e | 16.155 | d | 16.157 | c | 16.159 | c |

16.160 The increases in plasma volume and red cell mass in pregnancy occur at a ratio of approximately
a. 1:1
b. 3:1
c. 5:1
d. 7:1
e. 9:1

16.161 Iron deficiency anemia accounts for approximately what percent of anemias in pregnancy?
a. More than 90%
b. 90%
c. 75%
d. 60%
e. 45%

16.162 The initial laboratory evaluation of anemia in pregnancy should include
a. serum iron and total iron-binding capacity
b. serum folate and B_{12} levels
c. serum ferritin
d. all of the above
e. none of the above

16.163 The treatment of folate deficiency anemia during pregnancy is how many grams of folate per day?
a. 0.5
b. 1
c. 2
d. 4
e. 8

Answers

16.160 b	**16.161** b	**16.162** d	**16.163** b

Questions and Answers Chapter 17: Hypertension in Pregnancy

17.1 Hypertension in pregnancy is defined as a sustained systolic blood pressure at or above
   a. 130 mm Hg
   b. 140 mm Hg
   c. 150 mm Hg
   d. 160 mm Hg

17.2 Hypertension in pregnancy is defined as a sustained diastolic blood pressure at or above
   a. 90 mm Hg
   b. 100 mm Hg
   c. 110 mm Hg
   d. 120 mm Hg

17.3 A rise in the diastolic blood pressure of how many mm Hg is used to define hypertension in pregnancy?
   a. 5 mm Hg
   b. 10 mm Hg
   c. 15 mm Hg
   d. 20 mm Hg

17.4 A rise in the systolic blood pressure of how many mm Hg is used to define hypertension in pregnancy?
   a. 10 mm Hg
   b. 20 mm Hg
   c. 30 mm Hg
   d. 40 mm Hg

17.5 The blood pressure is lowest if measured when the patient is
   a. lying in the lateral position
   b. standing
   c. sitting
   d. lying in the prone position

17.6 During normal pregnancy, blood pressure follows which of the following patterns?
   a. Increases slightly during the second trimester
   b. Decreases slightly in the second trimester
   c. Fluctuates irregularly
   d. Increases gradually toward term

17.7 Pregnancy-induced hypertension develops in what percent of pregnancies that proceed beyond the first trimester?
   a. Less than 5%
   b. 5 to 10%
   c. 11 to 15%
   d. 16 to 20%
   e. 21 to 25%

17.8 Which of the following is characteristic of preeclampsia?
   a. Hypertension
   b. Proteinuria
   c. Edema
   d. All of the above

17.9 What is the most likely diagnosis of a patient who presents with hypertension in the twelfth week of pregnancy?
   a. Preeclampsia
   b. Eclampsia
   c. Chronic hypertension
   d. Hyperthyroidism

17.10 Approximately what percent of women with chronic hypertension develop superimposed preeclampsia or eclampsia?
   a. 25%
   b. 50%
   c. 75%
   d. 100%

Answers

17.1	b	17.3	c	17.5	a	17.7	b	17.9	c
17.2	a	17.4	c	17.6	c	17.8	d	17.10	c

17.11 The intrauterine growth restriction often associated with hypertensive disease in pregnancy is most likely related to
   a. chronic uteroplacental insufficiency
   b. congenital anomalies of the fetus
   c. anomalies of placental structure
   d. placental abruption

17.12 In the patient with preeclampsia, visual disturbances such as scotomata and persistent severe headache are usually caused by
   a. infarct
   b. vasospasm
   c. partial embolic occlusion
   d. demyelinization of nerves

17.13 The right upper quadrant pain seen in preeclampsia arises from
   a. hepatic infarction
   b. hepatic capsule distention
   c. hepatic rupture
   d. cholecystitis
   e. cholelithiasis

17.14 In a patient with preeclampsia, which of the following indicates a worsening disease process?
   a. Decreasing hematocrit
   b. Increasing hematocrit
   c. Increasing white blood cell count
   d. Increasing platelet count

17.15 All of the following are included in the definition of severe preeclampsia EXCEPT
   a. oliguria (500 mL or less in 24 hours) and a rising plasma creatinine level
   b. severe thrombocytopenia or overt intravascular hemolysis
   c. the development of convulsions in the absence of neurologic disease
   d. proteinuria of 5 g or more in 24 hours
   e. a persistent systolic blood pressure of at least 160 mm Hg or a diastolic blood pressure of at least 110 mm Hg

17.16 In general, antihypertensive therapy is indicated in preeclampsia when the diastolic blood pressure is repeatedly above
   a. 90 mm Hg
   b. 100 mm Hg
   c. 110 mm Hg
   d. 120 mm Hg
   e. 130 mm Hg

17.17 All of the following should be part of the management of a patient with mild preeclampsia who is being cared for at home EXCEPT
   a. bed rest
   b. recording of daily fetal movement
   c. daily dosing with magnesium sulfate
   d. daily weighing

17.18 Intravenous magnesium sulfate is used in the management of preeclampsia to
   a. prevent convulsions
   b. treat active convulsions
   c. lower blood pressure
   d. stabilize renal function

17.19 Muscular paralysis and respiratory difficulty occur when the serum concentration of magnesium is at least
   a. 4 to 7 mg/dL
   b. 8 to 12 mg/dL
   c. 15 to 17 mg/dL

17.20 Magnesium sulfate toxicity is treated with the slow intravenous administration of
   a. insulin
   b. calcium gluconate
   c. potassium hydroxide
   d. magnesium gluconate

17.21 Which of the following is the mechanism of action of thiazide?
   a. β-Adrenergic blocker
   b. Direct vasodilation, cardiac effects
   c. Decreased plasma volume and cardiac output
   d. Direct peripheral vasodilation

Answers

17.11	a	17.13	b	17.15	c	17.17	c	17.19	c	17.21	c
17.12	b	17.14	b	17.16	c	17.18	a	17.20	b		

17.22 Which of the following is the mechanism of action of methyldopa?
a. Calcium channel blocker
b. Direct vasodilation, cardiac effects
c. Decreased plasma volume and cardiac output
d. False neurotransmission, central nervous system effects
e. Direct peripheral vasodilation

17.23 Which of the following is the mechanism of action of hydralazine?
a. Direct peripheral vasodilation
b. Direct vasodilation, cardiac effects
c. Decreased plasma volume and cardiac output
d. False neurotransmission, central nervous system effects

17.24 Which of the following is the mechanism of action of propranolol?
a. Calcium channel blocker
b. β-Adrenergic blocker
c. α- and β-Adrenergic blockers
d. Decreased plasma volume and cardiac output
e. Direct peripheral vasodilation

17.25 Which of the following is the mechanism of action of labetalol?
a. Calcium channel blocker
b. β-Adrenergic blocker
c. α- and β-Adrenergic blockers
d. Direct vasodilation, cardiac effects

17.26 Which of the following is the mechanism of action of nifedipine?
a. Calcium channel blocker
b. β-Adrenergic blocker
c. α- and β-Adrenergic blockers
d. Direct vasodilation, cardiac effects

17.27 Which of the following is the mechanism of action of prazosin?
a. β-Adrenergic blocker
b. α- and β-Adrenergic blockers
c. Direct vasodilation, cardiac effects
d. Decreased plasma volume and cardiac output
e. Direct peripheral vasodilation

17.28 Magnesium sulfate given intravenously in a large dose for eclampsia may be associated with all of the following EXCEPT
a. transient loss of beat-to-beat variation
b. bone deposition of magnesium
c. hypermagnesia in the fetus
d. reduction in the glomerular filtration rate
e. diminished patellar reflex

17.29 In the postpartum period, reversal of the vasospastic process associated with preeclampsia is manifested by
a. decreased deep tendon reflexes
b. a rapid fall in blood pressure
c. brisk diuresis
d. continued weight gain

17.30 In a patient with hypertension, midepigastric pain in the last trimester is suggestive of
a. ruptured splenic aneurysm
b. impending eclampsia
c. Crohn's disease
d. hepatic hemorrhage
e. abruptio placentae

17.31 All of the following are elements of the HELLP syndrome EXCEPT
a. seizures
b. hemolysis
c. hepatic dysfunction
d. low platelet count

Answers

17.22	d	17.24	b	17.26	a	17.28	d	17.30	b
17.23	a	17.25	c	17.27	c	17.29	c	17.31	a

17.32 Platelet transfusion for the HELLP syndrome is usually indicated when the platelet count falls below
    a. 10,000/mm^3
    b. 20,000/mm^3
    c. 30,000/mm^3
    d. 40,000/mm^3
    e. 50,000/mm^3

17.33 For a 17-year-old patient at 32 weeks' gestation who presents to the hospital having an eclamptic seizure, the most appropriate management is
    a. an immediate vaginal delivery
    b. an immediate cesarean delivery
    c. administration of magnesium
    d. administration of Pitocin

17.34 Preeclampsia occurs in approximately what percent of deliveries?
    a. 3%
    b. 7%
    c. 10%
    d. 14%

17.35 Which of the following events is NOT characteristic of patients with chronic hypertension/preeclampsia?
    a. Fetal macrosomia
    b. Intrauterine growth restriction
    c. Oligohydramnios
    d. Dysmaturity

17.36 Which of the following is an appropriate fetal evaluation in patients suspected of having hypertension in pregnancy?
    a. Biophysical profile
    b. Amniotic fluid volume
    c. Fetal weight and growth evaluation
    d. All of the above

17.37 In patients with hypertension in pregnancy, which of the following tests is useful in evaluating a patient with suspected coagulopathy?
    a. Complete blood count
    b. Platelet count
    c. Fibrin split products
    d. Prothrombin time/partial thromboplastin time
    e. All of the above

17.38 Eclampsia occurs in what percent of deliveries?
    a. 0.01 to 0.1%
    b. 0.5 to 4%
    c. 4.5 to 6 %
    d. 6.5 to 8%

17.39 Perinatal mortality associated with preeclampsia increases progressively with increasing mean arterial pressure, primarily associated with uteroplacental insufficiency and
    a. disseminated intravascular coagulation
    b. renal failure
    c. abruptio placentae
    d. cardiomyopathy
    e. hepatoma

17.40 Which of the following most closely characterizes transient hypertension of pregnancy?
    a. Systolic blood pressure >140 mm or diastolic blood pressure >90 mm Hg
    b. Systolic blood pressure >140 mm or diastolic blood pressure >90 mm Hg and significant proteinuria or edema
    c. Systolic blood pressure >140 mm or diastolic blood pressure >90 mm Hg and oliguria
    d. Systolic blood pressure >140 mm or diastolic blood pressure >90 mm Hg and significant proteinuria or edema and convulsions

Answers

17.32	b	17.34	b	17.36	d	17.38	b	17.40	a
17.33	c	17.35	a	17.37	e	17.39	c		

17.41 Which of the following most closely characterizes preeclampsia?
a. Systolic blood pressure >140 mm or diastolic blood pressure >90 mm Hg
b. Systolic blood pressure >140 mm or diastolic blood pressure >90 mm Hg and significant proteinuria or edema
c. Systolic blood pressure >140 mm or diastolic blood pressure >90 mm Hg and oliguria
d. Systolic blood pressure >140 mm or diastolic blood pressure >90 mm Hg and significant proteinuria or edema and convulsions

17.42 Which of the following most closely characterizes eclampsia?
a. Systolic blood pressure >140 mm or diastolic blood pressure >90 mm Hg
b. Systolic blood pressure >140 mm or diastolic blood pressure >90 mm Hg and significant proteinuria or edema
c. Systolic blood pressure >140 mm or diastolic blood pressure >90 mm Hg and oliguria
d. Systolic blood pressure >140 mm or diastolic blood pressure >90 mm Hg and significant proteinuria or edema and convulsions

17.43 A 38-year-old G2 P1001 presents for prenatal care at 10 weeks of gestational age. She was given a disgnosis of essential hypertension 4 years ago and was placed on a diuretic and methyldopa. She reports that her blood pressure typically is 140/90. On physical examination, the patient weighs 280 pounds and her blood pressure, taken with a large cuff, is 135/85 supine and 140/95 sitting. She has mild arteriolar narrowing on fundoscopic examination, a normal cardiovascular examination, a 10-week size uterus, and 1+ lower extremity peripheral edema. Her urine sample dipstick shows 1+ protein and trace glucose. Your initial diagnosis should be
a. pregnancy-induced hypertension (PIH)
b. mild preeclampsia
c. severe preeclampsia
d. chronic hypertension
e. chronic hypertension with superimposed PIH

17.44 A 19-year-old G1 has had an unremarkable antepartum course since her first prenatal visit at 8 weeks. At the start of her 32nd week, she complains of swollen hands and feet and "puffy eyes," which have been getting worse for the past 2 days. Her blood pressure is 150/95, compared with her usual blood pressure of 130/70. After resting for 30 minutes, her blood pressure is 145/85. Her dipstick urinary protein is 1 to 2+. She reports daily fetal movement that has not changed and denies headache, abdominal pain,or dizzy spells. Your initial diagnosis is
a. PIH
b. mild preeclampsia
c. severe preeclampsia
d. chronic hypertension
e. chronic hypertension with superimposed PIH

Answers

| 17.41 | b | 17.42 | d | 17.43 | d | 17.44 | b |

17.45 A 26-year-old G1 at 39 weeks' gestational age presents in early labor, with contractions every 4 to 5 minutes, dilated to 5 cm, and effaced to 90% with the fetal head at zero station. She has been at home for 2 weeks on bed rest and with a diagnosis of mild preeclampsia (blood pressures ranging from 140 to 150/80 to 90 after the start of bed rest). Because of her mild preeclampsia and concerns about the quality of her uteroplacental function, a fetal scalp clip is placed and the fetal heart rate pattern is reassuring. Two hours after admission, the patient suddenly becomes unresponsive and seizes. Which of the following is NOT part of initial management for this patient?
a. Immediate cesarean delivery
b. Intravenous magnesium sulfate administration
c. Injury prevention precautions, including insertion of a tongue blade
d. Placement of a Foley catheter

17.46 Which of the following potential causes of maternal vasospasm is NOT associated with hypertensive disease in pregnancy?
a. Inadequate maternal vascular response
b. Increased platelet activation
c. Increased prostacyclin relative to thromboxane.
d. Decreased concentrations of nitric oxide.
e. Decreased levels of lipid peroxides and free radicals.

17.47 All of the following are associated with the common pathphysiologic changes in preeclamptics EXCEPT
a. persistent antiotensin II sensitivity
b. increased maternal plasma oncotic pressure
c. glomeular endotheliosis
d. pulmonary capillary leak
e. third spacing of fluid

17.48 The vasospastic process associated with preeclampsia generally begins to reverse itself in
a. 4 to 8 hours
b. 8 to 16 hours
c. 24 to 48 hours
d. 48 to 72 hours

17.49 Transient uterine activity typically spontaneously resolves up to how many minutes after an eclamptic seizure?
a. 5
b. 15
c. 35
d. 75
e. 155

17.50 Nonreassuring fetal heart rate changes continuing for more than how many minutes after an eclamptic seizure should engender emergency delivery?
a. 5
b. 10
c. 20
d. 40
e. 80

Answers

17.45	a	**17.46**	c	**17.47**	b	**17.48**	c	**17.49**	b	**17.50**	c

Questions and Answers Chapter 18: Multifetal Gestation

18.1 What is the incidence in the general population of monozygotic twins?
a. 1 in 3 pregnancies
b. 1 in 12 pregnancies
c. 1 in 90 pregnancies
d. 1 in 250 pregnancies
e. 1 in 500 pregnancies

18.2 What is the incidence in the general population of dizygotic twins?
a. 1 in 3 pregnancies
b. 1 in 12 pregnancies
c. 1 in 90 pregnancies
d. 1 in 250 pregnancies
e. 1 in 500 pregnancies

18.3 What is the incidence of twinning after clomiphene citrate induction of ovulation?
a. 1 in 3 pregnancies
b. 1 in 12 pregnancies
c. 1 in 90 pregnancies
d. 1 in 250 pregnancies
e. 1 in 500 pregnancies

18.4 What is the incidence of twinning after in vitro fertilization using several fertilized ova?
a. 1 in 3 pregnancies
b. 1 in 12 pregnancies
c. 1 in 90 pregnancies
d. 1 in 250 pregnancies
e. 1 in 500 pregnancies

18.5 The overall incidence of recognized twins in the United States is almost
a. 1%
b. 3%
c. 5%
d. 7%
e. 9%

18.6 The rate of twinning in the population is
a. increasing
b. stable
c. decreasing

18.7 Which of the following statements about monozygotic twinning is correct?
a. It results from two separate ova that are fertilized by two separate sperm
b. It results from the division of a single fertilized ovum
c. The incidence is variable around the world
d. Increasing parity is an independent factor

18.8 Which of the following statements about dyzygotic twinning is correct?
a. The incidence is fairly consistent around the world
b. The incidence, on average, is approximately 0.005%
c. Increasing age is an independent factor
d. Twinning follows the paternal lineage

18.9 Twinning within 3 days of fertilization will likely result in what organization of the fetal membranes?
a. Conjoined twins
b. Monoamniotic/monochorionic
c. Diamniotic/dichorionic
d. Diamniotic/monochorionic

18.10 Twinning between 4 and 8 days of fertilization will likely result in what organization of the fetal membranes?
a. Conjoined twins
b. Monoamniotic/monochorionic
c. Diamniotic/dichorionic
d. Diamniotic/monochorionic

18.11 Twinning between 9 and 12 days of fertilization will likely result in what organization of the fetal membranes?
a. Conjoined twins
b. Monoamniotic/monochorionic
c. Diamniotic/dichorionic
d. Diamniotic/monochorionic

Answers

18.1	d	**18.3**	b	**18.5**	b	**18.7**	b	**18.9**	c	**18.11**	b
18.2	c	**18.4**	a	**18.6**	a	**18.8**	c	**18.10**	d		

18.12 Twinning 12 days or more after fertilization will likely result in what organization of the fetal membranes?
a. Conjoined twins
b. Monoamniotic/monochorionic
c. Diamniotic/dichorionic
d. Diamniotic/monochorionic

18.13 Approximately what percent of twin pregnancies detected in the first trimester results in delivery of viable twins?
a. 30%
b. 50%
c. 70%
d. 90%

18.14 The percent of monozygotic gestations will result in a diamniotic monochorionic arrangement of the fetal membranes is about
a. 1 to 5%
b. 20 to 30%
c. 50 to 60%
d. 70 to 80%

18.15 Which of the following is NOT more commonly associated with multiple pregnancies?
a. Megaloblastic anemia
b. Fetal macrosomia
c. Vasa previa
d. Congenital anomalies
e. Polyhydramnios

18.16 Multifetal pregnancy is associated with an increased incidence of all of the following EXCEPT
a. perinatal morbidity
b. fetomaternal hemorrhage
c. intrauterine growth restriction
d. umbilical cord prolapse
e. postpartum hemorrhage

18.17 The perinatal morbidity in twin gestation is how many times higher than for a comparable singleton pregnancy?
a. 1 to 2 times
b. 3 to 4 times
c. 4 to 5 times
d. 5 to 6 times
e. 7 to 8 times

18.18 In monozygotic twins, oligohydramnios and anemia of one twin and hydramnios with polycythemia of the other twin are caused by
a. congenital anomalies of the fetus
b. vascular anastomoses between the fetuses
c. umbilical cord compression
d. maternal diabetes

18.19 A familial factor is present in twinning that follows the
a. maternal lineage
b. paternal lineage
c. both maternal and paternal lineages
d. neither the maternal nor the paternal lineages

18.20 The average time of delivery in a singleton pregnancy is
a. 25 weeks
b. 29 weeks
c. 33 weeks
d. 37 weeks
e. 40 weeks

18.21 The average time of delivery in a twin pregnancy is
a. 25 weeks
b. 29 weeks
c. 33 weeks
d. 37 weeks
e. 40 weeks

Answers

18.12	a	18.14	d	18.16	b	18.18	b	18.20	e
18.13	b	18.15	b	18.17	b	18.19	a	18.21	d

18.22 The average time of delivery in a triplet pregnancy is
a. 25 weeks
b. 29 weeks
c. 33 weeks
d. 37 weeks
e. 40 weeks

18.23 The average time of delivery in a quadruplet pregnancy is
a. 25 weeks
b. 29 weeks
c. 33 weeks
d. 37 weeks
e. 40 weeks

18.24 A twin pregnancy in which one twin is characterized by impaired growth, anemia, and hypovolemia and the other twin by hypervolemia, hypertension, polycythemia, and congestive heart failure is defined as
a. conjoined twin syndrome
b. twin–twin transfusion syndrome
c. single umbilical artery syndrome
d. congenital rubella syndrome
e. twin–twin isoimmunization syndrome

18.25 Multifetal pregnancy is associated with an increased risk of all of the following EXCEPT
a. maternal diabetes
b. preeclampsia
c. preterm labor
d. preterm delivery

18.26 The differential diagnosis for multifetal gestation at 34 weeks of gestational age by dates includes all of the following EXCEPT
a. polyhydramnios
b. hydatiform mole
c. uterine leiomyoma
d. ovarian mass

18.27 Diagnosis of multiple gestation is usually made by
a. ultrasound
b. Leopold maneuvers
c. pelvic examination
d. fundal height measurement
e. amniography

18.28 What is the chief antenatal assessment used to evaluate the progress of twin pregnancy?
a. Periodic fundal height measurements
b. Serial ultrasonography
c. Periodic pelvic examination
d. Serial urinary estriols

18.29 In multiple gestations, periodic ultrasonography is done approximately every 4 weeks beginning at
a. 16 weeks
b. 20 weeks
c. 24 weeks
d. 28 weeks
e. 32 weeks

18.30 What percent difference in weight between the larger and the smaller fetus defines discordant growth?
a. 10%
b. 20%
c. 30%
d. 40%

18.31 Antenatal concerns in twin pregnancies include all of the following EXCEPT:
a. adequate nutrition
b. pregnancy-induced hypertension
c. postterm morbidity
d. inadequate fetal growth

18.32 Intrapartum management of twin pregnancies at term is usually determined by
a. gestational age
b. presentation of the twins
c. local custom
d. size of the twins

Answers

18.22	c	18.24	b	18.26	b	18.28	b	18.30	b	18.32	b
18.23	b	18.25	a	18.27	a	18.29	b	18.31	c		

18.33 A single umbilical artery is seen in approximately what percent of twins?
a. 1 to 2%
b. 3 to 4%
c. 5 to 6%
d. 7 to 8%
e. 9 to 10%

18.34 The most significant cause of morbidity in multifetal pregnancy is
a. intrauterine growth restriction
b. placental and umbilical cord accidents
c. preterm labor and delivery
d. polyhydramnios
e. postpartum hemorrhage

18.35 In all twin deliveries, in what percent of cases is the presentation of the second twin NOT cephalic?
a. 10%
b. 20%
c. 30%
d. 40%
e. 50%

18.36 At 32 weeks of gestation, a 35-year-old G1 P0 with known twins is noted to have a fundal height not consistent with known gestational age. Her weight gain and blood pressure are normal, as are her antenatal laboratory studies. She says that the babies are moving normally and that she feels well, although "rather large." Which of the following interventions is indicated?
a. Oxytocin challenge test
b. Ultrasound and nonstress test
c. Induction of labor if there is a cephalic/cephalic presentation
d. Immediate cesarean delivery

18.37 Chorionicity can first be determined at approximately how many weeks of gestational age?
a. 5 to 6
b. 7 to 8
c. 9 to 10
d. 11 to 12
e. 13 to 14

18.38 Vanishing twin syndrome is seen in approximately what percent of twin pregnancies detected by ultrasound early in the first trimester?
a. <10%
b. 25%
c. 50%
d. 75%
e. >90%

18.39 In vitro fertilization programs, the percent of pregnancies with two or more fetuses is presently reported at
a. 5 to 10%
b. 15 to 20%
c. 25 to 30%
d. 35 to 40%
e. 45 to 50%

18.40 With each additional fetus in multifetal pregnancies, the length of gestation decreases by approximately how many weeks?
a. 2
b. 4
c. 6
d. 8
e. 10

Answers

18.33	b	18.35	d	18.37	c	18.39	d
18.34	c	18.36	b	18.38	c	18.40	b

Questions and Answers Chapter 19: Fetal Growth Abnormalities

19.1 Intrauterine growth restriction (IUGR) is defined as a fetus whose weight is at or below what percentile of the normal population?
a. Fifth
b. Tenth
c. Fifteenth
d. Twentieth

19.2 Intrauterine growth restriction is based on weight for a
a. given parity
b. specific gestational age
c. specific population
d. specific fetal gender

19.3 About what proportion of stillborn infants are growth-restricted?
a. 1 in 6
b. 1 in 3
c. 2 in 3
d. 5 in 6

19.4 The normal fetus grows throughout pregnancy, but the rate of growth falls off after what gestational age?
a. 39 weeks
b. 37 weeks
c. 35 weeks
d. 33 weeks
e. 31 weeks

19.5 The placenta grows early and rapidly compared with the fetus, reaching a maximum surface area at about how many weeks of gestational age?
a. 39 weeks
b. 37 weeks
c. 35 weeks
d. 33 weeks
e. 31 weeks

19.6 After the placenta has reached maximal surface area, there is a slow but steady decline, primarily because of
a. decreased distribution of cardiac output to the uterus at term
b. increased fetal vascular resistance
c. resorption of the placental collagen matrix
d. microinfarctions of the placental vascular system

19.7 A fetus with IUGR is at higher risk for all of the following EXCEPT
a. neonatal death
b. meconium aspiration
c. hyperglycemia
d. asphyxia during labor

19.8 Early onset IUGR is associated with all of the following EXCEPT
a. irreversible reduction in organ size
b. reversible decrease in cell size
c. genetic factors
d. immunologic abnormalities

19.9 Delayed onset IUGR is associated with
a. uteroplacental insufficiency
b. irreversible reduction in organ size
c. genetic factors
d. immunologic abnormalities

19.10 All of the following are causes of IUGR EXCEPT
a. recent onset of maternal diabetes
b. smoking
c. hypertension
d. fetal rubella

19.11 The most common maternal factor associated with IUGR is
a. hypertensive disease
b. inadequate nutrition
c. alcohol use
d. drug use
e. smoking

Answers

19.1	b	19.3	b	19.5	b	19.7	c	19.9	a	19.11 a
19.2	b	19.4	b	19.6	d	19.8	b	19.10	a	

19.12 Congenital anomalies account for what percent of all cases of IUGR?
a. 5%
b. 10%
c. 15%
d. 35%
e. 45%

19.13 Biparietal diameter appropriate for dates is associated with
a. asymmetric IUGR
b. symmetric IUGR
c. both asymmetric and symmetric IUGR

19.14 Normal or low amniotic fluid volume is associated with
a. asymmetric IUGR
b. symmetric IUGR
c. both asymmetric and symmetric IUGR

19.15 Head-to-abdominal circumference ratio (I IC/AC ratio) >95th percentile is associated with
a. asymmetric IUGR
b. symmetric IUGR
c. both asymmetric and symmetric IUGR

19.16 Biparietal diameter smaller than expected-for dates is associated with
a. asymmetric IUGR
b. symmetric IUGR
c. both asymmetric and symmetric IUGR

19.17 Low amniotic fluid volume is associated with
a. asymmetric IUGR
b. symmetric IUGR
c. both asymmetric and symmetric IUGR

19.18 Head-to-abdominal circumference ratio in normal range is associated with
a. asymmetric IUGR
b. symmetric IUGR
c. both asymmetric and symmetric IUGR

19.19 Asymmetrical IUGR is associated with
a. equal decrease in the size of structures
b. congenital anomalies
c. hypertension
d. early intrauterine infection

19.20 Assessment of IUGR by ultrasound includes all of the following EXCEPT
a. fetal Doppler measurement
b. evaluation of fetal growth
c. evaluation for fetal anomalies
d. percutaneous umbilical blood sampling for genetic evaluation
e. evaluation for amniotic fluid volume

19.21 Compared with asymmetric IUGR, morbidity with symmetrical IUGR is
a. greater
b. the same
c. less

19.22 An efficient screening procedure for IUGR is
a. clinical estimations of fetal weight
b. serial fundal height measurements
c. maternal weight gain
d. maternal blood pressure measurements

19.23 The most useful initial evaluation of IUGR is serial
a. obstetric ultrasound
b. maternal weight measurement
c. fundal height measurement
d. nonstress testing
e. biophysical profile testing

19.24 To monitor the extent of growth restriction, ultrasound evaluation should be carried out every
a. 1 to 2 weeks
b. 2 to 3 weeks
c. 3 to 4 weeks
d. 4 to 5 weeks
e. 5 to 6 weeks

Answers

19.12 b	19.15 a	19.18 b	19.21 a	19.24 c
19.13 a	19.16 b	19.19 c	19.22 b	
19.14 b	19.17 a	19.20 c	19.23 c	

19.25 In patients with suspected IUGR and uncertain dates, what ultrasonographic measurement may be useful in establishing gestational age?
a. Biparietal diameter
b. Intraorbital diameter
c. Cerebrum diameter
d. Cerebellum diameter
e. Femur length

19.26 Compared with IUGR alone, a case of IUGR with oligohydramnios is likely to have what type of outcome?
a. Worse
b. Unchanged
c. Improved

19.27 Amniocentesis allows which of the following direct studies to be accomplished?
a. Chromosomal analysis
b. Viral cultures
c. Immunoglobulin studies
d. Acid-base studies

19.28 Percutaneous umbilical blood sampling allows for all of the following direct fetal studies EXCEPT
a. chromosomal analysis
b. viral cultures
c. evaluation of free floating fibroblasts
d. immunoglobulin studies
e. oxygenation and acid-base studies

19.29 Chorionic villus sampling allows for which of the following direct fetal studies?
a. Chromosomal analysis
b. Viral culture
c. Oxygenation studies
d. Acid-base studies

19.30 Bed rest is often recommended for patients with IUGR to
a. regulate fetal heart rate
b. increase uteroplacental blood flow
c. decrease maternal metabolic activity
d. decrease maternal catecholamine release

19.31 Which of the following may be used to evaluate fetal well-being in cases of IUGR?
a. Fetal "kick-counts"
b. Nonstress test
c. Biophysical profile
d. Doppler ultrasound of blood flow through the umbilical cord
e. All of the above

19.32 Hyperviscosity syndrome associated with IUGR is defined as a fetal hematocrit of more than
a. 35%
b. 45%
c. 55%
d. 65%
e. 75%

19.33 Hyperviscosity syndrome in IUGR is associated with all of the following EXCEPT
a. a lower-than-normal fetal hematocrit
b. multiorgan thrombosis
c. heart failure
d. hyperbilirubinemia

19.34 Which of the following is useful in the treatment of fetal heart rate deceleration in a patient with IUGRand oligohydramnios?
a. Pitocin augmentation
b. Amnioinfusion
c. Intravenous fluids
d. Blood transfusion

19.35 Growth-restricted newborns have difficulty maintaining euglycemia because they
a. have less fat deposition in late pregnancy
b. have relative hyperthyroid status
c. have a low hematocrit
d. have hyperbilirubinemia

Answers

19.25 d	19.27 a	19.29 a	19.31 e	19.33 a	19.35 a
19.26 a	19.28 c	19.30 b	19.32 d	19.34 b	

19.36 Fetal macrosomia is defined as weight greater than how many grams?
a. 3,000
b. 4,000
c. 5,000

19.37 A definition of macrosomia is a fetal weight above what percentile for gestational age?
a. 70th
b. 80th
c. 90th

19.38 All of the following can be consequences of fetal macrosomia EXCEPT
a. prolonged second stage of labor
b. hypothermia
c. shoulder dystocia
d. intrapartum fetal injury

19.39 Which of the following should be included in the differential diagnosis of a larger-than-expected uterine size?
a. Large but normal fetus
b. Polyhydramnios
c. Uterine leiomyomata
d. Multiple pregnancy
e. All of the above

19.40 Recommended weight gain in pregnancy is approximately how many pounds?
a. 20 to 30
b. 25 to 35
c. 30 to 40
d. 35 to 45
e. 40 to 50

19.41 In a diabetic mother, the development of fetal macrosomia is thought to be caused by transfer of
a. glucose from mother to fetus
b. insulin from fetus to mother
c. growth hormone from mother to fetus
d. insulin from mother to fetus

19.42 Which of the following is NOT a risk factor for fetal macrosomia?
a. Preeclampsia
b. Maternal diabetes
c. Excessive maternal weight gain
d. Maternal obesity

19.43 Which of the following represents current American College of Obstetricians and Gynecologists recommendations for primary cesarean delivery based on sonographic estimation of fetal weight?
a. Greater than 4,500 g for a woman with diabetes; >5000 g for a woman without diabetes
b. Greater than 4,250 g for a woman with diabetes; >4500 g, for a woman without diabetes
c. Greater than 4,000 g for a woman with diabetes; >4500 g for a woman without diabetes

Answers

19.36 b	**19.38** b	**19.40** b	**19.42** a
19.37 c	**19.39** e	**19.41** b	**19.43** a

Questions and Answers Chapter 20: Third-Trimester Bleeding

20.1 Approximately what percent of women will experience bleeding at some time during the second or third trimesters of pregnancy?
a. 5%
b. 10%
c. 15%
d. 20%
e. 25%

20.2 Bleeding in the second half of pregnancy can come from which of the following sources?
a. Vaginal tears or lacerations
b. Cervical carcinoma
c. Cervicitis
d. All of the above

20.3 An 18-year-old primigravida at term, not in labor, has sudden onset of severe continuous lower abdominal pain with a rapid pulse, low blood pressure, fetal bradycardia, and a tender abdomen. Which of the following is the most likely diagnosis?
a. Abruptio placentae
b. Placenta previa
c. Uterine rupture
d. Amniotic fluid embolus
e. Supine hypotensive syndrome

20.4 A primigravida at term has profuse vaginal bleeding. Fetal heart tones are normal. The cervix is 2 to 3 cm dilated with an edge of placenta palpable. Which of the following is the most appropriate treatment?
a. Voorhees bag
b. Braxton Hicks version
c. Cesarean delivery
d. Rupture of the fetal membranes to stimulate delivery
e. Replace blood loss and await vaginal delivery

20.5 All of the following are associated with massive placental abruption EXCEPT
a. painless vaginal bleeding
b. uterine rigidity
c. uterine pain
d. maternal cardiovascular collapse
e. absent fetal heart sounds

20.6 Vasa previa diagnosed in early labor is best treated with
a. Voorhees bag
b. forceps delivery
c. spontaneous delivery
d. cesarean section
e. Willett clamp

20.7 Which of the following best describes complete or total placenta previa?
a. The margin of the placenta extends across part but not all of the internal os
b. The entire cervical os is covered by the placenta
c. The placenta is located near but not directly adjacent to the internal os
d. The edge of the placenta lies adjacent to the internal os

20.8 Which of the following best describes partial placenta previa?
a. The margin of the placenta extends across part but not all of the internal os
b. The entire cervical os is covered by the placenta
c. The placenta is located near but not directly adjacent to the internal os
d. The edge of the placenta lies adjacent to the internal os

Answers

20.1	a	20.3	a	20.5	a	20.7	b
20.2	d	20.4	c	20.6	d	20.8	a

20.9 Which of the following best describes marginal placenta previa?
a. The margin of the placenta extends across part but not all of the internal os
b. The entire cervical os is covered by the placenta
c. The placenta is located near but not directly adjacent to the internal os
d. The edge of the placenta lies adjacent to the internal os

20.10 Which of the following best describes low-lying placenta previa?
a. The margin of the placenta extends across part but not all of the internal os
b. The entire cervical os is covered by the placenta
c. The placenta is located near but not directly adjacent to the internal os
d. The edge of the placenta lies adjacent to the internal os

20.11 All of the following factors are associated with placenta previa EXCEPT
a. increasing maternal age
b. increasing parity
c. previous cesarean section
d. presence of a twin pregnancy
e. maternal hypertension

20.12 What is the frequency of placenta previa?
a. 1 in 100
b. 1 in 250
c. 1 in 500
d. 1 in 1,000
e. 1 in 1,500

20.13 Compared with multiparas, the incidence of placenta previa in nulliparas is
a. lower
b. the same
c. greater

20.14 In placenta previa, the first bleeding episode occurs most commonly at what gestational age?
a. 23 to 24 weeks
b. 25 to 26 weeks
c. 27 to 28 weeks
d. 29 to 30 weeks
e. 31 to 32 weeks

20.15 Placenta previa is coincident with abruptio placentae in approximately what percent of cases?
a. Less than 5%
b. 10%
c. 20%
d. 40%

20.16 Transvaginal ultrasonography is especially useful in the diagnosis of what type of placenta previa?
a. Anterior
b. Lateral
c. Posterior
d. All types of placenta previa

20.17 The initial management of a patient with placenta previa and a bleeding episode always includes which of the following?
a. Hospitalization
b. Immediate cesarean section
c. Immediate Pitocin induction of labor
d. Blood transfusion

20.18 Which of the following are criteria for outpatient care of a patient with known placenta previa?
a. Highly motivated patient
b. Evidence of understanding of and compliance with instructions
c. Immediate access to the hospital
d. All of the above

Answers

20.9	d	20.11	e	20.13	a	20.15	b	20.17	a
20.10	c	20.12	b	20.14	d	20.16	d	20.18	d

20.19 What is the current perinatal morality rate associated with placenta previa?
a. less than 10%
b. 15%
c. 20%
d. 30%
e. 40%

20.20 Vaginal delivery with known placenta previa may be indicated if
a. the fetus is dead
b. there are major fetal malformations, leading to likely fetal demise
c. the pregnancy is clearly previable
d. the placental location and stage of labor are such that it is anticipated that vaginal delivery can be accomplished with a relatively small blood loss
e. all of the above

20.21 Compared with that of all pregnancies, what is the incidence of congenital anomalies in cases of placenta previa?
a. The same
b. Twice as high
c. Three times as high
d. Four times as high

20.22 In placenta previa accreta, the trophoblastic tissue invades the
a. cervix
b. lower uterine segment
c. vaginal wall
d. mesosalpinx

20.23 Which of the following are common to both placenta previa and abruptio placentae?
a. Vaginal bleeding
b. Abdominal discomfort
c. Painful uterine contractions
d. Presence of a normal fetal heart rate

20.24 Placental abruption is defined as
a. abnormal position of the placenta
b. abnormal separation of the normally implanted placenta
c. abnormal morphology of the placenta

20.25 Placental abruption is associated with
a. maternal hypertension
b. polyhydramnios
c. maternal trauma
d. maternal cocaine use
e. all of the above

20.26 Couvelaire uterus is associated with
a. placenta previa
b. abruptio placentae
c. vasa previa
d. all of the above

20.27 The diagnosis of placental abruption is made primarily by
a. clinical presentation and evaluation
b. ultrasound
c. amniocentesis
d. laboratory evaluation

20.28 Which of the following is present in packed red blood cells (RBCs)?
a. Fibrinogen, factors VII and XIII
b. RBCs only
c. All procoagulants, no platelets
d. RBCs and all procoagulants

20.29 Which of the following is present on fresh-frozen plasma?
a. Fibrinogen, factors VII and XIII
b. RBCs only
c. All procoagulants, no platelets
d. RBCs and all procoagulants

20.30 Which of the following is present in cryoprecipitate?
a. Fibrinogen, factors VII and XIII
b. RBCs only
c. All procoagulants, no platelets
d. RBCs and all procoagulants

Answers

20.19	a	20.21	b	20.23	a	20.25	e	20.27	a	20.29	c
20.20	e	20.22	b	20.24	b	20.26	b	20.28	b	20.30	a

20.31 Which of the following is present in fresh whole blood?
  a. Fibrinogen, factors VII and XIII
  b. RBCs only
  c. All procoagulants, no platelets
  d. RBCs and all procoagulants

20.32 All of the following are included in the "classic clinical presentation" of abruptio placentae EXCEPT
  a. vaginal bleeding
  b. tender uterus
  c. frequent painful uterine contractions
  d. normal fetal heart rate

20.33 In vasa previa, the umbilical cord inserts into the
  a. central mass of the placenta
  b. membranes of the placenta
  c. internal os
  d. endocervix

20.34 Which of the following tests is useful in differentiating maternal blood from fetal blood?
  a. Kleihauer-Betke
  b. Coombs
  c. Venereal Disease Research Laboratory (VDRL)
  d. Lee-White

20.35 What is the appropriate treatment for ruptured vasa previa?
  a. Augmentation of labor
  b. Tocolysis
  c. Immediate cesarean delivery
  d. Periumbilical artery transfusion

20.36 In the absence of massive blood loss, coagulation defects are most common in which of the following?
  a. Abruptio placentae
  b. Placenta previa
  c. Vasa previa
  d. Routine labor

20.37 Which of the following is associated with uterine scar dehiscence?
  a. Fetal bradycardia
  b. Separation of the placenta
  c. Fetus remains in utero
  d. Nonreassuring fetal status

20.38 Which of the following is NOT characteristic of uterine rupture?
  a. Fetal bradycardia
  b. Nonreassuring fetal status
  c. Separation of the placenta
  d. Minimal bleeding

20.39 Uterine rupture is associated with nonreassuring fetal status in about what percent of cases?
  a. 1 to 25%
  b. 25 to 50%
  c. 50 to 75%
  d. 75 to 100%

20.40 Because of the risk of uterine rupture in a woman with a previous uterine rupture involving the upper uterine segment, repeat cesarean section is usually recommended at a gestational age of
  a. 30 to 31 weeks
  b. 33 to 34 weeks
  c. 36 to 37 weeks
  d. 39 to 40 weeks

20.41 What is the overall incidence of uterine rupture in a woman with a previous uncomplicated lower segment transverse cesarean section?
  a. 0.5%
  b. 2.5%
  c. 4.5%
  d. 6.5%

Answers

20.31	d	20.33	b	20.35	c	20.37	c	20.39	c	20.41	a
20.32	d	20.34	a	20.36	a	20.38	d	20.40	c		

20.42 A 26-year-old G1 at 26 weeks' gestation phones saying that she had an episode of bright red vaginal bleeding without other symptoms 2 hours ago. You have not seen her previously. What should be your instruction to her?

a. Call back if there is another bleeding episode
b. Come in now for an evaluation
c. Make an office appointment
d. Make an appointment for an ultrasound evaluation

20.43 The initial management of a patient with third-trimester bleeding should include all of the following EXCEPT

a. uterine contraction monitoring
b. fetal heart rate monitoring
c. utrasound evaluation
d. digital examination of the cervix
e. assessment of maternal vital signs

20.44 A 26-year-old G6 P5005 presents for a routine antepartum visit at 18 weeks' gestational age. At her ultrasound visit the day before, she was told by the technician that her placenta was partly over the cervix. You should tell the patient that she has a

a. placenta previa and will definitely require cesarean section
b. placenta previa and may require cesarean section
c. vasa previa and will definitely require cesarean section
d. vasa previa and may require cesarean section

20.45 A 31-year-old G3 P1011 who believes she is approximately 8 months pregnant presents complaining of bright red vaginal bleeding and some cramps for the last hour. On questioning, you learn she has had no prenatal care and was in a drug rehabilitation program but left a few weeks ago. On examination, she is normotensive, has a fundal height of 30 cm, and a slightly tender uterus. She has irregular uterine contractions and a baseline fetal heart rate of 150 with good beat-to-beat variability. Ultrasound shows a 30-week gestation with adequate amniotic fluid and a fundal placenta without evidence of placenta previa or abruptio placentae. Urine drug screen is positive for cocaine. Careful pelvic examination by speculum shows her cervix to be closed with minimal bleeding and no evidence of rupture of membranes. Your most likely diagnosis is

a. Labor
b. Abruptio placentae
c. Placenta previa
d. Cervicitis
e. Cervical carcinoma

Answers

| 20.42 | b | 20.43 | d | 20.44 | b | 20.45 | b |

Questions and Answers Chapter 21: Postterm Pregnancy

21.1 A normal pregnancy is defined to last from about 38 weeks to how many weeks?
a. 40
b. 41
c. 42
d. 43
e. 44

21.2 A patient is considered postterm if she has not delivered by the end of what week from the first day of the last menstrual period?
a. 40
b. 41
c. 42
d. 43
e. 44

21.3 If a patient's due date is November 11, she would be defined as postterm on
a. November 18
b. November 25
c. November 12
d. December 2

21.4 Postterm pregnancy occurs in what percent of pregnancies?
a. 8 to 10%
b. 11 to 13%
c. 14 to 16%
d. 17 to 19%
e. 20 to 22%

21.5 Approximately what percent of patients having one postterm pregnancy will have a prolonged pregnancy with their next gestation?
a. 0%
b. 25%
c. 50%
d. 75%
e. 100%

21.6 What is the most common "cause" of postterm pregnancy?
a. Anencephaly
b. Placental sulfatase deficiency
c. Inaccurate date
d. Extrauterine pregnancy

21.7 Which of the following "causes" of postterm pregnancy is associated with altered estrogen production?
a. Inaccurate dates
b. Anencephaly
c. Extrauterine pregnancy

21.8 Which of the following statements about the dysmaturity (postmaturity) syndrome is INCORRECT?
a. It occurs in approximately one-fifth of true postterm pregnancies
b. It is associated with fetal growth restriction
c. Integumentary changes (scaling epidermis, meconium staining) are seen
d. Increased amounts of subcutaneous fat are common

21.9 In macrosomia associated with postterm pregnancy, all of the following are likely to be present EXCEPT
a. hyperglycemia
b. hyperbilirubinemia
c. shoulder dystocia
d. fetopelvic disproportion

21.10 Postterm pregnancy may be associated with
a. increased incidence of fetal compromise
b. placental dysfunction
c. meconium aspiration
d. oligohydramnios
e. all of the above

Answers

| 21.1 | c | 21.3 | a | 21.5 | c | 21.7 | b | 21.9 | a |
| 21.2 | b | 21.4 | c | 21.6 | b | 21.8 | a | 21.10 | d |

21.11 Dysmature newborns may demonstrate altered glucose and bilirubin metabolism, and are at risk for:
a. hyperglycemia and hypobiliru-binemia
b. hyperglycemia and hyperbiliru-binemia
c. hypoglycemia and hypobiliru-binemia
d. hypoglycemia and hyperbiliru-binemia

21.12 If, after rupture of membranes, meconium-stained amniotic fluid is discovered in the intrapartum patient, the next management step should be
a. immediate cesarean section
b. periumbilical blood gas measurement
c. amnioinfusion
d. fetal scalp blood sampling
e. close electronic monitoring of fetal status

21.13 In utero meconium passage is seen in about what percent of term pregnancies?
a. 15%
b. 25%
c. 35%
d. 45%
e. 55%

21.14 An amniotic fluid index of less than what value is usually considered to be consistent with oligohydramnios?
a. 2
b. 5
c. 8
d. 11

21.15 Brachial plexus injury is reported in what proportion of term deliveries?
a. 1 in 250
b. 1 in 500
c. 1 in 750
d. 1 in 1,000

21.16 Approximately what percent of placentas from postterm pregnancies demonstrate anatomic changes consistent with decreased functional capability?
a. 20%
b. 40%
c. 60%
d. 80%
e. 100%

21.17 What percent of placentas from postterm pregnancies demonstrate placental infarcts, calcifications, and fibrosis?
a. 20%
b. 40%
c. 60%
d. 80%

21.18 The management options of inducing labor or continuing to monitor fetal well-being should be considered once the patient approaches how many weeks of gestation?
a. 38
b. 39
c. 40
d. 41
e. 42

21.19 All of the following may be used to assess fetal well-being during a postterm pregnancy EXCEPT
a. daily fetal movement counts
b. biweekly nonstress testing
c. biweekly biophysical profile testing
d. weekly oxytocin challenge testing
e. ultrasound for biparietal diameter

21.20 Cesarean birth should be considered when the estimated fetal weight exceeds how many grams?
a. 3,500 to 4,000
b. 4,000 to 4,500
c. 4,500 to 5,000
d. 5,000 to 5,500

Answers

21.11	d	21.13	b	21.15	b	21.17	d	21.19	c
21.12	a	21.14	b	21.16	b	21.18	e	21.20	d

21.21 Which of the following can be used to induce labor in the postterm pregnancy?
 a. Oxytocin
 b. Prostaglandin vaginal suppository
 c. Laminaria
 d. All of the above

21.22 Erb palsy results in paralysis of which of the following muscles?
 a. Deltoid
 b. Infraspinatus
 c. Flexor muscles of the forearm
 d. All of the above

21.23 Paralysis of the hand is also termed
 a. Erb palsy
 b. Duchenne palsy
 c. Bell palsy
 d. Klumpke paralysis

21.24 Which of the following conditions is NOT associated with postterm pregnancy?
 a. Meconium passage
 b. Shoulder dystocia
 c. Placental dysfunction
 d. Maternal hypertension
 e. Macrosomia

Answers

21.21	d	**21.22**	d	**21.23**	d	**21.24**	d

Questions and Answers Chapter 22: Preterm Labor

22.1 Labor occurring prior to the completion of how many weeks of gestation (counted from the last menstrual period) is considered preterm labor?
a. 35
b. 36
c. 37
d. 38
e. 39

22.2 Of neonatal deaths that are not the result of congenital malformations, what percent are associated with premature labor and birth?
a. 25%
b. 50%
c. 75%
d. 100%

22.3 All of the following are predisposing factors for respiratory distress syndrome EXCEPT
a. short gestation
b. cesarean section
c. inaccurate gestational age estimation
d. maternal diabetes
e. grand multiparity

22.4 The 10% of babies born prematurely in the United States account for what percent of all perinatal morbidity and mortality?
a. 30 to 45%
b. 45 to 60%
c. 60 to 75%
d. 75 to 90%

22.5 An infant born at 30 weeks of gestation and weighing 2,600 g would be defined as
a. low birth weight
b. preterm
c. both low birth weight and preterm
d. neither low birth weight nor preterm

22.6 Preterm labor is functionally defined as the presence of regular uterine contractions, between 20 and 36 weeks' gestation, occurring with a frequency of
a. 5 minutes or less and lasting at least 30 seconds
b. 5 minutes or less and lasting at least 60 seconds
c. 10 minutes or less and lasting at least 30 seconds
d. 10 minutes or less and lasting at least 60 seconds

22.7 Premature birth is associated with all of the following perinatal complications EXCEPT
a. respiratory distress syndrome
b. intraventricular hemorrhage
c. skeletal abnormalities
d. sepsis
e. seizures

22.8 All of the following factors have been associated with preterm birth EXCEPT
a. maternal infections
b. maternal age
c. uterine distortion
d. placental abnormalities
e. substance abuse

22.9 Multiple gestations account for about what percent of preterm births?
a. 10%
b. 20%
c. 30%
d. 40%

22.10 If a patient's first pregnancy ends in preterm labor and delivery, her risk of preterm labor in a subsequent pregnancy is
a. unchanged
b. increased twofold
c. increased fourfold
d. increased sixfold

Answers									
22.1	c	22.3	e	22.5	b	22.7	c	22.9	a
22.2	c	22.4	c	22.6	c	22.8	b	22.10	b

22.11 All of the following indicators often precede preterm birth EXCEPT
a. increased uterine irritability
b. increased frequency of contractions
c. rapid weight gain
d. feeling of pelvic pressure

22.12 Which of the following are recognized signs and symptoms associated with preterm labor?
a. Low, dull backache
b. Pelvic pressure
c. Abdominal cramps
d. Change in vaginal discharge
e. All of the above

22.13 All of the following should be included in the evaluation of suspected preterm labor EXCEPT
a. status of the cervix
b. computed axial tomography scan for gestational age
c. electronic fetal monitor for frequency of contractions
d. abdominal palpation for strength of contractions

22.14 Which of the following laboratory studies is useful in the evaluation of a patient at risk for preterm labor?
a. Urinalysis and urine culture
b. Culture for β-streptococcus
c. Culture for *Neisseria gonorrhoeae*
d. Wet preparation for bacterial vaginosis
e. All of the above

22.15 Which of the following statements about fetal fibronectin (fFN) is incorrect?
a. It has been associated with preterm labor.
b. It is an extracellular glycoprotein normally found in the amniotic fluid in early pregnancy and then again near term.
c. A rise in the concentration of fFN may be associated with the impending onset of preterm labor.
d. Its absence is an indicator that delivery is unlikely in the 7 days after the sample is taken.

22.16 Which of the following is the mechanism of action of magnesium sulfate?
a. Increases cyclic adenosine monophosphate (cAMP) in cells, which decreases free calcium
b. Competes with calcium for entry into cells
c. Prevents calcium entry into muscle cells
d. Decreases prostaglandin production

22.17 Which of the following is the mechanism of action of β-Adrenergic agents, such as ritodrine or terbutaline?
a. Increase cAMP in cells, which decreases free calcium
b. Compete with calcium for entry into cells
c. Prevent calcium entry into muscle cells
d. Decrease prostaglandin production

22.18 Which of the following is the mechanism of action of prostaglandin-synthetase inhibitors, such as indomethacin?
a. Increase cAMP in cells, which decreases free calcium
b. Compete with calcium for entry into cells
c. Prevent calcium entry into muscle cells
d. Decrease prostaglandin production

22.19 Which of the following is the mechanism of action of calcium channel blockers, such as nifedipine?
a. Increase cAMP in cells, which decreases free calcium
b. Compete with calcium for entry into cells
c. Prevent calcium entry into muscle cells
d. Decrease prostaglandin production

Answers

22.11	c	22.13	b	22.15	b	22.17	a	22.19	c
22.12	e	22.14	e	22.16	b	22.18	d		

22.20 Which of the following is a possible complication of magnesium sulfate?
a. Maternal hypertension, tachycardia, anxiety, chest tightening, and electrocardiogram (ECG) changes
b. Premature constriction of ductus arteriosus, especially after 34 weeks' gestation
c. Maternal flushing and headache, respiratory depression at high doses
d. Possible decrease in uteroplacental blood flow with fetal hypoxia and hypercarbia

22.21 Which of the following is a possible complication of β-Adrenergic agents (ritodrine or terbutaline)?
a. Maternal hypertension, tachycardia, anxiety, chest tightening, and ECG changes
b. Premature constriction of ductus arteriosus, especially after 34 weeks' gestation
c. Maternal flushing and headache, respiratory depression at high doses
d. Possible decrease in uteroplacental blood flow with fetal hypoxia and hypercarbia

22.22 Which of the following is a possible complication of prostaglandin-synthetase inhibitors (indomethacin)?
a. Maternal hypertension, tachycardia, anxiety, chest tightening, and ECG changes
b. Premature constriction of ductus arteriosus, especially after 34 weeks' gestation
c. Maternal flushing and headache, respiratory depression at high doses
d. Possible decrease in uteroplacental blood flow with fetal hypoxia and hypercarbia

22.23 Which of the following is a possible complication of calcium channel blockers?
a. Maternal hypertension, tachycardia, anxiety, chest tightening, and ECG changes
b. Premature constriction of ductus arteriosus, especially after 34 weeks' gestation
c. Maternal flushing and headache, respiratory depression at high doses
d. Possible decrease in uteroplacental blood flow with fetal hypoxia and hypercarbia

22.24 It is customary to stop tocolytic therapy at
a. 30 weeks
b. 32 weeks
c. 34 weeks
d. 36 weeks
e. 38 weeks

22.25 With regard to preterm labor, what is the tocolytic agent generally considered to have the highest degree of safety?
a. Terbutaline
b. Indomethacin
c. Magnesium sulfate
d. Nifedipine

22.26 In patients with preterm labor before 32 weeks' gestation, corticosteroids are often given to
a. decrease uterine activity
b. stabilize vascular membranes
c. enhance fetal lung maturity
d. prevent infection

22.27 What is the most common cause of perinatal morbidity and mortality?
a. Preterm birth resulting from preterm labor
b. Multiple gestation
c. Intrapartum asphyxia
d. Inadequate neonatal resuscitation

Answers

22.20	c	22.22	b	22.24	d	22.26	c	22.27	a
22.21	a	22.23	d	22.25	c				

22.28 Which of the following is NOT a surgically correctable cause of preterm birth?
a. incompetent cervix
b. uterine leiomyomas
c. septate uterus
d. vaginal stenosis

22.29 All of the following are related to excessive uterine enlargement that may lead to preterm birth EXCEPT
a. multiple gestation
b. leiomyomata uteri
c. hydramnios
d. incorrect menstrual dates

22.30 Which of the following are factors associated with preterm birth?
a. Placental abnormalities
b. Uterine distortion
c. Excessive uterine enlargement
d. All of the above

22.31 Which of the following statements about betamethasone therapy in preterm labor is incorrect?
a. It generally is administered when preterm delivery is expected within 7 days.
b. It generally is administered between 24 and 34 weeks of gestation.
c. It generally is administered as two 12-mg doses given 24 hours apart.
d. The benefits of administration include increased pulmonary volume and surfactant pool.

22.32 Which of the following is an indication for tocolysis?
a. Intrauterine infection
b. Multiple fetal anomalies
c. Regular uterine contractions and cervical effacement at 30 weeks' gestational age
d. Evidence of fetal maturity
e. All of the above

22.33 The presence of chorioamnionitis
a. is an indication for tocolysis
b. is contraindication to tocolysis
c. has no bearing on the decision to begin tocolysis

22.34 Maternal age greater than 35
a. is an indication for tocolysis
b. is a contraindication to tocolysis
c. has no bearing on the decision to begin tocolysis

22.35 A 29-year-old G4 P2103 presents at 30 weeks of gestational age complaining of painful uterine contractions for the past 2 hours and a sensation of pelvic fullness. Cervical examination shows that she is 3 cm dilated and 90% effaced. Her membranes are intact and there is cephalic presentation at zero station. On external fetal monitoring, she is having moderate-to-strong uterine contractions every 4 minutes. The fetal heart pattern is reassuring. Which of the following is NOT recommended at this time?
a. Perform an ultrasound to evaluate for fetal anomalies
b. Perform an amniocentesis
c. Perform UA, C&S, and cervical cultures
d. Administer intravenous fluids
e. Begin tocolysis with magnesium sulfate

22.36 Multiple gestations account for about what percent of births?
a. 1%
b. 2%
c. 4%
d. 8%

Answers

22.28	d	22.30	d	22.32	c	22.34	c	22.36	a
22.29	d	22.31	a	22.33	b	22.35	b		

Questions and Answers Chapter 23: Premature Rupture of Membranes

23.1 Amniotic fluid serves to protect against
   a. infection of the fetus
   b. fetal trauma
   c. umbilical cord compression
   d. all of the above

23.2 Premature rupture of membranes is defined as rupture of the chorioamniotic membrane
   a. before the onset of labor
   b. at the onset of labor
   c. during the active phase of labor
   d. before complete cervical effacement

23.3 Premature rupture of membranes occurs in what percent of all pregnancies?
   a. Less than 2%
   b. 2 to 5%
   c. 10 to 15%
   d. 20 to 25%

23.4 Premature rupture of membranes is associated with approximately what percent of term pregnancies (37 weeks' gestational age or more)?
   a. 10%
   b. 30%
   c. 50%
   d. 70%

23.5 Premature rupture of membranes is associated with approximately what percent of preterm deliveries?
   a. 15%
   b. 30%
   c. 45%
   d. 60%
   e. 75%

23.6 Midtrimester preterm premature rupture of membranes (between 16 and 26 weeks' gestational age) complicates about what percent of all pregnancies?
   a. 0.01%
   b. 0.1%
   c. 1.0%
   d. 10%

23.7 The most serious primary risk resulting from preterm premature rupture of membranes is
   a. chorioamnionitis
   b. cord compression
   c. preterm delivery
   d. abruptio placentae

23.8 Which of the following is NOT a risk factor for premature spontaneous rupture of membranes (PSROM)?
   a. Prior PSROM
   b. Prior preterm delivery
   c. Smoking
   d. Bleeding in early pregnancy
   e. Advanced maternal age

23.9 Which of the following can cause a false-negative Nitrazine test?
   a. Basic urine
   b. Presence of cervical mucus
   c. Blood contamination
   d. Earlier premature rupture of the membranes with no residual fluid
   e. All of the above

23.10 Which of the following is associated with a false-positive Nitrazine test?
   a. Presence of cervical mucus
   b. Presence of semen
   c. Blood contamination
   d. All of the above

23.11 The most common situation that can be confused at term with premature rupture of membranes is
   a. bloody show
   b. passage of cervical mucus
   c. intermittent urinary leakage
   d. yeast vaginitis

23.12 The Nitrazine test is used to assess for premature rupture of membranes based on the fact that amniotic fluid has
   a. a higher pH than vaginal secretions
   b. a lower pH than vaginal secretions
   d. a higher specific gravity than water
   e. a lower specific gravity than water

Answers

23.1	d	**23.3**	c	**23.5**	b	**23.7**	c	**23.9**	d	**23.11**	c
23.2	a	**23.4**	a	**23.6**	c	**23.8**	e	**23.10**	d	**23.12**	a

23.13 Of the following, which is the best indicator of intrauterine infection?
a. Presence of bacteria on Gram's stain of amniotic fluid
b. Presence of white cells in amniotic fluid
c. Decelerations of fetal heart tones
d. Onset of uterine contractions

23.14 Which of the following factors should be considered in developing a management plan for a patient with premature rupture of the membranes?
a. The gestational age at the time of rupture
b. The presence of uterine contractions
c. The amount of amniotic fluid around the fetus
d. All of the above

23.15 Premature rupture of the membranes presents the risks of pulmonary hypoplasia and amniotic band syndrome before what gestational age?
a. 25 weeks
b. 27 weeks
c. 29 weeks
d. 31 weeks

23.16 The expectant management of premature rupture of membranes in a fetus that is significantly preterm usually includes all of the following EXCEPT
a. daily white blood cell counts for the first few days
b. frequent ultrasound assessment for amniotic fluid volume
c. serial cervical digital examinations to detect the onset of labor
d. daily fetal movement monitoring
e. intermittent electronic monitoring

23.17 The diagnosis of rupture of membranes may be based on all of the following EXCEPT
a. Nitrazine test
b. patient history
c. white blood cell count
d. ultrasound findings

23.18 Which of the following mechanisms does NOT contribute to amniotic fluid production?
a. Fetal urine production
b. Fetal bowel movements
c. Fetal pulmonary effluent
d. Passage of fluid across the fetal membranes
e. Passage of fluid across the fetal skin

23.19 Between 28 weeks' gestational age and term, approximately what percent of patients with premature spontaneous rupture of membranes labor within 24 hours?
a. 40%
b. 50%
c. 60%
d. 70%
e. 80%

23.20 Between 28 weeks' gestational age and term, approximately what percent of patients with premature spontaneous rupture of membranes labor within 1 week?
a. 40%
b. 50%
c. 60%
d. 70%
e. 80%

23.21 Between 24 and 28 weeks' gestational age, approximately what percent of patients with premature spontaneous rupture of membranes labor within 1 week?
a. 40%
b. 50%
c. 60%
d. 70%
e. 80%

23.22 After 37 weeks' gestational age, spontaneous labor and delivery will occur in what percent of women within approximately 24 hours after premature rupture of the membranes?
a. 25%
b. 50%
c. 75%
d. 90%

Answers

23.13	a	23.15	a	23.17	b	23.19	b	23.21	b
23.14	d	23.16	c	23.18	b	23.20	e	23.22	d

23.23 Which of the following statements about premature rupture of membranes and chorioamnionitis is INCORRECT?
  a. Purulent discharge often precedes fever and uterine tenderness by several hours
  b. This situation often leads to tumultuous, spontaneous labor
  c. Fever >100.5°F is common
  d. This situation is often associated with fetal tachycardia
  e. Treatment consists of antibiotic therapy and prompt delivery

23.24 The differential diagnosis of premature rupture of the membranes includes
  a. urinary incontinence
  b. increased vaginal secretions in pregnancy
  c. vaginal discharge associated with vaginitis
  d. vesicovaginal fistula
  e. all of the above

23.25 Betamethasone therapy to enhance fetal lung maturity is generally recommended in preterm premature spontaneous rupture of membranes until approximately how many weeks of gestational age?
  a. 37 weeks
  b. 36 weeks
  c. 34 weeks
  d. 32 weeks
  e. 30 weeks

23.26 A 25-year-old G1 at 30 weeks of gestation presents with a history of "water leaking from my vagina" for the past 4 hours. Her pregnancy has been unremarkable except for a positive cervical culture of *Chlamydia trachomatis* at the time of her initial obstetric visit at 8 weeks of gestational age. The infection was treated and a repeat culture was negative. Which of the following should NOT be included in the initial evaluation of this patient?
  a. Sterile speculum examination
  b. Digital examination of the cervix
  c. External electronic fetal monitoring
  d. Cervical cultures for *Neisseria gonorrhoeae* and *C. trachomatis*
  e. Transabdominal ultrasonography

23.27 A 36-year-old infertility patient, who conceived after administration of clomiphene citrate and now is at 30 weeks of gestation presents with the history of a gush of fluid from her vagina about 1 hour ago. She now is feeling "little twinges" in her uterus. Speculum examination shows fluid coming from the cervical os, which is Nitrazine-positive. The cervix is approximately 1 cm dilated. On external fetal monitoring, the fetal heart rate is 170 and there are occasional uterine contractions. Her white blood count is 16,000/mm^3 and she is afebrile. Which of the following is NOT a likely problem in this case?
  a. Premature labor
  b. Intrauterine infection
  c. Pulmonary hypoplasia
  d. Fetal cord compression

Answers

23.23	a	23.24	e	23.25	d	23.26	b	23.27	c

Questions and Answers Chapter 24: Obstetric Procedures

24.1 Amniocentesis generally is associated with what risk of fetal loss?
a. 0.5%
b. 1.5%
c. 2.5%
d. 3.5%

24.2 Chorionic villus sampling is generally associated with what risk of fetal loss?
a. 0.5%
b. 1.5%
c. 2.5%
d. 3.5%

24.3 As compared with amniocentesis, chorionic villus sampling may first be performed
a. earlier in pregnancy
b. later in pregnancy
c. at the same time as amniocentesis

24.4 What is the role of obstetric forceps?
a. Replace the expulsive forces of the second stage of labor
b. Augment the expulsive forces of the second stage of labor
c. Augment the contractions of the first stage of labor
d. Overcome uterine inertia in the first stage of labor

24.5 Which type of obstetrical forceps is especially suited for a rotation of the fetal head?
a. Piper
b. Simpson
c. Kielland
d. All of the above

24.6 Which type of forceps is specially designed to facilitate the delivery of the "after-coming" head in vaginal breech deliveries?
a. Piper
b. Simpson
c. Kielland
d. All of the above

24.7 Which of the following tests may be performed by means of percutaneous umbilical blood sampling?
a. Blood count
b. Genetic status
c. Blood chemistries
d. All of the above

24.8 Currently, the cesarean delivery rate in the United States is about
a. 5 to 10%
b. 10 to 15%
c. 15 to 20%
d. 25 to 30%

24.9 Which type of uterine incision at the time of cesarean section is generally accepted to require cesarean section with subsequent pregnancies?
a. Low transverse
b. Low vertical
c. Classic

24.10 If there was a prior cesarean delivery with a classic incision, the risk of uterine rupture during labor in a subsequent pregnancy is approximately
a. 2%
b. 4%
c. 6%
d. 8%
e. 10%

24.11 The primary reason for circumcision of the male infant is
a. reduction of the prevalence of penile carcinoma
b. improved penile hygiene
c. social-religious considerations

24.12 Cesarean sections are generally classified by
a. the indication
b. the type of abdominal incision
c. the type of uterine incision
d. the stage of fetal maturity

Answers

24.1	a	24.3	a	24.5	c	24.7	d	24.9	c	24.11	c
24.2	a	24.4	b	24.6	c	24.8	d	24.10	d	24.12	c

24.13 When performed by an experienced, skilled operator, external cephalic version is successful about what percent of the time?
  a. 1 to 25%
  b. 25 to 50%
  c. 50 to 75%
  d. 75 to 100%

24.14 The criteria for vacuum-assisted vaginal delivery
  a. are the same as for forceps-assisted vaginal delivery
  b. similar to forceps-assisted vaginal delivery except that full dilation is not needed because the soft plastic cup does not tear the cervix as does the metallic forceps
  c. entirely different because of the nature of the soft vacuum cup allowing different placement than the rigid metallic forceps

24.15 Chorionic villus sampling carries approximately what percent risk of fetal loss?
  a. 0.01%
  b. 0.03%
  c. 0.05%
  d. 0.07%

Answers

24.13 c   **24.14** a   **24.15** c

Questions and Answers Chapter 25: Contraception

25.1 In assessing the effectiveness of various contraceptive methods, the "method failure rate" reflects the rate of failure when the method is
  a. used by a random sample of women
  b. tested in the laboratory
  c. used correctly 100% of the time
  d. compared with the use of no contraception at all

25.2 What is the primary mechanism of action of the interuterine device?
  a. Inhibit the development and release of the egg
  b. Impose a barrier between the sperm and the egg
  c. Alter the ability of the fertilized egg to implant and grow

25.3 What is the primary mechanism of action of contraceptive foam?
  a. Inhibit the development and release of the egg
  b. Impose a barrier between the sperm and the egg
  c. Alter the ability of the fertilized egg to implant and grow

25.4 What is the primary mechanism of action of oral contraceptives?
  a. Inhibit the development and release of the egg
  b. Impose a barrier between the sperm and the egg
  c. Alter the ability of the fertilized egg to implant and grow

25.5 What is the primary mechanism of action of the long-lasting progesterone injection?
  a. Inhibit the development and release of the egg
  b. Impose a barrier between the sperm and the egg
  c. Alter the ability of the fertilized egg to implant and grow

25.6 What is the primary mechanism of action of the diaphragm?
  a. Inhibit the development and release of the egg
  b. Impose a barrier between the sperm and the egg
  c. Alter the ability of the fertilized egg to implant and grow

25.7 Which of the following contraceptive methods does NOT provide some measure of protection from sexually transmitted diseases?
  a. Male condom
  b. Diaphragm
  c. Spermicidal jelly
  d. Female condom
  e. Intrauterine contraceptive device

25.8 The most common method of contraception among younger women in the United States is
  a. spermicidal foam
  b. male condom
  c. long-acting hormone (rod or injection)
  d. oral contraceptive
  e. intrauterine device (IUD)

25.9 The synthetic estrogen most frequently found in oral contraceptives is
  a. ethinyl estradiol
  b. β-estradiol
  c. mestranol
  d. levonorgestrel
  e. norethindrone

25.10 The hormone used in implantable contraceptive rods (Norplant) is
  a. ethinyl estradiol
  b. β-estradiol
  c. mestranol
  d. levonorgestrel
  e. norethindrone

Answers

25.1 c	25.3 b	25.5 a	25.7 e	25.9 a
25.2 c	25.4 a	25.6 b	25.8 d	25.10 d

25.11 Ethinyl estradiol is approximately how many times as potent as the same weight of mestranol?
a. 0.5
b. 1.0
c. 1.3
d. 1.7
e. 2.3

25.12 Which of the following progestins used in oral contraceptives has the LEAST biologic potency?
a. Norethindrone acetate
b. Norgestrel
c. Ethynodiol acetate
d. Norethindrone
e. Norethynodrel

25.13 Progesterone-only oral contraceptive agents are less widely used by younger women because they
a. cost more than monophasic oral contraceptives
b. cause breast tenderness
c. have a higher failure rate
d. raise serum high-density lipoprotein levels

25.14 Combination oral contraceptive pills mainly act to prevent pregnancy through
a. altering cervical mucus
b. inducing endometrial atrophy
c. causing elevated endometrial prostaglandin formation
d. suppressing follicle-stimulating hormone and luteinizing hormone release
e. altering tubal motility

25.15 The progestins used in most oral contraceptives tend to
a. increase the occurrence of acne
b. increase smooth muscle tone
c. decrease sebum production
d. decrease hair growth

25.16 Which of the following occurs in users of multiphasic (low-dose) oral contraceptives at a higher rate than it occurs in the general population?
a. Ovarian cancer
b. Intermenstrual bleeding
c. Ectopic pregnancy
d. Anemia
e. Dysmenorrhea

25.17 A 20-year-old G0P0 moderately obese patient consults you about the use of oral contraceptives. Her menarche was at age 15 and her period comes every 30 to 45 days and lasts 2 to 4 days. If this patient were to use an oral contraceptive agent, she would be at greater risk for
a. "postpill amenorrhea"
b. endometrial cancer
c. ectopic pregnancy
d. acne

25.18 When taken concurrently, which of the following will reduce the efficacy of oral contraceptives?
a. Insulin
b. Tricyclic antidepressants
c. Oral penicillin
d. Methyldopa
e. Aspirin

25.19 The most common side effect of injectable or implantable contraceptive steroids is
a. involuntary weight loss
b. dysmenorrhea
c. vaginal dryness
d. random vaginal bleeding

25.20 Which of the following is NOT an attribute of long-acting injectable and implantable progestins?
a. Good compliance
b. Patient-controlled reversibility
c. Low failure rate
d. Low incidence of major side effects

Answers

25.11 d	25.13 c	25.15 a	25.17 a	25.19 d
25.12 d	25.14 d	25.16 b	25.18 c	25.20 b

25.21 A couple wishes to use "natural family planning" for contraception. Her periods are regular, coming every 28 ± 3 days. This patient's "fertile" period would be days
a. 7 to 14
b. 7 to 17
c. 7 to 20
d. 10 to 17
e. 10 to 20

25.22 At the time of ovulation, basal body temperature typically
a. rises
b. remans unchanged
c. drops

25.23 Following unprotected coitus, it is recommended that high-dose estrogen preparations be given within a maximum of
a. 1 day
b. 2 days
c. 3 days
d. 4 days
e. 5 days

25.24 The pregnancy rate for a couple using no method of contraception typically is
a. 20
b. 25
c. 28
d. 40
e. 85

25.25 In the first year of use, the pregnancy rate for a woman using the combination pill typically is
a. 0.2
b. 0.3
c. <1
d. <2
e. 3

25.26 In the first year of use, the pregnancy rate for a woman using the progestin pill typically is
a. 0.2
b. 0.3
c. <1
d. <2
e. 3

25.27 In the first year of use, the pregnancy rate for a woman using Norplant typically is
a. 0.2
b. 0.3
c. <1
d. <2
e. 3

25.28 In the first year of use, the pregnancy rate for a woman using Depo-Provera typically is
a. 0.2
b. 0.3
c. <1
d. <2
e. 3

25.29 In the first year of use, the pregnancy rate for a woman using spermicides typically is
a. 3
b. 12
c. 18
d. 20
e. 25

25.30 In the first year of use, the pregnancy rate for couples using a condom typically is
a. 3
b. 12
c. 18
d. 20
e. 25

Answers

25.21 c	25.23 d	25.25 e	25.27 a	25.29 d
25.22 a	25.24 e	25.26 e	25.28 b	25.30 b

Review

25.31 In the first year of use, the pregnancy rate for a parous woman using a sponge typically is
  a. 18
  b. 20
  c. 25
  d. 28
  e. 40

25.32 In the first year of use, the pregnancy rate for a nulliparous woman using a sponge typically is
  a. 18
  b. 20
  c. 25
  d. 28
  e. 40

25.33 In the first year of use, the pregnancy rate for a woman using a cervical cap typically is
  a. 18
  b. 20
  c. 25
  d. 28
  e. 40

25.34 In the first year of use, the pregnancy rate for a woman using a diaphragm and spermicide typically is
  a. 18
  b. 20
  c. 25
  d. 28
  e. 40

25.35 In the first year of use, the pregnancy rate for a woman using an intrauterine device typically is
  a. 0.3
  b. <1
  c. <2
  d. 3
  e. 12

25.36 In the first year of use, the pregnancy rate for a couple using withdrawal typically is
  a. 12
  b. 18
  c. 20
  d. 25
  e. 28

25.37 In the first year of use, the pregnancy rate for a woman using a postcoital douche typically is
  a. 20
  b. 25
  c. 28
  d. 40
  e. 85

25.38 In the first year of use, the pregnancy rate for a couple using periodic abstinence typically is
  a. 20
  b. 25
  c. 28
  d. 40
  e. 85

25.39 In the first year of use, the pregnancy rate for a couple using the Yuzpe method typically is
  a. 20
  b. 25
  c. 28
  d. 40
  e. 85

25.40 What action should be taken when a woman using an oral contraceptive experiences diplopia?
  a. Continue oral contraceptive but evaluate immediately
  b. Discontinue oral contraceptive and evaluate immediately; start nonhormonal contraceptive method
  c. Take no action

Answers

25.31 d	25.33 a	25.35 d	25.37 d	25.39 b
25.32 a	25.34 a	25.36 b	25.38 a	25.40 b

25.41 What action should be taken when a woman using an oral contraceptive has hemoptysis?
  a. Continue oral contraceptive but evaluate immediately
  b. Discontinue oral contraceptive and evaluate immediately; start nonhormonal contraceptive method
  c. Take no action

25.42 What action should be taken when a woman using an oral contraceptive is discovered to have a hepatic mass?
  a. Continue oral contraceptive but evaluate immediately
  b. Discontinue oral contraceptive and evaluate immediately; start nonhormonal contraceptive method
  c. Take no action

25.43 What action should be taken when a woman using an oral contraceptive experiences a slurring of speech?
  a. Continue oral contraceptive but evaluate immediately
  b. Discontinue oral contraceptive and evaluate immediately; start nonhormonal contraceptive method
  c. Take no action

25.44 What action should be taken when a woman using an oral contraceptive has a severe headache?
  a. Continue oral contraceptive but evaluate immediately
  b. Discontinue oral contraceptive and evaluate immediately; start nonhormonal contraceptive method
  c. Take no action

25.45 What action should be taken when a woman using an oral contraceptive experiences severe chest/neck pain?
  a. Continue oral contraceptive but evaluate immediately
  b. Discontinue oral contraceptive and evaluate immediately; start nonhormonal contraceptive method
  c. Take no action

25.46 What action should be taken when a woman using an oral contraceptive experiences severe leg pain and tenderness?
  a. Continue oral contraceptive but evaluate immediately
  b. Discontinue oral contraceptive and evaluate immediately; start nonhormonal contraceptive method
  c. Take no action

25.47 The failure of oral contraceptives usually is related to
  a. an inherent problem in the estrogen-to-progesterone ratio
  b. interference by other medications that the patient is taking
  c. missed doses of the oral contraceptive
  d. altered gastrointestinal absorption of the oral contraceptive caused by hormonal influences

25.48 The estrogenic components of oral contraceptives preferentially inhibit
  a. follicle-stimulating hormone (FSH) and are dose-dependent
  b. FSH and are not dose-dependent
  c. luteinizing hormone (LH) and are dose-dependent
  d. LH and are not dose-dependent

25.49 Hormonal agents in oral contraceptives make cervical mucus
  a. thicker
  b. thinner
  c. unchanged

25.50 The use of oral contraceptives offers some protection against all of the following EXCEPT
  a. endometrial carcinoma
  b. asthma
  c. benign breast disease
  d. ovarian carcinoma
  e. ectopic pregnancy

Answers

25.41 b	25.43 b	25.45 b	25.47 c	25.49 a
25.42 b	25.44 a	25.46 b	25.48 a	25.50 b

25.51 Compared with low-dose oral contraceptives, high-dose oral contraceptives have a
   a. higher incidence of breakthrough bleeding
   b. similar incidence of breakthrough bleeding
   c. lower incidence of breakthrough bleeding

25.52 Approximately what percent of patients will experience postpill amenorrhea when discontinuing oral contraceptives after long-term use?
   a. 1%
   b. 3%
   c. 5%
   d. 7%
   e. 9%

25.53 Postpill amenorrhea is more likely to be experienced by
   a. older women
   b. younger women
   c. smokers
   d. nonsmokers
   e. women with regular menses

25.54 What is the dosage of Depo-Provera that is given every 3 months for the purpose of contraception?
   a. 50 mg
   b. 100 mg
   c. 150 mg
   d. 200 mg
   e. 250 mg

25.55 Most women who discontinue Depo-Provera injections will not become fertile for how many months?
   a. 1 to 2
   b. 2 to 3
   c. 3 to 4
   d. 4 to 5
   e. 5 to 6

25.56 Norplant is effective for how many years after insertion?
   a. 1
   b. 2
   c. 3
   d. 4
   e. 5
   f. 6

25.57 Injectable and implantable progestin contraceptive methods cause all of the following EXCEPT
   a. suppressed ovulation
   b. thickened cervical mucus
   c. thinned cervical mucus
   d. impeded sperm transport

25.58 Which of the following is NOT a positive attribute of barrier contraceptives?
   a. Requirement for good patient compliance
   b. Patient-controlled reversibility
   c. Low failure rate
   d. Low incidence of major side effects
   e. Low cost per month

25.59 In addition to the failure rate, which of the following is the most common problem associated with the use of condoms?
   a. Premature ejaculation
   b. Increased risk of vaginal yeast infection
   c. Contact dermatitis
   d. Urinary retention

25.60 When used for contraception, a diaphragm must be left in place following intercourse for at least
   a. 1 hour
   b. 2 to 3 hours
   c. 6 to 8 hours
   d. 12 to18 hours
   e. 24 or more hours

Answers

25.51 c	25.53 b	25.55 d	25.57 c	25.59 c
25.52 b	25.54 c	25.56 e	25.58 a	25.60 c

25.61 If a diaphragm is in place following intercourse (during the "waiting time" before diaphragm removal), what should be done before additional intercourse?
a. Delay intercourse until the waiting time has expired
b. Remove the diaphragm, reapply the contraceptive jelly, and restart the waiting time
c. Insert additional jelly without disturbing the diaphragm and restart the waiting time
d. Remove the diaphragm, reapply the contraceptive jelly, and remove the diaphragm at the end of the original waiting time
e. Remove the diaphragm and use an alternate method of contraception

25.62 When correctly fitted and worn, a contraceptive diaphragm should
a. completely cover the posterior vaginal wall
b. have its apex in the posterior fornix
c. rest firmly against the posterior fourchette
d. sit 1 to 2 cm below the symphysis

25.63 Susceptibility to urinary tract infections by women who use diaphragms is
a. slightly higher
b. about the same
c. slightly lower

25.64 Following intercourse using contraceptive foam, douching should be avoided for at least
a. 30 to 60 minutes
b. 1 to 2 hours
c. 4 to 6 hours
d. 8 to 10 hours
e. 12 or more hours

25.65 Spermicidal foam provides protection for
a. a single act of intercourse
b. 1 to 3 hours
c. 4 to 6 hours
d. 10 to 12 hours
e. up to 24 hours

25.66 How does the presence of a reservoir tip in a condom affect the likelihood of breakage during use?
a. Increases the likelihood
b. Does not affect the likelihood
c. Decreases the likelihood

25.67 The vaginal sponge acts as a contraceptive primarily by
a. acting as a barrier to sperm
b. delivering spermicide
c. irritating the vaginal wall

25.68 Following unprotected intercourse, an intrauterine contraceptive device may prevent pregnancy if it is inserted within
a. 12 hours
b. 24 hours
c. 36 hours
d. 72 hours
e. 5 days

25.69 The main contraceptive action of intrauterine contraceptive devices as a class is to
a. inhibit ovulation
b. cause cervical mucus thickening
c. alter tubal motility
d. prevent implantation
e. cause heavy metal poisoning of sperm

25.70 The most important factor in selection of patients for IUD use is
a. age
b. parity
c. risk of sexually transmitted diseases
d. history of dysmenorrhea

Answers

25.61 c	25.63 a	25.65 a	25.67 b	25.69 d
25.62 b	25.64 d	25.66 c	25.68 e	25.70 c

25.71 The relative ratio of extrauterine pregnancy to intrauterine pregnancy in an IUD user compared with an oral contraceptive user is
   a. greater
   b. the same
   c. less

25.72 The overall risk of ectopic pregnancy in users of IUDs is
   a. increased
   b. unchanged
   c. decreased

25.73 The spontaneous expulsion rate of IUDs in the first year following insertion is
   a. 5%
   b. 10%
   c. 15%
   d. 20%
   e. 25%

25.74 What is the best time for insertion of an IUD?
   a. At the time of ovulation
   b. In the time between the menstrual period and ovulation
   c. In the time between ovulation and the menstrual period
   d. At the time of the menstrual period

25.75 Increased vaginal bleeding and menstrual pain is experienced in what percent of women using an IUD?
   a. 1 to 5%
   b. 5 to 10%
   c. 10 to 15%
   d. 15 to 20%
   e. 20 to 25%

25.76 The increased vaginal bleeding and menstrual pain sometimes associated with IUD use may be lessened in some women by the use of what adjunctive regimen in the first few months of IUD use?
   a. Oral contraceptives
   b. Lupron
   c. Nonsteroidal anti-inflammatory drugs
   d. Doxycycline

Instructions for items 25.77 to 25.79: Match the type of IUD with the best description. An option may be used once, more than once, or not at all.

25.77 The ParaGard IUD is
   a. medicated
   b. unmedicated

25.78 The Progestasert IUD is
   a. medicated
   b. unmedicated

25.79 The Lippes Loop IUD is
   a. medicated
   b. unmedicated

25.80 For a woman with mild dysmenorrhea, which intrauterine device may offer advantages in addition to contraception?
   a. ParaGard
   b. Progestasert
   c. Lippes Loop

Answers

25.71 a	25.73 b	25.75 b	25.77 a	25.79 b
25.72 b	25.74 d	25.76 c	25.78 a	25.80 b

25.81 The copper from copper-containing IUDs may exert all the following additional contraceptive effects EXCEPT
    a. endometrial decidualization
    b. enhanced endometrial inflammatory response
    c. enhanced spermicidal effect in cervical mucus

25.82 Which of the following patients should not use IUDs for contraception?
    a. Adolescents
    b. Nulliparas
    c. Immunosuppressed individuals
    d. Individuals with uterine fibroids

25.83 The management of an asymptomatic woman with a positive cervical culture for gonorrhea and an IUD is
    a. removal of the IUD and treatment of the infection by standard protocol
    b. treatment of the infection without IUD removal and careful observation

25.84 Insertional infection (occurs within 6 to 8 weeks of insertion of an IUD) should be treated by
    a. Doxycycline 200 mg orally before insertion
    b. Ceftriaxone 25 mg intramuscularly and doxycycline 100 mg orally twice daily for 7 days

25.85 Delayed infection (occurs 3 or more months after insertion of an IUD) should be treated by
    a. Doxycycline 200 mg orally before insertion
    b. Ceftriaxone 25 mg intramuscularly and doxycycline 100 mg orally twice daily for 7 days

25.86 Women who are breast feeding and are given an IUD generally have a
    a. greater incidence of postinsertional discomfort/bleeding
    b. unchanged incidence of postinsertional discomfort/bleeding
    c. decreased incidence of postinsertional discomfort/bleeding

25.87 What percent of patients will spontaneously abort if they become pregnant while using an IUD?
    a. 20 to 30%
    b. 40 to 50%
    c. 60 to 70%
    d. 80 to 90%

25.88 Removal of an IUD in the first trimester of a pregnancy is associated with a spontaneous abortion rate of
    a. 10%
    b. 30%
    c. 50%
    d. 70%
    e. 90%

25.89 If an IUD is left in situ during pregnancy, there is an increased incidence of
    a. congenital facial anomalies in the fetus
    b. congenital trunk anomalies in the fetus
    c. placental implantation problems
    d. preterm labor and delivery
    e. intrauterine growth restriction

25.90 Which of the following is an effective postcoital antifertility method?
    a. Yuzpe method
    b. Postcoital douche
    c. Immediate uterine curettage
    d. Carbonic anhydrase
    e. Hydroxyzine hydrochloride

Answers

25.81 a	25.83 b	25.85 b	25.87 b	25.89 d
25.82 c	25.84 a	25.86 c	25.88 b	25.90 a

25.91 The two types of estrogen compounds present in oral contraceptives are
   a. estrone and mestranol
   b. ethinyl estradiol and mestranol
   c. estradiol and estrone
   d. estriol and mestranol

25.92 Which of the following has been implicated as the causative agent of thromboembolism in women using oral contraceptives?
   a. Estrogen
   b. Progesterone

25.93 Which of the following statements about the progestin-only minipill is INCORRECT?
   a. It is more effective in younger women
   b. It does not alter the quality of breast milk
   c. It does not alter the quantity of breast milk
   d. It may be started immediately postpartum
   e. It must be taken at the same time every day

25.94 Which of the following is NOT a mechanism of action of the progestin-only minipill?
   a. It makes the endometrium resistant to implantation
   b. It has a synergistic effect with lactation-associated prolactin effects
   c. It suppresses ovulation
   d. It causes a thickening of the cervical mucus

25.95 The failure rate of the Yuzpe method of postcoital contraception is approximately
   a. 5%
   b. 15%
   c. 25%
   d. 35%
   e. 45%

25.96 What is the dosage of Lo-Ovral in the Yuzpe method of postcoital contraception?
   a. two tablets followed by two tablets in 12 hours, administered within 72 hours of the unprotected coital event
   b. four tablets followed by four tablets in 12 hours, administered within 72 hours of the unprotected coital event

25.97 What is the dosage of Ovral in the Yuzpe method of postcoital contraception?
   a. two tablets followed by two tablets in 12 hours, administered within 72 hours of the unprotected coital event
   b. four tablets followed by four tablets in 12 hours, administered within 72 hours of the unprotected coital event

25.98 What is the dosage of Nordette in the Yuzpe method of postcoital contraception?
   a. two tablets followed by two tablets in 12 hours, administered within 72 hours of the unprotected coital event
   b. four tablets followed by four tablets in 12 hours, administered within 72 hours of the unprotected coital event

25.99 What is the dosage of Triphasil (yellow pills) in the Yuzpe method of postcoital contraception?
   a. two tablets followed by two tablets in 12 hours, administered within 72 hours of the unprotected coital event
   b. four tablets followed by four tablets in 12 hours, administered within 72 hours of the unprotected coital event

Answers

25.91 b	25.93 a	25.95 c	25.97 a	25.99 b
25.92 a	25.94 c	25.96 b	25.98 b	

25.100 About what percent of women who successfully use the Yuzpe method of emergency contraception will have a menstrual period within 3 weeks?
a. 100%
b. 75%
c. 50%
d. 25%

25.101 Is migraine headache a relative or absolute contraindication to the use of biphasic oral contraceptive therapy?
a. Relative contraindication
b. Absolute contraindication

25.102 Is thrombophlebitis or thromboembolic disease a relative or absolute contraindication to the use of biphasic oral contraceptive therapy?
a. Relative contraindication
b. Absolute contraindication

25.103 Is cerebral vascular disease a relative or absolute contraindication to the use of biphasic oral contraceptive therapy?
a. Relative contraindication
b. Absolute contraindication

25.104 Is coronary occlusion a relative or absolute contraindication to the use of biphasic oral contraceptive therapy?
a. Relative contraindication
b. Absolute contraindication

25.105 Is impaired liver function a relative or absolute contraindication to the use of biphasic oral contraceptive therapy?
a. Relative contraindication
b. Absolute contraindication

25.106 Is known or suspected breast cancer a relative or absolute contraindication to the use of biphasic oral contraceptive therapy?
a. Relative contraindication
b. Absolute contraindication

25.107 Is abnormal vaginal bleeding of unknown origin a relative or absolute contraindication to the use of biphasic oral contraceptive therapy?
a. Relative contraindication
b. Absolute contraindication

25.108 Is known or suspected pregnancy a relative or absolute contraindication to the use of biphasic oral contraceptive therapy?
a. Relative contraindication
b. Absolute contraindication

25.109 Is hypertension in a patient who is under the age of 35 a relative or absolute contraindication to the use of biphasic oral contraceptive therapy?
a. Relative contraindication
b. Absolute contraindication

25.110 Is diabetes mellitus a relative or absolute contraindication to the use of biphasic oral contraceptive therapy?
a. Relative contraindication
b. Absolute contraindication

25.111 Is gallbladder disease a relative or absolute contraindication to the use of biphasic oral contraceptive therapy?
a. Relative contraindication
b. Absolute contraindication

25.112 Is obstructive jaundice in a previous pregnancy a relative or absolute contraindication to the use of biphasic oral contraceptive therapy?
a. Relative contraindication
b. Absolute contraindication

Answers

25.100 a	25.103 b	25.106 b	25.109 a	25.112 a
25.101 a	25.104 b	25.107 b	25.110 a	
25.102 b	25.105 b	25.108 b	25.111 a	

25.113 Is epilepsy a relative or absolute contraindication to the use of biphasic oral contraceptive therapy?
a. Relative contraindication
b. Absolute contraindication

25.114 Is severe obesity a relative or absolute contraindication to the use of biphasic oral contraceptive therapy?
a. Relative contraindication
b. Absolute contraindication

25.115 Is being a smoker over the age of 35 a relative or absolute contraindication to the use of biphasic oral contraceptive therapy?
a. Relative contraindication
b. Absolute contraindication

25.116 Is congenital hyperlipidemia a relative or absolute contraindication to the use of biphasic oral contraceptive therapy?
a. Relative contraindication
b. Absolute contraindication

25.117 Is hepatic neoplasm a relative or absolute contraindication to the use of biphasic oral contraceptive therapy?
a. Relative contraindication
b. Absolute contraindication

25.118 Which of the following is NOT common in individuals using the Depo-Provera and Norplant systems?
a. Thickening of the cervical mucus
b. Decidualization of the endometrium
c. Inhibition of ovulation

25.119 What percent of women using Depo-Provera will resume normal menses within 6 months?
a. 25%
b. 50%
c. 75%
d. 100%

25.120 In which of the following cases should biphasic oral contraceptives be discontinued?
a. Amenorrhea
b. Galactorrhea
c. Right upper quadrant pain
d. Hepatic mass with tenderness

25.121 For purposes of contraception, injectable medroxyprogesterone and estradiol cyprionate are given every
a. month
b. 2 months
c. 6 months
d. year
e. 5 years

25.122 As compared with the Yuzpe method, Plan B emergency contraception has
a. an increased incidence of nausea
b. a similar incidence of nausea
c. a decreased incidence of nausea

25.123 The Yuzpe or Plan B contraceptive regimens are best used for all of the following indications EXCEPT
a. IUD expulsion
b. unintended unprotected intercourse
c. interval contraception
d. sexual assault when no contraceptive method is in use

Answers

25.113 a	25.115 b	25.117 b	25.119 b	25.121 a	25.123 c
25.114 a	25.116 b	25.118 c	25.120 d	25.122 c	

Questions and Answers Chapter 26: Sterilization

26.1 Among the methods used to control fertility in the United States, sterilization is the
a. most frequently used
b. second most frequently used
c. third most frequently used
d. least frequently used

26.2 Roughly what proportion of married couples in the United States use sterilization for contraception?
a. 1 in 8
b. 1 in 5
c. 1 in 3
d. 1 in 2

26.3 Despite careful counseling, what percent of patients will request sterilization reversal?
a. 1%
b. 3%
c. 5%
d. 8%
e. 12%

26.4 Successful reversal of sterilization is possible in approximately what percent of cases?
a. 5 to 10%
b. 20 to 30%
c. 40 to 60%
d. 70 to 80%
e. 90 to 95%

26.5 Vasectomy accounts for approximately what percent of all sterilization procedures?
a. 10 to 15%
b. 20 to 25%
c. 30 to 35%
d. 40 to 45%
e. 50 to 55%

26.6 Antibodies against sperm are found in what proportion of men who have undergone vasectomy?
a. 10 to 15%
b. 20 to 25%
c. 30 to 35%
d. 40 to 45%
e. 50 to 55%

26.7 When compared with female sterilization, which of the following is NOT an advantage of vasectomy?
a. Lower incidence of postoperative depression
b. Greater reversibility
c. Lower cost
d. Lower operative complication rate
e. The possibility of routine postoperative verification

26.8 Which of the following is the LEAST likely complication associated with vasectomy?
a. Hematoma formation
b. Wound infection
c. Femoral nerve damage
d. Continued bleeding at the operative site

26.9 The most common reason for pregnancy following a vasectomy is
a. recanalization
b. sexual activity too soon after surgery
c. ligation of the tunica albicans
d. operative hematoma formation

26.10 Sterilization after vasectomy usually is complete by
a. 24 to 36 hours
b. 3 to 5 days
c. 2 to 3 weeks
d. 4 to 6 weeks
e. 8 to 10 weeks

Answers

26.1	d	26.3	a	26.5	c	26.7	a	26.9	b
26.2	c	26.4	c	26.6	e	26.8	c	26.10	d

26.11 Which of the following anesthetic methods is NOT used for laparoscopic sterilization procedures?
  a. Local
  b. General
  c. Epidural
  d. Spinal
  e. Saddle

26.12 Which of the following female sterilization methods is most likely to result in future ectopic pregnancy?
  a. Hulka clip
  b. Falope ring
  c. Electrocautery
  d. Pomeroy tubal ligation
  e. Kroener fimbriectomy

26.13 Which of the following female sterilization methods is most likely to be successfully reversed?
  a. Hulka clip
  b. Falope ring
  c. Electrocautery
  d. Pomeroy tubal ligation
  e. Kroener fimbriectomy

26.14 Which of the following female sterilization methods is most likely to result in operative complications?
  a. Hulka clip
  b. Falope ring
  c. Electrocautery
  d. Pomeroy tubal ligation
  e. Kroener fimbriectomy

26.15 Which of the following female sterilization methods is most likely to result in postoperative pain requiring strong analgesics?
  a. Hulka clip
  b. Falope ring
  c. Electrocautery
  d. Pomeroy tubal ligation
  e. Kroener fimbriectomy

26.16 Which of the following best describes Madlener tubal ligation?
  a. Fimbriated end of tube excised
  b. Fimbriated end of tube buried in broad ligament
  c. Tube divided, proximal stump buried in uterine wall, distal stump buried in leaves of broad ligament
  d. Tube divided, proximal stump buried in round ligament, distal stump buried in leaves of broad ligament
  e. Tube elevated, base crushed in clamp, crushed area ligated with nonabsorbable suture
  f. Loop of tube from middle third of tube elevated, ligated with plain gut and excised

26.17 Which of the following best describes Pomeroy tubal ligation?
  a. Fimbriated end of tube excised
  b. Fimbriated end of tube buried in broad ligament
  c. Tube divided, proximal stump buried in uterine wall, distal stump buried in leaves of broad ligament
  d. Tube divided, proximal stump buried in round ligament, distal stump buried in leaves of broad ligament
  e. Tube elevated, base crushed in clamp, crushed area ligated with nonabsorbable suture
  f. Loop of tube from middle third of tube elevated, ligated with plain gut and excised

Answers

26.11 e	**26.13** a	**26.15** b	**26.17** f
26.12 c	**26.14** c	**26.16** e	

26.18 Which of the following best describes Irving tubal ligation?
a. Fimbriated end of tube excised
b. Fimbriated end of tube buried in broad ligament
c. Tube divided, proximal stump buried in uterine wall, distal stump buried in leaves of broad ligament
d. Tube divided, proximal stump buried in round ligament, distal stump buried in leaves of broad ligament
e. Tube elevated, base crushed in clamp, crushed area ligated with nonabsorbable suture
f. Loop of tube from middle third of tube elevated, ligated with plain gut and excised

26.19 Which of the following best describes Cook tubal ligation?
a. Fimbriated end of tube excised
b. Fimbriated end of tube buried in broad ligament
c. Tube divided, proximal stump buried in uterine wall, distal stump buried in leaves of broad ligament
d. Tube divided, proximal stump buried in round ligament, distal stump buried in leaves of broad ligament
e. Tube elevated, base crushed in clamp, crushed area ligated with nonabsorbable suture
f. Loop of tube from middle third of tube elevated, ligated with plain gut and excised

26.20 Which of the following best describes Kroener tubal ligation?
a. Fimbriated end of tube excised
b. Fimbriated end of tube buried in broad ligament
c. Tube divided, proximal stump buried in uterine wall, distal stump buried in leaves of broad ligament
d. Tube divided, proximal stump buried in round ligament, distal stump buried in leaves of broad ligament
e. Tube elevated, base crushed in clamp, crushed area ligated with nonabsorbable suture
f. Loop of tube from middle third of tube elevated, ligated with plain gut and excised

26.21 Which of the following best describes Aldridge tubal ligation?
a. Fimbriated end of tube excised
b. Fimbriated end of tube buried in broad ligament
c. Tube divided, proximal stump buried in uterine wall, distal stump buried in leaves of broad ligament
d. Tube divided, proximal stump buried in round ligament, distal stump buried in leaves of broad ligament
e. Tube elevated, base crushed in clamp, crushed area ligated with nonabsorbable suture
f. Loop of tube from middle third of tube elevated, ligated with plain gut and excised

Answers
26.18 c   26.19 d   26.20 a   26.21 b

26.22 Compared with electrocautery, the Hulka clip has a
a. higher failure rate
b. similar failure rate
c. lower failure rate

26.23 Which of the following is NOT required as part of vaginal tubal sterilization procedures?
a. Specialized equipment
b. Prophylactic antibiotics
c. Restrictions on intercourse
d. Restrictions on douching

26.24 The term "interval sterilization" refers to procedures that
a. remove a segment of the fallopian tube
b. destroy a portion of the fallopian tube
c. are performed after the immediate postpartum period
d. are performed during the immediate postpartum period

26.25 Compared with tubal ligation, vasectomy is
a. more easily reversed
b. as easily reversed
c. less easily reversed

26.26 A woman who becomes pregnant 3 months after tubal ligation most likely has
a. an ectopic pregnancy
b. an intrauterine pregnancy
c. a combined pregnancy

26.27 A patient who has undergone reversal of a tubal ligation and then exhibits signs of pregnancy should initially be presumed to have
a. a normal intrauterine pregnancy
b. an abnormal intrauterine pregnancy
c. an ectopic pregnancy
d. a false pregnancy

26.28 Which of the following statements about surgical sterilization is INCORRECT?
a. There is an approximately 1% chance of pregnancy after female tubal sterilization
b. The rate of permanent surgical sterilization has steadily risen in recent years
c. Approximately equal numbers of men and women request surgical sterilization

26.29 Postoperative complications of vasectomy such as bleeding, hematoma formation, and local skin infection occur in about what percent of cases?
a. <1%
b. 3 to 5%
c. 7 to 9%
d. 12 to 15%

26.30 Post-tubal ligation syndrome is considered to include
a. menstrual dysfunction
b. dysmenorrhea
c. disruption of blood flow in the area of the fallopian tubes
d. all of the above

26.31 What is the failure rate in the Pomeroy method of tubal ligation?
a. 1 in 100
b. 1 in 200
c. 1 in 300
d. 1 in 400
e. 1 in 500

26.32 The fatality rate in women from sterilization is what percent of the rate from childbearing?
a. 1%
b. 2%
c. 5%
d. 10%

Answers

26.22 a	26.24 c	26.26 b	26.28 c	26.30 d	26.32 d
26.23 a	26.25 a	26.27 c	26.29 b	26.31 e	

26.33 Compared with countries with a low vasectomy rate, the incidence of prostate cancer in countries where there is a high rate of vasectomy is
a. higher
b. the same
c. lower

26.34 During a routine prenatal visit, a 28-year-old G3 P2002 patient tells you that she and her husband of 8 years have decided that their family will be complete with the birth of their next child. They are interested in sterilization options that could be "done right away, if the baby is OK." Which of the following is NOT a possible option for this couple?
a. Pomeroy tubal ligation
b. Tubal electrocautery
c. Falope ring
d. Vaginal tubal cautery

Answers

26.33 b   **26.34** d

Questions and Answers Chapter 27: Vulvitis and Vaginitis

27.1 Complaints of vulvar irritation account for approximately what percent of gynecologic office visits?
a. 3%
b. 5%
c. 10%
d. 15%
e. 25%

27.2 Which of the following characterizes a physiologic discharge?
a. Few white blood cells with multiple, flat, polygonal small nuclei on microscopic examination
b. Positive whiff test
c. Vaginal pH of 5.5
d. Motile protozoa on microscopic examination

27.3 Which of the following is characteristic of bacterial vaginosis?
a. Vaginal pH less than 4.5
b. Curdy consistency
c. Greenish tinge
d. Fishy odor

27.4 Vaginal candidiasis is characterized by
a. white cells
b. foul odor
c. thin, homogeneous consistency
d. intense itching

27.5 Which of the following characterizes vaginal trichomoniasis?
a. Cervical ectropion
b. Vaginal dryness
c. Motile protozoa on microscopic examination
d. White discharge

27.6 What types of cells are characteristic of atrophic vaginitis?
a. Columnar cells
b. Parabasal cells
c. Ciliated cells
d. White blood cells

27.7 Vulvar ulceration characterizes which of the following?
a. Condyloma acuminatum
b. Psoriasis
c. Scabies
d. Herpes simplex

27.8 Most of the liquid portion of physiologic vaginal secretions in a woman of reproductive age comes from
a. the cervix
b. vaginal transudate
c. the Bartholin glands
d. the Skene glands

27.9 The creamy white portion of physiologic vaginal secretions in a woman of reproductive age comes from
a. cervical mucus
b. vaginal epithelium
c. the Bartholin glands
d. vaginal white blood cells

27.10 The average amount of vaginal secretion produced in 24 hours by a woman of reproductive age is approximately
a. 0.1 g
b. 0.5 g
c. 1.5 g
d. 3.0 g
e. 5.0 g

27.11 The normal pH of vaginal secretions of reproductive-aged women is
a. 3.5 to 4.5
b. 5.0 to 6.0
c. 6.5 to 7.5
d. 8.0 to 9.0

27.12 The normal pH of the vagina after the menopause but without estrogen replacement therapy is
a. 2.0 to 3.0
b. 3.5 to 5.5
c. 6.0 to 8.0
d. 9.0 to 11.0

Answers

27.1 c	27.3 d	27.5 c	27.7 d	27.9 b	27.11 a
27.2 a	27.4 d	27.6 b	27.8 a	27.10 c	27.12 c

27.13 The most common symptom associated with a vaginal infection is
a. fever
b. pain
c. pruritus
d. discharge

27.14 The most common cause of persistently increased vaginal secretions is
a. sexual arousal
b. microbiologic infection
c. contact vulvitis
d. hormonal variation

27.15 The most common cause of increased vaginal discharge is
a. candidiasis
b. trichomoniasis
c. bacterial vaginosis
d. human papillomavirus

27.16 A 25-year-old patient complains of vaginal discharge. The diagnosis is established by
a. odor
b. microscopic examination
c. symptoms
d. color of the discharge

27.17 In a 30-year-old patient with bacterial vaginosis, a foul odor after intercourse is most likely caused by
a. the alkaline pH of semen
b. colonization of the vagina by penile microorganisms
c. bacterial digestion of seminal proteins
d. liberation of prostaglandins from sperm

27.18 Which of the following best describes a "whiff test"?
a. Mixing of vaginal secretions with 10% potassium hydroxide to liberate amines
b. Testing for odor of undiluted secretions from the vaginal apex
c. Mixing of vaginal secretions with normal saline to determine color
d. Passing of the speculum under the nose to detect odor

27.19 Which of the following best describes a "clue cell"?
a. clumped white blood cells
b. immature vaginal epithelial cells
c. keratinized vaginal epithelial cells with adherent white blood cells
d. vaginal epithelial cells with adherent bacteria

27.20 *Trichomonas vaginalis* is a flagellate protozoan that can live in the
a. vagina
b. oropharynx
c. anus
d. bladder

27.21 Approximately what percent of sexual partners of women with *Trichomonas* infections also have the infections?
a. <10%
b. 20 to 30%
c. 40 to 50%
d. >60%

27.22 Approximately what percent of women with a *Trichomonas* infection of the vagina are symptomatic?
a. 10%
b. 25%
c. 50%
d. 75%
e. 90%

Answers

27.13 d	27.15 c	27.17 a	27.19 d	27.21 d
27.14 b	27.16 b	27.18 a	27.20 a	27.22 c

27.23 Which of the following characterizes the microscopic appearance of *Trichomonas*?
   a. multiple pseudopods
   b. circular shape
   c. slightly larger than a white blood cell
   d. fine stippling

27.24 Characteristic petechia, or strawberry patches, are found in the upper vagina or on the cervix of patients with *Trichomonas vaginalis* in approximately what percent of cases?
   a. 10%
   b. 30%
   c. 50%
   d. 70%
   e. 90%

27.25 A standard treatment for *Trichomonas* vaginal infection is
   a. metronidazole 2 g orally in one dose
   b. metronidazole 250 mg orally every day for 14 days
   c. clindamycin 1 g orally in one dose
   d. ampicillin 500 mg orally four times a day for 10 days

27.26 The standard treatment for *T. vaginalis* will generally give a cure rate of
   a. 100%
   b. 90%
   c. 80%
   d. 70%
   e. 60%

27.27 What percent of patients with *T. vaginalis* will also have bacterial vaginosis?
   a. 0%
   b. 25%
   c. 50%
   d. 75%
   e. 100%

27.28 When prescribing metronidazole for the treatment of *Trichomonas* infections, it is important to advise the patient to avoid alcohol intake because alcohol
   a. diminishes gastric uptake of metronidazole
   b. induces metronidazole resistance in *Trichomonas*
   c. decreases tissue levels of metronidazole
   d. may cause severe nausea and vomiting

27.29 The most common source of monilial infections of the vagina is from
   a. sexual contact with an infected partner
   b. airborne colonization
   c. contaminated clothing
   d. bath water retained in the vagina following bathing

27.30 Approximately 90% of vaginal "yeast" infections are caused by
   a. *Candida albicans*
   b. *Candida tropicalis*
   c. *Candida glabrata*
   d. *Torulopsis glabrata*

27.31 Which of the following is thought to increase the risk of vaginal "yeast" infection?
   a. nulliparity
   b. vitamin ingestion
   c. urinary tract infection
   d. use of spermicidal foam
   e. immunosuppression

27.32 Approximately what percent of women with vaginal "yeast" infections are symptomatic?
   a. 10%
   b. 25%
   c. 40%
   d. 60%
   e. 80%

Answers

27.23 c	27.25 a	27.27 b	27.29 b	27.31 e
27.24 a	27.26 b	27.28 d	27.30 a	27.32 e

27.33 The normal pH of vaginal secretions found in women with vaginal "yeast" infections is
a. 4.0 to 4.5
b. 5.5 to 6.0
c. 6.5 to 7.0
d. 8.0 to 9.0

27.34 The most common presenting complaint in women with vaginal "yeast" infections is
a. thick discharge
b. vulvar burning
c. dysuria
d. intense itching

27.35 A 10% potassium hydroxide solution is used for a wet preparation when "yeast" infection is suspected because this solution
a. renders *C. albicans* noninfective
b. causes lysis of white blood cells
c. liberates amines from solution
d. immobilizes *Trichomonas* organisms

27.36 Despite compliant therapy with an appropriate medication, the recurrence rate for vaginal yeast infections is
a. 5%
b. 10%
c. 25%
d. 40%
e. 60%

27.37 The primary treatment of candidal vaginitis is
a. topical synthetic imidazoles
b. systemic corticosteroids
c. topical cephalosporins
d. systemic penicillin

27.38 An appropriate treatment of *Pthirus pubis* (crab louse) is
a. ampicillin
b. gentamicin
c. sulfamethoxazole
d. clindamycin
e. γ-benzene hexachloride

27.39 The presence of "clue" cells is usually diagnostic of
a. tinea cruris
b. bacterial vaginosis
c. diabetic vulvitis
d. scabies

27.40 Which of the following is present in the vagina?
a. Apocrine glands
b. Sweat glands
c. Hair follicles
d. Sebaceous glands
e. Nonkeratinized squamous epithelium

27.41 Which of the following is characteristic of the vagina?
a. vulnerability to contact with external irritants
b. mucus-secreting epithelium
c. keratinized epithelium
d. sweat glands

27.42 Vulvitis in children is associated with
a. constipation
b. urinary retention
c. puberty
d. sexual abuse

27.43 In a patient with recurrent yeast infections, what concurrent disease should be suspected?
a. Systemic lupus erythematosus
b. Diabetes mellitus
c. Syphilis
d. Cushing syndrome

27.44 Which of the following accurately describes contact dermatitis?
a. Pale
b. Ulcerated
c. Hemorrhagic
d. Edematous

Answers

27.33 a	27.35 b	27.37 a	27.39 b	27.41 a	27.43 b
27.34 d	27.36 c	27.38 e	27.40 e	27.42 d	27.44 d

27.45 Which of the following conditions affects up to 3% of women and seems to have a familial pattern?
a. Contact dermatitis
b. Psoriasis
c. Seborrheic dermatitis
d. Hidradenitis suppurativa

27.46 Which of the following conditions often presents with deep painful scars, foul discharge, and may require wide surgical excision?
a. Hidradenitis suppurativa
b. Seborrheic dermatitis
c. Contact dermatitis
d. Psoriasis
e. Yeast vulvitis

27.47 Which type of bacteria in the lower genital tract of normal women break down glycogen to lactic acid?
a. *Gardnerella*
b. *Streptococcus*
c. *Trichomonas*
d. *Lactobacillus*

27.48 A wet preparation showing clumps of epithelial cells with adherent bacteria is associated with
a. *Trichomonas vaginalis*
b. Candidal vaginitis
c. Bacterial vaginosis
d. Cervical dysplasia

27.49 When does cytolytic vaginitis typically worsen?
a. Follicular phase
b. Puberty
c. Menopause
d. Luteal phase

27.50 Which of the following suggests desquamative inflammatory vaginitis?
a. Clear discharge
b. Vesicles
c. Overgrowth of gram negative bacilli
d. Purulent discharge

Answers

| 27.45 b | 27.46 a | 27.47 d | 27.48 c | 27.49 d | 27.50 d |

Questions and Answers Chapter 28: Sexually Transmitted Diseases

28.1 Approximately what percent of patients with a sexually transmitted disease (STD) have more than one STD?
a. Less than 3%
b. 5 to 10%
c. 20 to 50%
d. 60 to 80%
e. 95 to 100%

28.2 In approximately what percent of cases will a single sexual contact with a patient who has an active herpes infection result in transmission of the infection?
a. Less than 3%
b. 5 to 10%
c. 20 to 50%
d. 60 to 80%
e. 95 to 100%

28.3 The normal progression of symptoms in primary herpes infections is a prodromal phase followed by
a. ulcer, vesicle, crusting, resolution
b. ulcer, crusting, vesicle, resolution
c. crusting, vesicle, ulcer, resolution
d. vesicle, ulcer, crusting, resolution
e. vesicle, crusting, ulcer, resolution

28.4 What percent of genital herpes lesions are caused by the herpes simplex virus type II?
a. 95%
b. 85%
c. 75%
d. 65%
e. 55%

28.5 Approximately what percent of patients with an initial herpes genitalis infection will require hospitalization for pain control or management of urinary complications?
a. 10%
b. 20%
c. 30%
d. 40%
e. 50%

28.6 Primary herpes genitalis infections are characterized by malaise, low-grade fever, and inguinal adenopathy in approximately what percent of patients?
a. 20%
b. 40%
c. 60%
d. 80%

28.7 Herpes genitalis lesions recur in approximately what percent of patients?
a. 10%
b. 30%
c. 50%
d. 70%

28.8 Compared with primary genital lesions, recurrent herpes lesions are
a. longer in duration
b. more severe
c. milder
d. more systemic

28.9 A pregnant patient at term presents in active labor. Her membranes are intact. She has active herpetic lesions in the vagina. If vaginal delivery occurs, what is the likelihood that the newborn will be infected?
a. 25%
b. 50%
c. 75%
d. 100%

28.10 Neonatal herpes infection acquired at the time of delivery is associated with a mortality rate of approximately
a. 100%
b. 80%
c. 60%
d. 40%
e. 20%

Answers

28.1	c	28.3	d	28.5	a	28.7	b	28.9	b
28.2	d	28.4	b	28.6	b	28.8	c	28.10	b

28.11 An 18-year-old patient presents with a 5-day history of very painful vulvar ulcers that began as small "blisters." She is now complaining of a low-grade fever, headache, and meningismus. Large, painful vulvar and perineal ulcers and inguinal adenopathy are found on examination. The most likely diagnosis is
  a. disseminated gonococcal infection
  b. primary herpes vulvitis
  c. secondary syphilis
  d. lymphogranuloma venereum
  e. molluscum contagiosum

28.12 A 23-year-old G3 P2001 patient presents at term in early labor with an active herpes infection of the labia that has been present for the past 3 days. Membranes are intact. Contractions are regular at 3-minute intervals and have been present for the last 3 hours. Her last term labor was 3 years ago and lasted 12 hours, ending in a vaginal delivery of a normal 7-pound infant. Which of the following is the best management of this patient?
  a. Anticipate normal labor and delivery
  b. Anticipate normal labor and delivery, plan acyclovir prophylaxis for the infant
  c. Anticipate rapid labor and delivery but avoid episiotomy
  d. Tocolysis and intravenous acyclovir (200 mg)
  e. Immediate cesarean delivery

28.13 All of the following are caused by infection by *Chlamydia* species EXCEPT
  a. cervicitis
  b. pelvic inflammatory disease
  c. lymphogranuloma venereum
  d. granuloma inguinale

28.14 *Chlamydia* infections are frequently associated with co-infections by
  a. herpes simplex
  b. *Neisseria gonorrhoeae*
  c. human papillomavirus
  d. *Treponema pallidum*

28.15 Antibodies to *Chlamydia* are found in approximately what percent of sexually active women?
  a. 1 to 5%
  b. 10 to 15%
  c. 20 to 40%
  d. 60 to 80%
  e. Greater than 90%

28.16 How long does it take to confirm the diagnosis of *Chlamydia* using the culture technique?
  a. 12 to 24 hours
  b. 24 to 48 hours
  c. 48 to 72 hours
  d. 96 hours

28.17 Outpatient treatment with doxycycline or erythromycin for suspected or confirmed *Chlamydia* infection is associated with a cure rate of
  a. 95%
  b. 80%
  c. 65%
  d. 50%

28.18 A common sequela of infection by *Chlamydia trachomatis* is
  a. recurrent vulvar growths
  b. cyclic, migratory arthralgia
  c. involuntary infertility
  d. vaginismus

28.19 *Neisseria gonorrhoeae* is a
  a. gram-negative intracellular diplococcus
  b. gram-negative extracellular diplococcus
  c. gram-positive intracellular diplococcus
  d. gram-positive extracellular diplococcus

Answers

28.11 b	28.13 d	28.15 c	28.17 a	28.19 a
28.12 e	28.14 b	28.16 c	28.18 c	

28.20 Infection of the pharynx is found in what percent of heterosexual women with confirmed *Neisseria gonorrhoeae* infections?
a. 1 to 10%
b. 10 to 20%
c. 20 to 30%
d. 30 to 40%
e. 40 to 50%

28.21 For women, a single encounter with a partner infected with *Neisseria gonorrhoeae* is estimated to lead to infection in what percent of cases?
a. 20 to 30%
b. 40 to 50%
c. 60 to 70%
d. 80 to 90%
e. 100%

28.22 Following initial infection by *Neisseria gonorrhoeae*, symptoms first appear in
a. 1 to 2 days
b. 3 to 5 days
c. 1 to 2 weeks
d. 3 to 5 weeks

28.23 A 22-year-old G0P0 patient has just been successfully treated for *Neisseria gonorrhoeae* salpingitis and asks about her chances of infertility. Based on this single infection, her chances of involuntary infertility are approximately
a. <1%
b. 3 to 5%
c. 8 to 10%
d. 15 to 20%

28.24 A 22-year-old G0P0 patient has just been successfully treated for her third episode of *Neisseria gonorrhoeae* salpingitis and asks about her chances of infertility. Based on these infections, her chances of involuntary infertility are approximately
a. <10%
b. 20 to 25%
c. 40 to 50%
d. 70 to 80%

28.25 Lower genital tract infections by *Neisseria gonorrhoeae* are usually characterized by
a. malodorous, purulent vaginal or urethral discharge
b. firm, painless vulvar ulcer
c. inguinal adenopathy
d. fever, malaise, and labial swelling bilaterally

28.26 Which of the following is the most frequent site of gonorrheal infection in women?
a. Bartholin glands
b. Skene glands
c. Cervix
d. Urethra
e. Rectal crypts

28.27 Which of the following criteria is required to make a diagnosis of acute salpingitis?
a. fever >38°C
b. adnexal tenderness
c. mass on ultrasound
d. pus obtained via culdocentesis

28.28 All of the following are criteria for the hospitalization of patients with pelvic inflammatory disease EXCEPT
a. coexisting pregnancy
b. significant gastrointestinal symptoms
c. patient <20 years of age
d. white blood count greater than 20,000
e. nulliparity

28.29 The initiation of treatment for presumed pelvic inflammatory disease is based on
a. clinical suspicion
b. cervical Gram's stain
c. anaerobic culture
d. white blood cell count <8,000
e. rebound tenderness

Answers

28.20 b	28.22 b	28.24 d	28.26 c	28.28 c
28.21 d	28.23 d	28.25 a	28.27 b	28.29 a

28.30 The development of cervical cancer is associated with
a. *Chlamydia trachomatis* infections
b. herpes simplex type II infections
c. human papillomavirus (HPV) infections
d. herpes zoster infections

28.31 In approximately what percent of cases will a single sexual contact with an individual with an HPV infection result in transmission of the infection?
a. Less than 3%
b. 5 to 10%
c. 30 to 40%
d. 60 to 70%
e. 95 to 100%

28.32 Lesions caused by HPV may be confused with those of
a. early herpes simplex type II infections
b. late lymphogranuloma venereum
c. granuloma inguinale
d. secondary syphilis

28.33 Human papillomavirus infection is associated with
a. condyloma lata
b. cyst formation
c. deep ulcers
d. kissing lesions
e. tender vesicles

28.34 The HPV is found in approximately what percent of women?
a. 2.5 to 4%
b. 6.5 to 7%
c. 8.5 to 10%
d. 12 to 15%

28.35 All of the following modalities are used to treat simple condylomata acuminata EXCEPT
a. podophyllin in tincture of benzoin
b. trichloracetic acid
c. 5-fluorouracil
d. acyclovir

28.36 Which of the following does NOT make a patient more resistant to therapy for condylomata acuminata?
a. pregnant
b. immunosuppressed
c. smoker
d. overweight

28.37 Vaginal delivery of a patient with extensive condylomata acuminata of the vulva may result in
a. infant herpes encephalopathy
b. maternal hemorrhage
c. maternal febrile morbidity
d. infant laryngeal papillomas

28.38 Transplacental spread of *Treponema pallidum* can occur
a. only during the first trimester of pregnancy
b. only during the third trimester of pregnancy
c. at any time during pregnancy
d. only after rupture of membranes

28.39 The chancre of primary syphilis will
a. spontaneously heal in 3 to 9 weeks
b. coalesce to form running sores
c. transform into raised, fleshy growths that persist indefinitely
d. result in regional adenopathy and abscess formation within 2 weeks

28.40 Which of the following is characteristic of primary syphilis?
a. Chancre appears 3 to 5 days after infection
b. Chancre is often asymptomatic
c. Serologic testing usually is positive
d. Accompanying low-grade fever and anorexia are common

28.41 The most contagious stage of syphilis is
a. primary
b. secondary
c. tertiary
d. latent

Answers

28.30 c	28.32 d	28.34 a	28.36 d	28.38 c	28.40 b
28.31 d	28.33 d	28.35 d	28.37 d	28.39 a	28.41 b

28.42 The mucous patches of secondary syphilis will
a. spontaneously heal in 2 to 6 weeks
b. progress to coalesced running sores
c. progress to raised, fleshy growths that persist indefinitely
d. progress with regional adenopathy and abscess formation

28.43 Which of the following is a nontreponemal test?
a. Rapid plasma reagin (RPR)
b. Venereal Disease Research Laboratory (VDRL)
c. Automated reagin test
d. All of the above

28.44 Which of the following is the approximate sensitivity of the VDRL test in detecting primary syphilis?
a. 45%
b. 55%
c. 65%
d. 75%
e. 85%

28.45 Which of the following is the sensitivity of the RPR test in detecting primary syphilis?
a. 45%
b. 55%
c. 65%
d. 75%
e. 85%

28.46 Which of the following is the sensitivity of the fluorescent treponemal antibody absorption (FTA-ABS) test in detecting primary syphilis?
a. 45%
b. 55%
c. 65%
d. 75%
e. 85%

28.47 Which of the following is the sensitivity of the microhemagglutination assay-*Treponema pallidum* (MHA-TP) test in detecting primary syphilis?
a. 45%
b. 55%
c. 65%
d. 75%
e. 85%

28.48 Which of the following serologic tests for syphilis has a sensitivity of approximately 100% for secondary syphilis?
a. VDRL
b. RPR
c. Fluorescent treponemal antibody absorption (FTA-ABS)
d. Microhemagglutination assay-*Treponema pallidum* (MHA-TP)
e. All of the above

28.49 Which if the following does NOT result in a false-positive VDRL or RPR test?
a. gonorrhea
b. malaria
c. systemic lupus erythematosus
d. connective tissue disease

28.50 Which of the following is characteristic of secondary syphilis?
a. Asymptomatic chancre that is often missed
b. Noninfectious mucous patches
c. Low-grade fever, headache, malaise, sore throat, anorexia, and generalized lymphadenopathy
d. Serologic testing for syphilis generally negative

28.51 Without intervention, the risk of transmission of the HIV to a fetus is approximately
a. 25%
b. 50%
c. 75%
d. 100%

Answers

28.42 a	28.44 d	28.46 e	28.48 e	28.50 c
28.43 d	28.45 e	28.47 d	28.49 a	28.51 b

28.52 The diagnosis of HIV infection is established on the basis of
- a. serum immunoassay
- b. Western blot testing
- c. CD_4 white blood cell counts
- d. presence of clinical symptoms

28.53 Painless, ulcerated vulvar lesions are characteristic of infections with
- a. herpes simplex, type II
- b. *Chlamydia trachomatis*
- c. *Treponema pallidum*
- d. *Haemophilus ducreyi*

28.54 Which of the following conditions has an incubation period (from infection to clinical symptoms) of >1 month?
- a. Genital herpes
- b. Condyloma acuminata
- c. Chancroid
- d. Lymphogranuloma venereum

28.55 Multiple vulvar vesicles are typical of which of the following infections?
- a. Genital herpes
- b. Condyloma acuminata
- c. Chancroid
- d. Lymphogranuloma venereum

28.56 Which of the following is the incubation period for herpes?
- a. 3 to 7 days
- b. 1 to 8 months
- c. 10 to 60 days
- d. 1 to 4 weeks
- e. 8 to 12 weeks

28.57 Which of the following is the incubation period for genital warts?
- a. 3 to 7 days
- b. 1 to 8 months
- c. 10 to 60 days
- d. 1 to 4 weeks
- e. 8 to 12 weeks

28.58 Which of the following is the incubation period for syphilis?
- a. 3 to 7 days
- b. 1 to 8 months
- c. 10 to 60 days
- d. 1 to 4 weeks
- e. 8 to 12 weeks

28.59 Which of the following is the causative agent for genital warts?
- a. Human papillomavirus
- b. *Haemophilus ducreyi*
- c. *Calymmatobacterium granulomatis*
- d. *Chlamydia trachomatis*
- e. *Treponema pallidum*

28.60 Which of the following is the causative agent for syphilis?
- a. Human papillomavirus
- b. *Haemophilus ducreyi*
- c. *Calymmatobacterium granulomatis*
- d. *Chlamydia trachomatis*
- e. *Treponema pallidum*

28.61 Which of the following is the causative agent for chancroid?
- a. Human papillomavirus
- b. *Haemophilus ducreyi*
- c. *Calymmatobacterium granulomatis*
- d. *Chlamydia trachomatis*
- e. *Treponema pallidum*

28.62 Which of the following is the causative agent for lymphogranuloma venereum?
- a. Human papillomavirus
- b. *Haemophilus ducreyi*
- c. *Calymmatobacterium granulomatis*
- d. *Chlamydia trachomatis*
- e. *Treponema pallidum*

28.63 Which of the following is the causative agent for granuloma inguinale?
- a. Human papillomavirus
- b. *Haemophilus ducreyi*
- c. *Calymmatobacterium granulomatis*
- d. *Chlamydia trachomatis*
- e. *Treponema pallidum*

Answers

28.52 b	28.54 b	28.56 a	28.58 c	28.60 e	28.62 d
28.53 c	28.55 a	28.57 b	28.59 a	28.61 b	28.63 c

28.64 Which of the following STDs is generally NOT associated with lymphadenopathy?
a. Herpes
b. Genital warts
c. Syphilis
d. Chancroid
e. Lymphogranuloma venereum

28.65 Which of the following STDs is associated with a purulent, hemorrhagic secretion?
a. Granuloma inguinale
b. Lymphogranuloma venereum
c. Chancroid
d. Syphilis
e. Genital warts

28.66 Which of the following STDs is characteristically associated with multiple vesicular lesions that often coalesce?
a. Herpes
b. Genital warts
c. Syphilis
d. Chancroid
e. Lymphogranuloma venereum

28.67 Which of the following is NOT associated with acute cervicitis?
a. There is polymorphonuclear infiltration of the mucosa
b. The presenting symptom is often leukorrhea
c. It may be caused by acute *Neisseria gonorrhoeae* infection
d. Treatment in the acute phase is surgical
e. Patients may have associated acute salpingitis

28.68 What percent of normal women with *Neisseria gonorrhoeae* cervicitis will develop acute pelvic inflammatory disease?
a. 5%
b. 15%
c. 25%
d. 35%
e. 45%

28.69 A Word catheter being used to drain a Bartholin gland abscess should be left in place for a minimum of
a. 24 hours
b. 48 hours
c. 3 days
d. 1 week

28.70 Condyloma acuminata that exceed 2 cm in size are best treated with
a. Podofilox
b. Trichloroacetic acid
c. Laser therapy
d. Interferon injections

28.71 The initial involvement in pelvic tuberculosis typically is
a. ovarian
b. tubal
c. endometrial
d. vulvar

28.72 A false-positive screening test for AIDS is more likely in what women who
a. are White
b. are over age 30
c. are taking oral contraceptives
d. have a history of syphilis

Answers

28.64 b	28.66 a	28.68 b	28.70 c	28.72 c
28.65 c	28.67 d	28.69 d	28.71 b	

28.73 Measures to prevent HIV include use of latex condoms containing
a. Nonoxynol 9
b. Doxycycline
c. Azithromycin
d. HAART (highly active antiretroviral therapy)

28.74 When neurosyphilis is clinically suspected, a VDRL should be obtained on what fluid?
a. Peritoneal fluid
b. Cerebrospinal fluid
c. Serum
d. Urine
e. Gastric secretions

28.75 What is the additional risk for ectopic pregnancy in patients with a history of salpingitis?
a. Twofold
b. Fourfold
c. Eightfold
d. 20-fold

Answers

28.73 a	**28.74** b	**28.75** c

Questions and Answers Chapter 29: Pelvic Relaxation, Urinary Incontinence, and Urinary Tract Infection

29.1 Which of the following is NOT a characteristic symptom of pelvic relaxation?
a. Pelvic pressure
b. Dyspareunia
c. Stress incontinence (urinary)
d. Intermittent diarrhea

29.2 What percent of women will have loss of urine during coughing, laughing, or other stress at some time in their lives?
a. 5%
b. 20%
c. 50%
d. 70%
e. 90%

29.3 Approximately what percent of women suffer significant, recurrent urinary incontinence in the presence of increased intra-abdominal pressure?
a. Less than 5%
b. 10 to 15%
c. 20 to 25%
d. 30 to 35%
e. 40 to 45%

29.4 Which of the following structures does NOT provide direct support to the pelvic organs?
a. Pelvic floor muscles
b. Fascia
c. Bony pelvis
d. Ligaments

29.5 In a patient with enterocele, there is a descent or herniation of the
a. uterus
b. apex of the vagina
c. bladder
d. urethra
e. rectum

29.5 A 45-year-old patient complains of frequent loss of urine when she coughs, laughs, or strains. The volume lost is small, but it occurs frequently. She does not report any dysuria. This patient's problem is most appropriately defined as
a. stress incontinence
b. urgency incontinence
c. overflow incontinence
d. behavioral incontinence
e. enuresis

29.7 A 45-year-old diabetic patient complains of frequent loss of urine. The volume lost is small, but it occurs almost continuously. She does not report any sense of fullness, urgency, or dysuria and she voids frequently but in small amounts. She does not ever feel "full" but also never has the sense that she has completely emptied her bladder. This patient's problem is most appropriately defined as
a. stress incontinence
b. urgency incontinence
c. overflow incontinence
d. behavioral incontinence
e. enuresis

29.8 A 22-year-old patient complains of occasional loss of urine. The volume lost is large when it occurs. She reports a sense of intense fullness and urgency just before the urine is lost. She voids infrequently but in large amounts. She does not ever feel that she "gets enough warning" to get to the bathroom. This patient's problem is most appropriately defined as
a. stress incontinence
b. urgency incontinence
c. overflow incontinence
d. behavioral incontinence
e. enuresis

Answers

29.1 d	29.3 b	29.5 b	29.7 c
29.2 c	29.4 c	29.6 a	29.8 b

29.9 A 22-year-old patient complains of occasional loss of urine. The volume lost is large when it occurs. She reports that the loss occurs primarily when she changes position (e.g., rising from a chair) or when she is around running water. This patient's problem is most appropriately defined as
a. stress incontinence
b. urgency incontinence
c. overflow incontinence
d. behavioral incontinence
e. enuresis

29.10 A symptomatic rectocele is often characterized by
a. loss of urine during stress
b. urinary retention
c. intermittent diarrhea
d. difficulty passing stools

29.11 A cystocele may best be demonstrated clinically by
a. use of a Valsalva maneuver with the patient supine
b. use of a Sims speculum to retract the anterior vaginal wall
c. gentle traction on the cervix
d. observing posterior rotation of the anterior vaginal wall in response to change in position

29.12 What condition is most likely in a patient who needs to press on the back of her vagina with her fingers to facilitate having a bowel movement?
a. Rectocele
b. Cystocele
c. Urethral prolapse (urethrocele)
d. Enterocele

29.13 A patient who loses urine when she coughs or sneezes most likely has a(n)
a. rectocele
b. cystocele
c. urethral prolapse (urethrocele)
d. enterocele

29.14 Small bowel herniation is found in
a. rectocele
b. cystocele
c. urethral prolapse (urethrocele)
d. enterocele

29.15 Which of the following is lined with peritoneum, making it a true hernia?
a. Rectocele
b. Cystocele
c. Urethral prolapse (urethrocele)
d. Enterocele

29.16 Which of the following is NOT a manifestation of pelvic relaxation?
a. Uterine prolapse
b. Procidentia
c. Vaginal vault prolapse
d. Uterine retroversion

29.17 A cough causes genuine stress incontinence when the bladder pressure is
a. less than the urethral pressure
b. the same as the urethral pressure
c. greater than the urethral pressure

29.18 Which of the following conditions is associated with urinary incontinence?
a. Bladder atony
b. Bladder spasm
c. Psychosis
d. Fistulous tract
e. All of the above

29.19 When the structure (e.g., the cervix) descends to the upper third of the vagina, the prolpase is defined as
a. first-degree prolapse
b. second-degree prolapse
c. third-degree prolapse
d. procidentia

29.20 Whan the structure (e.g., the cervix) descends to the vaginal introitus, the prolapse is defined as
a. first-degree prolapse
b. second-degree prolapse
c. third-degree prolapse
d. procidentia

Answers

29.9 b	**29.11** a	**29.13** c	**29.15** d	**29.17** c	**29.19** a
29.10 d	**29.12** a	**29.14** d	**29.16** d	**29.18** e	**29.20** b

29.21 When the structure (e.g., the cervix) descends to outside the vaginal opening, the prolapse is defined as
a. first-degree prolapse
b. second-degree prolapse
c. third-degree prolapse
d. procidentia

29.22 A "Q-tip test" is used to evaluate the
a. presence of residual urine
b. support for the posterior vaginal wall
c. degree of cervical descent down the vaginal canal
d. amount of urethral mobility
e. degree of urethral sensitivity

29.23 When performing a "Q-tip test," incontinence is generally associated with upward rotation of
a. <5°
b. 10°
c. 20°
d. 30°

29.24 The key anatomic abnormality in stress incontinence is
a. a urethrovesical angle of <90°
b. the urethra prolapsing at times of increased intra-abdominal pressure
c. the pressure of bladder herniation
d. the urethra dropping outside the influence of intra abdominal pressure and the bladder remaining within

29.25 Which of the following may result from the vaginal mucosa prolapsing beyond the introitus?
a. Bleeding
b. Ulceration
c. Infection
d. All of the above

29.26 Pelvic relaxation is best demonstrated with the patient
a. at rest, supine
b. at rest, upright
c. straining
d. under anesthesia

29.27 While a speculum is retracting the posterior vaginal wall, a 51-year-old patient is asked to strain down. There is a bulge from the anterior vaginal wall. This is most likely
a. a rectocele
b. a cystocele
c. an enterocele
d. a vaginal vault prolapse

29.28 Which of the following is associated with procidentia?
a. Fecal incontinence
b. Constipation
c. Ureteral obstruction
d. Bladder atony

29.29 Anticholinergic. This category of drug is represented by which medications?
a. Oxybutynin chloride (Ditropan)
b. Metaproterenol sulfate (Alupent)
c. Flavoxate hydrochloride (Urispas)
d. Diazepam (Valium)
e. Imipramine hydrochloride (Tofranil)

29.30 Which of the following is an example of a musculotropic drug?
a. Oxybutynin chloride (Ditropan)
b. Metaproterenol sulfate (Alupent)
c. Flavoxate hydrochloride (Urispas)
d. Diazepam (Valium)
e. Imipramine hydrochloride (Tofranil)

29.31 Which of the following is an example of an antidepressant drug?
a. Oxybutynin chloride (Ditropan)
b. Metaproterenol sulfate (Alupent)
c. Flavoxate hydrochloride (Urispas)
d. Diazepam (Valium)
e. Imipramine hydrochloride (Tofranil)

Answers

29.21 c	29.23 d	29.25 d	29.27 b	29.29 a	29.31 e
29.22 d	29.24 d	29.26 c	29.28 c	29.30 c	

29.32 Which of the following is the LEAST effective treatment for urgency incontinence?
a. Biofeedback
b. Surgery
c. Bladder training
d. Medical therapy

29.33 Bladder training programs have which of the following goals?
a. Increasing the amount of time between voiding
b. Decreasing the duration of urine flow
c. Decreasing bladder volume
d. Increasing midstream urine flow

29.34 The purpose of Kegel exercises is to
a. strengthen pelvic floor muscles
b. improve bladder capacity and control
c. tighten uterine ligaments
d. increase bladder awareness

29.35 Kegel exercises may be useful in a patient with
a. second-degree prolapse of the uterus
b. symptomatic rectocele
c. mild stress incontinence
d. dyspareunia

29.36 The main function of pessaries is to
a. obstruct the urethra
b. provide mechanical support to the vagina
c. focus intra-abdominal pressure toward the introitus
d. decrease bladder capacity

29.37 Hysterectomy is used to repair
a. vaginal vault prolapse
b. stress incontinence
c. uterine prolapse
d. rectocele

29.38 Colpocleisis is used to repair
a. vaginal vault prolapse
b. stress incontinence
c. uterine prolapse
d. rectocele

29.39 Posterior colporrhaphy is used to repair
a. vaginal vault prolapse
b. stress incontinence
c. uterine prolapse
d. rectocele

29.40 Paravaginal repair is used to repair
a. vaginal vault prolapse
b. stress incontinence
c. uterine prolapse
d. rectocele

29.41 Which of the following surgical procedures does not require an abdominal incision?
a. Marshall-Marchetti-Krantz
b. Burch
c. Pereyra
d. LeFort
e. Moskowitz

29.42 Which of the following surgical procedures obliterates the vaginal canal?
a. Marshall-Marchetti-Krantz
b. Burch
c. Pereyra
d. LeFort
e. Moskowitz

29.43 Which of the following surgical procedures provides a sling for the vagina?
a. Marshall-Marchetti-Krantz
b. Burch
c. Pereyra
d. LeFort
e. Moskowitz

Answers

29.32 b	29.34 a	29.36 b	29.38 a	29.40 b	29.42 d
29.33 a	29.35 c	29.37 c	29.39 d	29.41 d	29.43 c

29.44 Which of the following surgical procedures decreases the possibility of future
enterocele formation?
a. Marshall-Marchetti-Krantz
b. Burch
c. Pereyra
d. LeFort
e. Moskowitz

29.45 The first step in the treatment of a vesicovaginal fistula first noted 4 days after
an abdominal hysterectomy is
a. catheter drainage of the bladder
b. insertion of a vaginal pessary
c. surgical dissection of the fistulous
tract
d. irradiation to create scarring

29.46 Approximately what percent of women
will suffer a urinary tract infection at
some point in their lives?
a. Less than 5%
b. 10 to 15%
c. 20 to 25%
d. 30 to 35%
e. 40 to 45%

29.47 The relative ratio of urinary tract infections in men and women (M:F) is
a. 10:1
b. 5:1
c. 1:1
d. 1:5
e. 1:10

29.48 In women, most urinary tract infections
occur through
a. hematogenous seeding
b. lymphatic spread
c. ascending contamination from the
urethra
d. retained urine

29.49 Which of the following factors is associated with a higher risk of bladder infection in women as compared with men?
a. Relatively shorter urethra in
women
b. Estrogen effects
c. Sexual activity
d. Trauma
e. All of the above

29.50 Asymptomatic bacteriuria is found in
approximately what percent of postmenopausal women?
a. Less than 5%
b. 10 to 15%
c. 20 to 25%
d. 30 to 35%
e. 40 to 45%

29.51 First urinary tract infections in women
are most commonly caused by
a. β-streptococcus
b. *Proteus mirabilis*
c. *Escherichia coli*
d. *Clostridium perfringes*

29.52 Irritation of the trigone (trigonitis)
causes which of the following
symptoms?
a. Frequency
b. Urgency
c. Nocturia
d. All of the above

29.53 A single drop of uncentrifuged urine is
examined under the microscope and 2
white blood cells per high-power field
are found. What is the likelihood that
this patient has a bladder infection?
a. 15%
b. 30%
c. 50%
d. 70%
e. 90%

Answers

29.44 e	29.46 b	29.48 c	29.50 b	29.52 d
29.45 a	29.47 e	29.49 e	29.51 c	29.53 e

29.54 The culture of a urine sample is reported to show >100,000 colonies of "mixed flora." This is most likely indicative of
  a. infection of the proximal urethra
  b. trigonitis
  c. upper urinary tract infection
  d. a contaminated specimen

29.55 In a symptomatic patient, which of the following is indicative of lower urinary tract infection?
  a. 10,000 colonies of *Escherichia coli*
  b. 10,000 colonies of *Staphylococcus aureus*
  c. More than 100,000 colonies of mixed flora
  d. 1,000 colonies of *Bacteroides* species

29.56 When treating an uncomplicated first episode of lower urinary tract infection, which of the following is most likely to precipitate a concomitant vaginal yeast infection?
  a. Ascorbic acid
  b. Phenazopyridine hydrochloride (Pyridium)
  c. Nitrofurantoin (Macrodantin)
  d. Ampicillin

29.57 Which is the LEAST likely finding in a patient with cystitis?
  a. Frequency
  b. Dysuria
  c. Fever
  d. Suprapubic tenderness

29.58 Which of the following provides urinary analgesia?
  a. Ascorbic acid
  b. Phenazopyridine hydrochloride (Pyridium)
  c. Nitrofurantoin (Macrodantin)
  d. Ampicillin

29.59 In the region where the urethra joins the bladder, the urethra is surrounded by circular smooth muscle fibers called
  a. the pubovesicocervical neck
  b. the external sphincter
  c. Retzius angle
  d. the internal sphincter

29.60 Urethrocele is best defined as
  a. herniation of the top of the vagina
  b. descent or prolapse of urethra
  c. descent or prolapse of rectum
  d. descent or prolapse of bladder

29.61 Cystocele is best defined as
  a. herniation of the top of the vagina
  b. descent or prolapse of urethra
  c. descent or prolapse of rectum
  d. descent or prolapse of bladder

29.62 Rectocele is best defined as
  a. herniation of the top of the vagina
  b. descent or prolapse of urethra
  c. descent or prolapse of rectum
  d. descent or prolapse of bladder

29.63 Enterocele is best defined as
  a. herniation of top of vagina
  b. descent or prolapse of urethra
  c. descent or prolapse of rectum
  d. descent or prolapse of bladder

29.64 Procidentia describes uterine descent beyond the
  a. plane of the pelvic inlet
  b. level of the uterine artery
  c. vaginal introitus
  d. vulva

Answers

29.54 d	29.56 d	29.58 b	29.60 b	29.62 c	29.64 d
29.55 a	29.57 c	29.59 d	29.61 d	29.63 a	

Questions and Answers Chapter 30: Endometriosis

30.1 All of the following symptoms are associated with endometriosis EXCEPT
a. infertility
b. dysmenorrhea
c. incontinence
d. dyspareunia
e. chronic pelvic pain

30.2 The diagnosis of endometriosis is suspected on the basis of
a. culture and sensitivity
b. histology
c. typical history
d. family history

30.3 The diagnosis of endometriosis is confirmed on the basis of
a. culture and sensitivity
b. histology
c. typical history
d. pelvic examination
e. family history

30.4 Which of the following is thought to be associated with an increased risk of endometriosis?
a. Early menopause
b. Multiparity
c. First-degree relative with endometriosis
d. Middle-to-upper income socioeconomic status

30.5 About what percent of women in the general population have endometriosis?
a. 1 to 2%
b. 4 to 5%
c. 7 to 8%
d. 10 to 11%
e. 13 to 14%

30.6 About what percent of infertile women have endometriosis?
a. 10 to 30%
b. 30 to 50%
c. 50 to 70%
d. 80 to 90%

30.7 A first-degree relative of a woman with endometriosis has an approximately what percent chance of being similarly affected?
a. 3%
b. 7%
c. 11%
d. 15%
e. 19%

30.8 Sampson's theory of the development of endometriosis is based on the occurrence of
a. retrograde menstruation
b. multipotent coelomic cells
c. vascular and lymphatic dissemination
d. a viral DNA vector

30.9 The occurrence of distant implants of endometriosis (such as in the pleural cavity or kidney) supports the theory of endometriosis development based on
a. retrograde menstruation
b. multipotent coelomic cells
c. vascular and lymphatic dissemination
d. a viral DNA vector

30.10 Which of the following is the most common site in which endometriosis is found?
a. Posterior cul-de-sac
b. Uterosacral ligaments
c. Ovary
d. Fallopian tube

Answers

30.1 c	30.3 b	30.5 a	30.7 b	30.9 c
30.2 c	30.4 c	30.6 b	30.8 a	30.10 c

30.11 All of the following findings at the time of laparoscopy are consistent with the diagnosis of mild endometriosis EXCEPT
- a. 1-mm vascular hemorrhagic area in the posterior cul-de-sac
- b. multiple rust-colored spots on the peritoneal surfaces, 1 to 2 mm in diameter
- c. small, puckered white lesions on the uterosacral ligaments
- d. small, firm, yellow nodules on the anterior surface of the uterus

30.12 What percent of women with endometriosis have ovarian involvement?
- a. 10%
- b. 20%
- c. 40%
- d. 60%
- e. 80%

30.13 The term "endometrioma" refers to
- a. an isolated collection of endometriosis involving an ovary and creating a tumor
- b. any endometrial implant >5 mm
- c. endometrial tissue found deep within the wall of the uterus
- d. endometrial implants that are symptomatic

30.14 The histologic diagnosis of endometriosis requires the presence of all the following findings EXCEPT
- a. glands
- b. stroma
- c. decidual reaction
- d. hemosiderin-laden macrophages

30.15 What percent of cases with a clinical diagnosis of endometriosis can be supported by histologic findings?
- a. 95%
- b. 85%
- c. 70%
- d. 50%

30.16 The presence of endometrial glands and stroma within the wall of the uterus is termed
- a. endometriosis
- b. adenomyosis
- c. endometrial hyperplasia
- d. endometrioma

30.17 It is estimated that approximately what percent of women with adenomyosis are asymptomatic?
- a. 5%
- b. 15%
- c. 40%
- d. 60%
- e. 85%

30.18 All of the following symptoms are consistent with the clinical diagnosis of endometriosis EXCEPT
- a. cyclic pelvic pain
- b. "deep thrust" dyspareunia
- c. vaginal bleeding between periods
- d. intermittent fever
- e. painful bowel movements

30.19 What is the most common cause for infertility in patients with endometriosis?
- a. pelvic scarring
- b. persistent anovulation
- c. elevated levels of follicle-stimulating hormone (FSH)
- d. increased macrophage activity

30.20 What is the estimated overall incidence of endometriosis in women in the general population?
- a. 0.1%
- b. 1%
- c. 10%
- d. 20%
- e. 35%

Answers

30.11 d	30.13 a	30.15 c	30.17 c	30.19 a
30.12 d	30.14 c	30.16 b	30.18 d	30.20 b

30.21 The prevalence of endometriosis in infertile women is approximately
  a. 5%
  b. 10 to 15%
  c. 20 to 25%
  d. 35 to 40%
  e. 60 to 65%

30.22 In which age group is endometriosis most likely to be diagnosed?
  a. Prepubertal (<12 years of age)
  b. Adolescent (13 to 17 years)
  c. 20 to 35 years
  d. Perimenopausal (45 to 52 years)
  e. Postmenopausal (63 to 68 years)

30.23 Endometriosis is discovered in about what proportion of teenagers undergoing laparoscopy for evaluation of chronic pelvic pain or dysmenorrhea?
  a. 1 in 4
  b. 1 in 2
  c. 3 in 4
  d. almost all

30.24 Intermenstrual bleeding occurs in approximately what proportion of women with endometriosis?
  a. 1 in 6
  b. 1 in 3
  c. 2 in 3
  d. 3 in 4

30.25 Vaginal bleeding between periods occurs in approximately what percent of women with endometriosis?
  a. Less than 5%
  b. 10 to 15%
  c. 20 to 25%
  d. 30 to 35%
  e. 40 to 45%

30.26 Which of the following best describes the dysmenorrhea associated with endometriosis?
  a. It is not necessarily proportional to the extent of the disease
  b. It is caused by a fixed, retroverted uterus
  c. It is a result of uterosacral involvement
  d. It is worse in patients who are infertile
  e. It is indicative of ovarian involvement

30.27 What is a typical finding on pelvic examination of patients with adenomyosis?
  a. There is retroversion of the uterus
  b. There is reduced mobility of the uterus
  c. There is adnexal thickening
  d. There is nodularity of the cul-de-sac
  e. There is firm, symmetrical enlargements of the uterus

30.28 All of the following physical findings are consistent with a clinical diagnosis of endometriosis EXCEPT
  a. retroversion of the uterus
  b. reduced mobility of the uterus
  c. adnexal thickening
  d. nodularity of the cul-de-sac
  e. firm, symmetrical enlargements of the uterus

30.29 According to the American Fertility Society classification of endometriosis, a patient with complete obliteration of the cul-de-sac by adhesions has
  a. minimal disease
  b. mild disease
  c. moderate disease
  d. severe disease

Answers

30.21 d	30.23 b	30.25 d	30.27 e	30.29 d
30.22 c	30.24 b	30.26 a	30.28 e	

30.30 According to the American Fertility Society classification of endometriosis, a patient with extensive ovarian adhesions enclosing two thirds of both ovaries but no other signs of disease has
a. minimal disease
b. mild disease
c. moderate disease
d. severe disease

30.31 Infertility in the presence of minimal endometriosis is a result of
a. adhesions
b. tubal obstruction
c. autoantibodies
d. prostaglandin overproduction
e. unknown causes

30.32 What type of abnormal bleeding is associated with endometriosis?
a. Menorrhagia
b. Intermenstrual bleeding
c. Amenorrhea
d. Hypermenorrhea

30.33 A 25-year-old patient is found to have minimal endometriosis at the time of laparoscopy for infertility. What is appropriate treatment for this patient?
a. Administration of oral contraceptives
b. Administration of a gonadotropin-releasing hormone (GnRH) agonist
c. Laser surgery
d. Expectant management

30.34 In a patient that has undergone total abdominal hysterectomy and bilateral salpingo-oophorectomy for endometriosis, estrogen-replacement therapy should be
a. begun immediately
b. begun after follow-up laparoscopy 1 year later
c. begun only after 5 symptom-free years
d. avoided indefinitely

30.35 Continuous administration of combination oral contraceptives is effective in treating endometriosis because they
a. lower FSH and luteinizing hormone (LH) levels
b. induce anovulation
c. reduce endometrial prostaglandin production
d. induce a decidual reaction in the endometrial implants

30.36 Medical therapy for endometriosis can be expected to accomplish all of the following EXCEPT
a. improvement of dyspareunia
b. reduction of adhesions
c. reduction of cyclic pain
d. reduction of menstrual flow

30.37 Which of the following drugs induces "pseudopregnancy"?
a. Oral contraceptives
b. Danazol (17α-ethinyl testosterone derivative)
c. Gonadotropin-releasing hormone (GnRH) agonist
d. Medroxyprogesterone acetate

30.38 Which of the following drugs has side effects that include hot flashes and alterations of lipoprotein metabolism?
a. Oral contraceptives
b. Danazol (17α-ethinyl testosterone derivative)
c. Gonadotropin-releasing hormone (GnRH) agonist
d. Medroxyprogesterone acetate

30.39 Gonadotropin-releasing hormone (GnRH) agonists act by
a. suppression of endometrial responsiveness
b. down-regulation of the pituitary gland
c. hyperstimulation of the ovary
d. stimulation of the metabolism of progesterone

Answers

30.30 c	30.32 b	30.34 a	30.36 b	30.38 b
30.31 e	30.33 d	30.35 d	30.37 a	30.39 b

30.40 Definitive surgical therapy for
endometriosis includes
a. total abdominal hysterectomy
b. bilateral salpingo-oophorectomy
c. lysis of adhesions
d. removal of endometriotic implants
e. all of the above

30.41 After conservative surgical therapy,
what is the average pregnancy rate
for patients who have had severe
endometriosis?
a. 80%
b. 60%
c. 40%
d. 20%

30.42 In danazol-induced pseudomenopause,
which of the following statements
about FSH and LH levels is correct?
a. Both are suppressed
b. Both are elevated
c. FSH is elevated and LH is
suppressed
d. FSH is suppressed and LH is
elevated

Answers

30.40 e   **30.41** c   **30.42** a

Questions and Answers Chapter 31: Dysmenorrhea and Chronic Pelvic Pain

31.1 What is the most common cause of dysmenorrhea in a 19-year-old patient?
 a. anovulation
 b. excess prostaglandin production
 c. adenomyosis
 d. endometriosis
 e. pelvic congestion syndrome

31.2 Which of the following is NOT a physiologic mechanism responsible for the generation of a neurologic signal that is perceived as pain?
 a. Ischemia
 b. Stretch
 c. Inflammation
 d. Spasm
 e. Perforation

31.3 It is uncommon for primary dysmenorrhea to occur
 a. after the birth of a child
 b. after tubal ligation
 c. during breast feeding
 d. during the first three to six menstrual cycles of reproductive life

31.4 Childbearing affects
 a. both the occurrence of primary and secondary dysmenorrhea
 b. neither the occurrence of primary nor secondary dysmenorrhea
 c. the occurrence of primary but not secondary dysmenorrhea
 d. the occurrence of secondary but not primary dysmenorrhea

31.5 What is the agent thought to be responsible for causing primary dysmenorrhea?
 a. Estrogen
 b. Progesterone
 c. Prostaglandin E_2.
 d. Prostaglandin F_{2a}.

31.6 Prostaglandin production in the uterus associated with dysmenorrhea normally increases under the influence of
 a. progesterone only
 b. both estrogen and progesterone
 c. estrogen only
 d. prolactin

31.7 Primary and secondary dysmenorrhea cause significant disability for approximately what percent of women?
 a. 1 to 2%
 b. 5 to 8%
 c. 10 to 15%
 d. 20 to 25%
 e. 30 to 35%

31.8 During primary dysmenorrhea, intrauterine pressures may reach a maximum of
 a. 50 mm Hg
 b. 80 mm Hg
 c. 125 mm Hg
 d. 250 mm Hg
 e. 4,000 mm Hg

31.9 The uterine contractions associated with primary dysmenorrhea result in baseline intrauterine pressures in excess of
 a. 30 mm Hg
 b. 50 mm Hg
 c. 80 mm Hg
 d. 110 mm Hg
 e. 140 mm Hg

31.10 Which of the following would establish a diagnosis of secondary dysmenorrhea?
 a. Crampy, episodic pain
 b. Pain that begins on the first day of menstrual flow
 c. Patient began to experience pain at age 20
 d. Presence of an abnormal pelvic examination
 e. Presence of a heavy menstrual flow

Answers

| 31.1 | b | 31.3 | d | 31.5 | d | 31.7 | c | 31.9 | c |
| 31.2 | d | 31.4 | b | 31.6 | a | 31.8 | e | 31.10 | d |

31.11 A patient is referred for evaluation of possible primary dysmenorrhea. Which of the following would cause suspicion of secondary dysmenorrhea?
  a. Dyspareunia
  b. Presence of blood clots in menstrual flow
  c. Nausea and vomiting during period
  d. Irregular periods

31.12 Compared with primary dysmenorrhea, secondary dysmenorrhea tends to be
  a. more common in older women
  b. as common in older women
  c. less common in older women

31.13 In secondary dysmenorrhea, intrauterine resting pressure is typically
  a. decreased
  b. unchanged
  c. increased

31.14 Which of the following is an action of prostaglandin F_{2a}?
  a. Vasodilation
  b. Hyperemia
  c. Smooth muscle contraction
  d. Hypomotility of the intestines

31.15 A 23-year-old G0P0 patient complains of increasing pelvic heaviness and cyclic lower abdominal pain that begins 1 day before her menstrual flow and lasts for 3 days. Periods are regular, but are heavy with clots. She has been attempting pregnancy for the past 3 years. Which of the following is NOT a likely diagnosis for this patient?
  a. Primary dysmenorrhea
  b. Adenomyosis
  c. Uterine myomas
  d. Endometriosis

31.16 A 23-year-old G0P0 patient complains of increasing pelvic heaviness and cyclic lower abdominal pain that begins 1 day before her menstrual flow and lasts for 3 days. Periods are regular, but are heavy with clots. She has been attempting pregnancy for the past 3 years. Pelvic examination is normal except for painful nodules posterior to the cervix. Which of the following is the most likely diagnosis for this patient?
  a. Primary dysmenorrhea
  b. Adenomyosis
  c. Uterine myomas
  d. Endometriosis

31.17 An 18-year-old G0P0 patient complains of cyclic, sharp, crampy, lower abdominal pain that begins on the day of her menstrual flow and lasts for 2 to 3 days. Periods are regular and heavy, with clots. She has been attempting pregnancy for the past year. Pelvic examination is normal. Which of the following is the most likely diagnosis for this patient?
  a. Primary dysmenorrhea
  b. Adenomyosis
  c. Uterine myomas
  d. Endometriosis

31.18 An 18-year-old G0P0 patient complains of cyclic, sharp, crampy, lower abdominal pain that begins on the day of her menstrual flow and lasts for 2 to 3 days. Periods are regular and heavy, with clots. She has been attempting pregnancy for the past year. Pelvic examination is normal. The most appropriate therapy for this patient would be
  a. low-dose, monophasic oral contraceptive pills
  b. an acetaminophen/codeine combination
  c. a nonsteroidal anti-inflammatory agent
  d. an injectable progestin contraceptive agent

Answers

31.11 a	**31.13** b	**31.15** a	**31.17** a	**31.18** c
31.12 a	**31.14** c	**31.16** d		

31.19 An identifiable cause is found in what percent of patients who undergo diagnostic laparoscopy for pelvic pain?
a. 10 to 15%
b. 30 to 40%
c. approximately 50%
d. 60 to 70%
e. 90 to 95%

31.20 Thickening in the adnexae is consistent with
a. pelvic inflammatory disease
b. leiomyoma uteri
c. endometritis
d. adenomyosis uteri

31.21 The term "chronic pelvic pain" is applied to pain that has been present for
a. three consecutive menstrual periods
b. at least 6 months
c. three or more of a woman's first six menstrual cycles
d. more than 21 days in a given month

31.22 The term "chronic pelvic pain" is generally applied to pelvic discomfort
a. not solely associated with menstruation and that lasts more than 6 months
b. solely associated with menstruation and that lasts more than 6 months
c. not solely associated with menstruation and that lasts more than 12 months
d. solely associated with menstruation and that lasts more than 12 months

31.23 The Rome criteria for the diagnosis of irritable bowel syndrome include the presence of abdominopelvic pain in the past 12 months that cannot be explained by known disease and which persists for how many weeks (not necessarily consecutive)?
a. 3
b. 6
c. 9
d. 12

31.24 Which of the following complaints is not used to categorize irritable bowel syndrome for purposes of treatment?
a. Pain
b. Blood in the stool
c. Diarrhea
d. Constipation
e. Alternating constipation and diarrhea

31.25 Which of the following would not contribute to a diagnosis of irritable bowel syndrome?
a. Pain relieved by defecation
b. Change in the frequency of bowel movements
c. Change in appetite
d. Change in the form of stool

31.26 The pathophysiology of irritable bowel syndrome may include all of the following EXCEPT
a. altered bowel mobility
b. visceral insensitivity
c. psychosocial factors (especially stress)
d. an imbalance of neurotransmitters (especially serotonin)
e. infection (often indolent or subclinical)

31.27 Which of the following statements about the diagnosis of irritable bowel syndrome is incorrect?
a. The diagnosis relies heavily on the history.
b. The diagnosis relies on colonoscopy plus barium enema in women under approximately 50 years of age.
c. The diagnosis relies on flexible sigmoidoscopy in women under approximately 50 years of age.
d. The diagnosis relies on biopsy of the mucosae of the descending colon when diarrhea is a predominant symptom.

Answers

31.19 d	31.21 b	31.23 d	31.25 c	31.27 b
31.20 a	31.22 a	31.24 b	31.26 b	

31.28 Which of the following would not be part of the management of a patient whose irritable bowel syndrome has constipation as the predominant sympton?
a. Keeping a food diary
b. Fiber
c. Lactulose
d. Loperamide

31.29 Depending on the patient's situation, which of the following is an appropriate goal in the management of chronic pelvic pain?
a. Alleviation of the cause of the pain
b. Management of pain symptoms
c. Both of the above

31.30 In the treatment of chronic pelvic pain, analgesics are best administered on
a. a fixed time schedule that is independent of symptoms
b. a fixed schedule that is dependent on symptoms
c. an as-needed schedule that is independent of symptoms
d. an as-needed schedule that is dependent on symptoms

Answers

31.28 d	**31.29** c	**31.30** a

Questions and Answers Chapter 32: Disorders of the Breast

32.1 In which quadrant of the breast is glandular tissue disproportinately distributed?
a. Upper inner
b. Upper outer
c. Lower inner
d. Lower outer

32.2 As a malignancy in women, breast cancer ranks where in frequency?
a. First
b. Second
c. Third
d. Fourth
e. Fifth

32.3 Collecting ducts arising from breast lobes terminate (drain) at the
a. areola
b. nipple
c. Montgomery ducts
d. chest wall lymphatics

32.4 What is the most common benign breast condition?
a. Ductal ectasia
b. Fibroadenoma
c. Fibrocystic change
d. Intraductal papilloma
e. Galactocele

32.5 What is the benign breast condition most commonly mistaken for cancer?
a. Fat necrosis
b. Fibrocystic change
c. Ductal ectasia
d. Intraductal papilloma

32.6 What is the most common presenting complaint of women with fibrocystic breast change?
a. Solitary breast mass
b. Localized breast tenderness
c. Bilateral, cyclic pain
d. Nipple discharge
e. Multiple breast masses

32.7 What is the usual sequence of events in the development of fibrocystic breast change?
a. Obstruction of ducts, cyst formation, fibrosis
b. Fibrosis, ductal expansion, cyclic breast pain
c. Ductal atrophy, fibrosis, cyst formation
d. Proliferation of stroma, adenosis, cyst formation

32.8 A 23-year-old patient presents with a 2- to 3-cm firm, painless, freely movable mass in her left breast. She reports that the mass does not change during her menstrual cycle and has grown slowly over the past year. The patient found the mass during breast self-examination. What is the most likely diagnosis?
a. Intraductal carcinoma
b. Fibroadenoma
c. Ductal ectasia
d. Fibrocystic change

32.9 Multiple fibroadenomas develop in approximately what percent of patients?
a. Less than 5%
b. 5 to 10%
c. 15 to 20%
d. 25 to 30%
e. 35 to 40%

Answers

32.1 b	32.3 b	32.5 a	32.7 d	32.9 c
32.2 b	32.4 c	32.6 c	32.8 b	

32.10 A 34-year-old patient complains of cyclic breast tenderness and diffuse nodularity on monthly breast self-examination. Your examination finds multiple firm, mobile masses, predominantly in the upper outer quadrants of each breast. You aspirate one of these masses and obtain clear, straw-colored fluid. What is the best initial management of this condition?
   a. Mechanical support of the breast
   b. Danazol sodium therapy
   c. Progesterone-only oral contraceptives
   d. Gonadotropin-releasing hormone (GnRH) agonist therapy
   e. Excisional biopsy

32.11 During what decade of life is a patient most likely to develop mammary duct ectasia?
   a. Sixth
   b. Fifth
   c. Fourth
   d. Third

32.12 Fibroadenomas occur in about what percent of all women?
   a. 1 to 2%
   b. 10 to 20%
   c. 30 to 40%
   d. 50 to 60%

32.13 Which of the following statements about the management of suspected fibroadenomas is INCORRECT?
   a. Ultrasound is not useful in distinguishing fibroadenomas from breast cysts.
   b. Surgical excision is indicated if the breast mass is painful.
   c. Surgical indication is indicated if the breast mass is rapidly growing.
   d. Fine-needle aspiration may provide sufficient information to allow management by frequent examination and mammographic evaluation.

32.14 Breast self-examination should be performed
   a. following menstruation
   b. at 2-week intervals, on the same day of the week
   c. weekly, on the same day of the week
   d. 3 to 5 days before menstruation

32.15 Approximately what percent of breast cancers are found by the patient herself?
   a. 10%
   b. 30%
   c. 50%
   d. 70%
   e. 90%

32.16 Currently, a woman living in the United States has what lifetime risk of developing breast cancer?
   a. 1 in 2
   b. 1 in 4
   c. 1 in 6
   d. 1 in 8
   e. 1 in 10

32.17 What is the risk of developing breast cancer for a woman over the age of 60?
   a. 1 in 120
   b. 1 in 90
   c. 1 in 60
   d. 1 in 30
   e. 1 in 3

32.18 What is the relative risk for developing cancer in a patient whose menarche occurs at <12 years of age?
   a. 0 to 1.0
   b. 1.1 to 2.0
   c. 2.1 to 4.0
   d. Greater than 4
   e. Greater than 8

Answers

32.10 a	32.12 b	32.14 a	32.16 d	32.18 b
32.11 b	32.13 a	32.15 e	32.17 d	

32.19 What is the relative risk for cancer in a patient with one first-degree relative with breast cancer (with pre-menopausal or postmenopausal, unilateral disease)?
a. 0 to 1.0
b. 1.1 to 2.0
c. 2.1 to 4.0
d. Greater than 4
e. Greater than 8

32.20 What is the relative risk for breast cancer in a patient with a personal history of cancer of major salivary glands?
a. 0 to 1.0
b. 1.1 to 2.0
c. 2.1 to 4.0
d. Greater than 4
e. Greater than 8

32.21 What is the relative risk for breast cancer in a patient with a personal history of cancer of the endometrium, ovary, or colon?
a. 0 to 1.0
b. 1.1 to 2.0
c. 2.1 to 4.0
d. Greater than 4
e. Greater than 8

32.22 What is the relative risk for developing breast cancer in a patient whose menarche occurs after 17 years of age?
a. 0 to 1.0
b. 1.1 to 2.0
c. 2.1 to 4.0
d. Greater than 4
e. Greater than 8

32.23 What is the relative risk for developing breast cancer in a patient whose menopause occurs before age 45?
a. 0 to 1.0
b. 1.1 to 2.0
c. 2.1 to 4.0
d. Greater than 4
e. Greater than 8

32.24 The relative risk for breast cancer in a patient who delivers a term pregnancy before age 35 is
a. 0 to 1.0
b. 1.1 to 2.0
c. 2.1 to 4.0
d. >4
e. >8

32.25 The relative risk to develop breast cancer in a patient who has a pre-menopausal first-degree relative with bilateral breast cancer is
a. 0 to 1.0
b. 1.1 to 2.0
c. 2.1 to 4.0
d. >4
e. >8

32.26 The relative risk for breast cancer in a woman who is over 65 years of age is
a. 0 to 1.0
b. 1.1 to 2.0
c. 2.1 to 4.0
d. >4
e. >8

32.27 The relative risk for breast cancer in a woman with inherited genetic mutations for breast cancer is
a. 0 to 1.0
b. 1.1 to 2.0
c. 2.1 to 4.0
d. >4
e. >8

32.28 The relative risk for breast cancer in a woman with a personal history of breast cancer is
a. 0 to 1.0
b. 1.1 to 2.0
c. 2.1 to 4.0
d. >4
e. >8

Answers

32.19 c	**32.21** d	**32.23** a	**32.25** e	**32.27** d
32.20 c	**32.22** a	**32.24** a	**32.26** d	**32.28** d

32.29 The relative risk for breast cancer in a woman who has never breast fed a child is
a. 0 to 1.0
b. 1.1 to 2.0
c. 2.1 to 4.0
d. >4
e. >8

32.30 The relative risk for breast cancer in a woman with no full-term pregnancies (for cancer diagnosed after age 40) is
a. 0 to 1.0
b. 1.1 to 2.0
c. 2.1 to 4.0
d. >4
e. >8

32.31 What is the relative risk for breast cancer in a woman with a first full-term pregnancy after age 35?
a. 0 to 1.0
b. 1.1 to 2.0
c. 2.1 to 4.0
d. >4
e. >8

32.32 The relative risk for breast cancer in a woman whose menopause occurs after age 55 is
a. 0 to 1.0
b. 1.1 to 2.0
c. 2.1 to 4.0
d. >4
e. >8

32.33 The relative risk for breast cancer if a woman has had an atypical hyperplasia on breast biopsy is
a. 0 to 1.0
b. 1.1 to 2.0
c. 2.1 to 4.0
d. >4
e. >8

32.34 The relative risk for breast cancer in a woman with two or more first-degree relatives with breast cancer is
a. 0 to 1.0
b. 1.1 to 2.0
c. 2.1 to 4.0
d. >4
e. >8

32.35 A 33-year-old patient asks about her risk for breast cancer in light of her mother having breast cancer. She should be told that her relative risk is
a. 0 to 1.0
b. 1.2 to 3.0
c. 4.0 to 6.0
d. >8

32.36 At her annual examination, a 40-year-old woman inquires about her risk for breast cancer because she had taken oral contraceptives for a year in high school. Her relative risk is
a. 0 to 1.0
b. 1.2 to 3.0
c. 4.0 to 6.0
d. >8

32.37 The relative risk for breast cancer in a patient who tried estrogen replacement therapy for a month is
a. 0 to 1.0
b. 1.2 to 3.0
c. 4.0 to 6.0
d. >8

32.38 A 50-year-old patient with breast cancer asks about her chances of developing cancer in the other breast. She should be told that her relative risk for contralateral breast cancer is
a. 0 to 1.0
b. 1.2 to 3.0
c. 4.0 to 6.0
d. >8

Answers

32.29 b	32.31 b	32.33 c	32.35 b	32.37 a
32.30 b	32.32 b	32.34 d	32.36 a	32.38 c

32.39 A patient with atypical hyperplasia on breast biopsy is being counseled regarding her risk of breast cancer. She should be told that her relative risk is
a. 0 to 1.0
b. 1.2 to 3.0
c. 4.0 to 6.0
d. 5.0

32.40 Historical risk factors identify what percent of breast cancer patients?
a. 10%
b. 25%
c. 40%
d. 55%
e. 70%

32.41 What proportion of patients 30 to 54 years of age with breast cancer are identified by specific risk factors?
a. 1:5
b. 2:5
c. 3:5
d. 4:5

32.42 What percent of all breast cancer occurs after the age of 40?
a. 95%
b. 85%
c. 75%
d. 65%

32.43 Breast pain is a presenting symptom in approximately what percent of patients with breast cancer?
a. 10%
b. 30%
c. 50%
d. 70%
e. 90%

32.44 What is the average doubling time of breast cancer cells?
a. 35 days
b. 100 days
c. 175 days
d. 300 days
e. 450 days

32.45 Mutations or alterations in the breast cancer susceptibility genes (such as BRCA1 and BRCA2) appear in what percent of the general population?
a. Less than 1%
b. Approximately 5%
c. Approximately 10%
d. Approximately 25%
e. Approximately 40%

32.46 What is the most common form of breast cancer?
a. Cystosarcoma phylloides
b. Infiltrating intraductal carcinoma
c. Noninfiltrating intraductal carcinoma
d. Lobular carcinoma
e. Paget disease

32.47 Paget disease accounts for approximately what percent of breast cancers?
a. 1%
b. 10%
c. 15%
d. 20%
e. 35%

32.48 Compared with detection of breast cancer by self-examination, breast cancer is detectable by mammography
a. significantly earlier
b. at about the same time
c. significantly later

32.49 Approximately what percent of breast cancers present as a mass?
a. 20%
b. 40%
c. 60%
d. 80%
e. 100%

Answers

32.39 c	**32.41** a	**32.43** a	**32.45** a	**32.47** a	**32.49** d
32.40 b	**32.42** b	**32.44** b	**32.46** b	**32.48** a	

32.50 A 30-year-old patient with a family history of breast cancer undergoes a needle aspiration of a cystic breast mass. The fluid obtained is clear. Your next step in the management of this patient would be to
a. send the fluid for cytology
b. obtain a mammogram
c. check the site for recurrence of the mass
d. perform a needle biopsy of the cyst wall

32.51 The advantage of mammography is that it can
a. identify suspicious lesions 2 or more years before they are palpable
b. assess the degree of spread of malignancy
c. differentiate between benign and malignant conditions
d. provide reassurance about suspicious masses

32.52 The accuracy of mammography in diagnosing breast cancer is approximately
a. 45%
b. 65%
c. 85%
d. 100%

32.53 The current use of mammography has been credited with reducing the overall mortality rate of breast cancer by
a. 5%
b. 15%
c. 30%
d. 45%
e. 60%

32.54 Current mammography techniques result in radiation exposure that approximates
a. 0.5 to 1 rad
b. 3 to 5 rad
c. 8 to 10 rad
d. 12 to 15 rad

32.55 A BI-RADS Category 0 report is defined as what type of finding?
a. Negative
b. Benign finding
c. Additional imaging needed
d. Probably benign
e. Suspicious abnormality

32.56 BI-RADS Category 1 report is defined as what type of finding?
a. Negative
b. Benign finding
c. Additional imaging needed
d. Probably benign
e. Suspicious abnormality

32.57 A Category 2 BI-RADS report is defined as what type of finding?
a. Negative
b. Benign finding
c. Additional imaging needed
d. Probably benign
e. Suspicious abnormality

32.58 A Category 3 on a BI-RADS mammography report is defined as what type of finding?
a. Negative
b. Benign finding
c. Additional imaging needed
d. Probably benign
e. Suspicious abnormality

32.59 A Category 4 on a BI-RADS mammography report is defined as what type of finding?
a. Negative
b. Benign finding
c. Additional imaging needed
d. Probably benign
e. Suspicious abnormality

32.60 A Category 5 on a BI-RADS mammography report is defined as what type of finding?
a. Negative
b. Benign finding
c. Additional imaging evaluation needed
d. Probably benign finding
e. Highly suggestive of malignancy

Answers

32.50 c	**32.52** c	**32.54** a	**32.56** a	**32.58** d	**32.60** e
32.51 a	**32.53** c	**32.55** c	**32.57** b	**32.59** e	

32.61 Which of the following most closely matches a Category 0 BI-RADS report?
   a. Lesions are noted that do not have the characteristic morphologies of breast cancer but have a definite probability of being malignant
   b. The finding has a high probability of being benign, but the mammographer would prefer to establish its mammographic stability over a short interval
   c. A finding is noted that warrants further imaging
   d. Breasts are symmetrical, and masses, architectural disturbances, or suspicious calcifications are not noted
   e. A mammographer wishes to describe a finding while concluding that there is no mammographic evidence of malignancy

32.62 The recurrence rate of fibroadenomas of the breast is approximately
   a. 1 to 3%
   b. 5 to 8%
   c. 12 to 15%
   d. 18 to 20%
   e. 30 to 33%

32.63 A 42-year-old woman presents with a firm, nontender mass in her right breast. You perform fine-needle aspiration, which is reported as "negative for malignancy." The next step in the management of this patient should be
   a. open biopsy
   b. immediate mammography
   c. repeat fine-needle aspiration
   d. mammography in 6 months
   e. reassurance and mammography as per routine

32.64 What is the most common presenting complaint of patients with intraductal papillomas of the breast?
   a. unilateral bloody nipple discharge
   b. unilateral cyclic pain
   c. subareolar palpable mass
   d. bilateral milky discharge

32.65 Nipple discharge associated with burning, itching, or nipple discomfort in older patients is suggestive of
   a. intraductal papilloma
   b. fibroadenoma
   c. ductal ectasia
   d. papillary carcinoma

32.66 Cytologic evaluation of nipple discharge is associated with a false-negative rate of approximately
   a. 3%
   b. 8%
   c. 12%
   d. 20%

32.67 In patients with hormonally responsive breast tumors, the medication LEAST appropriate for the treatment menopausal hot flashes is
   a. estrogen
   b. SSRI (selective serotonin reuptake inhibitor) antidepressants
   c. Bellergal
   d. Clonidine

32.68 Which of following has the most effect on the endometrium?
   a. Fluoxetine
   b. Bellergal
   c. Clonidine
   d. Tamoxifen
   e. Black cohosh

Answers

32.61 c	32.63 a	32.65 c	32.67 a	32.68 d
32.62 d	32.64 a	32.66 d		

Questions and Answers Chapter 33: Gynecologic Procedures

33.1 Which of the following is the LEAST accurate statement about ultrasound?
   a. The technique uses high-energy sound waves to directly image organs
   b. Ultrasound should not be used to replace the pelvic examination
   c. There may be interference from substances such as bowel gas
   d. In Doppler mode, ultrasound may be useful in evaluating blood flow patterns

33.2 Which of the following is the LEAST appropriate use for ultrasonography?
   a. To differentiate solid from cystic mass
   b. To routinely confirm findings from the pelvic examination
   c. To measure size of uterine fibroids
   d. To identify possible cause of pelvic pain
   e. To locate possible causes of abnormal bleeding

33.3 Which of the following is the LEAST appropriate for magnetic resonance imaging technology?
   a. Visualization of pelvic adhesions
   b. Imaging of bony structures
   c. Staging of cervical malignancy
   d. Evaluation of breast lesions

33.4 Hysterosalpingography is LEAST appropriate for the evaluation of
   a. the size of the uterine cavity
   b. the configuration of the uterine cavity
   c. fallopian tube patency
   d. pelvic endometriosis

33.5 Vulvar biopsy is performed using which of the following?
   a. Novak biopsy
   b. Keyes biopsy
   c. Pipelle biopsy
   d. Kevorkian biopsy
   e. Vabra biopsy

33.6 Vaginal biopsy requires what type of anesthesia?
   a. General
   b. Regional
   c. Conscious sedation
   d. Local

33.7 Biopsy of which organ is least likely to require the assistance of colposcopy?
   a. Vulva
   b. Vagina
   c. Cervix
   d. Endometrium

33.8 Which of the following conditions is least likely to be diagnosed with a hysteroscope?
   a. Endometriosis
   b. Polyp
   c. Myoma
   d. Septum
   e. Carcinoma

33.9 A profuse watery vaginal discharge is most commonly associated with which therapy for cervical dysplasia?
   a. Colposcopy
   b. Cryotherapy
   c. Laser therapy
   d. Conization

33.10 Which of the following is the LEAST appropriate indication for cervical conization?
   a. A two-step discrepancy between Pap smear and colposcopically directed biopsy
   b. A colposcopy in which the squamocolumnar junction cannot be visualized
   c. Therapy for cervical dysplasia
   d. Abnormal bleeding

Answers

33.1	a	33.3	a	33.5	b	33.7	d	33.9	b
33.2	b	33.4	d	33.6	d	33.8	a	33.10	d

33.11 Total abdominal hysterectomy refers to the removal of the
   a. uterus
   b. ovaries
   c. fallopian tubes
   d. bladder

33.12 Which term refers to the surgical removal of the uterine corpus?
   a. Total hysterectomy
   b. Subtotal hysterectomy
   c. Radical hysterectomy
   d. Laparoscopically assisted hysterectomy

33.13 Which of the following is an advantage of abdominal hysterectomy over vaginal hysterectomy?
   a. Ability to visualize associated pelvic pathology
   b. Shorter recovery period
   c. Repair of rectocele more readily accessible
   d. Fewer incisional complications

33.14 Hysteroscopy is LEAST appropriate for which of the following?
   a. Polypectomy
   b. Endometrial ablation
   c. Myomectomy
   d. Uterosacral nerve ablation

33.15 Biopsy of what organ is usually performed with an aspiration technique?
   a. Vulva
   b. Vagina
   c. Cervix
   d. Endometrium

33.16 In the initial evaluation of a possible adnexal mass, the most appropriate imaging technique is
   a. computed axial tomography scanning
   b. magnetic resonance imaging
   c. ultrasound
   d. flat plate of the abdomen

33.17 Colposcopy is most commonly used to evaluate an abnormality of what organ?
   a. Cervix
   b. Breast
   c. Endometrium
   d. Ovary

33.18 In which condition is transabdominal ultrasound preferable to transvaginal?
   a. 20-week-size uterine fibroids
   b. Ectopic pregnancy
   c. 4-cm ovarian cyst
   d. 6-week intrauterine pregnancy

33.19 Sonohysterography is most useful in evaluation of which of the following conditions?
   a. Endometriosis
   b. Pelvic inflammatory disease
   c. Ovarian cyst
   d. Abnormal uterine bleeding

33.20 What is the most appropriate biopsy for a 35-year-old woman with vaginal bleeding for 5 days and a normal physical examination?
   a. Vulva
   b. Vagina
   c. Cervix
   d. Endometrium

33.21 A 25-year-old patient had an intrauterine device inserted last year, but no longer feels the string. Which of the following is the most appropriate first step in management?
   a. Hysteroscopy
   b. Dilation and curettage
   c. Ultrasound
   d. Magnetic resonance imaging
   e. Colposcopy

33.22 Endometrial ablation is most appropriate for which of the following indications?
   a. Menorrhagia
   b. Amenorrhea
   c. Pelvic pain
   d. Sterilization

Answers

33.11 a	**33.13** a	**33.15** d	**33.17** a	**33.19** d	**33.21** c
33.12 b	**33.14** d	**33.16** c	**33.18** a	**33.20** d	**33.22** a

33.23 A patient who is having a LEEP (loop electrosurgical excision) procedure is likely being treated for
a. vulvar disease
b. abnormal Pap smear
c. abnormal uterine bleeding
d. pelvic pain
e. endometriosis

33.24 A 25-year-old patient does not recall why she had a laparoscopy 3 years ago. The condition that she most likely was being treated for was
a. abnormal bleeding
b. recurrent cystitis
c. pelvic pain
d. abnormal Pap smear

33.25 Which of the following is the LEAST appropriate indication for hysterectomy?
a. Pelvic pain
b. Abnormal uterine bleeding
c. Symptomatic uterine fibroids
d. Sterilization

33.26 A radical hysterectomy is most appropriate for treatment of
a. severe endometriosis
b. pelvic pain
c. extensive pelvic adhesions
d. cancer

33.27 The primary advantage of laparoscopically assisted vaginal hysterectomy over vaginal hysterectomy is
a. visualization of adnexal structures
b. recovery time
c. hospital costs
d. extent and duration of pain

Answers
33.23 b   **33.24** c   **33.25** d   **33.26** d   **33.27** a

Questions and Answers Chapter 34: Reproductive Cycle

34.1 At what average age is a regular, predictable reproductive cycle established in women?
   a. 11 years
   b. 13 years
   c. 15 years
   d. 17 years

34.2 At what average age does the female reproductive cycle become inefficient?
   a. 30 years
   b. 35 years
   c. 40 years
   d. 45 years

34.3 A woman's optimal reproductive time occupies approximately how many years?
   a. 10
   b. 15
   c. 20
   d. 30

34.4 On average, how many times during the year will a healthy, nonpregnant woman ovulate?
   a. 6 to 8 times
   b. 10 to 12 times
   c. 13 to 14 times
   d. 16 to 18 times

34.5 What is the average length of the female reproductive cycle?
   a. 26 days
   b. 28 days
   c. 30 days
   d. 32 days

34.6 What is the name of the pulse generator that secretes gonadotropin-releasing hormone?
   a. Arcuate nucleus of the anterior hypothalamus
   b. Anterior lobe of the pituitary gland
   c. Posterior lobe of the pituitary gland
   d. Third ventricle

34.7 Gonadotropin-releasing hormone flows from the hypothalamus to the anterior pituitary gland through the
   a. cerebrospinal fluid
   b. lymphatic system
   c. pituitary portal venous plexus
   d. cerebral venous drainage

34.8 What is the pulse frequency of hypothalamic gonadotropin-releasing hormone secretion?
   a. Every 50 to 60 minutes
   b. Every 70 to 90 minutes
   c. Every 100 to 120 minutes
   d. Every 6 to 8 hours
   e. Every 2 to 3 days

34.9 Given a woman with the inability to secrete gonadotropin-releasing hormone (GnRH; Kallmann syndrome), at what pulse frequency should an external GnRH pump be set?
   a. Every 50 to 60 minutes
   b. Every 70 to 90 minutes
   c. Every 100 to 120 minutes
   d. Every 6 to 8 hours
   e. Every 2 to 3 days

34.10 The hormone that stimulates the granulosa cells of the primary ovarian follicle is
   a. follicle-stimulating hormone (FSH)
   b. luteinizing hormone (LH)
   c. progesterone
   d. estradiol
   e. testosterone

34.11 The hormone that triggers ovulation is
   a. thyrotropin (TSH)
   b. androstenedione
   c. estrone
   d. estradiol
   e. LH

Answers

34.1	c	34.3	d	34.5	b	34.7	c	34.9	b	34.11	e
34.2	d	34.4	c	34.6	a	34.8	b	34.10	a		

34.12 The principal sex steroid secreted by the granulosa cells of the ovarian follicle is
a. estradiol
b. estrone
c. estriol
d. progesterone
e. testosterone

34.13 The hormone that stimulates the pre-granulosa cells of the primordial follicle to become granulosa cells is
a. FSH
b. LH
c. TSH
d. prolactin
e. melanocyte-stimulating hormone

34.14 The hormone that facilitates preparation of the endometrium for implantation of the blastocyst following fertilization is
a. estradiol
b. estriol
c. estrone
d. progesterone
e. testosterone

34.15 The hormone that has the greatest effect on the hypothalamic thermoregulatory center is
a. estradiol
b. progesterone
c. testosterone
d. androstenedione
e. estriol

34.16 The hormone that is associated with the development of the secretory endometrium is
a. estriol
b. estradiol
c. estrone
d. progesterone
e. testosterone

34.17 The hormone that stimulates the ductal elements of the breast (nipples, areolae, and ducts) is
a. estriol
b. estradiol
c. estrone
d. progesterone
e. testosterone

34.18 The hormone that stimulates the acinar elements of the breast (milk-producing glands) is
a. testosterone
b. progesterone
c. androstenedione
d. dehydroepiandrosterone sulfate
e. prolactin

34.19 The hormone associated with the development of a proliferative endometrium is
a. progesterone
b. estradiol
c. testosterone
d. prolactin
e. androstenedione

34.20 Which of the following reflects the activity of the arcuate nucleus?
a. Gonadotropin-releasing hormone
b. Prolactin
c. TSH
d. FSH
e. LH

34.21 The hormone that is most heavily secreted in response to a perceived estrogen deficiency is
a. estradiol
b. LH
c. FSH
d. progesterone
e. prolactin

Answers

34.12 a	34.14 d	34.16 d	34.18 b	34.20 a
34.13 a	34.15 b	34.17 b	34.19 b	34.21 c

34.22 Which is the principal sex steroid hormone secreted by the theca lutein cells?
   a. Estradiol
   b. Testosterone
   c. Progesterone
   d. Estriol

34.23 Which of the following is secreted by the theca lutein cells during the follicular phase of the cycle and acts as a precursor in the synthesis of sex steroid hormone by granulosa cells?
   a. Androgens
   b. Prostaglandins
   c. Estrogens
   d. Endorphins

34.24 The oocyte in the primordial follicle is arrested in what stage of division?
   a. Prophase of meiosis
   b. Metaphase of meiosis
   c. Prophase of mitosis
   d. Metaphase of mitosis

34.25 Which of the following stimulates the arrested oocyte to complete maturation?
   a. A critical level of FSH
   b. The LH surge
   c. An FSH:LH ratio of 3:1
   d. A critical level of estradiol

34.26 What endocrine event initiates the onset of menstruation?
   a. Luteinizing hormone surge
   b. Estradiol peak
   c. Involution of the corpus luteum
   d. An FSH:LH ratio of 3:1

34.27 What is the average volume of blood lost each menstrual cycle?
   a. 10 to 25 mL
   b. 30 to 50 mL
   c. 70 to 90 mL
   d. 120 to 150 mL

34.28 Where do the prostaglandins that initiate uterine contractions during menstruation originate?
   a. Ovary
   b. Endocervix
   c. Uterine musculature
   d. Endometrium
   e. Pituitary

34.29 What is the clinical condition associated with symptomatic uterine contractions during menstruation?
   a. Primary dysmenorrhea
   b. Secondary dysmenorrhea
   c. Dyspareunia
   d. Dyschezia
   e. Menorrhagia

34.30 What is the preferred form of treatment for women who suffer from menstrual pain?
   a. β-Blockers
   b. Calcium channel blockers
   c. Prostaglandin synthetase inhibitors
   d. Narcotics

34.31 When does the pituitary gland begin to secrete FSH to initiate a new reproductive cycle?
   a. Just before ovulation
   b. Just after ovulation
   c. 24 to 48 hours before the onset of menstruation
   d. 24 to 48 hours after the onset of menstruation

34.32 What is the consequence of an androgen-to-estrogen ratio of greater than one in a follicle that is undergoing stimulation?
   a. Multiple gestation
   b. Atretic follicle
   c. Chromosomal abnormalities
   d. Spontaneous abortion

Answers

34.22 c	34.24 a	34.26 c	34.28 d	34.30 c	34.32 b
34.23 a	34.25 b	34.27 b	34.29 a	34.31 c	

34.33 What is the presumed chemical stimulus for extrusion of the oocyte from the follicle at the time of ovulation?
a. Metabolism of endorphins
b. Release of progesterone
c. Synthesis of prostaglandins
d. Liberation of intrafollicular prostaglandins

34.34 What is the consequence if prostaglandin synthetase inhibitors are administered at the expected time of ovulation?
a. The oocyte will be retained in the follicle
b. Mittelschmerz is intensified
c. Progesterone synthesis is enhanced
d. The corpus luteum is ruptured

34.35 What term is given to the pain associated with ovulation?
a. Premenstrual syndrome
b. Dysmenorrhea
c. Dyspareunia
d. Mittelschmerz

34.36 The clinical term for insufficient progesterone production by the corpus luteum is
a. secondary dysmenorrhea
b. primary dysmenorrhea
c. inadequate luteal phase
d. premenstrual syndrome
e. spontaneous abortion

34.37 Which hormone is necessary to sustain the corpus luteum beyond 14 days?
a. Progesterone
b. Human chorionic gonadotropin
c. Estradiol
d. Human chorionic somatomammotropin

34.38 At approximately what age will a woman begin to notice changes in her reproductive cycle associated with perimenopause?
a. 30 to 32 years
b. 34 to 36 years
c. 38 to 42 years
d. 45 to 48 years
e. 50 to 52 years

34.39 What is the first evidence of diminished reproductive efficiency in a woman?
a. A change in the length of the reproductive cycle
b. Hot flushes
c. Vaginal atrophy
d. Premenstrual mood changes

34.40 What is the clinical condition when the few remaining ovarian follicles are resistant to stimulation by FSH?
a. Polycystic ovarian disease
b. Menopause
c. Kallmann's syndrome
d. Premenstrual syndrome

34.41 What procedure is used for endometrial dating, to diagnose inadequate luteal phase?
a. Transvaginal ultrasound
b. Hysteroscopy
c. Endometrial biopsy
d. Hysterosalpingogram
e. Serum estrogen measurement

34.42 What is the common condition characterized by breast tenderness, mood changes, fluid retention, abdominal bloating, and weight gain?
a. Primary dysmenorrhea
b. Secondary dysmenorrhea
c. Premenstrual syndrome
d. Perimenopause

Answers

34.33 d	34.35 d	34.37 b	34.39 a	34.41 c
34.34 a	34.36 c	34.38 c	34.40 b	34.42 c

34.43 A 20-year-old patient inquires about a watery, thin mucus that seems to come and go. She should be told that it occurs at the time of
a. ovulation
b. impending menstruation
c. fertilization
d. prostaglandin release

34.44 Endocervical glands play a critical role in
a. ovulation
b. fertilization
c. menstruation
d. puberty

34.45 A 35-year-old woman who complains of vaginal dryness with intercourse should be told that lubrication of the vagina during the sexual response cycle comes from the
a. endometrium
b. endocervix
c. vagina
d. Bartholin glands

34.46 In counseling a patient regarding the basal body temperature chart, she should be told to take her temperature
a. after breakfast
b. before dinner
c. at bedtime
d. first thing in the morning

34.47 A 40-year-old woman inquires about the changes in her menstrual periods that are likely to occur. Which of the following is the most accurate?
a. They will stay regular until menopause, at which time they will cease suddenly
b. They will be accompanied by increasing pain
c. Ovulation will occur before every period she experiences
d. The changes will reflect those of her mother
e. The luteal phase will likely be maintained at normal length

Answers

34.43 a	**34.44** b	**34.45** c	**34.46** d	**34.47** e

Questions and Answers Chapter 35: Puberty

35.1 The event that triggers puberty is
   a. achieving a critical body weight
   b. adequate sun exposure
   c. reaching a critical height
   d. having a specific body surface area

35.2 The hypothalamic-pituitary axis is first known to function
   a. in utero
   b. at birth
   c. at 1 year of age
   d. at 13 years of age

35.3 What is the first endocrine event associated with secondary sexual maturation?
   a. Secretion of dehydroepiandrosterone by the adrenal glands
   b. Ovarian hormone secretion
   c. Pituitary development
   d. Hypothalamus down-regulation

35.4 What is the usual length of time from the first physical signs of secondary sexual maturation until sexual maturation is complete?
   a. 1 year
   b. 2 years
   c. 3 years
   d. 4 years
   e. 5 years

35.5 What is the expected sequence of secondary sexual development in girls?
   a. Adrenarche, growth spurt, thelarche, menarche, ovulation
   b. Menarche, growth spurt, thelarche, adrenarche, ovulation
   c. Growth spurt, menarche, adrenarche, thelarche, ovulation
   d. Thelarche, adrenarche, growth spurt, menarche, ovulation

35.6 Which of the following is required for timely secondary sexual maturation?
   a. Sufficient body fat
   b. Sufficient sleep
   c. Sufficient height
   d. Exposure to adequate levels of light
   e. Sufficient body fat AND sleep AND light

35.7 What is the baseline percentage of body fat needed to sustain female reproductive function?
   a. 6%
   b. 12%
   c. 24%
   d. 36%

35.8 What is the earliest sign of delayed puberty in girls?
   a. Failure of growth spurt by age 10
   b. Failure of menarche by age 12
   c. Failure of breast budding by age 13
   d. Failure of ovulation by age 17

35.9 When adrenarche occurs first, what is the expected interval to the onset of thelarche?
   a. 4 to 5 months
   b. 6 to 9 months
   c. 12 to 15 months
   d. 24 months

35.10 Which of the following may cause premature sexual development in adolescent girls?
   a. Turner syndrome (45X karyotype)
   b. Deletion of the long arm of the X chromosome
   c. Ovarian neoplasm
   d. Alkylating chemotherapy

35.11 What is the most common genital tract cause of primary amenorrhea?
   a. Congenital absence of the uterus
   b. Imperforate hymen
   c. Asherman syndrome
   d. Premature ovarian failure

Answers

35.1	b	35.3	a	35.5	d	35.7	c	35.9	b	35.11	b
35.2	a	35.4	d	35.6	e	35.8	c	35.10	c	

35.12 Which of the following is a method for treating vaginal agenesis?
a. Vaginal vault suspension
b. Vulvectomy
c. Vulvar flap
d. Vaginal marsupialization
e. Pressure dilation of the vaginal space

35.13 What is the simple, definitive treatment for imperforate hymen?
a. Hymenectomy
b. Hymenotomy
c. Vaginal reconstruction
d. Administration of a gonadotropin-releasing hormone agonist
e. Topical estrogen therapy

35.14 What is the definitive chemical evidence of ovarian failure?
a. Depressed estradiol
b. Elevated prolactin
c. Elevated follicle-stimulating hormone
d. Depressed testosterone
e. Absent gonadotropin-releasing hormone

35.15 Genetic information that regulates the rate of ovarian follicular atresia is located on
a. the short arm of the X chromosome
b. the long arm of the X chromosome
c. chromosome 21
d. chromosome 18

35.16 Genetic information that determines height and somatic characteristics is located on
a. the short arm of the X chromosome
b. the long arm of the X chromosome
c. chromosome 21
d. chromosome 18

35.17 Which of the following hormones must be replaced in girls with premature ovarian failure?
a. Prolactin
b. Progesterone
c. Estradiol-17β
d. Testosterone
e. Gonadotropin-releasing hormone

35.18 What is the risk of administering excessive estradiol-17β (or other estrogens) in girls with pubertal failure?
a. Endometrial cancer
b. Short stature
c. Hirsutism
d. Vaginal agenesis
e. Amenorrhea

35.19 What is the risk of delaying administration of estradiol-17β in girls with pubertal failure?
a. Short stature
b. Mental retardation
c. Osteoporosis
d. Clinical depression
e. Endometrial cancer

35.20 Alteration of the gonadotropin-releasing hormone pulse frequency in adolescent girls will result in
a. ovarian hyperstimulation
b. ovarian atrophy
c. ovarian neoplasm
d. no pituitary stimulation of the ovary

35.21 What condition is associated with olfactory tract hypoplasia and failure of gonadotropin-releasing hormone secretion?
a. Turner syndrome
b. Cushing syndrome
c. Kallmann syndrome
d. Swyer syndrome

Answers

35.12 e	35.14 c	35.16 a	35.18 b	35.20 d
35.13 b	35.15 b	23.17 c	35.19 c	35.21 c

35.22 What condition is associated with failure to establish secondary sexual development, a webbed neck, and short stature?
a. Turner syndrome
b. Cushing syndrome
c. Kallmann syndrome
d. Swyer syndrome

35.23 During clinical evaluation, Kallmann syndrome can be recognized by
a. serum estradiol levels
b. visual field evaluation
c. serum follicle-stimulating hormone
d. olfactory challenge

35.24 How could a patient with Kallmann syndrome be treated to help her conceive?
a. Artificial insemination
b. Pulsatile administration of gonadotropin-releasing hormone
c. Administration of clomiphene citrate
d. Administration of sequential estrogen and progesterone

35.25 In adolescents, what would be evidence of incomplete puberty that is caused by marijuana use?
a. Elevated estradiol
b. Elevated testosterone
c. Suppressed gonadotropins (follicle stimulating hormone and luteinizing hormone)
d. Suppressed prolactin

35.26 What is the prognosis for adolescent girls who have delayed puberty or secondary amenorrhea resulting from participation in competitive athletics?
a. Increased incidence of congenital anomalies in offspring can be anticipated
b. Infertility can be anticipated
c. Normal secondary sexual development can be anticipated
d. Reduced reproductive capacity can be anticipated
e. Early menopause can be anticipated

35.27 Isosexual precocious puberty is defined as
a. premature sexual maturation following the normal sequence
b. premature sexual maturation following an abnormal sequence
c. sexual maturation on time but following an abnormal sequence
d. sexual maturation on time but following a prolonged sequence

35.28 What is the most common cause of inappropriate hormone secretion leading to precocious puberty in girls?
a. Cushing syndrome
b. Addison syndrome
c. Adrenal hyperplasia, 21-hydroxylase type
d. Adrenal hyperplasia, 11-hydroxylase type

35.29 What is the treatment of choice for children with isosexual precocious puberty?
a. Steroids
b. Estrogen alone
c. Gonadotropin-releasing hormone agonist
d. Oral contraceptives

35.30 Isosexual precocious puberty generally results in
a. infertility
b. secondary menorrhea
c. obesity
d. short stature
e. disordered pubertal (developmental) sequence

35.31 A woman with uterine and vaginal agenesis can have her own genetic child through
a. sequential administration of estrogen and progesterone for three reproductive cycles
b. tonic administration of estrogen alone
c. pelvic reconstructive surgery
d. ovum donation
e. insemination with donor sperm

Answers

35.22 a	35.24 b	35.26 c	35.28 c	35.30 d
35.23 d	35.25 c	35.27 a	35.29 c	35.31 d

35.32 Premature ovarian failure is characterized by
   a. lower estrogen level, lower
      gonadotropin levels
   b. elevated estrogen level, lower
      gonadotropin levels
   c. lower estrogen level, elevated
      gonadotropin levels
   d. elevated estrogen level, elevated
      gonadotropin levels

35.33 In patients with premature ovarian
failure, the daily dose of conjugated
estrogen to initiate secondary sexual
maturation is
   a. 0.3 mg
   b. 1.25 mg
   c. 2.5 mg
   d. 5.0 mg

35.34 In patients with premature ovarian
failure, the daily dose of conjugated
estrogen to induce menarche is
   a. 0.3 mg
   b. 0.625 mg
   c. 1.25 mg
   d. 2.5 mg

35.35 In patients with premature ovarian
failure, induction of cyclic bleeding is
accomplished with the cyclic administration of
   a. estrogen
   b. progestin
   c. gonadotropin-releasing hormone
   d. testosterone

Answers

35.32 c	**35.33** a	**35.34** c	**35.35** b

Questions and Answers Chapter 36: Amenorrhea and Dysfunctional Uterine Bleeding

36.1 At what average chronological age is a regular, predictable reproductive cycle established?
a. 9 years
b. 11 years
c. 13 years
d. 15 years

36.2 Dysfunctional uterine bleeding is defined as
a. menstruation beyond the age of 50
b. failure to menstruate because of anatomic obstruction
c. irregular menstruation without anatomic lesions of the uterus
d. failure to menstruate within 6 months of a previous menstrual cycle

36.3 Which of the following do amenorrhea and dysfunctional uterine bleeding have in common?
a. Both are associated with endometriosis
b. Both can result from anovulation
c. Both have similar levels of testosterone
d. Both have similar amounts of bleeding
e. Both carry a risk of cancer

36.4 What is the most common cause of secondary amenorrhea?
a. Ovarian failure
b. Cervical stenosis
c. Pregnancy
d. Vaginal agenesis
e. Outflow obstruction

36.5 What is the most common cause of pathologic amenorrhea?
a. Outflow obstruction
b. Disruption of the hypothalamic–pituitary axis
c. Asherman syndrome
d. Kallmann syndrome
e. Turner syndrome

36.6 Which of the following distinguishes secondary from primary amenorrhea?
a. Absence of anatomic defects
b. History of prior menses
c. Chance of future fertility
d. Amount of bleeding at times other than menses
e. Follicle-stimulating hormone (FSH) levels

36.7 Disruption of the pulsatile secretion of gonadotropin-releasing hormone directly interferes with the secretion of
a. FSH
b. estradiol
c. catecholamines
d. prolactin
e. adrenocorticotropic hormone

36.8 What tests can help differentiate hypothalamic–pituitary amenorrhea from ovarian failure?
a. Measurement of FSH levels
b. Measurement of serum estradiol
c. Pregnancy test
d. Measurement of testosterone

36.9 Ovarian failure is associated with
a. oligomenorrhea
b. hypomenorrhea
c. menorrhagia
d. amenorrhea
e. dysmenorrhea

36.10 The most common anatomic abnormality to cause secondary amenorrhea is
a. cervical stenosis
b. vaginal septum
c. Asherman syndrome
d. intact hymen
e. labial adhesions

Answers

36.1	c	36.3	b	36.5	b	36.7	a	36.9	d
36.2	c	36.4	c	36.6	b	36.8	a	36.10	c

36.11 What is the typical cause of the endometrial scarring that characterizes Asherman syndrome?
   a. Cervical infection
   b. Dilation and curettage
   c. Intrauterine device use
   d. Hysterosalpingography
   e. Pelvic inflammatory disease

36.12 Which of the following patients would be classified as having oligomenorrhea?
   a. A 16-year-old patient who has never menstruated
   b. A 22-year-old woman with periods that occur every 35 days and last 5 days
   c. A 26-year-old woman with periods that occur every 28 days and last 2 days
   d. A 45-year-old woman with periods that occur every 45 days and last 8 to 10 days
   e. A 36-year-old woman with periods that occur every 8 to 10 months and last 3 to 5 days

36.13 Estrogen is the primary therapy for which of the following conditions?
   a. Dysfunctional uterine bleeding
   b. Menopausal vaginal atrophy
   c. Precocious puberty
   d. Oligomenorrhea
   e. Secondary amenorrhea

36.14 What is the endocrine environment that leads to dysfunctional uterine bleeding?
   a. Falling prolactin
   b. Chronic progesterone secretion
   c. Chronic estrus
   d. Fluctuating testosterone

36.15 What causes irregular bleeding in women with dysfunctional uterine bleeding?
   a. Subclinical infection
   b. Progesterone withdrawal
   c. Endometrial polyps
   d. Outgrowth of endometrial blood supply
   e. Progestin effects

36.16 What is the medical treatment of choice for immediate management of dysfunctional uterine bleeding?
   a. Daily oral contraceptives
   b. Progestin for 10 days
   c. Progesterone in oil for 1 month
   d. Gonadotropin-releasing hormone agonist

36.17 What is the medical treatment of choice for long-term management of dysfunctional uterine bleeding?
   a. Daily oral contraceptives
   b. Progestin for 10 days
   c. Progesterone in oil for 1 month
   d. Gonadotropin-releasing hormone agonist

36.18 In luteal phase defect, the endometrium is not maintained because there is insufficient
   a. estrogen
   b. progesterone
   c. prolactin
   d. FSH
   e. LH

36.19 In evaluating the patient with amenorrhea, in what situation is serum prolactin elevated?
   a. Pituitary adenoma
   b. Weight loss
   c. Obesity
   d. Hyperthyroidism
   e. Ovarian neoplasm

36.20 In patients with hypothalamic amenorrhea, what is the typical pattern of FSH and LH?
   a. FSH high, LH high
   b. FSH low, LH low
   c. FSH high, LH low
   d. FSH low, LH high

Answers

36.11 b	36.13 b	36.15 d	36.17 a	36.19 a
36.12 d	36.14 c	36.16 b	36.18 b	36.20 b

36.21 What is the best treatment for mild cases of intrauterine scarring?
a. Systemic estrogen administration
b. Dilation and curettage
c. Vaginal estrogen administration
d. Laparoscopy

36.22 In cases of Asherman syndrome, the regeneration of endometrium in previously denuded areas is stimulated by what hormone?
a. Estrogen
b. Progesterone
c. Testosterone
d. Androstenedione

36.23 Hyperprolactinemia caused by a pituitary adenomas is frequently associated with amenorrhea and
a. hirsutism
b. vaginal atrophy
c. hot flushes
d. galactorrhea

36.24 What percent of pituitary tumors secrete prolactin?
a. 5%
b. 20%
c. 50%
d. 80%

36.25 Which of the following conditions is commonly associated with chronic anovulation?
a. Obesity
b. Anorexia nervosa
c. Leiomyomata uteri
d. Cervicitis

36.26 What type of bleeding pattern is characteristic of polycystic ovarian syndrome?
a. Menorrhagia
b. Amenorrhea
c. Hypomenorrhea
d. Dysfunctional uterine bleeding

36.27 In patients with dysfunctional uterine bleeding, the lack of predictable ovulation results in the lack of
a. estrogen
b. prolactin
c. progesterone
d. testosterone

36.28 What phenomenon do amenorrhea and dysfunctional uterine bleeding share?
a. Anovulation
b. Pain
c. Vaginal discharge
d. Molimina
e. Premenstrual syndrome

36.29 Which of the following is an example of dysfunctional uterine bleeding in the presence of ovulation?
a. Midcycle spotting
b. Postcoital spotting
c. Metrorrhagia
d. Postmenopausal bleeding

36.30 A patient with luteal phase defect would typically experience
a. irregular periods
b. shortened interval between periods
c. unpredictable spotting
d. postcoital bleeding

36.31 Premenstrual syndrome should be absent in which of the following conditions?
a. Primary dysmenorrhea
b. Polycystic ovary syndrome
c. Secondary dysmenorrhea
d. Menorrhagia

36.32. In which condition is the menstrual cycle totally unpredictable?
a. Leiomyomata uteri
b. Cervical cancer
c. Dysfunctional uterine bleeding
d. Endometritis

Answers

36.21 b	**36.23** d	**36.25** a	**36.27** c	**36.29** a	**36.31** b
36.22 a	**36.24** d	**36.26** d	**36.28** a	**36.30** b	**36.32** c

36.33. What is a likely finding on endometrial biopsy of a patient with dysfunctional uterine bleeding (chronic anovulation)?

    a. Secretory endometrium
    b. Atrophic endometrium
    c. Endometritis
    d. Endometrial hyperplasia

36.34 A patient with dysfunctional uterine bleeding is at greater risk for developing what type of cancer?

    a. Vaginal
    b. Cervical
    c. Endometrial
    d. Ovarian
    e. Gestational trophoblastic disease

36.35 Which of the following mimics the physiologic hormonal event that induces normal menstrual bleeding?

    a. Administering estrogen
    b. Administering progestin
    c. Discontinuing estrogen
    d. Discontinuing progestin

Answers

36.33 d   **36.34** c   **36.35** d

Questions and Answers Chapter 37: Hirsutism and Virilization

37.1 Which of the following is a common cause of hirsutism and virilization?
a. Hilus cell tumor
b. Polycystic ovarian disorder
c. Sertoli-Leydig tumor
d. Exogenous testosterone administration

37.2 Hirsutism and virilization are characterized as
a. estrogen-excess disorders
b. androgen-excess disorders
c. progesterone-excess disorders
d. prolactin-excess disorders

37.3 Which of the following is a major function of androgens in women?
a. Control of blood pressure
b. Determinant of adult weight
c. Precursor for estrogen biosynthesis
d. Modulator of anxiety disorders

37.4 The treatment for androgen-excess disorders is directed at
a. suppression of source of androgen
b. stimulation of production of feminizing hormones
c. induction of estrogen receptors
d. reduction of hair growth

37.5 What histologic structure is characteristic of the hilus cell tumor?
a. Signet cell
b. Clue cell
c. Reinke crystalloid
d. Donovan body

37.6 Hirsutism is most frequently associated with
a. temporal balding
b. development of acne
c. enlargement of the clitoris
d. remodeling of the limb-shoulder girdle

37.7 Which is the first event usually associated with virilization?
a. Involution of the breasts
b. Deepening of the voice
c. Enlargement of the clitoris
d. Terminal hair growth
e. Temporal balding

37.8 In adipose tissue, there is extraglandular production of testosterone from
a. dehydroepiandrosterone
b. androstenedione
c. estrone
d. estriol

37.9 In hair follicles, dihydrotestosterone is produced by the local action of 5α-reductase on
a. dehydroepiandrosterone
b. testosterone
c. estrone
d. prolactin

37.10 What percent of testosterone is not bound to sex hormone–binding globulin (SHBG)?
a. 1 to to 3%
b. 5 to to 7%
c. 10 to to 15%
d. 20 to to 25%

37.11 The hepatic production of sex hormone–binding globulin is stimulated by
a. testosterone
b. dihydrotestosterone
c. estrogen
d. adrenocorticotropic hormone

37.12 In women, the most common cause of hirsutism associated with androgen excess is
a. luteinizing hormone excess
b. genetic predisposition
c. obesity
d. polycystic ovarian disease

Answers

37.1	b	37.4	a	37.6	b	37.9	b	37.12	d
37.2	b	37.4	a	37.7	c	37.10	a		
37.3	c	37.5	c	37.8	b	37.11	c		

37.13 Which of the following is inconsistent with the diagnosis of polycystic ovarian disease?
a. Oligomenorrhea
b. Amenorrhea
c. Anovulation
d. Acne
e. Virilization

37.14 Which of the following is a characteristic finding in women with polycystic ovarian disease?
a. Decreased luteinizing hormone-to-follicle-stimulating hormone ratio
b. Estradiol in greater concentration than estrone
c. Androstenedione at the upper limits of normal or increased
d. Testosterone at or below normal limits

37.15 Successful treatment of polycystic ovarian syndrome with oral contraceptives should result in
a. increased luteinizing hormone production
b. increased production of androstenedione
c. increased production of testosterone
d. decreased ovarian androgen secretion
e. decreased incidence of endometrial hyperplasia

37.16 An example of virilization caused by polycystic ovarian syndrome is
a. hyperthecosis
b. androgen insensitivity syndrome
c. hyperandrogenic syndrome
d. acanthosis nigricans

37.17 Sertoli-Leydig cell tumors are characterized by increased
a. testosterone secretion
b. estrogen production
c. follicle-stimulating hormone levels
d. luteinizing hormone levels
e. menstrual bleeding

37.18 Patients with Sertoli-Leydig cell tumors typically have
a. an increased level of follicle-stimulating hormone
b. an increased level of luteinizing hormone
c. a high plasma androstenedione level
d. an elevated level of testosterone

37.19 The surgical removal of a unilateral Sertoli-Leydig cell tumor should result in the reversal of which symptom?
a. Amenorrhea
b. Hirsutism
c. Clitormegaly
d. Deepening of the voice

37.20 Which of the following is characteristic of gynandroblastoma?
a. Overgrowth of mature hilus cells or cells from the ovarian mesenchyme
b. Small tumor containing sheets of round, clear, pale staining cells
c. Granulosa cell and arrhenoblastoma components
d. Contains Reinke crystalloids

37.21 Which of the following is characteristic of lipid (lipoid) cell tumors?
a. Overgrowth of mature hilus cells or cells from the ovarian mesenchyme
b. Small tumor containing sheets of round, clear, pale staining cells
c. Granulosa cell and arrhenoblastoma components
d. Contain Reinke crystalloids

37.22 Which of the following is most likely to be positively affected following medical treatment of adrenal hyperplasia with prednisone?
a. Facial acne
b. Ovulation
c. New terminal hair growth
d. Hirsutism

Answers

37.13 e	**37.15** d	**37.17** a	**37.19** a	**37.21** b
37.14 c	**37.16** d	**37.18** d	**37.20** c	**37.22** b

37.23 Which of the following is characteristic of 11β-hydroxylase deficiency?
  a. Severe hypertension
  b. Severe hirsutism
  c. Increased serum desoxycorticos-terone
  d. Reduced conversion of proges-terone to cortisol

37.24 Women with constitutional hirsutism are characterized by
  a. anovulation
  b. greater activity of 5α-reductase
  c. abnormal estrogen levels
  d. coexistent acne

37.25 The potent metabolite of testosterone that is produced in genital skin and hair follicles is
  a. dehydroepiandrosterone
  b. dihydrotestosterone
  c. androstenedione

37.26 Which of the following is associated with hirsutism?
  a. Excess body hair
  b. Involution of the breasts
  c. Deepening voice
  d. Remodeling of limb-shoulder girdle

37.27 An elevated 24-hour-free cortisol level is suggestive of what condition?
  a. Cushing disease
  b. Polycystic ovarian disease
  c. Sarcoidosis
  d. Porphyria

Answers
37.23 c   **37.24** b   **37.25** b   **37.26** a   **37.27** a

Questions and Answers Chapter 38: Menopause

38.1 The climacteric is defined as the
  a. time of the last menstrual flow
  b. time when the symptoms of menopause first begin
  c. transition from the reproductive to the nonreproductive years
  d. last five regular menstrual cycles

38.2 The average age of menopause is approximately
  a. 40 years
  b. 45 years
  c. 50 years
  d. 55 years
  e. 60 years

38.3 Ovarian function ceases by 55 years of age in what percent of women?
  a. 80%
  b. 85%
  c. 90%
  d. 95%
  e. 99%

38.4 Between infancy and the time of menopause, the number of oocytes in the ovary
  a. steadily increases
  b. increases and then decreases
  c. steadily decreases
  d. remains constant

38.5 Approximately how many oocytes will a woman ovulate during her reproductive years?
  a. 100
  b. 200
  c. 300
  d. 400
  e. 500

38.6 Approximately how many oocytes does a woman have at the time of puberty?
  a. 4,000
  b. 40,000
  c. 400,000
  d. 4 million

38.7 As a woman approaches menopause, there is
  a. increased sensitivity of granulosa cells to testosterone
  b. reduced sensitivity of oocytes to follicle-stimulating hormone (FSH)
  c. increased sensitivity of theca luteal cells to estrogen
  d. reduced sensitivity of ovarian stromal cells to gonadotropin-releasing hormone

38.8 Which hormone is the major product of the postmenopausal ovary?
  a. Luteinizing hormone
  b. Estradiol-17β
  c. Testosterone
  d. Estrone

38.9 The plasma concentration of FSH begins to increase
  a. approximately 10 years before menopause
  b. approximately 3 years before menopause
  c. at the time of menopause
  d. approximately 3 years after menopause
  e. approximately 10 years after menopause

38.10 What is the typical FSH level in childhood?
  a. >30 mIU/mL
  b. 14 to 24 mIU/mL
  c. 6 to 10 mIU/mL
  d. <4 mIU/mL

38.11 What is the typical FSH level during a women's prime reproductive years?
  a. >30 mIU/mL
  b. 14 to 24 mIU/mL
  c. 6 to 10 mIU/mL
  d. <4 mIU/mL

Answers

38.1	c	**38.3**	d	**38.5**	d	**38.7**	b	**38.9**	b
38.2	c	**38.4**	c	**38.6**	c	**38.8**	c	**38.10**	d

38.11	c

38.12 What is the typical FSH level during perimenopause?
a. >30 mIU/mL
b. 14 to 24 mIU/mL
c. 6 to 10 mIU/mL
d. <4 mIU/mL

38.13 What is the typical FSH level during menopause?
a. >30 mIU/mL
b. 14 to 24 mIU/mL
c. 6 to 10 mIU/mL
d. <4 mIU/mL

38.14 Which of the following is generally the first physical manifestation of ovarian failure?
a. Sleep disturbance
b. Vaginal dryness
c. Hot flushes
d. Mood changes
e. Skin thickening

38.15 Decrease in the level of which of the following hormones is responsible for the vasomotor symptoms of menopause?
a. Progesterone
b. Estrogen
c. Testosterone
d. FSH
e. Androstenedione

38.16 Which of the following statements about hot flushes is INCORRECT?
a. Over 95% of perimenopausal and menopausal women experience hot flushes (vasomotor instability).
b. As a woman approaches menopause, the frequency and intensity of hot flushes increases.
c. Hot flushes may be associated with disabling diaphoresis.
d. If a menopausal woman does not receive estrogen therapy, hot flushes will resolve within 6 to 9 months.

38.17 What is the effect of decreasing estrogen on the sleep cycle?
a. Latent phase shortened, sleep period shortened
b. Latent phase shortened, sleep period lengthened
c. Latent phase lengthened, sleep period shortened
d. Latent phase lengthened, sleep period lengthened

38.18 Which of the following statements about vaginal atrophy associated with menopause is INCORRECT?
a. The vaginal epithelium becomes thin.
b. Cervical secretions increase in quantity.
c. Many patients experience dyspareunia.
d. Vaginal tissue is more likely to become infected by local flora.

38.19 Which of the following is an effect of estrogen deficiency on paravaginal tissue?
a. Bladder prolapse
b. Uterine retroversion
c. Urinary retention
d. Vaginal vault prolapse

38.20 Which of the following is NOT a consequence of estrogen deficiency?
a. Acne
b. Thinning of the skin
c. Brittle nails
d. Synchronous hair shedding

38.21 Which of the following is NOT a sign or symptom common to menopausal women who are not taking estrogen therapy?
a. Dyspareunia
b. Urinary frequency and urgency
c. Increased breast size
d. Altered libido
e. Vasomotor symptoms

Answers

38.12 b	38.14 c	38.16 d	38.18 b	38.20 a
38.13 a	38.15 b	38.17 c	38.19 a	38.21 c

38.22 Approximately what percent of women experience vasomotor symptoms (hot flushes) in the perimenopausal and menopausal period?
   a. 35%
   b. 55%
   c. 75%
   d. 95%

38.23 Increased facial hair in menopausal women results from
   a. increased testosterone production
   b. increased dihydrotestosterone production
   c. increased dehydroepiandrosterone sulfate production
   d. reduced sex hormone-binding - globulin

38.24 What is the expected rate of bone loss in perimenopausal women?
   a. 0.1% per year
   b. 0.5% per year
   c. 1% per year
   d. 5% per year

38.25 What is the expected rate of bone loss in postmenopausal women who are not receiving estrogen?
   a. 0.1 to 0.2% per year
   b. 0.5% per year
   c. 1 to 2% per year
   d. 5% per year

38.26 Which of the following is NOT a risk factor for osteoporosis?
   a. Reduced height for weight
   b. Family history of osteoporosis
   c. Late menopause
   d. Low calcium intake
   e. Cigarette smoking

38.27 Which of the following is MOST effective in reducing postmenopausal bone loss?
   a. Weight-bearing exercise
   b. Calcium supplementation
   c. Estrogen therapy
   d. Vitamin D supplementation
   e. Calcitonin therapy

38.28 Compared with normal women, the number of ovarian follicles in women with Savage syndrome is
   a. increased
   b. unchanged
   c. reduced

38.29 Cigarette smoking has what effect on the timing of menopause?
   a. Smokers experience menopause 3 to 5 years earlier than nonsmokers.
   b. Smokers experience menopause at about the same time as nonsmokers.
   c. Smokers experience menopause 3 to 5 years later than nonsmokers.
   d. Smokers experience a longer period of menopausal symptoms.

38.30 Individuals who smoke
   a. do not respond as well as non-smokers to estrogen therapy
   b. respond equally as well as non-smokers to estrogen therapy
   c. respond better than nonsmokers to estrogen therapy

38.31 Approximately what percent of women will experience menopause before the age of 40?
   a. 1%
   b. 5%
   c. 10%
   d. 15%

38.32 Which of the following has NOT been found to be a factor in premature menopause?
   a. Chromosomal abnormalities
   b. Follicle resistance to FSH
   c. Production of autoantibodies
   d. Obesity

Answers

38.22 d	**38.24** b	**38.26** c	**38.28** b	**38.30** a	**38.32** d
38.23 d	**38.25** c	**38.27** c	**38.29** a	**38.31** a	

38.33 Climara/Estraderm patch contains which of the following hormones?
   a. Estradiol-17β
   b. Conjugated estrogens
   c. Esterified estrogen
   d. Estropipate (piperazine estrone sulfate)
   e. Ethinyl estradiol
   f. Medroxyprogesterone acetate
   g. Micronized estradiol
   h. Norethindrone acetate

38.34 Ogen contains which of the following hormones?
   a. Estradiol-17β
   b. Conjugated estrogens
   c. Esterified estrogen
   d. Estropipate (piperazine estrone sulfate)
   e. Ethinyl estradiol
   f. Medroxyprogesterone acetate
   g. Micronized estradiol
   h. Norethindrone acetate

38.35 Premarin contains which of the following hormones?
   a. Estradiol-17β
   b. Conjugated estrogens
   c. Esterified estrogen
   d. Estropipate (piperazine estrone sulfate)
   e. Ethinyl estradiol
   f. Medroxyprogesterone acetate
   g. Micronized estradiol
   h. Norethindrone acetate

38.36 Estrace contains which of the following hormones?
   a. Estradiol-17β
   b. Conjugated estrogens
   c. Esterified estrogen
   d. Estropipate (piperazine estrone sulfate)
   e. Ethinyl estradiol
   f. Medroxyprogesterone acetate
   g. Micronized estradiol
   h. Norethindrone acetate

38.37 Depo-Provera contains which of the following hormones?
   a. Estradiol-17β
   b. Conjugated estrogens
   c. Esterified estrogen
   d. Estropipate (piperazine estrone sulfate)
   e. Ethinyl estradiol
   f. Medroxyprogesterone acetate
   g. Micronized estradiol
   h. Norethindrone acetate

38.38 Provera (oral) contains which of the following hormones?
   a. Estradiol-17β
   b. Conjugated estrogens
   c. Esterified estrogen
   d. Estropipate (piperazine estrone sulfate)
   e. Ethinyl estradiol
   f. Medroxyprogesterone acetate
   g. Micronized estradiol
   h. Norethindrone acetate

38.39 Norlutate contains which of the following hormones?
   a. Estradiol-17β
   b. Conjugated estrogens
   c. Esterified estrogen
   d. Estropipate (piperazine estrone sulfate)
   e. Ethinyl estradiol
   f. Medroxyprogesterone acetate
   g. Micronized estradiol
   h. Norethindrone acetate

38.40 Women with a history of thromboembolic disease
   a. should not receive estrogen therapy
   b. may receive oral or injectable estrogen therapy
   c. may receive transdermal estrogen therapy

Answers

38.33 a	38.35 b	38.37 f	38.39 h	38.40 c
38.34 d	38.36 g	38.38 f		

38.41 Which of the following is a known risk of unopposed estrogen therapy?
a. Endometrial hyperplasia
b. Leiomyoma uteri
c. Endocervical adenocarcinoma
d. Squamous cell carcinoma of the cervix

38.42 If estrogen is administered alone for menopausal hormone therapy because of unacceptable side effects of progestins, then the patient should specifically be counseled as to the need for which of the following tests?
a. Yearly Pap smear
b. Yearly endometrial biopsy
c. Yearly complete blood count
d. Yearly fecal occult blood test

38.43 Alendronate has which mechanism of action?
a. Inhibition of osteoclast bone resorption
b. Estrogen receptor inhibition
c. Osteoclast bone resorption

38.44 Raloxifene has which mechanism of action?
a. Inhibition of osteoclast bone resorption
b. Estrogen receptor inhibition
c. Osteoclast bone resorption

38.45 Risedronate has which mechanism of action?
a. Inhibition of osteoclast bone resorption
b. Estrogen receptor inhibition
c. Osteoclast bone resorption

Answers
38.41 a   **38.42** b   **38.43** a   **38.44** b   **38.45** c

Questions and Answers Chapter 39: Infertility

39.1 Approximately what percent of couples will conceive within 1 year?
a. 50%
b. 60%
c. 70%
d. 80%
e. 90%

39.2 Infertility is defined as a couple's failure to conceive following unprotected sexual intercourse for
a. 6 months
b. 1 year
c. 2 years
d. 3 years
c. 4 years

39.3 Infertility affects what percent of reproductive-age couples in the United States?
a. 1%
b. 5%
c. 10%
d. 15%
e. 25%

39.4 What percent of couples with a clinical diagnosis of infertility may expect to have a child following specific diagnosis and treatment?
a. 55%
b. 65%
c. 75%
d. 85%
e. 95%

39.5 Fertility is decreased by approximately how much between about years 37 and 45 of a woman's life?
a. 25%
b. 50%
c. 75%
d. 90%

39.6 Anovulation, anatomic defects of the female genital tract, and abnormal spermatogenesis together account for what percent of reproductive dysfunction?
a. 65%
b. 75%
c. 85%
d. 95%

39.7 The characteristic biphasic temperature shift associated with ovulation occurs in what percent of ovulating women?
a. 60%
b. 70%
c. 80%
d. 90%
e. 99%

39.8 A rise in basal body temperature typically occurs
a. 2 to 3 days before ovulation
b. at the time of ovulation
c. 2 to 3 days after ovulation
d. immediately before menstruation

39.9 If a woman does not conceive, how many days after ovulation will her basal body temperature return to preovulatory levels?
a. 8
b. 10
c. 14
d. 18
e. 22

39.10 There is a strong possibility of pregnancy if basal body temperature remains elevated at least
a. 10 days
b. 14 days
c. 16 days
d. 20 days
e. 24 days

Answers

39.1 e	39.3 d	39.5 b	39.7 d	39.9 c
39.2 b	39.4 d	39.6 d	39.8 b	39.10 c

39.11 What portion of an ejaculate contains the greatest density of sperm?
a. First quarter
b. Second quarter
c. Third quarter
d. Last quarter

39.12 After a semen specimen is collected, semen analysis should be performed within
a. 1 hour
b. 2 hours
c. 4 hours
d. 6 hours
e. 8 hours

39.13 In a normal semen specimen, abnormal sperm forms constitute less than what percent of the total?
a. 10%
b. 15%
c. 20%
d. 25%
e. 30%

39.14 A normal semen analysis contains at least what percent of motile sperm?
a. 40%
b. 50%
c. 60%
d. 70%
e. 80%

39.15 A normal semen analysis excludes a male cause for infertility in what percent of cases?
a. 50%
b. 60%
c. 70%
d. 80%
e. 90%
f. 100%

39.16 A normal semen analysis is characterized by full liquefaction within
a. 15 minutes
b. 60 minutes
c. 90 minutes
d. 120 minutes

39.17 In detecting abnormalities of the genital tract, a hysterosalpingogram has a diagnostic accuracy of approximately
a. 30%
b. 50%
c. 70%
d. 90%

39.18 On average, the menstrual cycle of a healthy woman between the ages of 18 and 36 is characterized by
a. ovulation 13 to 14 times per year
b. ovulation occurring on the tenth day
c. menstruation beginning on the thirtieth day
d. menstruation lasting approximately 3 days

39.19 Following ovulation, the basal body temperature
a. increases by 0.6°F
b. increases by 0.2°F
c. does not change
d. decreases by 0.2°F
e. decreases by 0.6°F

39.20 Which of the following is typical of the luteal phase of the menstrual cycle?
a. Improvement of mood
b. Presence of a proliferative endometrium
c. Appearance of sticky cervical mucus
d. Proliferation of the breast ducts

39.21 Which of the following is NOT associated with abnormal sperm morphology?
a. Varicocele
b. Infection
c. Immunologic factors, including antisperm antibodies
d. Stress

39.22 Capacitation of sperm occurs in the
a. fallopian tube
b. endometrial cavity
c. endocervix
d. vagina

Answers

39.11 a	**39.13** d	**39.15** e	**39.17** c	**39.19** a	**39.21** c
39.12 b	**39.14** c	**39.16** b	**39.18** a	**39.20** c	**39.22** c

39.23 The generation time of sperm is approximately
   a. 33 days
   b. 53 days
   c. 73 days
   d. 93 days
   e. 113 days

39.24 Normal sperm production typically occurs at a temperature that is approximately
   a. 3°F above body temperature
   b. 1°F above body temperature
   c. at body temperature
   d. 1°F below body temperature
   e. 3°F below body temperature

39.25 Which of the following does NOT result in decreased sperm production resulting from thermal shock?
   a. Spending excessive time in hot tubs or hot baths
   b. Sitting on the testicles for long periods of time with poor heat dispersion
   c. Wearing tight clothing
   d. Living in a climate where the temperature exceeds 90°F for long periods

39.26 Which of the following is the MOST appropriate initial test for infertility in the case of a 32-year-old G2P2002 who has recently married a 35-year-old man with no children?
   a. Antisperm antibodies
   b. Basal body temperature record
   c. Diagnostic laparoscopy
   d. Endometrial biopsy
   e. Hysterosalpingogram
   f. Hysteroscopy
   g. Luteal phase progesterone
   h. Postcoital test
   i. Semen analysis
   j. Urinary luteinizing hormone detection kit

39.27 Which of the following is the MOST appropriate initial test for infertility in the case of a 21-year-old G1P0010 who has had amenorrhea since an elective abortion that was followed by infection?
   a. Antisperm antibodies
   b. Basal body temperature record
   c. Diagnostic laparoscopy
   d. Endometrial biopsy
   e. Hysterosalpingogram
   f. Hysteroscopy
   g. Luteal phase progesterone
   h. Postcoital test
   i. Semen analysis
   j. Urinary luteinizing hormone detection kit

39.28 Which of the following is the MOST appropriate initial test for infertility in the case of a 28-year-old G1P1001 who wishes to increase her chance of pregnancy by the timing of intercourse?
   a. Antisperm antibodies
   b. Basal body temperature record
   c. Diagnostic laparoscopy
   d. Endometrial biopsy
   e. Hysterosalpingogram
   f. Hysteroscopy
   g. Luteal phase progesterone
   h. Postcoital test
   i. Semen analysis
   j. Urinary luteinizing hormone detection kit

Answers

39.23 c	**39.24** d	**39.25** d	**39.26** i	**39.27** e	**39.28** b

39.29 Which of the following is the MOST appropriate initial test for infertility in the case of a 32-year-old G0 with a history of chronic pelvic pain and dysmenorrhea whose partner has a normal semen analysis?
  a. Antisperm antibodies
  b. Basal body temperature record
  c. Diagnostic laparoscopy
  d. Endometrial biopsy
  e. Hysterosalpingogram
  f. Hysteroscopy
  g. Luteal phase progesterone
  h. Postcoital test
  i. Semen analysis
  j. Urinary luteinizing hormone detection kit

39.30 Which of the following is the MOST appropriate initial test for infertility in the case of a 26-year-old G0 with a history of irregular periods, who works several jobs, and has unpredictable sleeping patterns?
  a. Antisperm antibodies
  b. Basal body temperature record
  c. Diagnostic laparoscopy
  d. Endometrial biopsy
  e. Hysterosalpingogram
  f. Hysteroscopy
  g. Luteal phase progesterone
  h. Postcoital test
  i. Semen analysis
  j. Urinary luteinizing hormone detection kit

39.31 Which of the following is the MOST appropriate initial test for infertility in the case of a couple undergoing infertility evaluation who demonstrate clumping of sperm on the Huhner-Sims test?
  a. Antisperm antibodies
  b. Basal body temperature record
  c. Diagnostic laparoscopy
  d. Endometrial biopsy
  e. Hysterosalpingogram
  f. Hysteroscopy
  g. Luteal phase progesterone
  h. Postcoital test
  i. Semen analysis
  j. Urinary luteinizing hormone detection kit

39.32 Which of the following statements about clomiphene citrate is correct?
  a. It acts by stimulating estrogen production and binding
  b. It should be administered in conjunction with progesterone
  c. It results in an increase in the release of follicle-stimulating hormone from the pituitary
  d. Dosage should not exceed 50 mg/day

39.33 What is the success rate of clomiphene citrate in inducing spermatogenesis?
  a. 5%
  b. 10%
  c. 15%
  d. 20%
  e. 25%

Answers

39.29 c	**39.30** g	**39.31** a	**39.32** c	**39.33** d

39.34 The expected success rate of in vitro fertilization in properly selected couples is approximately
  a. 13 to 17% per cycle
  b. 18 to 22% per cycle
  c. 23 to 27% per cycle
  d. 28 to 32% per cycle
  e. 33 to 37% per cycle

39.35 How many days after the completion of therapy with clomiphene citrate will presumptive signs of ovulation occur?
  a. 1 to 3 days
  b. 4 to 6 days
  c. 7 to 11 days
  d. 12 to 14 days
  e. 15 to 17 days

39.36 "Spinnbarkeit" is a term that means
  a. mucus secretion of the cervix
  b. thinning of the cervical mucus
  c. threading of cervical mucus
  d. crystallization of the cervical mucus

39.37 Luteal phase failure as a cause of infertility is treated by
  a. thyroid hormone
  b. estrogens and progestins combined
  c. progestins alone
  d. Pergonal

39.38 A serum progesterone level above what level is 80% accurate in distinguishing a normal from an abnormal cycle?
  a. 15 ng/mL
  b. 25 ng/mL
  c. 35 ng/mL
  d. 45 ng/mL

39.39 A serum progesterone level below what level is rarely associated with normal cycles?
  a. 40 ng/mL
  b. 30 ng/mL
  c. 20 ng/mL
  d. 10 ng/mL

Answers

39.34 b	39.35 c	39.36 c	39.37 c	39.38 a	39.39 d

Questions and Answers Chapter 40: Premenstrual Syndrome

40.1 Which of the following statements is LEAST descriptive of premenstrual syndrome (PMS)?
  a. It occurs in a regular, cyclical relationship to the luteal phase of the menstrual cycle
  b. It can resemble certain psychiatric conditions
  c. Its onset may occur in a woman's fourth decade of life
  d. The severity tends to increase over time

40.2 The symptoms of PMS typically resolve
  a. at ovulation
  b. 2 weeks before the onset of menses
  c. near the end of menses
  d. about 2 weeks after the start of menses

40.3 In PMS, there is a symptom-free interval of at least
  a. 1 week per cycle
  b. 2 weeks per cycle
  c. 2 cycles per year
  d. 1 of 4 cycles

40.4 The maximum estimated incidence of women with some physical or emotional PMS is
  a. 30%
  b. 50%
  c. 70%
  d. 90%

40.5 Premenstrual syndrome that is severe and debilitating occurs in what percent of women?
  a. 5%
  b. 25%
  c. 50%
  d. 75%

40.6 Premenstrual syndrome tends to be more common in women in which of the following age groups?
  a. Teens and 20s
  b. 20s and 30s
  c. 30s and 40s
  d. 40s and 50s

40.7 In making the diagnosis of PMS, the characteristic that is most important is the
  a. severity of symptoms
  b. duration of symptoms
  c. cyclic occurrence of symptoms
  d. degree of disability in the patient
  e. association with exogenous therapy

40.8 The psychiatric basis for PMS is supported by
  a. response to antidepressants
  b. laboratory findings
  c. physical examination findings
  d. success with dietary management

40.9 The endocrinologic basis for PMS is best demonstrated by symptom
  a. severity
  b. variability
  c. cyclicity
  d. type

40.10 The dietary modification that is LEAST likely to help patients with PMS is
  a. eating three meals a day
  b. reducing carbohydrates
  c. reducing sodium
  d. eating fresh fruits
  e. eating more vegetables

40.11 The role of endorphins in PMS is best demonstrated by
  a. sedentary patients
  b. patients who exercise
  c. patients who take analgesics
  d. premenarchal patients

Answers

40.1	d	40.3	a	40.5	a	40.7	c	40.9	c	40.11 b
40.2	c	40.4	d	40.6	c	40.8	a	40.10	a	

40.12 Which of the following is most likely related to the underlying cause of PMS?
   a. Norepinephrine
   b. Progesterone
   c. Dopamine
   d. Serotonin
   e. Estrogen

40.13 Data supporting the endorphin basis of PMS comes from patients who report alleviation of symptoms with
   a. aspirin consumption
   b. exercise
   c. caffeine consumption
   d. bed rest
   e. sexual arousal

40.14 The most useful diagnostic tool with respect to PMS is
   a. serial progesterone levels
   b. serial blood glucose determinations
   c. a menstrual diary
   d. cyclic vaginal wall cytology
   e. a symptom list

40.15 Which of the following is LEAST likely to be effective in a patient with PMS?
   a. fluoxetine
   b. nortriptyline
   c. sertraline
   d. paroxetine
   e. escitalopram

40.16 Modification of which of the following dietary components appears to have the LEAST effect in patients with PMS?
   a. Carbohydrates
   b. Fat
   c. Protein
   d. Caffeine

40.17 In a patient with PMS who responds to use of gonadotropin-releasing hormone agonist, what surgical procedure would be most appropriate?
   a. Hysterectomy
   b. Endometrial ablation
   c. Oophorectomy
   d. Dilation and curettage

40.18 Which of the following is useful to confirm the diagnosis of premenstrual syndrome?
   a. Tetracycline
   b. Premarin
   c. Bromocriptine
   d. Gonadotropin-releasing hormone agonist
   e. Prostaglandin F2α

40.19 Which of the following is most likely to help a patient's PMS symptoms?
   a. Transdermal estrogen
   b. Vaginal progesterone
   c. Combined oral contraceptives
   d. Oral medroxyprogesterone acetate

40.20 Which of the following is a "core" symptom in establishing a diagnosis of premenstrual dysphoric disorder?
   a. Persistent anger
   b. Headache
   c. Lack of energy
   d. Difficulty with concentration

40.21 Which of the following reflects the method of diagnosing PMS?
   a. Criteria established by DSM-IV
   b. Requires only one symptom
   c. Requires a prospective calendar of symptoms
   d. Patient must be functionally impaired

40.22 Which of the following is the LEAST important aspect of PMS/premenstrual dysphoric disorder?
   a. Work
   b. School
   c. Usual activities
   d. Libido

Answers

40.12 d	40.14 c	40.16 c	40.18 d	40.20 a	40.22 d
40.13 b	40.15 b	40.17 c	40.19 c	40.21 b	

Questions and Answers Chapter 41: Cell Biology and Principles of Cancer Therapy

41.1 Cells are especially vulnerable to anti-cancer therapies during what portion of the cell cycle?
a. The portion of the cycle when cells are dividing
b. The portion of time when cells are in the resting stage
c. Both the dividing and resting stages
d. When the cells are degenerating

41.2 In the cell cycle, the major event of G0 is
a. synthesis of RNA and protein in preparation for DNA synthesis
b. DNA synthesis
c. additional RNA, protein, and specialized DNA synthesis
d. cell division occurs
e. resting phase

41.3 In the cell cycle, the major event of G1 is
a. synthesis of RNA and protein in preparation for DNA synthesis
b. DNA synthesis
c. additional RNA, protein, and specialized DNA synthesis
d. cell division occurs
e. resting phase

41.4 In the cell cycle, the major event of G2 is
a. synthesis of RNA and protein in preparation for DNA synthesis
b. DNA synthesis
c. additional RNA, protein, and specialized DNA synthesis
d. cell division occurs
e. resting phase

41.5 In the cell cycle, the major event of S is
a. synthesis of RNA and protein in preparation for DNA synthesis
b. DNA synthesis
c. additional RNA, protein, and specialized DNA synthesis
d. cell division occurs
e. resting phase

41.6 In the cell cycle, the major event of M is
a. synthesis of RNA and protein in preparation for DNA synthesis
b. DNA synthesis
c. additional RNA, protein, and specialized DNA synthesis
d. cell division occurs
e. resting phase

41.7 Anticancer therapies specifically designed to affect cells engaged in synthetic activities are LEAST effective during which stage of the cell cycle?
a. G0
b. G1
c. G2
d. S

41.8 The phase of the cell cycle that is the most variable in length is
a. G1.
b. S
c. G2.
d. M

41.9 The growth fraction is the number of cells in a tumor that are NOT in the
a. G0 phase
b. S phase
c. G1 phase
d. G2 phase

41.10 As a tumor enlarges in size, the growth fraction
a. increases
b. remains the same
c. decreases

41.11 Cytoreductive debulking surgery has what effect on the remaining tumor cells?
a. Causes tumor cells to enter the G0 phase
b. Causes tumor cells to leave the G0 phase
c. Causes the growth fraction of tumor cells to decrease
d. The surgery has no effect on the remaining tumor cells

Answers

41.1 a	41.3 a	41.5 b	41.7 a	41.9 a	41.11 b
41.2 e	41.4 c	41.6 d	41.8 a	41.10 c	

41.12 Which of the following is characteristic of alkylating agents?
- a. Affects assembly of microtubules
- b. Structural analogs of normal molecules necessary for cell function
- c. Inhibits DNA-directed RNA synthesis
- d. Interferes with base pairs, producing cross links, causing single-strand and double-strand breaks

41.13 Which of the following is characteristic of antitumor antibiotics?
- a. Affects assembly of microtubules
- b. Structural analogs of normal molecules necessary for cell function
- c. Inhibits DNA-directed RNA synthesis
- d. Interferes with base pairs, producing cross links, causing single-strand and double-strand breaks

41.14 Which of the following is characteristic of antimetabolites?
- a. Affects assembly of microtubules
- b. Structural analogs of normal molecules necessary for cell function
- c. Inhibits DNA-directed RNA synthesis
- d. Interferes with base pairs, producing cross links, causing single-strand and double strand breaks

41.15 Which of the following is characteristic of plant alkaloids?
- a. Affects assembly of microtubules
- b. Structural analogs of normal molecules necessary for cell function
- c. Inhibits DNA-directed RNA synthesis
- d. Interferes with base pairs, producing cross links, causing single-strand and double-strand breaks

41.16 Alkylating agents are active during which phase of the cell cycle?
- a. G1
- b. S
- c. G2
- d. M
- e. Phase nonspecific

41.17 Antitumor antibiotics act during which phase of the cell cycle?
- a. G1
- b. S
- c. G2
- d. M
- e. Phase nonspecific

41.18 Antimetabolites act during which phase of the cell cycle?
- a. G1
- b. S
- c. G2
- d. M
- e. Phase nonspecific

41.19 Plant alkaloids act during which phase of the cell cycle?
- a. G1
- b. S
- c. G2
- d. M
- e. Phase nonspecific

41.20 Suppression of blood cell formation is a common side effect of
- a. alkylating agents
- b. antitumor antibiotics
- c. plant alkaloids
- d. antimetabolites
- e. all of the above

41.21 Impaired renal function is most often associated with which antineoplastic drug?
- a. Methotrexate
- b. Cisplatin
- c. Busulfan
- d. Hydroxyurea

Answers

41.12 d	41.14 b	41.16 a	41.18 b	41.20 e
41.13 c	41.15 a	41.17 e	41.19 d	41.21 b

41.22 Which of the following is an alkylating agent?
- a. Chlorambucil
- b. Bleomycin
- c. Actinomycin D
- d. Methotrexate

41.23 An example of an antitumor antibiotic is
- a. actinomycin D
- b. cisplatin
- c. vincristine
- d. vinblastine

41.24 Which of the following is an antimetabolite?
- a. Methotrexate
- b. Cyclophosphamide
- c. Ifosfamide
- d. Cisplatin

41.25 An example of a plant alkaloid is
- a. vincristine
- b. chlorambucil (Leukeran)
- c. bleomycin (Blenoxane)
- d. actinomycin D

41.26 Which of the following is NOT a criterion that must be met for antineoplastic drugs to be used in combination?
- a. They must be effective when used singularly.
- b. They must have different mechanisms of action.
- c. They must be additive in action.
- d. They must not lead to drug resistance.

41.27 An additive interaction between chemotherapeutic agents results in
- a. improved antitumor activity or decreased toxicity compared with each agent alone
- b. enhanced antitumor activity equal to the sum of each of the individual agents
- c. less antitumor activity than each individual agent

41.28 An antagonistic interaction between antineoplastic drugs results in
- a. improved antitumor activity or decreased toxicity compared with each agent alone
- b. enhanced antitumor activity equal to the sum of each of the individual agents
- c. less antitumor activity than each individual agent

41.29 A synergistic action between anticancer agents is defined as
- a. improved antitumor activity or decreased toxicity compared with each agent alone
- b. enhanced antitumor activity equal to the sum of each of the individual agents
- c. less antitumor activity than each individual agent

41.30 In sequential blockade combination chemotherapy, the drugs
- a. interfere with different steps in the synthesis of DNA or RNA
- b. attack parallel biochemical pathways leading to the same end product
- c. block enzymes in a single biochemical pathway

41.31 Which of the following best describes the purpose of adjuvant chemotherapy?
- a. Cure
- b. Palliation
- c. Cytoreduction
- d. Symptomatic relief

41.32 Induction chemotherapy is used to bring about
- a. palliation
- b. symptomatic relief
- c. remission
- d. reduction of side effects of other treatment

Answers

41.22 a	41.24 a	41.26 d	41.28 c	41.30 c	41.32 c
41.23 a	41.25 a	41.27 b	41.29 a	41.31 a	

41.33 Maintenance chemotherapy is
  a. a short course of combination chemotherapy given in high doses for the purpose of eliminating residual cancer cells
  b. long-term and low-dose therapy designed to keep a patient in remission by inhibiting the growth of remaining cancer cells
  c. high-dose combination chemotherapy with the goal of causing remission
  d. designed to bring pain relief

41.34 Radiation therapy kills cells according to
  a. zero order kinetics
  b. first order kinetics
  c. second order kinetics

41.35 Compared with fractionated small doses, a single, large focused dose of radiation is
  a. more likely to be effective in destroying a tumor
  b. as likely to be effective in destroying a tumor
  c. less likely to be effective in destroying a tumor

41.36 How does the presence of oxygen affect tumor cells' vulnerability to radiation?
  a. Oxygen increases vulnerability
  b. Oxygen does not affect vulnerability
  c. Oxygen decreases vulnerability

41.37 Local irradiation of tumor cells is termed
  a. teletherapy
  b. brachytherapy
  c. maintenance therapy

41.38 One gray equals
  a. 1 rad
  b. 10 rads
  c. 100 rads
  d. 1,000 rads

41.39 One gray is defined as one joule per
  a. kilogram
  b. $meter^2$
  c. meter
  d. rad

41.40 Tamoxifen acts as a competitive inhibitor of
  a. progesterone binding
  b. estrogen binding
  c. prolactin binding
  d. follicle-stimulating hormone binding

Answers

41.33 b	41.35 c	41.37 b	41.39 a
41.34 b	41.36 a	41.38 c	41.40 b

Questions and Answers Chapter 42: Gestational Trophoblastic Disease

42.1 Approximately what percent of patients with gestational trophoblastic disease will develop persistent or malignant disease?
a. 10%
b. 20%
c. 30%
d. 40%
e. 60%

42.2 The incidence of gestational trophoblastic disease in the United States is approximately one in how many pregnancies?
a. 500
b. 1,000
c. 1,500
d. 2,000
e. 2,500

42.3 Genetically, complete moles are of
a. paternal origin only
b. maternal origin only
c. mixed paternal and maternal origin

42.4 Approximately what percent of molar pregnancies are of the complete mole type?
a. 50%
b. 60%
c. 70%
d. 80%
e. 90%

42.5 Complete molar pregnancy is characterized by
a. a karyotype of 69, XXY
b. a chromosomally abnormal fetus
c. proliferation from the cytotrophoblast
d. absent fetal membranes

42.6 Incomplete molar pregnancy is characterized by
a. a karyotype of 69,XXY
b. absent fetal membranes
c. proliferation of the syncytiotrophoblast
d. all villi edematous

42.7 Compared with a partial mole, what is the potential for malignant transformation in a complete mole?
a. Higher
b. The same
c. Lower

42.8 Abnormal bleeding during a complete molar pregnancy most commonly occurs early in which trimester?
a. First
b. Second
c. Third

42.9 A discrepancy between the uterine size and the gestational age is seen in approximately what percent of patients with complete molar pregnancy?
a. 30%
b. 50%
c. 70%
d. 90%

42.10 Which of the following is NOT a sign or symptom commonly seen in molar pregnancy?
a. Pregnancy-induced hypertension
b. Severe nausea
c. Bradycardia
d. Visual disturbances

Answers

42.1	b	42.3	a	42.5	d	42.7	a	42.9	c
42.2	d	42.4	e	42.6	a	42.8	b	42.10	c

42.11 Which of the following statements about invasive mole is INCORRECT?
 a. It is a complete mole invading the myometrium without any intervening endometrial stroma.
 b. It often is diagnosed months after evacuation of a complete mole following evaluation for human chorionic gonadotropin (hCG) levels that do not fall appropriately.
 c. It may be diagnosed on curettage at the time of initial molar evacuation.
 d. Its natural course includes local invasion and, on occasion, vascular invasion and metastasis.
 e. It follows after 35 to 45% of complete hydatidiform moles.

42.12 A molar pregnancy is confirmed through
 a. serial measurement of hCG levels
 b. use of ultrasound imaging
 c. bimanual pelvic examination

42.13 Compared with patients with complete molar pregnancy, patients with partial molar pregnancy typically present at
 a. an earlier gestational age
 b. the same gestational age
 c. a later gestational age

42.14 The determination of hCG) titers associated with molar pregnancy is NOT useful for
 a. classifying the risk category for the tumor
 b. serving as a tumor marker in follow-up of therapy
 c. ascertaining whether the pregnancy is a partial or complete mole

42.15 Which of the following is NOT characteristic of high-risk gestational trophoblastic disease?
 a. Uterus greater than 16-week size
 b. Presence of a large theca lutein cyst
 c. Marked trophoblastic proliferation and/or anaplasia
 d. Hyperthyroidism
 e. 46,XX karyotype

42.16 What is the basic treatment of molar pregnancy?
 a. Evacuation of the uterine contents
 b. Abdominal hysterectomy
 c. Abdominal hysterectomy with bilateral salpingo-oophorectomy
 d. Radiation therapy
 e. Chemotherapy

42.17 In the follow-up of a molar pregnancy, serum hCG levels should be obtained monthly for how many months?
 a. 6 months
 b. 12 months
 c. 18 months
 d. 24 months

42.18 Following molar pregnancy, what is the incidence of placental accreta?
 a. Increased
 b. Unchanged
 c. Decreased

42.19 In the United States, what is the incidence of choriocarcinoma?
 a. 1 in 40 normal pregnancies
 b. 1 in 5,000 normal pregnancies
 c. 1 in 15,000 normal pregnancies
 d. 1 in 150,000 normal pregnancies

42.20 In the United States, what is the incidence of choriocarcinoma associated with molar pregnancy?
 a. 1 in 40 molar pregnancies
 b. 1 in 5,000 molar pregnancies
 c. 1 in 15,000 molar pregnancies
 d. 1 in 150,000 molar pregnancies

Answers

42.11 e	42.13 c	42.15 e	42.17 b	42.19 d
42.12 b	42.14 c	42.16 a	42.18 a	42.20 a

42.21 In the United States, what is the incidence of choriocarcinoma associated with abortion?
   a. 1 in 40 abortions
   b. 1 in 5,000 abortions
   c. 1 in 15,000 abortions
   d. 1 in 150,000 abortions

42.22 In the United States, what is the incidence of choriocarcinoma associated with ectopic pregnancy?
   a. 1 in 40 ectopic pregnancies
   b. 1 in 5,000 ectopic pregnancies
   c. 1 in 15,000 ectopic pregnancies
   d. 1 in 150,000 ectopic pregnancies

42.23 Which of the following is NOT an indication for chemotherapy in trophoblastic disease?
   a. Histologic diagnosis of choriocarcinoma
   b. Evidence of metastatic disease
   c. Plateaued or rising hCG titers after evacuation
   d. β-hCG titer that has returned to normal after 12 weeks' postevacuation
   e. Increased β-hCG titer after a normal level has been obtained, exclusive of a normal pregnancy

42.24 The recurrence rate for gestational trophoblastic disease is approximately
   a. 2%
   b. 4%
   c. 6%
   d. 8%

42.25 The treatment of a patient with a hydatidiform mole could include all of the following EXCEPT
   a. periodic assays of serum β-hCG
   b. periodic clinical examinations for the detection of malignant changes
   c. radiotherapy
   d. prophylactic chemotherapy
   e. evacuation of the uterus

42.26 Eclampsia in the first trimester is most frequently associated with
   a. abruptio placenta
   b. acute glomerulonephritis
   c. molar degeneration
   d. pregnancy-induced hypertension
   e. berry aneurysm

42.27 What is a serious complication of choriocarcinoma?
   a. Intestinal obstruction
   b. Uterine perforation and massive bleeding
   c. Cardiac arrhythmia
   d. Multifocal seizures

42.28 Which of the following statements about placental site tumors is incorrect?
   a. The tumor is composed of monomorphic populations of intermediate cytotrophoblast cells that are locally invasive at the site of placental implantation.
   b. The tumor secretes placental lactogen.
   c. The tumor is rarely metastatic.
   d. The tumor is sensitive to standard chemotherapy.

Answers

42.21 c	**42.23** d	**42.25** c	**42.27** b
42.22 b	**42.24** a	**42.26** c	**42.28** d

Questions and Answers Chapter 43: Vulvar and Vaginal Disease and Neoplasia

43.1 Lichen simplex chronicus is best described as
   a. yellow-pink in color
   b. a raised patch with a silvery scale
   c. ulcerative
   d. diffusely reddened

43.2 A description of lichen planus would include
   a. an oily appearance
   b. raised patches on an erythematous base
   c. white lacy bands of keratosis
   d. diffuse redness with hyperpigmented plaques

43.3 Psoriasis has what characteristic appearance?
   a. Oily-appearing, scaly crust
   b. Silver scale
   c. Whitish lacy band
   d. Hyperpigmented plaque

43.4 Seborrheic dermatitis has what characteristic appearance?
   a. Lesions are pale to red to yellow–pink and may be covered by an oily-appearing, scaly crust
   b. Lesions are typically slightly raised, round, or ovoid patches with a silver scale appearance atop an erythematous base
   c. Areas of whitish lacy bands of keratosis near reddish ulcerated-like lesions
   d. Diffusely reddened areas with occasional hyperplastic or hyperpigmented plaques of red to reddish-brown

43.5 Lichen simplex chronicus is best treated with
   a. antipruritic at night and topical steroid cream
   b. topical steroid with stronger fluorinated steroid for hyperkeratosis
   c. cold tar preparation and exposure to ultraviolet light
   d. Burrow solution soaks

43.6 Lichen planus should be treated with
   a. antipruritic at night and topical steroid cream
   b. topical steroid with stronger fluorinated steroid for hyperkeratosis
   c. cold tar preparation and exposure to ultraviolet light
   d. Burrow solution soaks

43.7 Of the following, which is the most appropriate treatment for psoriasis?
   a. Antipruritc at night with topical steroid during the day
   b. Topical steroids alone
   c. Cold tar preparation and exposure to ultraviolet light
   d. Burrow solution soaks

43.8 Seborrheic dermatitis management should include
   a. antipruritic to inhibit nighttime itching and topical steroid creams
   b. topical steroid preparations, but stronger fluorinated steroid preparations may be used in the presence of hyperkeratosis
   c. topical cold tar preparations, followed by exposure to ultraviolet light
   d. Burrow solution soaks, followed by topical corticosteroid lotions or creams

Answers

43.1 d	43.3 b	43.5 a	43.7 c
43.2 c	43.4 a	43.6 b	43.8 d

43.9 Which of the following is the LEAST accurate statement about vulvar vestibulitis?

a. Vulvar vestibulitis involves the vestibular glands located just inside the vaginal introitus near the hymenal ring.

b. Patients often report a progressive worsening of the condition

c. Light touch of a moistened cotton tip applicator to the proper anatomic areas will duplicate the pain of the complaint.

d. The affected areas often appear as small, reddened patches.

e. Treatment with hydrocortisone ointments and topical Xylocaine jelly is uniformly successful.

43.10 A 28-year-old happily married woman presents with new onset insertional dyspareunia. The most likely diagnosis is:

a. chronic cervicitis

b. vulvar dysplasia

c. vestibulitis

d. Bartholin abscess

43.11 Which of the following is most characteristic of an inclusion cyst?

a. It may become pedunculated

b. It is associated with a hernia

c. It contains cheesy material

d. It arises from sweat glands

43.12 A hydrocele is associated with

a. vulvar neoplasms

b. canal of Nuck

c. cystocele

d. condyloma

43.13 A fibroma may become

a. pedunculated

b. malignant

c. liquefied

d. incarcerated

43.14 A hidradenoma is associated with

a. nerve cells

b. the bladder

c. hernias

d. sweat glands

43.15 A description of nevi would include

a. usually small size, although occasionally may become large and pedunculated

b. a cyst of the canal of Nuck

c. small, smooth nodular masses containing cheesy material

d. typically benign and arises from the sweat glands on the inner surface of the labia majora

e. pigmented lesions that must be distinguished from a common malignant lesion, occurring on the external genitalia

43.16 Which of the following conditions may be associated with high urinary oxalic acid concentrations?

a. Hidradenoma

b. Seborrheic dermatitis

c. Lichen simplex chronicus

d. Vestibulitis

e. Psoriasis

43.17 Lichen sclerosis and hyperplastic dystrophy without atypia carry what estimated risk of vulvar carcinoma?

a. 0 to 1%

b. 2 to 3%

c. 4 to 5%

d. 6 to 7%

e. 8 to 9%

Answers

43.9 e	43.11 c	43.13 a	43.15 e	43.17 b
43.10 c	43.12 b	43.14 d	43.16 d	

43.18 Mixed dystrophy–lichen sclerosis admixed with areas of hyperplastic dystrophy–is treated by
a. corticosteroid cream alone
b. testosterone appropionate cream alone
c. corticosteroid cream for 2 TO 3 weeks, then topical testosterone propionate
d. topical testosterone appropionate for 2 TO 3 weeks, then corticosteroid cream
e. laser ablation

43.19 Which of the following is characteristic of hyperplastic dystrophy?
a. Unlikely to resolve totally
b. High risk for malignancy
c. Thin, white epithelium
d. Secondary excoriation

43.20 Lichen sclerosis is characterized by which of the following statements?
a. The lesion is unlikely to totally resolve, requiring intermittent treatment for an indefinite period
b. The lesion is likely to be pre-malignant
c. The vulva is only rarely termed "onion-skinned" in appearance
d. There is obviously hyperkeratotic skin with secondary excoriation

43.21 Which of the following is characteristic of vulvar intraepithelial neoplasia I and II?
a. It should be treated like a cancer
b. It is associated with colon cancer
c. It may be associated with human papillomavirus
d. There is full-thickness loss of maturation

43.22 Vulvar intraepithelial neoplasia III (VIN III, carcinoma in situ) is characterized by
a. an association with breast cancer
b. an association with colon cancer
c. pain as a presenting complaint
d. pruritus as a presenting complaint

43.23 Which of the following is LEAST associated with Paget disease?
a. breast cancer
b. colon cancer
c. skin cancer
d. cervical cancer

43.24 Melanoma is most commonly associated with which characteristic?
a. Pigmentation
b. Pain
c. Papillomavirus
d. Pruritus

43.25 When vulvar melanoma invades to the depth of the subcutaneous tissue, survival is generally
a. 0 to 20%
b. 20 to 40%
c. 40 to 60%
d. 60 to 80%

43.26 Extended vulvar intraepithelial neoplasia I and II lesions are best treated by
a. cryocautery
b. electrodesiccation
c. laser cautery, using local anesthetic
d. laser ablation, using general anesthetic

43.27 Vulvar carcinoma accounts for approximately what percent of all gynecologic malignancies?
a. 4%
b. 8%
c. 12%
d. 20%

Answers

43.18 c	43.20 a	43.22 d	43.24 a	43.26 d
43.19 d	43.21 c	43.23 d	43.25 a	43.27 a

43.28 What percent of all squamous vulvar malignancies are found in women <40 years old?
a. Less than 1%
b. 5%
c. 10%
d. 15%
e. 20%

43.29 What percent of vulvar carcinomas are of the squamous cell type?
a. 30%
b. 50%
c. 70%
d. 90%

43.30 In patients with vulvar carcinoma, what is the most common presenting complaint?
a. An exophytic ulcerative lesion on a labium majus
b. Vulvar pruritus
c. Dysuria
d. Dyspareunia

43.31 The spread of squamous cell carcinoma of the vulva is best characterized by which of the following?
a. Metastasis occurs early in the disease course
b. Spread of the disease is usually predictable
c. Spread depends on patient age
d. Lesions in the posterior aspect of the vulva may spread directly to the deep pelvic nodes.

43.32 The overall incidence of lymph node metastasis in squamous cell carcinoma of the vulva is approximately
a. 10%
b. 20%
c. 30%
d. 40%

43.33 For patients with negative inguinal and femoral lymph nodes, the 5-year survival rate for patients with vulvar carcinoma is approximately
a. 30%
b. 50%
c. 70%
d. 90%

43.34 Treatment of cancer of the Bartholin gland is
a. radiation
b. simple excision
c. radical vulvectomy and bilateral lymphadenectomy
d. simple vulvectomy

43.35 A Gartner duct cyst is related to
a. remnants of the wolffian duct
b. episiotomy scarring
c. vaginal cancer
d. urinary incontinence

43.36 An inclusion cyst
a. arises from vestigial remnants of the wolffian or mesonephric system
b. arises from imperfect alignment of childbirth lacerations or episiotomy
c. is lined with columnar epithelium
d. is premalignant

43.37 Which of the following does NOT increase the likelihood of vaginal carcinoma in situ?
a. A preexisting lower genital tract neoplasia
b. Previous hysterectomy for cervical carcinoma in situ
c. Radiation therapy for another gynecologic malignancy
d. Exposure to diethylstilbestrol in utero

Answers

43.28 c	43.30 b	43.32 c	43.34 d	43.36 b
43.29 d	43.31 b	43.33 d	43.35 a	43.37 d

43.38 Invasive vaginal cancer accounts for approximately what percent of gynecologic malignancies?
a. 1 to 2%
b. 3 to 4%
c. 5 to 6%
d. 7 to 8%
e. 9 to 10%

43.39 Squamous cell carcinoma accounts for what percent of vaginal carcinoma?
a. 35%
b. 55%
c. 75%
d. 95%

43.40 Stage 0 vaginal carcinoma is characterized by
a. carcinoma involving the subvaginal tissue but not extending onto the pelvic wall
b. carcinoma extending onto the pelvic side wall
c. carcinoma limited to the vaginal mucosa
d. carcinoma in situ
e. carcinoma extending into the bladder mucosa or distant metastases

43.41 Stage 1 vaginal carcinoma is characterized by
a. carcinoma involving the subvaginal tissue but not extending onto the pelvic wall
b. carcinoma extending onto the pelvic side wall
c. carcinoma limited to the vaginal mucosa
d. carcinoma in situ
e. carcinoma extending into the bladder mucosa or distant metastases

43.42 Stage 2 vaginal carcinoma is characterized by
a. carcinoma involving the subvaginal tissue but not extending onto the pelvic wall
b. carcinoma extending onto the pelvic side wall
c. carcinoma limited to the vaginal mucosa
d. carcinoma in situ
e. carcinoma extending into the bladder mucosa or distant metastases

43.43 Stage 3 vaginal carcinoma is characterized by
a. carcinoma involving the subvaginal tissue but not extending onto the pelvic wall
b. carcinoma extending onto the pelvic side wall
c. carcinoma limited to the vaginal mucosa
d. carcinoma in situ
e. carcinoma extending into the bladder mucosa or distant metastases

43.44 Stage 4 vaginal carcinoma is characterized by
a. carcinoma involving the subvaginal tissue but not extending onto the pelvic wall
b. carcinoma extending onto the pelvic side wall
c. carcinoma limited to the vaginal mucosa
d. carcinoma in situ
e. carcinoma extending into the bladder mucosa or distant metastases

Answers

43.38 a	**43.40** d	**43.42** a	**43.44** e
43.39 d	**43.41** c	**43.43** b	

43.45 Approximately what fraction of patients with vaginal carcinoma in situ will have an antecedent or coexistent neoplasm of the lower genital tract?
 a. 1/5 to 1/3
 b. 1/3 to 1/2
 c. 1/2 to 2/3
 d. 3/4 to 4/5

43.46 Which of the following statements about sarcoma botryoides is INCORRECT?
 a. Presents as a mass of polyps protruding from the introitus of young girls and infants.
 b. Arises from the undifferentiated mesenchyme of the lamina propria of the anterior vaginal wall.
 c. Often associated with a bloody discharge
 d. Treated in almost all cases by radical pelvic exenteration.

43.47 Screening for the recognition of potential malignancy of the cervix is best accomplished by
 a. self-investigation of the vagina
 b. Papanicolaou (Pap) smear
 c. cervical canal curettage
 d. aspiration of endocervical mucus
 e. posterior fornix aspiration

43.48 Diethylstilbestrol administered to a pregnant woman is associated with which condition in the female offspring?
 a. Clear cell adenocarcinoma of the vagina
 b. Endometrial carcinoma
 c. Hidradenitis
 d. Carcinoma in situ of the vagina
 e. Embryonal rhabdomyosarcoma

43.49 What is the recommended procedure for the evaluation of a chronic vulvar ulcer?
 a. Darkfield examination
 b. Biopsy
 c. Pap smear
 d. Culture of lesion
 e. Lymphangiography

43.50 The most common cause of the delay in diagnosing vulva carcinoma is the
 a. unreliability of a Pap smear of the vulva
 b. equivocal histology of early lesions
 c. failure to obtain a biopsy of lesions
 d. lack of visibility of most lesions

Answers
43.45 b   **43.46** d   **43.47** b   **43.48** a   **43.49** b   **43.50** c

Questions and Answers Chapter 44: Cervical Neoplasia and Carcinoma

44.1 Which of the following is not a risk factor associated with cervical neoplasia?
a. Multiple sexual partners
b. Low socioeconomic status
c. Previous pelvic inflammatory disease
d. Cigarette smoking

44.2 Which of the following statements best describes cervical "erosion"?
a. Cervical tissue exposed to *Trichomonas vaginalis*
b. Exocervical tissue undergoing squamous metaplasia
c. Normal endocervical tissue that has moved to the cervical surface
d. Endocervical tissue undergoing squamous metaplasia
e. Endocervical tissue associated with mechanical abrasion

44.3 The transformation zone develops
a. before puberty
b. during puberty and adolescence
c. during pregnancy
d. at the time of menopause

44.4 In the menopausal years, the location of the squamocolumnar junction shifts
a. into the endocervical canal
b. to just outside the external os
c. onto the cervical surface
d. onto the vaginal side wall

44.5 What percent of squamous intraepithelial neoplasia and cervical cancer arise from within the transformation zone?
a. 55%
b. 65%
c. 75%
d. 85%
e. 95%

44.6 Which of the following statements about human papillomavirus is correct?
a. The human papillomavirus is a direct cervical carcinogen.
b. The human papillomavirus may serve as a cofactor in the abnormal maturation and division of epithelial cells.
c. The great majority of women who harbor the human papillomavirus have accompanying abnormal cytologic changes.

44.7 Which of the following types of human papillomavirus is LEAST associated with a high risk of squamous intraepithelial neoplasia?
a. 16
b. 18
c. 21
d. 31

44.8 A virginal 21-year-old patient undergoes her first Pap smear which is reported as ASCUS (atypical squamous cells of undetermined significance). Which of the following is the most appropriate next step?
a. Colposcopy
b. Loop electrical excision procedure (LEEP)
c. Repeat Pap smear
d. Topical antibiotics

44.9 According to the American College of Obstetricians and Gynecologists, Pap smears should be obtained
a. yearly
b. every 2 years
c. every 3 years
d. at no set interval

Answers

44.1	c	44.3	b	44.5	e	44.7	c	44.9 a
44.2	c	44.4	a	44.6	b	44.8	c	

44.10 A Class I Pap smear would be considered
- a. normal
- b. inflammation
- c. mild dysplasia
- d. moderate dysplasia

44.11 A Class II Pap smear would be considered
- a. normal
- b. inflammation
- c. mild dysplasia
- d. moderate dysplasia

44.12 A Class III Pap smear would be considered
- a. normal
- b. inflammation
- c. mild dysplasia
- d. moderate dysplasia

44.13 A Class IV Pap smear suggests
- a. squamous cell cancer
- b. carcinoma in situ
- c. moderate dysplasia
- d. inflammation

44.14 Squamous cell cancer of the cervix is most closely linked to what class of Pap smear?
- a. V
- b. IV
- c. III
- d. II

44.15 A Bethesda system Pap smear that reads "Within normal limits" is most compatible with which of the following?
- a. Inflammation
- b. Mild dysplasia
- c. Moderate dysplasia
- d. Severe dysplasia

44.16 A Bethesda system Pap smear report that reads "Low-grade squamous intraepithelial lesion (LGSIL)" is most consistent with
- a. inflammation
- b. mild dysplasia
- c. moderate dysplasia
- d. severe dysplasia

44.17 High-grade SIL (HGSIL) on a Bethesda system Pap smear report is least likely to suggest
- a. inflammation
- b. mild dysplasia
- c. moderate dysplasia
- d. severe dysplasia

44.18 If squamous cell cancer is suspected and a visible lesion is present, the next step should be
- a. Pap smear
- b. colposcopy
- c. biopsy
- d. LEEP procedure

44.19 Carcinoma in situ of the cervix becomes classified as invasive cervical cancer when the dysplastic cells traverse the
- a. transformation zone
- b. squamocolumnar junction
- c. basement membrane
- d. endocervical canal
- e. canal of Nuck

44.20 What percent of all cases of mild dysplasia of the cervix [low-grade squamous intraepithelial lesion (LGSIL)] will spontaneously regress?
- a. 25%
- b. 35%
- c. 45%
- d. 55%
- e. 65%

Answers

44.10 a	**44.12** b	**44.14** a	**44.16** c	**44.18** c	**44.20** e
44.11 b	**44.13** b	**44.15** a	**44.17** a	**44.19** c	

44.21 What percent of all cases of mild dysplasia of the cervix [low-grade squamous intraepithelial lesion (LGSIL)] will progress to worsening disease?
   a. 5%
   b. 15%
   c. 25%
   d. 30%
   e. 45%

44.22 A single Pap smear reading of "Atypical squamous cells of undetermined significance" should be followed up with
   a. repeat Pap smear
   b. colposcopy
   c. endometrial biopsy
   d. endocervical curettage

44.23 A Pap smear reading of "Low-grade squamous intraepithelial lesions (LGSIL)" should be followed by
   a. repeat Pap smear
   b. colposcopy
   c. endometrial biopsy
   d. LEEP procedure

44.24 Management of a Pap smear report of "High-grade SIL (HGSIL)" includes
   a. repeat Pap
   b. testing for high-risk human papillomavirus subtypes
   c. colposcopy
   d. conization

44.25 In a patient who presents with a Pap smear reading of "Atypical glandular cells of undetermined significance," management would include
   a. Repeat Pap every 4 to 6 months for 2 years until there are three consecutive negative smears
   b. Colposcopy with endocervical curettage and directed biopsies
   c. Repeat Pap smear after treatment for candida vaginitis and bacterial vaginosis
   d. In postmenopausal patient, repeat Pap smear following course of vaginal estrogen therapy
   e. Repeat Pap smear with endocervical curettage and endometrial sampling

44.26 A colposcopy is considered to be satisfactory when the entire
   a. squamocolumnar junction is visualized
   b. external cervical os is visualized
   c. internal cervical os is visualized
   d. vesicouterine reflection is visualized
   e. erosive zone is visualized

44.27 Which of the following is NOT an indication for conization of the cervix?
   a. Unsatisfactory colposcopy
   b. ASCUS
   c. Positive endocervical curettage
   d. Two-step discrepancy between Pap smear and cervical biopsy results

44.28 The acetic acid solution used to wash the cervix before colposcopy functions as a
   a. stain
   b. emulsifier
   c. desiccant
   d. antiseptic

Answers

44.21 b	**44.23** b	**44.25** e	**44.27** b
44.22 a	**44.24** c	**44.26** a	**44.28** c

44.29 The endocervical curettage will be positive for dysplasia in what percent of women with a dysplastic Pap smear?
a. Less than 5%
b. 5 to 10%
c. 11 to 15%
d. 16 to 20%
e. 21 to 25%

44.30 Approximately what percent of colposcopically directed biopsies and endocervical curettages will demonstrate a significant discrepancy between the screening Pap smear and the histologic data?
a. 1%
b. 5%
c. 10%
d. 15%
e. 20%

44.31 To ensure adequate evaluation of a cervix from which an abnormal Pap smear has been obtained, biopsies should be taken from what location(s) at the time of colposcopy?
a. At least two quadrants of the cervix
b. At least three quadrants of the cervix
c. From areas of colposcopic abnormality and at least one other quadrant of the cervix
d. From areas of colposcopic abnormality

44.32 For a conization specimen to be considered satisfactory, it is NOT necessary that the specimen encompass
a. the entire cervix
b. the entire squamocolumnar junction
c. the entire extent of identified lesions
d. a portion of the endocervical canal

44.33 Which of the following techniques is NOT commonly used for conization of the cervix?
a. Scalpel and scissors
b. Heated electric wire
c. Super-cooled electric probe
d. Laser

44.34 Which of the following is NOT a risk factor for a woman undergoing conization of the cervix who desires future childbearing?
a. Incompetent cervical os
b. Abnormal cervical contours impeding coitus
c. Reduced cervical capacity to facilitate sperm transport
d. Loss of uterus secondary to hysterectomy associated with hemorrhage

44.35 Characteristics of cryocautery include
a. use for focal areas of abnormality
b. applied with a wire loop
c. use of liquid nitrogen
d. appropriate for high-grade lesions

44.36 Laser therapy characteristics include
a. precise control
b. watery discharge after treatment
c. confined to use for low-grade lesions
d. provides optimal surgical specimen

44.37 Cervical conization is associated with
a. both diagnostic and therapeutic applicability
b. watery discharge postoperatively
c. precise control of depth of specimen
d. high incidence of rectum and bladder injury

Answers

44.29 b	44.31 d	44.33 c	44.35 c	44.37 a
44.30 c	44.32 a	44.34 b	44.36 a	

44.38 Excisional biopsy of cervical intraepithelial neoplasia is characterized by which of the following?
   a. May be considered for the treatment of specific focal areas of abnormality
   b. Procedure is associated postoperatively with profuse watery discharge admixed with necrotic cellular debris
   c. May involve the use of "mushroom-tip" stainless steel probe, super-cooled with circulating liquid nitrogen or carbon dioxide
   d. Associated with cervical stenosis

44.39 The average age of diagnosis of invasive cervical carcinoma is approximately
   a. 20 years
   b. 30 years
   c. 40 years
   d. 50 years
   e. 60 years

44.40 Advanced cervical intraepithelial neoplasia is thought to precede the occurrence of invasive cervical carcinoma by an average of
   a. 1 year
   b. 5 years
   c. 10 years
   d. 15 years
   e. 20 years

44.41 What percent of cervical cancer is of the squamous cell variety?
   a. 45%
   b. 55%
   c. 65%
   d. 75%
   e. 85%
   f. 95%

44.42 Approximately what percent of cervical carcinoma is adenocarcinoma arising from the cervical glands?
   a. 5%
   b. 15%
   c. 25%
   d. 35%
   e. 45%
   f. 55%

44.43 Clear cell carcinoma of the cervix is associated with intrauterine exposure to
   a. progesterone
   b. estrone
   c. dehydroepiandrosterone
   d. diethylstilbestrol
   e. cigarette smoke

44.44 The 5-year survival for stage I cervical carcinoma is
   a. 91%
   b. 64%
   c. 25%
   d. 5%

44.45 The 5-year survival for stage IIA cervical carcinoma is
   a. 83%
   b. 64%
   c. 45%
   d. 5%

44.46 The 5-year survival for stage IIIA cervical carcinoma is
   a. 5%
   b. 14%
   c. 25%
   d. 45%

44.47 The 5-year survival for stage IV cervical carcinoma is
   a. 5%
   b. 14%
   c. 25%
   d. 45%
   e. 64%

Answers

44.38 a	44.40 c	44.42 b	44.44 a	44.46 d
44.39 d	44.41 e	44.43 d	44.45 a	44.47 b

44.48 Which of the following is present in all patients with invasive cervical cancer?
a. Postcoital bleeding
b. Pain
c. Abnormal uterine bleeding
d. Presence of dysplastic cells below the basement membrane

44.49 Stage I AI is characterized by
a. carcinoma involves the lower third of the vagina, but there is no extension to the pelvic wall
b. carcinoma extends beyond the cervix but not to the pelvic wall; there is no obvious parametrial involvement
c. all cases of stage I cancer not included in other classifications or divisions
d. minimal evidence of stromal invasion on microscopic examination
e. microscopic lesion(s) no more than 5 mm in depth measured from base of epithelial surface or glandular surface from which it originates, and horizontal spread not to exceed 7 mm

44.50 Stage I AII is characterized by
a. carcinoma involves the lower third of the vagina, but there is no extension to the pelvic wall
b. carcinoma extends beyond the cervix but not to the pelvic wall; there is no obvious parametrial involvement
c. all cases of stage I cancer not included in other classifications or divisions
d. minimal evidence of stromal invasion on microscopic examination
e. microscopic lesion(s) no more than 5 mm in depth measured from base of epithelial surface or glandular surface from which it originates, and horizontal spread not to exceed 7 mm

44.51 Stage IB is characterized by
a. carcinoma involves the lower third of the vagina, but there is no extension to the pelvic wall
b. carcinoma extends beyond the cervix but not to the pelvic wall; there is no obvious parametrial involvement
c. all cases of stage I cancer not included in other classifications or divisions
d. minimal evidence of stromal invasion on microscopic examination
e. microscopic lesion(s) no more than 5 mm in depth measured from base of epithelial surface or glandular surface from which it originates, and horizontal spread not to exceed 7 mm

44.52 Stage IIA is defined as
a. carcinoma involves the lower third of the vagina, but there is no extension to the pelvic wall
b. carcinoma extends beyond the cervix but not to the pelvic wall; there is no obvious parametrial involvement
c. all cases of stage I cancer not included in other classifications or divisions
d. minimal evidence of stromal invasion on microscopic examination
e. microscopic lesion(s) no more than 5 mm in depth measured from base of epithelial surface or glandular surface from which it originates, and horizontal spread not to exceed 7 mm

Answers

44.48 d	**44.49** d	**44.50** e	**44.51** c	**44.52** b

44.53 Stage IIB is characterized by
a. carcinoma extends beyond cervix with obvious parametrial involvement
b. carcinoma extends to pelvic side wall
c. carcinoma has spread to adjacent pelvic organs
d. carcinoma has spread to distant organs

44.54 The definition of Stage IIIA is
a. carcinoma involves the lower third of the vagina, but there is no extension to the pelvic wall
b. carcinoma extends beyond the cervix but not to the pelvic wall; there is no obvious parametrial involvement
c. all cases of stage I cancer not included in other classifications or divisions
d. minimal evidence of stromal invasion on microscopic examination
e. microscopic lesion(s) no more than 5 mm in depth measured from base of epithelial surface or glandular surface from which it originates, and horizontal spread not to exceed 7 mm

44.55 Stage IIIB is characterized by
a. carcinoma extends beyond cervix with obvious parametrial involvement
b. carcinoma extends to pelvic side wall
c. carcinoma has spread to adjacent pelvic organs
d. carcinoma has spread to distant organs

44.56 Stage IVA is characterized by
a. carcinoma extends beyond cervix with obvious parametrial involvement
b. carcinoma extends to pelvic side wall
c. carcinoma has spread to adjacent pelvic organs
d. carcinoma has spread to distant organs

44.57 Stage IVB is defined as
a. carcinoma extends beyond cervix with obvious parametrial involvement
b. carcinoma extends to pelvic side wall
c. carcinoma has spread to adjacent pelvic organs
d. carcinoma has spread to distant organs

44.58 All patients with cervical carcinoma with hydronephrosis or a nonfunctioning kidney should be included in at least stage
a. I
b. II
c. III
d. IV

44.59 In general, surgical therapy for cervical carcinoma is indicated for most patients with
a. stage I
b. stage II
c. stage III
d. stage IV

44.60 Which of the following is the least likely complication noted after radiation therapy for cervical carcinoma?
a. Radiation cystitis
b. Radiation proctitis
c. Dyspareunia
d. Fistulae
e. Hemorrhage

Answers

44.53 a	**44.55** b	**44.57** d	**44.59** a
44.54 a	**44.56** c	**44.58** c	**44.60** e

44.61 A 31-year-old woman who has three living children and has had a tubal ligation has a Pap smear reported as high-grade squamous intraepithelial lesion. There are no macroscopic lesions. The management should involve which of the following?

a. Hysterectomy
b. Radiotherapy
c. Local chemotherapy
d. Colposcopically directed cervical biopsies
e. Systemic chemotherapy

44.62 What are the primary lymph nodes involved in the spread of cervical carcinoma?

a. Paracervical and obturator
b. Sacral and inguinal
c. Common iliac and aortic
d. Perineal
e. Femoral

44.63 Metastatic cervical carcinoma is least likely to cause

a. hydronephrosis
b. paraplegia
c. hematemesis
d. colon obstruction
e. cardiomyopathy

44.64 The healing process after cervical cryotherapy usually is complete after

a. 1 month
b. 2 months
c. 3 months
d. 4 months

44.65 Repeat Pap smears after ablative surgical therapy of the cervix are usually started after

a. 4 weeks
b. 8 weeks
c. 12 weeks
d. 16 weeks

44.66 When is serotyping of human papillomavirus most useful?

a. After radical hysterectomy
b. Before cryotherapy
c. Before conization
d. After the menopause
e. After an ASCUS Pap smear

Answers

44.61 d	**44.62** a	**44.63** e	**44.64** b	**44.65** c	**44.66** e

Questions and Answers Chapter 45: Uterine Leiomyoma and Neoplasia

45.1 Which of the following statements about leiomyoma uteri is INCORRECT?
  a. Approximately 70% of American women have these benign tumors.
  b. The majority of women with leiomyoma do not require hysterectomy.
  c. Leiomyoma is an indication in approximately one third of hysterectomies performed.
  d. Histologically, leiomyomas are benign tumors with localized proliferation of smooth muscle cells surrounded by a pseudocapsule.
  e. Leiomyomas grow in response to estrogen.

45.2 All of the following are common symptoms or clinical manifestations of uterine fibroids EXCEPT
  a. pain
  b. pressure
  c. anemia
  d. bleeding
  e. constipation

45.3 Estrogen may cause leiomyoma growth by stimulation of the production of
  a. progesterone receptors in the myometrium, where progesterone binding to these sites stimulates the production of several growth factors causing the growth of myomas
  b. estrogen receptors in the myometrium, where estrogen binding to these sites stimulates the production of several growth factors causing the growth of myomas
  c. estrogen receptors in the myometrium, where estrogen binding to these sites directly stimulates myometrial cell growth
  d. prolactin receptors in the myometrium, where prolactin binding to these sites stimulates the production of several growth factors causing the growth of myomas

45.4 Sensitive DNS studies suggest that each myoma arises from a
  a. single smooth muscle cell
  b. single vascular endothelial cell
  c. single connective tissue cell
  d. dormant leiomyoma cell present at birth

45.5 Which of the following statements about leiomyoma is INCORRECT?
  a. Pelvic examination is the most cost-effective means of identification and evaluation of uterine myomas.
  b. Cystic-appearing areas in an image consistent with a leiomyoma are commonly associated with areas of degeneration.
  c. Endometrial sampling usually does not provide additional information toward making the diagnosis of leiomyoma of the uterus.
  d. Irregular uterine bleeding in a woman with known uterine myomas does not require endometrial sampling.

45.6 Leiomyosarcomas occur in what percent of leiomyoma?
  a. 0.01%
  b. 0.1%
  c. 1.0%
  d. 10%

45.7 Which of the following statements about leiomyosarcoma is CORRECT?
  a. Leiomyosarcoma arises from degeneration of a normal fibroid.
  b. This malignancy is more common in patients under the age of 40.
  c. Patients typically present with a rapidly enlarging uterine mass, unusual vaginal discharge, and pelvic pain.
  d. Leiomyosarcoma consists of a cell type found only in the uterus.

Answers

45.1 a	45.3 a	45.5 d	45.7 c
45.2 c	45.4 a	45.6 b	

45.8 Which statement applies to intra-venous leiomyomatosis?
   a. Has been found in cardiac, pulmonary, and lymphatic nodules
   b. Has been found in pelvic veins and the vena cava
   c. Implants on peritoneal surfaces

45.9 Which statement applies to benign metastasizing leiomyoma?
   a. Has been found in cardiac, pulmonary, and lymphatic nodules
   b. Has been found in pelvic veins and the vena cava
   c. Implants on peritoneal surfaces

45.10 Leiomyomatosis peritonealis dissemi-nata is described by which statement?
   a. Has been found in cardiac, pulmonary, and lymphatic nodules
   b. Has been found in pelvic veins and the vena cava
   c. Implants on peritoneal surfaces

45.11 Postmenopausal patients who present with rapidly enlarging uterine masses should be considered at high risk for
   a. uterine leiomyoma
   b. uterine leiomyosarcoma
   c. intravenous leiomyomatosis
   d. benign metastasizing leiomyoma
   e. leiomyomatosis peritonealis disseminata

45.12 What is the most common change occurring in myomas during pregnancy?
   a. Red degeneration
   b. Calcification
   c. Liquefaction
   d. Hyalinization
   e. Parasitic growth

45.13 Red degeneration of uterine leiomy-oma refers to
   a. hyalinization of the smooth muscle elements
   b. calcification of the smooth muscle stroma
   c. hemorrhagic changes in the my-ometrium associated with rapid growth
   d. inflammatory changes in the sur-rounding smooth muscle stroma

45.14 Menorrhagia associated with uterine leiomyoma is characterized by an increased
   a. amount of menstrual flow only
   b. duration of menstrual flow only
   c. amount and duration of menstrual flow
   d. amount and frequency of menstrual flow
   e. frequency of menstrual flow

45.15 Menorrhagia associated with uterine leiomyoma is defined as menstrual blood loss of greater than
   a. 40 mL
   b. 80 mL
   c. 120 mL
   d. 160 mL
   e. 200 mL

Answers

45.8 b	**45.10** c	**45.12** a	**45.14** c
45.9 a	**45.11** b	**45.13** c	**45.15** b

45.16 Which of the following is NOT a generally accepted mechanism to explain the increased bleeding associated with uterine fibroids?
   a. Alteration of normal myometrial contractile function in the small arteries and the arteriolar blood supply underlying the endometrium
   b. Inability of the overlying endometrium to respond to the normal estrogen–progesterone menstrual phases
   c. Pressure necrosis of the overlying endometrial bed exposing vascular surfaces that bleed excessively with endometrial sloughing
   d. Increased proliferation of small blood vessels in the endometrium under the influence of hormonal stimulation

45.17 What is the type of leiomyoma most commonly associated with abnormal uterine bleeding?
   a. Subserosal
   b. Intramural
   c. Submucosal
   d. Parasitic
   e. Disseminated

45.18 Of the following, which is the least likely clinical complication of large uterine leiomyoma?
   a. Hydroureter
   b. Hydronephrosis
   c. Costovertebral angle tenderness
   d. Colon or rectal obstruction
   e. Small bowel obstruction

45.19 Which of the following statements about the physical examination and physical diagnosis of uterine fibroids is INCORRECT?
   a. There is characteristic presence of a large midline mobile mass with an irregular contour.
   b. The mass usually has a "hard-feel" or solid quality.
   c. Subserosal pedunculated myomas are easily distinguishable from solid adnexal masses.
   d. Uterine fibroids are usually appreciable on abdominal examination when they are >14 to 16 weeks of equivalent gestational size.

45.20 Which of the following has the highest cost-benefit for diagnosing uterine myomas?
   a. Magnetic resonance imaging
   b. Computerized axial tomography
   c. Ultrasound
   d. Pelvic examination

45.21 Which of the following statements about the ultrasound evaluation of presumed uterine leiomyoma is INCORRECT?
   a. Ultrasound is commonly used for confirmation of uterine myomas.
   b. Ultrasound can usually demonstrate hypoechogenicity amid otherwise normal myometrial patterns.
   c. Ultrasound can usually resolve the presence of a distorted endometrial stripe.
   d. Ultrasound cannot usually distinguish a myoma from a solid adnexal mass.

Answers

45.16 d	45.17 c	45.18 e	45.19 c	45.20 d	45.21 d

45.22 According to current data, what percent of patients undergoing hysteroscopic removal of submucous leiomyoma will require additional therapy within 10 years?
  a. 10%
  b. 20%
  c. 30%
  d. 40%
  e. 50%

45.23 Which of the following statements about the management of patients with uterine fibroids is INCORRECT?
  a. The majority of patients with uterine leiomyoma do not require surgical treatment.
  b. Assessment of uterine growth requires regular computerized axial tomography scans.
  c. Uterine bleeding may be minimized by intermittent progestin supplementation if significant endometrial cavity distortion is not present.
  d. Myomectomy may be warranted in young patients whose fertility is being compromised by intracavitary distortion.
  e. Periodic physical examination generally provides adequate follow-up.

45.24 Which of the following statements about the use of gonadotropin-releasing hormone agonists analogs is correct?
  a. They may be used as follow-up treatment (3 to 6 months) after surgery.
  b. They may be used for relatively long-term therapy (12 to 36 months) to bring about major reduction in large tumor size.
  c. Treatment is often associated with reduction in uterine masses by as much as 40 to 60%.
  d. Treatment will permanently reduce the size of myomas.

45.25 Which of the following statements about pregnancy associated with leiomyoma uteri is INCORRECT?
  a. The overall course of pregnancy is usually unremarkable.
  b. There is usually a normal labor and delivery.
  c. Myomas typically shrink during pregnancy.
  d. Pregnancy is sometimes associated with red or carneous degeneration of myomas.

45.26 Which of the following statements about the relationship of leiomyomas and pregnancy is INCORRECT?
  a. Leiomyomas are a significant cause of infertility.
  b. Pregnancy with leiomyomas is usually unremarkable.
  c. Bed rest and analgesia usually suffice in the management of carneous degeneration.
  d. Myomas located in the lower uterine segment are a rare cause of soft tissue dystocia.

45.27 Adenomyosis is found in coexistence with leiomyoma in approximately what percent of hysterectomy specimens?
  a. 10%
  b. 20%
  c. 30%
  d. 40%
  e. 50%

45.28 What is a common treatment for adenomyosis of the uterus?
  a. Therapy with estrogens
  b. Therapy of gonadotropin-releasing hormone agonists
  c. "Watchful waiting"
  d. Hysterectomy

Answers

45.22 b	45.24 c	45.26 a	45.28 d
45.23 b	45.25 c	45.27 c	

45.29 The virulence of uterine sarcoma is related to
 a. patient age
 b. number of mitotic figures
 c. endometrial histology
 d. size of the uterus

45.30 Which of the following statements about uterine sarcomas is INCORRECT?
 a. Uterine sarcoma should be suspected with the enlargement of a previously known myomatous uterus in a postmenopausal woman.
 b. Postmenopausal bleeding is associated with uterine adenocarcinoma, not uterine sarcomas.
 c. The virulence of uterine sarcoma is directly related to the number of mitotic figures and cellular proliferation as defined histologically.
 d. Uterine sarcoma is more likely to spread hematogenously than is endometrial adenocarcinoma.

45.31 Vaginal birth after myomectomy is
 a. the standard of care
 b. contraindicated
 c. best decided on a case-by-case basis
 d. advisable only in multiparous patients

45.32 The overall 5-year survival rate for patients with leiomyosarcoma is approximately
 a. 30%
 b. 50%
 c. 70%
 d. 90%

45.33 What is the most reliable method for the diagnosis of leiomyosarcoma?
 a. Pap smear
 b. Endocervical curretage
 c. Pipelle endometrial biopsy
 d. Dilation and curettage
 e. Histology of a hysterectomy specimen

45.34 Which of the following statements about the management of uterine sarcomas is INCORRECT?
 a. The staging for uterine sarcoma is surgical and identical to that for endometrial adenocarcinoma.
 b. The overall rate of survival for patients with uterine sarcoma is essentially equivalent stage-for-stage to that for endometrial adenocarcinoma.
 c. Adjunctive radiation therapy and chemotherapy provide little additional benefit as primary adjuvant therapy or as therapy for recurrent disease.
 d. Unlike endometrial adenocarcinoma, uterine sarcomas are not responsive to hormonal treatment with high-dose progestins.

45.35 Of the following indications and actions, which is least important prior to myomectomy in an infertility patient?
 a. The presence of leiomyoma of sufficient size or location to be a probable factor in infertility
 b. The absence of a more likely explanation for the failure to conceive
 c. Evidence of normal ovarian function
 d. Evidence of normal fallopian tube function
 e. History of a pregnancy loss at 6 weeks of gestation

45.36 Which of the following would be the strongest single criterion for hysterectomy for leiomyoma?
 a. The presence of asymptomatic leiomyoma that are palpable abdominally
 b. The presence of uterine bleeding that is uncomfortable for the patient, but without anemia
 c. The presence of acute or severe pelvic discomfort caused by myoma
 d. Patient concern in the presence of asymptomatic leiomyoma

Answers

45.29 b	45.31 c	45.33 e	45.35 e
45.30 b	45.32 b	45.34 b	45.36 c

45.37 Which of the following actions is NOT necessary before hysterectomy for leiomyoma uteri?
   a. Confirmation of the absence of cervical malignancy
   b. Elimination of anovulation or other causes of abnormal bleeding
   c. Confirmation of the absence of endometrial malignancy by endometrial biopsy in all patients over the age of 25
   d. Assessment of surgical risk from anemia and the need for presurgical treatment
   e. Consideration of psychological risk associated with hysterectomy

45.38 Which of the following is NOT a sign or symptom of uterine myomata?
   a. Bladder irritability with urinary frequency
   b. Heavy periods
   c. Amenorrhea
   d. Pressure on the rectum with pain on defecation
   e. A palpable pelvic mass

45.39 Adenomyosis is characterized by
   a. invasion of the myometrium with benign endometrial cells
   b. infiltration of the myometrium with lymphocytes secondary to endometritis
   c. invasion of the myometrium with endometrial adenocarcinoma
   d. invasion of pelvic tissues with endometrial adenocarcinoma
   e. invasion of the myometrium with squamous cell carcinoma of the cervix

45.40 Uterine sarcomas may originate from all of the following tissues EXCEPT
   a. blood vessels
   b. uterine fibroids (myomata)
   c. endometrium
   d. nerve fibers
   e. myometrium

45.41 What is the most common malignant nonepithelial tumor of the uterus?
   a. Leiomyosarcoma
   b. Hemangiopericytoma
   c. Fibrosarcoma
   d. Endometrial sarcoma
   e. Mixed mesodermal tumor

Answers

45.37 c	45.38 c	45.39 a	45.40 d	45.41 a

Questions and Answers Chapter 46: Endometrial Hyperplasia and Cancer

46.1 Among female genital tract malignancies, endometrial carcinoma ranks where in frequency?
   a. First
   b. Second
   c. Third
   d. Fourth
   e. Fifth

46.2 Not including skin cancer, endometrial carcinoma ranks where in frequency among all cancers?
   a. Second
   b. Third
   c. Fourth
   d. Fifth
   e. Sixth

46.3 About what percent of all women will develop endometrial carcinoma?
   a. 1 to 2%
   b. 2 to 3%
   c. 3 to 4%
   d. 4 to 5%
   e. 5 to 6%

46.4 What percent of endometrial carcinoma is found in women who are perimenopausal?
   a. 1 to 5%
   b. 5 to 10%
   c. 10 to 15%
   d. 15 to 20%
   e. 20 to 25%

46.5 Approximately what percent of patients with endometrial carcinoma are diagnosed in the postmenopausal years?
   a. 25%
   b. 50%
   c. 75%
   d. 100%

46.6 In a premenopausal woman, endometrial carcinoma can best be ruled out using
   a. transvaginal ultrasound
   b. endometrial sampling
   c. transabdominal ultrasound
   d. magnetic resonance imaging
   e. computed tomographic scan

46.7 The likelihood that complex hyperplasia will progress to cancer is
   a. 1%
   b. 3%
   c. 30%
   d. 50%

46.8 The likelihood that simple hyperplasia will progress to cancer is
   a. 1%
   b. 3%
   c. 30%
   d. 50%

46.9 The likelihood that atypical hyperplasia will progress to cancer is
   a. 1%
   b. 3%
   c. 30%
   d. 50%

46.10 Endometrial hyperplasia and endometrial carcinoma are often overgrowths of the endometrium in response to
   a. progesterone
   b. estrogen
   c. prolactin
   d. prostaglandin
   e. testosterone

46.11 Conversion of androstenedione to estrogen occurs mainly in
   a. peripheral tissue stroma
   b. peripheral muscular tissue
   c. peripheral fat tissue
   d. centers of bone marrow activity

Answers

46.1	a	46.3	b	46.5	c	46.7	b	46.9	c	46.11	c
46.2	c	46.4	d	46.6	b	46.8	a	46.10	b		

46.12 Endometrial hyperplasia is defined as abnormal proliferation of
a. both glandular and stromal elements, with altered histologic architecture
b. only glandular elements, with altered histologic architecture
c. only stromal elements, with altered histologic architecture
d. both glandular and stromal elements, with normal histologic architecture

46.13 Cystic hyperplasia is comparable to
a. complex hyperplasia
b. atypical hyperplasia
c. simple hyperplasia
d. adenomatous hyperplasia

46.14 Adenomatous hyperplasia is best treated with
a. progestin
b. dilation and curettage
c. endometrial ablation
d. hysterectomy

46.15 Atypical adenomatous hyperplasia in a postmenopausal woman is best treated with
a. radical hysterectomy
b. hysterectomy
c. endometrial ablation
d. dilation and curettage
e. oral progestins

46.16 If no clinical intervention occurs, which of the following histologic variations of endometrial hyperplasia is least likely to become endometrial carcinoma?
a. Cystic glandular hyperplasia
b. Adenomatous hyperplasia
c. Atypical adenomatous hyperplasia

46.17 If no clinical intervention occurs, which of the following histologic variations of endometrial hyperplasia presents the highest risk for the development of endometrial carcinoma?
a. Cystic glandular hyperplasia
b. Adenomatous hyperplasia
c. Atypical adenomatous hyperplasia

46.18 Estrogen-dependent endometrial carcinoma is characterized by
a. originates from atrophic endometrium
b. occurs in a slender patient
c. generally well differentiated
d. has a poor prognosis

46.19 Aspects of estrogen-independent endometrial carcinoma include
a. arises from atrophic endometrium
b. well-differentiated histology
c. obese body habitus
d. good prognosis

46.20 Which of the following patient groups is NOT at increased risk for endometrial hyperplasia?
a. Patients exposed to exogenous estrogen only
b. Patients who have a history of regular ovulation
c. Obese postmenopausal women
d. Women with menopause at more than 55 years of age

46.21 Cystic endometrial hyperplasia (simple hyperplasia) is typified by
a. Significant numbers of glandular elements exhibiting cytologic atypia
b. Increased gland: stroma ratio giving a "crowded" or "back-to-back" appearance
c. Simple tubules, with marked variation in size from small to enlarged, cystic dilated glands
d. carcinoma in situ of the endometrium

Answers

46.12 a	**46.14** a	**46.16** a	**46.18** c	**46.20** b
46.13 c	**46.15** b	**46.17** c	**46.19** a	**46.21** c

46.22 Adenomatous hyperplasia (complex hyperplasia) has a microscopic appearance that includes
   a. significant numbers of glandular elements exhibiting cytologic atypia
   b. increased gland: stroma ratio giving a "crowded" or "back-to-back" appearance
   c. simple tubules, with marked variation in size from small to enlarged, cystic dilated glands
   d. carcinoma in situ of the endometrium

46.23 Atypical adenomatous hyperplasia (atypical hyperplasia with cytologic atypia) is characterized by
   a. increased gland: stroma ratio giving a "crowded" or "back-to-back" appearance
   b. simple tubules, with marked variation in size from small to enlarged, cystic dilated glands
   c. carcinoma in situ of the endometrium
   d. abnormal proliferation of primarily glandular elements without substantial proliferation of stromal elements

46.24 What is the relative risk for a menopausal woman to develop endometrial hyperplasia/adenocarcinoma?
   a. 1
   b. 2 to 3
   c. 4 to 6
   d. >6

46.25 The relative risk to develop endometrial hyperplasia/adenocarcinoma in a woman who is on unopposed estrogen therapy is
   a. 1
   b. 2 to 3
   c. 4 to 8
   d. >8

46.26 What is the relative risk for endometrial hyperplasia/adenocarcinoma in a nulliparous patient?
   a. 1
   b. 2 to 3
   c. 4 to −8
   d. >8

46.27 Obesity confers a relative risk for endometrial hyperplasia/adenocarcinoma of
   a. 1 to 2
   b. 3 to 10
   c. 20 to 25
   d. >25

46.28 Tamoxifen therapy is associated with what relative risk for endometrial neoplasia?
   a. 1
   b. 2 to 3
   c. 4 to 5
   d. >5

46.29 A woman with diabetes mellitus has what relative risk for developing endometrial hyperplasia/adenocarcinoma?
   a. >10
   b. 6 to 8
   c. 5
   d. 3

46.30 Which of the following has an approximately 20 to 30% risk for malignant transformation?
   a. Cystic endometrial hyperplasia
   b. Adenomatous hyperplasia
   c. Atypical adenomatous hyperplasia

46.31 If a woman is more than 50 pounds over her ideal weight, what is her relative risk of developing endometrial carcinoma?
   a. 2
   b. 5
   c. 10
   d. 15
   e. 25

Answers

46.22 b	46.24 b	46.26 b	46.28 b	46.30 c
46.23 c	46.25 c	46.27 b	46.29 d	46.31 c

46.32 The relative risk for developing endometrial carcinoma is 2.4 times higher when a woman goes through menopause
  a. before age 49
  b. between ages 49 and 52
  c. after age 52

46.33 Tamoxifen increases the relative risk of developing endometrial carcinoma because it acts like
  a. progestin
  b. estrogen
  c. prolactin
  d. insulinase
  e. testosterone

46.34 The mean length of time for progression from endometrial hyperplasia without atypia to endometrial carcinoma is estimated to be
  a. 2 years
  b. 4 years
  c. 6 years
  d. 8 years
  e. 10 years

46.35 When compared with the findings of dilation and curettage or hysterectomy, what is the diagnostic accuracy of office endometrial sampling techniques?
  a. 90 to 98%
  b. 80 to 89%
  c. 70 to 79%
  d. 60 to 69%
  e. 50 to 59%

46.36 What is the main theoretical disadvantage of the "office endometrial biopsy" technique?
  a. Significant patient discomfort
  b. Associated cost
  c. Need for cervical dilation and instrumentation to perform this procedure
  d. Small part of the endometrial surface that is sampled

46.37 About what percent of patients with endometrial carcinoma may be expected to have abnormal Pap smear results?
  a. 10 to 20%
  b. 30 to 40%
  c. 50 to 60%
  d. 70 to 80%
  e. 90 to 100%

46.38 Abnormal vaginal bleeding or discharge is the only presenting complaint in what percent of women with endometrial carcinoma?
  a. 80 to 90%
  b. 60 to 70%
  c. 40 to 50%
  d. 20 to 30%

46.39 Approximately what percent of women found to have endometrial carcinoma were asymptomatic prior to diagnosis?
  a. 5%
  b. 15%
  c. 25%
  d. 35%
  e. 45%

46.40 The endometrial biopsy of a healthy, thin, postmenopausal woman not on estrogen replacement therapy and without medical problems or substantial risk factors for endometrial carcinoma is reported as "insufficient tissue for diagnosis." What should be the follow-up testing for this patient?
  a. Dilation and curettage
  b. Hysteroscopic evaluation
  c. No follow-up testing needed

46.41 What is the minimum hormone needed to treat simple endometrial hyperplasia?
  a. Cyclic medroxyprogesterone acetate (Provera)
  b. Oral contraceptives
  c. Continuous megestrol acetate (Megace)
  d. Continuous medroxyprogesterone acetate (Provera)

Answers

46.32 c	46.34 e	46.36 d	46.38 a	46.40 c
46.33 b	46.35 a	46.37 b	46.39 a	46.41 a

46.42 Atypical adenomatous hyperplasia is best treated medically with which of the following?
a. Cyclic medroxyprogesterone acetate (Provera)
b. Continuous progesterone vaginal suppository
c. Cyclic combined oral contraceptives
d. Continuous megestrol acetate (Megace)

46.43 Treatment of cystic endometrial hyperplasia is most appropriately accomplished with megestrol acetate (Megace) administered in what fashion?
a. In a cyclic fashion
b. Continuously
c. For 14 days once
d. For 10 days once

46.44 Of the following, which is the least appropriate treatment to treat adenomatous endometrial hyperplasia?
a. Cyclic oral medroxyprogesterone acetate (Provera)
b. High-dose intramuscular medroxyprogesterone acetate (Depo-Provera)
c. Continuous oral megestrol acetate (Megace)
d. progesterone vaginal suppository

46.45 Patients with endometrial polyps most commonly present with
a. abrupt onset pelvic pain
b. abnormal bleeding
c. abnormal vaginal discharge
d. pelvic pressure

46.46 Approximately what percent of endometrial polyps show malignant change?
a. 5%
b. 10%
c. 20%
d. 30%
e. 40%

46.47 Compared with polyps in menstrual-aged women, those in postmenopausal women are
a. more likely to be associated with endometrial carcinoma
b. as likely to be associated with endometrial carcinoma
c. less likely to be associated with endometrial carcinoma

46.48 Approximately what percent of postmenopausal women with bleeding have uterine malignancy?
a. 5 to 15%
b. 15 to 25%
c. 30 to 40%
d. 50 to 60%

46.49 Atrophy of the endometrium is associated with postmenopausal bleeding in what percentage of cases?
a. 2 to 12%
b. 5 to 10%
c. 10 to 15%
d. 15 to 25%
e. 60 to 80%

46.50 Hormone replacement therapy is associated with postmenopausal bleeding in what percent of cases?
a. 2 to 12%
b. 5 to 10%
c. 10 to 15%
d. 15 to 25%
e. 60 to 80%

46.51 What is the percent frequency with which endometrial carcinoma is associated with postmenopausal bleeding?
a. 2 to 12%
b. 5 to 10%
c. 10 to 15%
d. 15 to 25%
e. 60 to 80%

Answers

46.42 d	46.44 d	46.46 a	46.48 b	46.50 d
46.43 b	46.45 b	46.47 a	46.49 e	46.51 c

46.52 Endometrial polyps are associated with postmenopausal bleeding in what percent of cases?
a. 2 to 12%
b. 5 to 10%
c. 10 to 15%
d. 15 to 25%
e. 60 to 80%

46.53 The incidence of postmenopausal bleeding in cases of endometrial hyperplasia is what percent?
a. 2 to 12%
b. 5 to 10%
c. 10 to 15%
d. 15 to 25%
e. 60 to 80%

46.54 Endometrioid cell type represents what percentage of all endometrial cancers?
a. <1%
b. 3 to 4%
c. 5%
d. 80 to 85%

46.55 Mucinous cell type represents what percentage of all endometrial cancers?
a. <1%
b. 3 to 4%
c. 5%
d. 80 to 85%

46.56 Papillary serous cell type represents what percentage of all endometrial cancers?
a. <1%
b. 3 to 4%
c. 5%
d. 80 to 85%

46.57 Clear cell type represents what percentage of all endometrial cancers?
a. <1%
b. 3 to 4%
c. 5%
d. 80 to 85%

46.58 Squamous cell type represents what percentage of all endometrial cancers?
a. <1%
b. 3 to 4%
c. 5%
d. 80 to 85%

46.59 Mixed cell type represents what percentage of all endometrial cancers?
a. <1%
b. 3 to 4%
c. 5%
d. 80 to 85%

46.60 "Benign-appearing squamous areas" describes what type of endometrial cancer?
a. Mucinous
b. Adenoacanthoma
c. Villoglandular
d. Papillary serous

46.61 "Intracytoplasmic mucin" refers to what type of endometrial cancer?
a. Mucinous
b. Adenoacanthoma
c. Villoglandular
d. Papillary serous

46.62 "Resembles an ovarian and fallopian tube carcinoma" is a description that best fits which type of endometrial cancer?
a. Mucinous
b. Adenoacanthoma
c. Villoglandular
d. Papillary serous

46.63 Fibrovascular papillary stalks are related to what type of endometrial neoplasm?
a. Mucinous
b. Adenoacanthoma
c. Villoglandular
d. Papillary serous

Answers

46.52 a	46.54 d	46.56 b	46.58 a	46.60 b	46.62 c
46.53 b	46.55 c	46.57 c	46.59 a	46.61 a	46.63 d

46.64 Which grade of endometrial carcinoma is characterized by more than 50% of the tumor showing solid growth?
a. G1
b. G2
c. G3

46.65 Stage IA endometrial carcinoma is associated with
a. tumor limited to the endometrium
b. vaginal metastases
c. endocervical gland involvement
d. tumor invading the bladder

46.66 Stage IB endometrial carcinoma is associated with
a. tumor invasion to less than half of the myometrium
b. pelvic lymph node involvement
c. vaginal metastases
d. tumor invading rectum

46.67 Stage IC endometrial carcinoma is associated with
a. pelvic node involvement
b. periaortic node involvement
c. tumor involves more than half of the myometrium
d. vaginal metastases

46.68 Stage IIA endometrial carcinoma is associated with
a. vaginal metastases
b. cervical stromal invasion
c. endocervical gland involvement
d. tumor to bladder

46.69 Stage IIB endometrial carcinoma is associated with
a. Vaginal metastases
b. Cervical stromal invasion
c. Endocervical glandular involvement only
d. Invasion to more than half of the myometrium

46.70 Stage IIIA endometrial carcinoma is associated with
a. Vaginal metastases
b. Cervical stromal invasion
c. Endocervical glandular involvement only
d. Invasion to more than half of the myometrium
e. Tumor invades serosa, adnexa, or both; and/or positive peritoneal cytology

46.71 Stage IIIB endometrial carcinoma is associated with
a. Vaginal metastases
b. Cervical stromal invasion
c. Endocervical glandular involvement only
d. Invasion to more than half of the myometrium
e. Tumor invades serosa, adnexa, or both; and/or positive peritoneal cytology

46.72 Stage IIIC endometrial carcinoma is associated with
a. Vaginal metastases
b. Cervical stromal invasion
c. Endocervical glandular involvement only
d. Invasion to more than half of the myometrium
e. Metastases to pelvic and/or periaortic nodes

46.73 Stage IVA endometrial carcinoma is associated with
a. bladder invasion
b. lung metastases
c. renal failure
d. bowel obstruction

Answers

46.64 c	46.66 a	46.68 c	46.70 e	46.72 e
46.65 a	46.67 c	46.69 b	46.71 a	46.73 a

46.74 Stage IVB endometrial carcinoma is associated with
  a. Vaginal metastases
  b. Cervical stromal invasion
  c. Endocervical glandular involvement only
  d. Invasion to more than half of the myometrium
  e. Distant metastases, including intra-abdominal and/or inguinal lymph nodes

46.75 The term "adenoacanthoma" refers to the situation in which the squamous element of the tumor comprises more than what percent of the histologic image?
  a. 5%
  b. 10%
  c. 15%
  d. 20%
  e. 25%

46.76 The diagnosis of endometrial carcinoma is most frequently made by
  a. Pap smear
  b. endometrial sampling
  c. laparoscopy

46.77 Special consideration should be given to endometrial sampling in patients who present with abnormal uterine bleeding and who are over the age of
  a. 25
  b. 35
  c. 45
  d. 55

46.78 One indication for endometrial sampling is an endometrial thickness of more than how many millimeters on transvaginal ultrasound?
  a. 3 mm
  b. 5 mm
  c. 7 mm
  d. 9 mm
  e. 11 mm

46.79 An endometrial thickness of less than how many millimeters excludes the possibility of endometrial carcinoma?
  a. 3 mm
  b. 5 mm
  c. 7 mm
  d. 9 mm
  e. No thickness excludes the possibility of endometrial carcinoma

46.80 Compared with cervical or ovarian carcinoma, hematogenous spread in endometrial carcinoma occurs
  a. more frequently
  b. as frequently
  c. less frequently

46.81 Compared with adenocarcinoma of the endometrium, papillary serous adenocarcinoma tends to be
  a. more aggressive in abdominal pelvic spread
  b. equally aggressive in abdominal pelvic spread
  c. less aggressive in abdominal pelvic spread

46.82 What is the most important prognostic factor for endometrial carcinoma?
  a. the depth of invasion of the myometrium
  b. the cytologic grade of the carcinoma
  c. the patient's age at the time of diagnosis

46.83 The International Federation of Gynecology and Obstetrics (FIGO) guidelines for staging of endometrial carcinoma suggests the need for sampling of the periaortic and pelvic lymph nodes when the depth of invasion of the myometrium is:
  a. more than one third of the myometrial thickness
  b. more than two thirds of the myometrial thickness
  c. the total myometrial thickness

Answers

46.74 e	46.76 b	46.78 b	46.80 a	46.82 b
46.75 b	46.77 b	46.79 e	46.81 a	46.83 a

46.84 G1 endometrial cancer is
a. predominantly solid or entire undifferentiated carcinoma
b. mildly differentiated adenomatous carcinoma with partly solid areas
c. highly differentiated adenomatous carcinoma

46.85 G2 endometrial cancer is
a. predominantly solid or entire undifferentiated carcinoma
b. mildly differentiated adenomatous carcinoma with partly solid areas
c. highly differentiated adenomatous carcinoma

46.86 G3 endometrial cancer is
a. predominantly solid or entire undifferentiated carcinoma
b. mildly differentiated adenomatous carcinoma with partly solid areas
c. highly differentiated adenomatous carcinoma

46.87 The 5-year survival rate for grade 1 tumors of the endometrium is approximately
a. 95%
b. 85%
c. 75%
d. 65%
e. 55%

46.88 What is the incidence of vaginal apex recurrence when simple hysterectomy is used for the treatment of endometrial carcinoma?
a. Less than 5%
b. 5 to 10%
c. 15 to 20%
d. 25 to 30%

46.89 What is the primary surgical treatment of endometrial carcinoma?
a. Total abdominal hysterectomy alone
b. Total abdominal hysterectomy with bilateral salpingo-oophorectomy
c. Vaginal hysterectomy
d. Radical hysterectomy
e. Pelvic exenteration

46.90 What is the first line of treatment for recurrent endometrial carcinoma?
a. Debulking surgery
b. Hormonal therapy, usually progestins
c. Radiation therapy
d. Chemotherapy

46.91 Endometrial carcinoma is often associated with
a. chronic pelvic inflammatory disease
b. feminizing ovarian neoplasms
c. endometriosis
d. mesonephroma

46.92 Endometrial carcinoma is most closely associated with which ovarian tumor?
a. Serous cystadenoma
b. Sertoli-Leydig cell
c. Mucinous cystadenoma
d. Granulosa-theca cell
e. Arrhenoblastoma

46.93 Approximately what percent of recurrent endometrial carcinoma appears within 3 to 4 years of initial treatment?
a. 25%
b. 50%
c. 75%
d. 100%

Answers

46.84 c	46.86 a	46.88 b	46.90 b	46.92 d
46.85 b	46.87 a	46.89 b	46.91 b	46.93 c

Review

Questions and Answers Chapter 47: Ovarian and Adnexal Disease

47.1 Coelomic epithelium (epithelial) tumors include
a. Sertoli-Leydig cell
b. lymphoma
c. mucinous
d. endodermal sinus

47.2 An example of a gonadal stroma is
a. Sertoli-Leydig cell
b. endometrioid
c. dysgerminoma
d. serous cystadenoma

47.3 Germ cell tumors include
a. teratoma
b. lymphoma
c. Brenner cell
d. endometrioid

47.4 Miscellaneous cell line tumors include all of the following EXCEPT
a. metastatic tumor
b. sarcoma
c. lymphoma
d. lipid cell fibroma

47.5 Serous tumors of the ovary may include the following variations EXCEPT
a. cystadenoma with low malignant potential
b. cystadenoma
c. cystadenocarcinoma
d. endometrioid

47.6 Which of the mucinous tumors of the ovary should always be treated with hysterectomy, bilateral salpingo-oophorectomy and staging?
a. Cystadenoma
b. Cystadenoma with low malignant potential
c. Cystadenocarcinoma

47.7 Which of the following is not considered an endometrioid tumor of the ovary?
a. Endometrioma
b. Endometrioid benign cysts
c. Adenocarcinoma
d. Endometrioid tumors of low malignant potential

47.8 Stage I carcinoma of the ovary is defined by International Federation of Gynecology and Obstetrics (FIGO) as
a. growth involving one or both ovaries with pelvic extension
b. tumor involving one or both ovaries with peritoneal implants outside the pelvis and/or positive retroperitoneal or inguinal nodes
c. growth limited to the ovaries
d. Growth involving one or both ovaries with distant metastasis

47.9 Stage II carcinoma of the ovary is defined by FIGO as
a. growth involving one or both ovaries with pelvic extension
b. tumor involving one or both ovaries with peritoneal implants outside the pelvis and/or positive retroperitoneal or inguinal nodes
c. growth limited to the ovaries
d. growth involving one or both ovaries with distant metastasis

47.10 Stage III carcinoma of the ovary is defined by FIGO as
a. growth involving one or both ovaries with pelvic extension
b. tumor involving one or both ovaries with peritoneal implants outside the pelvis and/or positive retroperitoneal or inguinal nodes
c. growth limited to the ovaries
d. growth involving one or both ovaries with distant metastasis

Answers

47.1 c	47.3 a	47.5 d	47.7 a	47.9 a
47.2 a	47.4 d	47.6 c	47.8 c	47.10 b

47.11 Stage IV carcinoma of the ovary is defined by FIGO as
  a. growth involving one or both ovaries with pelvic extension
  b. tumor involving one or both ovaries with peritoneal implants outside the pelvis and/or positive retroperitoneal or inguinal nodes
  c. growth limited to the ovaries
  d. growth involving one or both ovaries with distant metastasis

47.12 Which of the following structures is not contained within the adnexae?
  a. Fallopian tubes
  b. Appendix
  c. Ovaries
  d. Upper portion of the broad ligament
  e. Mesosalpinx

47.13 Which structure in the genitourinary system may mimic a solid adnexal mass?
  a. Bladder
  b. Pelvic kidney
  c. Ureter
  d. Urethra
  e. Renal pelvis

47.14 In which age group of women is it most likely that the ovaries will be palpable?
  a. Premenarchal
  b. Reproductive
  c. Postmenopausal

47.15 Compared with reproductive age patients, palpable ovarian enlargement in the postmenopausal patient is:
  a. more likely to be the result of a malignancy
  b. as likely to be the result of a malignancy
  c. less likely to be the result of a malignancy

47.16 The use of oral contraceptives makes the ovaries
  a. more likely to be palpable
  b. as likely to be palpable
  c. less likely to be palpable

47.17 A small, unilocular ovarian mass in a patient within 3 years of natural menopause is managed by
  a. surgical removal of the mass
  b. observation through serial transvaginal ultrasound examinations

47.18 Functional ovarian cysts are
  a. neoplasms
  b. anatomic variations
  c. malignant tumors

47.19 Which of the following statements about ovarian follicular cysts is INCORRECT?
  a. They arise from the failure of an ovarian follicle to rupture.
  b. They are associated with a shortening of the follicular phase.
  c. They are lined with normal granulosa cells.
  d. They are filled with estrogen-rich fluid.

47.20 Alterations in the menstrual cycle associated with follicular cysts can be caused by
  a. mechanical pressure by the enlarged cyst
  b. stimulation by the large amount of estradiol produced by the granulosa cells within the follicle
  c. large concentrations of progesterone produced by the ovary in response to cyst growth

Answers

47.11 d	47.13 b	47.15 a	47.17 b	47.19 b
47.12 b	47.14 b	47.16 c	47.18 b	47.20 b

47.21 Follicular cysts usually are followed for how many weeks, with or without accompanying oral contraceptive treatment, before surgical evaluation is considered?

a. 2 to 4
b. 6 to 8
c. 10 to 12
d. 14 to 16

47.22 A patient not using oral contraceptives, with regular periods, presents with acute pain late in the luteal phase. This clinical picture is most consistent with

a. serous cystadenoma
b. mucinous cystadenoma
c. corpus hemorrhagicum
d. dermoid cyst
e. follicular cyst

47.23 Corpus luteum cysts are often associated with a delay in menstruation for 1 to 2 weeks and dull lower quadrant pain. Which of the following must be measured before consideration of conservative management of this situation?

a. Progesterone
b. Estrogen
c. Estradiol
d. β-Human chorionic gonadotropin
e. Follicle-stimulating hormone

Instructions for items 47.24 to 47.26: Match the site of origin with the resulting ovarian neoplasm. An option may be used once, more than once, or not at all.

47.24 Coelomic epithelium gives rise to what ovarian neoplasm?

a. teratoma
b. granulos-theca
c. serous
d. choriocarcinoma

47.25 Gonadal stroma gives rise to what ovarian tumor?

a. teratoma
b. granulosa-theca
c. mucinous
d. choriocarcinoma
e. serous

47.26 Germ cells result in what ovarian neoplasm?

a. teratoma
b. granulosa-theca
c. serous
d. mucinous

47.27 Approximately what percent of serous cystadenomas are benign?

a. 10%
b. 30%
c. 50%
d. 70%
e. 90%

47.28 Serous cystadenoma characteristics include

a. bilateral 5% of the time
b. most common in perimenopausal and postmenopausal women
c. large amount of stroma and fibrotic tissue surrounds the epithelial cells
d. cyst-lined by well-differentiated endometrial-like glandular tissue

Answers

47.21 b	47.23 d	47.25 b	47.27 d
47.22 c	47.24 c	47.26 a	47.28 b

47.29 Mucinous cystadenoma characteristics include
a. bilateral 5% of the time
b. most common in perimenopausal and postmenopausal women
c. large amount of stroma and fibrotic tissue surrounds the epithelial cells
d. cyst-lined by well-differentiated endometrial-like glandular tissue

47.30 Endometrioid tumor characteristics include
a. bilateral approximately 15% of the time
b. bilateral 5% of the time
c. most common in perimenopausal and postmenopausal women
d. large amount of stroma and fibrotic tissue surrounds the epithelial cells
e. cyst-lined by well-differentiated endometrial-like glandular tissue

47.31 Brenner cell tumor characteristics include
a. bilateral approximately 15% of the time
b. bilateral 5% of the time
c. most common in perimenopausal and postmenopausal women
d. large amount of stroma and fibrotic tissue surrounds the epithelial cells
e. cyst-lined by well-differentiated endometrial-like glandular tissue

47.32 Hyperthyroidism is associated with what ovarian neoplasm?
a. Mucinous cystadenoma
b. Serous cystadenoma
c. Stroma ovarii
d. Benign cystic teratoma

47.33 Which of the following is not characteristic of benign cystic teratomas?
a. They contain derivatives from all of the embryonic germ layers.
b. The most common elements are mesodermal in origin.
c. Ten to 20% are bilateral.
d. Diagnosis can be confirmed on ultrasound.
e. They often are felt anterior to the broad ligament on physical examination.

47.34 Granulosa-theca cell tumor characteristics include all of the following EXCEPT
a. produces hormones
b. may contribute to precocious puberty
c. produces androgenic components
d. produces estrogenic components

47.35 Sertoli-Leydig cell tumor characteristics include
a. produces estrogenic components
b. may contribute to hirsutism or virilizing symptoms
c. may result in feminization
d. may be associated with ascites

47.36 A unique finding of ovarian fibroma is
a. produces androgenic components
b. produces estrogenic components
c. may contribute to hirsutism or virilizing symptoms
d. may result in feminization
e. may be associated with ascites

47.37 Compared with malignant tumors, for women of all ages benign ovarian neoplasms are
a. more common
b. as common
c. less common

Answers

47.29 a	47.31 d	47.33 b	47.35 b	47.37 a
47.30 e	47.32 c	47.34 c	47.36 e	

47.38 A woman's risk of developing ovarian cancer during her lifetime is approximately
- a. 1%
- b. 3%
- c. 5%
- d. 7%
- e. 9%

47.39 Ovarian cancer presents most commonly in which decades of life?
- a. 30s and 40s
- b. 50s and 60s
- c. 70s and 80s

47.40 Approximately what percent of patients with ovarian cancer have metastatic disease at the time of diagnosis?
- a. 20%
- b. 30%
- c. 40%
- d. 50%
- e. 60%

47.41 Which ovarian tumor has the highest malignant potential?
- a. Cystadenofibroma
- b. Brenner tumor
- c. Mucinous cystadenoma
- d. Serous cystadenoma
- e. Dermoid

47.42 Which of the following has not been associated with a risk of developing ovarian cancer?
- a. Use of hormone replacement therapy
- b. Low parity
- c. Delayed childbearing
- d. Familial predisposition

47.43 Malignant ovarian epithelial cell tumors spread primarily by
- a. direct extension within the peritoneal cavity
- b. lymphatic dissemination
- c. hematogenous dissemination

47.44 The combination of benign ovarian fibroma and ascites and right unilateral hydrothorax is termed
- a. Sertoli-Leydig syndrome
- b. familial cancer syndrome
- c. Meigs syndrome
- d. hydrops tubae profluens

47.45 What percent of all ovarian malignancies are of the epithelial cell type?
- a. 90%
- b. 70%
- c. 50%
- d. 30%

47.46 Malignant serous epithelial tumors of the ovary are characterized by
- a. pseudomyxomatous peritonei
- b. most common malignant epithelial tumor
- c. 5% bilaterality
- d. histologically similar to endometrial carcinoma

47.47 Malignant mucinous epithelial tumors of the ovary have which of the following characeristics?
- a. pseudomyxomatous peritonei
- b. most common epithelial malignancy
- c. 50% bilaterality
- d. hypertension

47.48 Malignant endometrioid tumors are characterized by
- a. 10 to 15% bilateral
- b. 30% bilateral
- c. histologic features similar to endometrial carcinoma
- d. may be associated with widespread peritoneal extensions

47.49 What is the most common ovarian cancer in women under the age of 20?
- a. Malignant serous cystadenocarcinoma
- b. Malignant mucinous cystadenocarcinoma
- c. Clear cell carcinoma
- d. Germ cell tumor

Answers

47.38 a	47.40 e	47.42 a	47.44 c	47.46 b	47.48 c
47.39 b	47.41 d	47.43 a	47.45 a	47.47 a	47.49 d

47.50 What is the primary surgical approach involved in the treatment of ovarian carcinoma?
a. Total abdominal hysterectomy
b. Cytoreductive surgery or "tumor debulking"
c. Radical hysterectomy
d. Laparoscopically assisted vaginal hysterectomy

47.51 Which of the following statements about dysgerminomas is correct?
a. They are most commonly bilateral
b. They are less likely than epithelial cell tumors to spread via lymphatic channels
c. The tumors are radiosensitive
d. The survival rate for patients with small, unilateral tumors is approximately 50%

47.52 Which of the following statements about treatment of dysgerminomas is INCORRECT?
a. If tumor size is <10 cm and there is no evidence of extraovarian spread, treatment may include only the removal of the affected ovary.
b. Pelvic and periaortic nodes must be assessed at the time of surgery.
c. In all cases, there should be postoperative irradiation to the abdomen and pelvis.
d. Chemotherapy usually is reserved for primary treatment failures.

47.53 Granulosa cell tumor characteristics include all of the following EXCEPT
a. secretes testosterone
b. secretes estrogen
c. may result in endometrial hyperplasia
d. occurs in patients of all ages

47.54 Which statement characterizes Sertoli-Leydig tumors?
a. Secretes estrogen
b. May result in endometrial hyperplasia
c. Occurs in patients of all ages
d. More common in older patients

47.55 Which of the following tumors is metastatic to the ovary from other sites?
a. Krukenberg tumors
b. Malignant mesodermal sarcomas
c. Fibrosarcomas

47.56 What is the rarest carcinoma of the female genital tract?
a. Carcinoma of the fallopian tube
b. Bartholin gland carcinoma
c. Vulvar carcinoma
d. Leiomyosarcoma

47.57 Which of the following statements about fallopian tube carcinoma is INCORRECT?
a. The most common primary fallopian tube carcinomas are adenosquamous carcinoma and sarcoma.
b. Primary fallopian tube carcinoma may be associated with a profuse serosanguineous discharge, hydrotubae profluens.
c. Overall 5-year survival rate for primary fallopian tube carcinoma is 35 to 45%.
d. Carcinoma metastatic to the fallopian tube is more common than primary fallopian tube carcinoma.

47.58 What is a "pathognomonic sign" of tubal carcinoma?
a. Secondary amenorrhea coupled with intermittent pelvic pain
b. A pelvic mass
c. Profuse serosanguineous vaginal discharge
d. Colicky abdominal pain

Answers

47.50 b	47.52 c	47.54 d	47.56 a	47.58 c
47.51 c	47.53 a	47.55 a	47.57 a	

47.59 Which of the following is appropriate when clinically palpable ovarian enlargement is detected in a post-menopausal woman?
a. Take a Pap smear and review in 6 weeks
b. Treat with parenteral progestins
c. Radiography to evaluate osteoporosis and collect urine for 24-hour total estrogen excretion
d. Take a Pap smear and review in 6 months
e. Take a sonogram of pelvis and consider surgical evaluation

47.60 Which of the following is not a complication of functional ovarian cysts (follicular or luteal)?
a. Hemorrhage into the cyst
b. Rupture with hemoperitoneum
c. Rupture with brief acute pelvic pain
d. Pseudomyxoma peritonei
e. Torsion

47.61 Granulosa-theca cell ovarian tumors are seen most frequently
a. before puberty
b. during the childbearing years
c. postmenopausal

47.62 Abnormal uterine bleeding due to an ovarian neoplasm is secondary to
a. pressure
b. increased vascularity
c. metastasis
d. biologic activity of the hormones produced

47.63 Physiologic enlargement of the ovaries can be caused by
a. follicle cysts
b. corpus luteum cysts
c. theca lutein cysts
d. all of the above

47.64 Which of the following is the most common masculinizing ovarian tumor?
a. Arrhenoblastoma
b. Gynandroblastoma
c. Adrenal rest tumor
d. Leydig cell tumor

47.65 What is the hormone responsible for the findings in arrhenoblastoma?
a. Androstenedione
b. Androsterone
c. Testosterone
d. Estriol

47.66 What is the treatment of Brenner tumors of the ovary?
a. Simple excision
b. Excision and exploration of the other ovary
c. Excision and hysterectomy

47.67 The presence of a signet-ring cell type in ovarian tumors is most characteristic of
a. hilus cell tumors
b. adrenal rest tumors
c. Brenner tumors
d. Krukenberg tumors
e. serous adenoma

47.68 In autopsy data, breast cancer metastatic to the ovary is found in what proportion of cases?
a. 1/4
b. 1/2
c. 3/4
d. Most

47.69 Krukenberg tumors account for what percent of cancers metastatic to the ovary?
a. 10 to 20%
b. 30 to 40%
c. 50 to 60%
d. 70 to 80%

Answers

47.59	e	47.61	c	47.63	d	47.65	c	47.67	d	47.69	b
47.60	d	47.62	d	47.64	a	47.66	a	47.68	a		

47.70 Approximately what percent of epithelial ovarian carcinomas occur in familial or hereditary patterns?
a. 5%
b. 15%
c. 25%
d. 35%
e. 45%

47.71 Site-specific familial ovarian cancer is characterized by which of the following?
a. There is an increased risk of bilaterality of breast cancer and of developing ovarian tumors at a younger age.
b. The risk depends on the number of first- or second-degree relatives with a history of epithelial ovarian cancer.
c. The condition is associated with the BRCA1 gene, a locus on the 17q chromosome.
d. The condition occurs in families with first- and second-degree members with combinations of colon, ovarian, endometrial, and breast cancers.

47.72 Which of the following describes breast/ovarian familial cancer syndrome?
a. There is an increased risk of bilaterality of breast cancer and of developing ovarian tumors at a younger age.
b. The risk depends on the number of first- or second-degree relatives with a history of epithelial ovarian cancer.
c. The condition is associated with the BRCA1 gene, a locus on the 14 chromosome.
d. The condition occurs in families with first- and second-degree members with combinations of colon, ovarian, endometrial, and breast cancers.

47.73 A description of Lynch II syndrome includes which of the following?
a. There is an increased risk of bilaterality of breast cancer and of developing ovarian tumors at a younger age.
b. The risk depends on the number of first- or second-degree relatives with a history of epithelial ovarian cancer.
c. The condition is associated with the BRCA1 gene, a locus on the 17q chromosome.
d. The condition occurs in families with first- and second-degree members with combinations of colon, ovarian, endometrial, and breast cancers.

47.74 Women with the BRAC1 gene mutation have a cumulative lifetime risk for ovarian cancer of
a. 10%
b. 30%
c. 50%
d. 70%
c. 90%

47.75 Compared with the general population, what is the increased risk of women of Ashkenazi Jewish extraction for carrying the BRAC1 gene?
a. Twofold
b. Fivefold
c. 10-fold
d. 15-fold
e. 20-fold

47.76 Of the new cases of ovarian cancer yearly, what percent will die within 5 years?
a. 20%
b. 40%
c. 60%
d. 80%

Answers

47.70 a	**47.72** a	**47.74** a	**47.76** c
47.71 b	**47.73** d	**47.75** c	

47.77 The classic triad of symptoms associated with fallopian tube carcinoma (watery vaginal discharge, pain, and pelvic mass) is noted in less than what percent of cases?
a. 15%
b. 25%
c. 35%
d. 45%

47.78 Para-aortic lymph node spread occurs in what proportion of fallopian tube cancers?
a. One-fifth
b. One-fourth
c. One-third
d. One-half

47.79 Which of the following statements about tumors of low malignant potential is INCORRECT?
a. They usually remain confined to the ovary.
b. They are about equally common in premenopausal and menopausal women.
c. Approximately one-fifth show spread beyond the ovary.
d. They may be managed by unilateral oophorectomy if histologic and surgical criteria for borderline tumors are met.

47.80 The risk of torsion for mature cystic teratomas is approximately:
a. 5%
b. 15%
c. 25%
d. 35%
e. 45%

47.81 Which of the following statements about theca lutein cysts is INCORRECT?
a. They are the least common functional cysts.
b. They are more commonly unilateral.
c. They are usually multicystic.
d. They are more common with multiple gestation.

47.82 A corpus luteum greater than how many centimeters in diameter is usually designated a corpus luteum cyst?
a. 1 cm
b. 3 cm
c. 5 cm
d. 7 cm
e. 9 cm

47.83 In children and adolescents, mature cystic teratomas account for what proportion of benign ovarian neoplasms?
a. One-fourth
b. One-half
c. Three-fourths
d. Most

Answers

47.77 a	47.79 b	47.81 b	47.83 b
47.78 c	47.80 b	47.82 b	

Questions and Answers Chapter 48: Human Sexuality

48.1 What percent of women report some kind of sexual complaint?
a. 5 to 15%
b. 25 to 35%
c. 35 to 45%
d. 45 to 55%
e. 55 to 65%

48.2 Determinants of healthy sexuality include
a. sense of one's self as a sexual being
b. one's overall health status
c. one's general perception of well-being
d. the quality of an individual's previous sexual experiences
e. all of the above

48.3 Among couples who are not experiencing sexual dysfunctions, each partner will estimate that the sexual component of their relationship accounts for approximately what percent of their overall happiness?
a. 10%
b. 30%
c. 50%
d. 70%
e. 90%

48.4 All of the following are thought to have positive sexual effects except
a. norepinephrine
b. dopamine
c. oxytocin
d. prolactin
e. none of the above

48.5 The American Foundation of Urologic Disease classification of female sexual dysfunction includes all EXCEPT
a. hypoactive sexual desire disorder
b. hyperactive sexual desire disorder
c. female sexual arousal disorder
d. female orgasmic disorder
e. the pain disorder

48.6 Women who do not initiate sexual contact but are responsive to their partner's overtures do not have
a. hypoactive sexual desire disorder
b. female sexual arousal disorder
c. female orgasmic disorder
d. dyspaurenia
e. vaginismus

48.7 The persistent or recurrent deficiency or absence of sexual fantasies, thoughts, and/or desire for or receptivity to sexual activity is
a. hypoactive sexual desire disorder
b. female sexual arousal disorder
c. female orgasmic disorder
d. female pain disorder

48.8 The persistent or recurrent inability to attain or maintain sufficient sexual excitement, causing personal distress, is
a. hypoactive sexual desire disorder
b. female sexual arousal disorder
c. female orgasmic disorder
d. female pain disorder

48.9 Persistent or recurrent difficulty, delay, or absence of attaining orgasm following sufficient stimulation or arousal, which causes personal distress, is
a. hypoactive sexual desire disorder
b. female sexual arousal disorder
c. female orgasmic disorder
d. female pain disorder

48.10 Decreased sexual desire is associated with
a. paroxetine
b. sertraline
c. fluoxetine
d. escitalopram
e. all of the above

Answers

48.1	c	48.3	a	48.5	b	48.7	a	48.9	c
48.2	e	48.4	d	48.6	a	48.8	b	48.10	e

48.11 The human sexual response depends on
  a. a physical and emotional system sufficiently functional to allow the sexual response
  b. a sustained and sufficient sexual stimulation
  c. both a and b
  d. neither a nor b

48.12 The first stage of the human sexual response according to Masters and Johnson is
  a. orgasmic phase
  b. plateau phase
  c. resolution phase
  d. excitement phase

48.13 The second stage of the human sexual response according to Masters and Johnson is
  a. orgasmic phase
  b. plateau phase
  c. resolution phase
  d. excitement phase

48.14 The third stage of the human sexual response according to Masters and Johnson is
  a. orgasmic phase
  b. plateau phase
  c. resolution phase
  d. excitement phase

48.15 The fourth stage of the human sexual response according to Masters and Johnson is
  a. orgasmic phase
  b. plateau phase
  c. resolution phase
  d. excitement phase

Answers
48.11 c   **48.12** d   **48.13** b   **48.14** a   **48.15** c

Questions and Answers Chapter 49: Sexual Assault and Domestic Violence

49.1 What percent of women and children in the United States are victims of sexual assault?
a. Less than 1%
b. 5%
c. 15%
d. 25%

49.2 What percent of victims of sexual assault seek help of any kind?
a. 50%
b. 25%
c. 10%
d. 5%
e. Less than 1%

49.3 In caring for a victim of sexual assault, which of the following is NOT a direct responsibility of the health care team?
a. Care of the victim's emotional needs
b. Identification of the perpetrator
c. Collection of forensic specimens
d. All of the above

49.4 What is the most serious emotional problem faced by the sexual assault victim?
a. Gender identity conflict
b. Fear of infection
c. Loss of control
d. Uncontrolled anger

49.5 Threatened or actual violence is an integral part of sexual assault
a. always
b. sometimes
c. never

49.6 Which of the following is NOT characteristic of the acute phase of the rape trauma syndrome?
a. May not be fully manifested until time of initial disclosure
b. May be associated with cognitive dysfunction
c. Safety and regaining control are the victim's main emotional needs during this time
d. Retreat to routine activities
e. May be associated with drastic changes in lifestyle, friends, and work

49.7 Which of the following is characteristic of the middle phase of the rape trauma syndrome?
a. Unrealistic plans to avoid further sexual assault
b. May not be fully manifested until time of initial disclosure
c. May be associated with cognitive dysfunction
d. Safety and regaining control are the victim's main emotional needs during this time
e. Retreat to routine activities

49.8 Which of the following is characteristic of the late phase of the rape trauma syndrome?
a. Unrealistic plans to avoid further sexual assault
b. Rationalization that the victim should or could have prevented the assault
c. May be associated with cognitive dysfunction
d. Retreat to routine activities
e. May be associated with drastic changes in lifestyle, friends, and work

---

Answers

49.1	d	**49.3**	b	**49.5**	a	**49.7**	a
49.2	c	**49.4**	c	**49.6**	e	**49.8**	e

49.9 A woman's retreat to routine activities after a rape is misinterpreted by health care team members and police as evidence that a sexual assault did not actually occur
  a. always
  b. often
  c. sometimes
  d. never

49.10 The rape trauma syndrome
  a. has a common presentation in all victims
  b. has a predictable onset
  c. is involuntary in nature
  d. is typically of short duration

49.11 The presence or absence of retreat to routine activities is directly related to
  a. the severity of the victim's assault experience
  b. the timing of the sexual assault
  c. the identity of the attacker
  d. none of the above

49.12 The inability of the patient to think clearly after an assault typically is
  a. a manifestation of an underlying psychosis
  b. not usually recognized by the patient
  c. involuntary in nature
  d. relatively rare in occurrence

49.13 Which of the following is not part of the initial care of the sexual assault victim?
  a. The provision of a safe environment
  b. The treatment of serious or life-threatening trauma
  c. The avoidance of discussion of the details of the assault
  d. A gentle encouragement to work with the police

49.14 Minor trauma is seen in approximately what percent of sexual assault victims?
  a. 1%
  b. 10%
  c. 25%
  d. 50%

49.15 Victims of sexual assault perceive themselves as guilty and responsible for their assault
  a. often
  b. sometimes
  c. never

49.16 Which of the following statements about the physical examination of a sexual assault victim is INCORRECT?
  a. A general complete physical examination is not required as it would be too traumatic for the patient
  b. Forensic specimens should be collected and cultures sent to test for sexually transmitted disease
  c. Forensic specimens should be kept in the health professional's possession or control until turned over to an appropriate representative of the police laboratory
  d. Genital and rectal evaluations are mandatory in the evaluation of a sexual assault victim

49.17 Antibiotic prophylaxis for sexually transmitted disease should be offered to child victims of sexual assault
  a. if there is evidence that the assailant is infected
  b. if follow-up compliance is unlikely
  c. if the assailant is a stranger
  d. in all of the above situations

49.18 Which of the following is routinely required as part of laboratory testing following sexual assault?
  a. Complete blood count
  b. Liver function tests
  c. Renal function tests
  d. Hepatitis screen

Answers

49.9 b	49.11 b	49.13 c	49.15 a	49.17 d
49.10 c	49.12 c	49.14 c	49.16 a	49.18 d

49.19 If diethylstilbestrol is used as a post-coital contraceptive method following sexual assault, it should be combined with an antiemetic such as Compazine (prochlorperazine)
a. always
b. sometimes
c. never

49.20 If a female victim of sexual assault of menstrual age is using an effective method of contraception, a pregnancy test should be included as part of the sexual assault evaluation
a. always
b. sometimes
c. never

49.21 Which of the following antibiotics is appropriate to administer prophylactically following sexual assault?
a. Penicillin
b. Doxycycline
c. Cephalexin
d. Cipro Floxin

49.22 Under what circumstances should ceftriaxone (Rocephin) be offered to victims of sexual assault?
a. For all patients whose culture is positive for *Neisseria gonorrhoeae*
b. If the patient is penicillin-allergic
c. When the prevalence rate of antibiotic-resistant strains of *N. gonorrhoeae* exceeds 1%
d. If the victim is pregnant

49.23 What is the appropriate dose of diethylstilbestrol for postcoital contraception?
a. Two tablets twice a day for 3 days
b. Two tablets every day for 3 days
c. Two tablets twice a day for 5 days
d. Two tablets every day for 5 days

49.24 Which of the following statements about child sexual victimization is correct?
a. Victimization is most commonly by parents, family members, or family friends
b. Rape by a stranger is relatively uncommon in children
c. It is best to interview child victims apart from parents and other family members
d. The use of anatomically correct dolls is a useful routine adjunct to history-taking in young children
e. All of the above are correct

49.25 In examination of a small child, sedation should be used
a. always
b. sometimes
c. rarely

49.26 Suspected child sexual abuse should be reported to the authorities
a. always
b. sometimes
c. rarely

49.27 Whose responsibility is it to determine if a child may safely return home after evaluation of sexual assault, or if the risk of ongoing abuse requires foster home placement or hospitalization?
a. Health care team
b. Department of Social Work
c. Police
d. State's Attorney General

Answers

49.19 a	49.21 b	49.23 a	49.25 c	49.27 a
49.20 a	49.22 c	49.24 e	49.26 b	

49.28 A child who displays knowledge of sexual matters, anatomy, or function beyond that expected for her years
a. always is a victim of sexual abuse
b. may be a victim of sexual abuse
c. rarely is a victim of sexual abuse

49.29 Domestic violence is experienced by approximately what percent of women during their lives?
a. 1 to 25%
b. 25 to 50%
c. 50 to 75%
d. 75 to 99%

49.30 Approximately what proportion of women presenting to an emergency department have been injured by their partners?
a. 1 in 5
b. 2 in 5
c. 3 in 5
d. 4 in 5

49.31 Which of the following is NOT one of the common presentations of domestic violence?
a. Substance abuse
b. Physical abuse
c. Sexual assault
d. Emotional abuse

49.32 In the acronym SAFE, which of the following best defines the "S"?
a. Has the patient felt abused in a relationship? In her present relationship? How? When someone is angry in the patient's home, what is it like and what is likely to happen?
b. Are there friends or family, or clergy, who can help? Who can the patient turn to for support?
c. Does the patient have a plan, or idea, of what she would do in an emergency? If she has children, do they know where to go for and how to get help?
d. Does the patient feel safe? At home? At school? In the workplace? If not, who or what does she fear, and why?

49.33 In the acronym SAFE, which of the following best defines the "A"?
a. Has the patient felt abused in a relationship? In her present relationship? How? When someone is angry in the patient's home, what is it like and what is likely to happen?
b. Are there friends or family, or clergy, who can help? Who can the patient turn to for support?
c. Does the patient have a plan, or idea, of what she would do in an emergency? If she has children, do they know where to go for and how to get help?
d. Does the patient feel safe? At home? At school? In the workplace? If not, who or what does she fear, and why?

Answers

49.28 b	**49.29** b	**49.30** a	**49.31** a	**49.32** d	**49.33** a

49.34 In the acronym SAFE, which of the following best defines the "F"?

a. Has the patient felt abused in a relationship? In her present relationship? How? When someone is angry in the patient's home, what is it like and what is likely to happen?

b. Are there friends or family, or clergy, who can help? Who can the patient turn to for support?

c. Does the patient have a plan, or idea, of what she would do in an emergency? If she has children, do they know where to go for and how to get help?

d. Does the patient feel safe? At home? At school? In the workplace? If not, who or what does she fear, and why?

49.35 In the acronym SAFE, which of the following best defines the "E"?

a. Has the patient felt abused in a relationship? In her present relationship? How? When someone is angry in the patient's home, what is it like and what is likely to happen?

b. Are there friends or family, or clergy, who can help? Who can the patient turn to for support?

c. Does the patient have a plan, or idea, of what she would do in an emergency? If she has children, do they know where to go for and how to get help?

d. Does the patient feel safe? At home? At school? In the workplace? If not, who or what does she fear, and why?

Answers

49.34 b   49.35 c

Page numbers in italics denote figures; those followed by a "t" denote tables.

Index

Index

Index

Index

diagnostic procedures for, *385*, 389t
　basal body temperature, 384–385, *385, 386*
　hysterosalpingogram, 384–386, *385,* 389t
　　for anatomic disorders, 389–390, *390, 391*
　hysteroscopy, *385,* 386, 389t, 390
　laparoscopy, *385,* 386, 389t, 390
　semen analysis, 384–385, *385,* 387t, 388t
　serum progesterone levels, 385
emotional issues in, 384
with endometriosis, 303
evaluation scheme for, 384, *385*
history taking for, 11, 12t
prevalence of, 383
reproductive age in, 383
treatment of, 392
Inflammatory bowel disease, adnexal space and, 465
Inflammatory disorders, of hypothalamus, abnormal
　pubertal development related to, 354–355
Influenza vaccine, 8t
Informed consent, 24
　collaborative responsibility for, 9, 24
　for sterilization, 266
Injectable contraception
　contraindications for, 252, 253t
　indications for, 252, 253t
　preparations of, 244, 246, 251–252
　rate of release of, 251, *252*
Innominate bones, in pelvic anatomy, 33, *34*
Inpatient care, for postpartum period, 125
Insertional dyspareunia, 486
　new onset, 421
Inspection
　of breasts, 11–12, *14,* 15
　　teaching patient to do, 15–16, *17*
　in pelvic examination, 17–18
Inspiratory capacity, during pregnancy, 53, 53t
Inspiratory reserve, during pregnancy, 53, 53t
Insulinase, 58
Insulin resistance, during pregnancy, 58–60
Insulin secretion, during pregnancy, 58–60
Insulin sensitizers, polycystic ovarian syndrome and,
　369
Insulin therapy, for diabetes mellitus
　during labor, 178
　during pregnancy, 176–177
Insurance companies
　influence on clinical practice, 24
　reimbursement, for inpatient postpartum care, 125
Intercourse (*see* Sexual intercourse)
Internal podalic version, of multifetal gestation, 201,
　201
Internal rotation, fetal, during labor, 85, *86,* 87
International Federation of Gynecology and
　Obstetrics (FIGO)
　cervical cancer staging, 443–444, 443t
　endometrial cancer staging, 460–462, 461t
　ovarian carcinoma staging, 470–471, 471t
　vulvar cancer staging, 426, 427t
International Society for the Study of Vulvar Disease
　(ISSVD), vulvar neoplasia classification, 422,
　422t

Interpersonal factors, of sexuality, 480, 485
Interstitial implants, for radiation therapy, 410
Interviewing patients (*see* Patient history)
Intestinal transit time, during pregnancy, 52t, 53
Intimacy, physical, 480, 485
Intracavity devices, for radiation therapy, 410, 445,
　446
Intraductal papillomas, of breasts, 319–320, 327
Intraepithelial neoplasia
　cervical, 20–21, 431–442
　ovarian, 471
　vaginal, 426, 428
　vulvar, 423–424
Intraocular pressure, during pregnancy, 57
Intraoperative radiation therapy, 410
Intrapartum care
　of cardiac patients, 185
　for fetal macrosomia, 208
　fetal surveillance, 108–117
　　in abnormal labor, 97, 98–99, 103
　　electronic, 87–88, 110–111
　for intrauterine growth restriction, 207–208, 207t
　maternal diabetes and, 177–178
　maternal labor, 79–94 (*see also* Labor)
　　abnormal, 95–107 (*see also* Abnormal labor)
　　changes before onset of, 80, *81*
　　delivery, 90–93, *91–92*
　　evaluation for, 80–84, *82–84*
　　first stage of, 84–85, 85t
　　fourth stage of, 85, 93–94
　　management of, 87–90, *89–90*
　　mechanism of, 85–87, *86,* 96
　　positions for, 87, 90
　　process defined, 80
　　second stage of, 85, 85t, 89–90, 98
　　　management of prolonged, 98, 103
　　stages of, 84–85, *85,* 85t
　　third stage of, 85, 93, *93,* 94t
　for multifetal gestation, 201, *201*
　for postterm pregnancy, 219–220
Intrauterine circulation, transition to extrauterine
　circulation, *60,* 60–61
Intrauterine devices (IUDs)
　commonly used, 256, *256*
　contraindications to, 257
　decision tree for, 244, *246*
　ectopic pregnancy related to, 162
　insertion of, 257–258, *258*
　　post-coital/emergency, 259
　　prophylactic antibiotics for, 257
　method of action, 256
　pregnancy rates within first year, 245t
　sexually transmitted infections and, 257
　side effects of, 256–257
Intrauterine growth restriction (IUGR), 203–208
　asymmetric versus symmetric, 206
　causes of, 203–204, 204t
　with cytomegalovirus, 183–184
　delayed-onset, 203
　description of, 203
　early-onset, 203

Index

Index